SLEEP
PSYCHIATRY

SLEEP
PSYCHIATRY

Edited by

Alexander Z. Golbin, MD, PhD

Sleep and Behavior Medicine Institute
University of Illinois, Chicago, Illinois, USA

Howard M. Kravitz, DO, MPH

Rush University Medical Center
Chicago, Illinois, USA

Louis G. Keith, MD, PhD

Feinberg School of Medicine
Northwestern University, Chicago, Illinois, USA

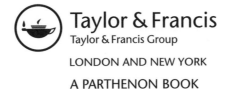

Taylor & Francis
Taylor & Francis Group

LONDON AND NEW YORK

A PARTHENON BOOK

© 2004 Taylor & Francis, an imprint of the Taylor & Francis Group

First published in the United Kingdom in 2004
by Taylor & Francis,
an imprint of the Taylor & Francis Group,
2 Park Square, Milton Park
Abingdon, Oxon OX14 4RN

Tel.:   +44 (0) 1235 828600
Fax.:   +44 (0) 1235 829000
Website; www.tandf.co.uk

British Library Cataloguing in Publication Data

Data available on application

Library of Congress Cataloging-in-Publication Data

Data available on application

ISBN 1-84214-145-7

Distributed in North and South America by

Taylor & Francis
2000 NW Corporate Blvd
Boca Raton, FL 33431, USA

Within Continental USA
Tel.: 800 272 7737; Fax.: 800 374 3401
Outside Continental USA
Tel.: 561 994 0555; Fax.: 561 361 6018
E-mail: orders@crcpress.com

Distributed in the rest of the world by
Thomson Publishing Services
Cheriton House
North Way
Andover, Hampshire SP10 5BE, UK
Tel.: +44 (0) 1264 332424
E-mail: salesorder.tandf@thomsonpublishingservices.co.uk

Composition by Siva Math Setters, Chennai, India
Printed and bound by CPI Bath, UK

Contents

Section 1: Psychobiology of sleep through the life span

Section 2: The effect of sleep disorders on health and mental function

Disclaimer

Every effort has been made to ensure that drug doses and other information are prescribed accurately. However, we make no representation that expresses or implies that this information is correct. Readers must check the information themselves. The authors and publisher do not accept responsibility or legal liability for any errors in the text, or misuse or misapplication of materials provided in this book.

List of contributors

Robert L. Barkin, MBA, PharmD
Departments of Pharmacology,
  Anesthesiology, Family Medicine
Rush North Shore Medical Center
Rush Medical College
9701 Knox Avenue, Suite 103
Skokie, IL 60076, USA
Tel: (847) 933-6974
Fax: (847) 933-6044

Joel Bornstein, PsyD
Adler School of Professional Psychology
Chicago, Illinois
Sleep and Behavior Medicine Institute
9700 N. Kenton Avenue, Suite 205
Skokie, IL 60076, USA
Tel: (847) 673-8005
Fax: (847) 673-8719

Peter Dodzik, PsyD
Department of Clinical Psychology and
  Behavioral Sciences
Illinois School of Professional Psychology –
  Chicago Northwest
Rolling Meadows, Illinois
Sleep and Behavior Medicine Institute
9700 N. Kenton Avenue, Suite 205
Skokie, IL 60076, USA
Tel: (847) 673-8005
Fax: (847) 673-8719
Email: Dodzik@mindspring.com

Neil S. Freedman, MD, FCCP
Sleep and Behavior Medicine Institute and
  Pulmonary Physicians of the North Shore
2151 Waukegan Avenue
Bannockburn, IL 60015, USA
Tel: (847) 236-1300
Fax: (847) 236-9677
Email: Neilfreedm@aol.com

Elbert Geuze, MD
Department of Military Psychiatry
Central Military Hospital and
  Brain Division
University Medical Centre
Mailbox BO1206
Heidelberglaan 100
3584 CX Utrecht, The Netherlands
Tel: 030 2509 585
Fax: 030 250 2586

Julian Gojer, MD
Department of Psychiatry
University of Toronto
10 Easson Avenue
Toronto, Ontario M6S3W5
Canada
Tel: (416) 603-5765
Fax: (416) 603-6919

Alexander Z. Golbin, MD, PhD
Department of Psychiatry
University of Illinois, Chicago
Sleep and Behavior
  Medicine Institute
9700 N. Kenton Avenue, Suite 205
Skokie, IL 60076, USA
Tel: (847) 673-8005
Fax: (847) 673-8719
Email: golbina@aol.com

Raed Hawa, MD
Department of Psychiatry
University of Toronto
10 Easson Avenue
Toronto, Ontario M6S3W5
Canada
Tel: (416) 603-5765
Fax: (416) 603-6919

Victor Kagan, MD, PhD, Sci
Vice President, VeriCare, San Diego,
   California
Sleep and Behavior Medicine Institute
9700 N. Kenton Avenue, Suite 205
Skokie, IL 60076, USA
Tel: (847) 673-8005
Fax: (847) 673-8719

Leonid Kayumov, PhD, DABSM
Department of Psychiatry
University of Toronto
10 Easson Avenue
Toronto, Ontario M6S3W5, Canada
Tel: (416) 603-5765
Fax: (416) 603-6919
Email: lkayumov@uhmres.utoronto.ca.com

Louis G. Keith, MD, PhD
Department of Obstetrics and
   Gynecology
Feinberg School of Medicine
Northwestern University
333 East Superior Street, Suite 465
Chicago, IL 60611, USA
Email: lgk395@northwestern.edu

Howard M. Kravitz, DO, MPH
Departments of Psychiatry and Preventative
   Medicine
Rush North Shore Medical Center
Skokie, IL 60076, USA
Email: hkravitz@rush.edu

Howard D. Kurland, MD
Department of Psychiatry
Northwestern University Medical School
Evanston, Illinois
500 Green Bay Road
Kenilworth, IL 60043, USA

Henry W. Lahmeyer, MD
Department of Psychiatry
Chicago Medical School
The Sleep Clinic
North Chicago, Illinois
778 Frontage Road, Suite 121
Northfield, IL 60093, USA
Tel: (847) 446-3531
Fax: (847) 446-3573

Jamie K. Lilie, PhD
Center for Psychological Services, LLC
Northfield, Illinois
778 Frontage Road, Suite 121
Northfield, IL 60093, USA
Tel: (847) 446-3531
Fax: (847) 446-3573

Bill McCarberg, MD
Chronic Pain Management Program
Kaiser Permanente
3033 Bunker Hill Street
San Diego, CA 92109, USA
Email: bill.h.mccarberg@kp.org

Sharon L. Merritt, RN, MSN, EdD
Department of Medical-Surgical Nursing
Center for Narcolepsy Research College of
   Nursing, M/C 802
University of Illinois at Chicago
845 S. Damen Avenue, Room 215
Chicago, IL 60612-7350, USA
Tel: 312-996-5175
Fax: 312-996-7008
Email: slm624@uic.edu
Homepage: www.uic.edu/depts/cnr

Joost Mertens, MD
Royal Netherlands Navy
Social Medicine Service
Department of Mental Health
Driehuis, The Netherlands
Department of Military Psychiatry
Central Military Hospital and Brain Division
University Medical Centre
Mailbox BO1206
Heidelberglaan 100
3584 CX Utrecht, The Netherlands
Tel: 030 2502 585
Fax: 030 250 2586

Steven L. Meyers, MD
Department of Neurology
Rush North Shore Medical Center
Rush Medical College
Chicago, IL 9669, USA
Kenton – Suite 203
Skokie, IL 60076, USA
Tel: (847) 677-2980
Fax: (847) 677-0231

Roberta Murphy, MD
Department of Psychiatry, University of
    Toronto
10 Easson Avenue
Toronto, Ontario M6S3W5, Canada
Tel: (416) 603-5765
Fax: (416) 603-6919

Marc Oster, PsyD
Adler School of Professional Psychology
Chicago, Illinois
Sleep and Behavior Medicine Institute
9700 N. Kenton Avenue, Suite 205
Skokie, IL 60076, USA
Tel: (847) 673-8005
Fax: (847) 673-8719

Rick Peticca, MD
Adler School of Professional Psychology
Chicago, Illinois
Sleep and Behavior Medicine Institute
9700 N. Kenton Avenue, Suite 205
Skokie, IL 60076, USA
Tel: (847) 673-8005
Fax: (847) 673-8719

Emma Robinson-Rossi, MD
Feinberg School of Medicine
Northwestern University
303 East Chicago Avenue
Chicago, IL 60611, USA

Vadim S. Rotenberg, MD, PhD, DSc
Tel-Aviv University
Abarbanel Mental Health Center
Keren Kayemet
15 Bat-Yam, Israel
Email: vadir@post.tau.ac.il

Jianhua Shen, MD, MSc
Department of Psychiatry
University of Toronto
10 Easson Avenue
Toronto, Ontario M6S3W5, Canada
Tel: (416) 603-5765
Fax: (416) 603-6919

Colin M. Shapiro, PhD
Department of Psychiatry
University of Toronto
10 Easson Avenue
Toronto, Ontario M6S3W5, Canada
Tel: (416) 603-5765
Fax: (416) 603-6919

Alexander N. Shepovalnikov, MD, DSc
Sechenov's Institute of Evolutionary
    Physiology and Biochemistry
Russian Academy of Science
Sestroreskaya 7, Suite 111
St. Petersburg, 197183, Russia
Email: rashep@mail.ru

Eric Vermetten, MD, PhD
Department of Military Psychiatry
Central Military Hospital and Brain Division
University Medical Centre
Mailbox BO1206
Heidelberglaan 100
3584 CX Utrecht, The Netherlands
Tel: 030 2502 585
Fax: 030 250 2586

Preface

Sleep psychiatry – a new field of sleep medicine

This book is published at a time when sleep medicine is celebrating its 50th Anniversary. The 'modern era' of sleep research and the beginning of sleep disorder medicine dates back to 1953 when Aserinsky and Kleitman first described the stages of sleep characterized by rapid eye movements (REM). This particular stage of sleep is often called 'paradoxical sleep', because everything we thought we knew about sleep at that time turned out to be just the opposite; eye balls start to jerk rapidly, heart rate increases without apparent reason, brain waves resemble those of active thinking and the metabolism speeds up. In short, during the REM stage of sleep all body functions become irregular and desynchronized. This stage of sleep is surprisingly 'active'.

Since then, new discoveries have been made about the mechanisms of sleep and wakefulness, their normal development and pathology. Among these was the finding that some hormones are released during different stages of sleep. Specific sleep disorders such as sleep apnea syndrome, narcolepsy, restless leg syndrome, REM behavior disorder and unusual parasomnias were described. Slowly but surely our understanding of their nature continues to grow and successful treatments are discovered.

The most important of all discoveries was the recognition that sleep is not a passive state of rest, but a complicated and active cyclic process. Of equal importance, normal sleep was recognized as the foundation for normal alertness and abnormal sleep as the foundation for abnormal alertness.

Psychological phenomena, represented by dreams, as well as the relationship of sleep to different psychiatric conditions, became the focus of direct physiological research, in ways not previously considered. Sleep became recognized by psychiatrists and psychologists as the neurobiological substrate for many emotional and behavioral disorders.

More recently, increased awareness about the high frequency of sleep-alertness disorders and their dramatic consequences led to their recognition as a public health problem. For example, transportation accidents caused by sleep deprivation range from missing stop signs to the thousands of fatalities occuring on the road, in the water, on trains, and even in space. Recent studies have uncovered the possibility that one of the causes of the Challenger tragedy may have been human error secondary to fatigue and sleep deprivation.

Sleep medicine is a growing field. New subdivisions have appeared, including sleep dentistry and forensic sleep medicine. Research and clinical evidence concerning the associations of sleep disorders with psychiatric problems is growing quickly. As is often the case in any new field, the literature has become abundant and often controversial. At the same time, specialized textbooks, manuals, periodicals and papers are not easily accessible and are difficult to interpret and apply to the practical needs of general practitioners, psychiatrists and other health professionals. There is an urgent need to summarize established facts regarding the conceptual basis for the relationships between physiology and pathology in the development and maintenance of daytime alertness, attention, concentration, habits, personality traits and psychiatric disorders in children and adults, in short, the field of sleep psychiatry.

The concepts reviewed in this book include but are not limited to:

(1) Sleep as a physiological basis for daytime mental and emotional functions;

(2) Physiological sleep mechanisms as the foundation for the development of alertness, attention and productive wakefulness;

(3) Sleep deviations as the basis for alertness/ attention problems;

(4) Sleep as a compensatory and recovery state;

(5) Sleep state as a trigger of sickness and death;

(6) Effective control of sleep mechanisms as a means to prevent and treat some medical and psychiatric problems.

In an attempt to be clear and keeping in mind the interests of different specialties, the book is divided into six sections:

(1) *Psychobiology of sleep throughout a person's life span*. This section is devoted to physiological mechanisms of sleep and wakefulness in relation to the mechanisms of psychiatric disorders.

(2) *The effect of sleep disorders on health and mental functions*. This section is devoted to psychiatric consequences of sleep disorders.

(3) *The relationships of parasomnias to mental health*. This section describes the relationships between parasomnias and mental health issues.

(4) *Neuropsychiatric disorders and sleep aberrations*. This section describes sleep abnormalities in psychiatric pathology.

(5) *Forensic sleep psychiatry*. This section discusses the complex and complicated legal issues associated with forensic sleep psychiatry.

(6) *Treatment methods in sleep psychiatry*. This section is devoted to traditional and alternative treatment methods in sleep psychiatry.

We have attempted to write this book in a reader-friendly style with a desire to be both interesting and useful for general physicians, psychiatrists, psychologists and other health professionals.

Many definitions of health exist, but the essence of health, by any definition, should include good sleep followed by productive alertness.

If you are interested – this book points the way.

Alexander Z. Golbin, MD, PhD
Howard M. Kravitz, DO, MPH
Louis G. Keith, MD, PhD

Foreword

It is strange that we had to wait until the end of the 20th century to begin to question the impact of sleep on diseases and the impact of diseases on sleep. However, there were a few exceptions to this. Hippocrates examined dreams for indications of certain diseases. Thomas Willis (1762) gave the first description of restless legs syndrome. The term 'pick wicklian' was coined to describe an obese somnolent patient in 1889 during the clinical presentation of a patient with sleep apnea. Freud and psychoanalysts were interested in dreams as a means of understanding psychopathology. Nonetheless, the medical community was not and still is not concerned – the proof of this being the limited number of physicians and nurses in hospitals at night, and then for emergency purposes only, the closing of almost all laboratories at night and the unfortunate tendency of providing patients with hypnotic drugs at night to keep them quiet. Furthermore, what would be said of the chief of a department who invited his medical staff to make a round of the patients at night? There can be no interest in diseased subjects while they are asleep[1].

It was not until 1979 that sleep-related pathologies such as sleep-related asthma, sleep-related cardiovascular symptoms and sleep-related epileptic seizures were listed in 'the Diagnostic Classification of Sleep and Arousal Disorders', and not until the 1990s that sleep disorders were associated with mental disorders included in the 'International Classification of Sleep Disorders' (1990) and the *Diagnostic and Statistical Manual of Mental Disorders* (4th edition) (1994). Today the ground is fertile. An increasing number of psychiatrists, neurologists, chest physicians and pediatricians are interested in the interplay between sleep and the disorders of their own field. Thus, this book *Sleep Psychiatry* is very timely and we must thank the editors. Indeed, a number of questions are continuously raised which need answers.

(1) How does sleep impact on general functioning, attention and vigilance, memory, and cerebral and motor functions?

(2) To what degree do sleep curtailment, insomnia or excessive daytime sleepiness result in loss of performance, mood disorders, alcoholism or generalized anxiety?

(3) Do nightmares in depressed patients add to the risk of suicide? Is there any unveiled psychiatric abnormality in adults with pavor nocturnus, sleep-walking or nightmares?

(4) What are the consequences of schizophrenia, mood disorders and anxiety disorders and alcohol dependence on sleep behavior? Are they responsible for insomnia, hypersomnia or disorders of the sleep–wake schedule? Do they result in alterations of sleep continuity or architecture? Can the study of sleep modifications help in the positive diagnosis of mental conditions?

(5) Pavor nocturnus and somnambulism may lead to injury and sometimes even to the killing of a spouse or roommate. How can it be demonstrated that the subject was asleep when this occurred? Is the subject responsible or not?

(6) Is the prescription of psychotropic drugs harmless or harmful in relation to sleep? What is the best therapeutic approach towards insomnia or excessive daytime sleepiness in mental disorder patients?

(7) Are sleep manipulations, such as sleep deprivation, sleep curtailment, chronotherapy, and so on, relevant to the treatment of sleep disorders or psychiatric conditions?

The questions are numerous. No doubt this book will help specialists and non-specialists alike to find the answers.

Michel Billard, MD
Department of Neurology
Gui de Chauliac Hospital
Montpellier, France
Email: mbilliard@wanadoo.fr

Acknowledgements

Writing a book, especially one summarizing a field of medicine, is similar to climbing a high mountain. From a distance, the top of the mountain is attractive and appears nearby. The difficulty, however, increases exponentially with each step toward the goal.

As in mountain climbing, writing a book requires an excellent team. Many promising authors drop out, but the result is worth the pain. Some names are already renowned, some are rising stars, but all share a passion for the field, devotion to finishing the task and a great sense of responsibility for bringing the latest news, the freshest ideas and the most practical advice.

This is an opportunity to express our deep gratitude to all those authors involved in preparing individual chapters.

Special thanks and appreciation go to our dear assistants Marci Givan, Barbara Stern and Erin Buhl for typing and retyping, and attempting to organize and clarify endless data and complex concepts.

This book is not the first for many of the authors, but the first where we experienced such friendly, gentle and always available support from Parthenon Publishing and personally from David Bloomer.

Last, but not least, deep thanks go to our families, our wives and children who have been so patient, supportive and understanding throughout.

Alexander Z. Golbin, MD, PhD
2004

Section 1:

Psychobiology of sleep through the life span

1

Basic neurophysiological changes in sleep and wakefulness

Alexander Z. Golbin, Neil S. Freedman and Howard M. Kravitz

Theories may become obsolete, even while the validity of the experiments on which they are based, remain unchallenged.

Morruzzi, 1972

INTRODUCTION

Sleep is a reversible behavioral state of perceptual disengagement from and unresponsiveness to the environment[1]. Sleep is defined electroencephalographically and behaviorally by two states: non-rapid eye movement (NREM) sleep and rapid eye movement (REM) sleep. NREM sleep is characterized by four sleep stages (1–4), with increasing arousal thresholds correlating with successive sleep stages. Brain activity as measured by the electroencephalogram (EEG) demonstrates relatively slow synchronous waveforms[1], and predominance of stages 2, 3 and 4, usually called slow-wave sleep (SWS) or NREM (Figures 1.1–1.4). REM sleep, by contrast, is identified in activation by EEG criteria, relative muscle atonia and episodic bursts of rapid eye movements (Figure 1.5). REM sleep tends to cycle every 90 to 120 min throughout the night becoming more prominent in the early morning hours[1,2] (Figure 1.1). The abundance of theories about the nature

of sleep and especially about its function are the best evidence of how little we know about sleep–wake mechanisms.

Theories of NREM/REM sleep regulation

The anatomic and physiological processes that control NREM and REM sleep are not clearly understood. Currently, the regulatory mechanisms of NREM sleep are believed to reside within diencephalic structures, while those regulating REM sleep appear to reside mainly in the pontine brainstem[1].

Although the exact mechanisms controlling NREM and REM sleep are still not clear, several theories of NREM and REM sleep regulation have been proposed. In the 1970s Jouvet proposed the monoaminergic theory of the sleep–wake cycle based on pharmacological and brainstem transection studies[3]. Jouvet's theory[3] suggested that the catecholaminergic system of the brain plays the executive role in REM sleep. The caudal two-thirds of the locus ceruleus (LC) complex (locus ceruleus, subceruleus and parabrochialis) act as the trigger for REM sleep. One-third of the LC complex controls the total inhibition of muscle tone, whereas the medial third of the coeruleus complex is responsible for pontogeniculo-occipital (PGO) activity

3

and both phasic and tonic components of REM sleep. The contemporary version of the monoaminergic theory is Hernandez-Peon's[4] cholinergic theory of sleep–wake regulation. According to this theory, the sleep–wake cycle is regulated by two antagonistic cholinergic systems: the sleep system and the waking system. Recently Jouvet[1] suggested that serotonin is the major neuromodulator of sleep, whereas Radulovacki presented data regarding the major role of adenosine in sleep–wake regulation[5].

In 1975 Hobson and colleagues offered a new explanation proposing a reciprocal interaction model of sleep–wake cycle control in an attempt to explain the sleep–wake cycle on a cellular level[6]. This concept, based on the interaction of multiple and widely distributed distinct groups of neurons, replaced the previous hypothesis of a single 'sleep center'. A simplified version of the reciprocal interaction model may be explained as follows: REM-ON cholinergic nuclei activate reticular formation neurons in a positive feedback interaction to produce REM sleep. When REM sleep is 'on', this excites REM 'off' neurons in the raphe and locus ceruleus systems. As the REM-OFF neurons become active at the end of REM sleep, they terminate REM and the NREM period starts, which inhibits REM-OFF cells, owing to self-inhibiting feedback, and then the cycle repeats itself.

One of the common features of the molecular and cellular theories is the idea of a single form of NREM and a single form of REM. Alternative approaches to the single NREM–REM model such as the sequential hypothesis of the sleep function were described by Ambrozini and co-workers[7]. They suggested that the functions of the sleeping brain depend on the nature of the previous waking experience. This theory also considered NREM and REM as a unitary process as in the original Hernandez-Peon theory[4]. Other interesting theories (see Drucker and Merchant[1]) attempting to unite several states of human experiences suggested that sleep after feeding, stress, coitus, fatigue

or infection, etc. is not the same sleep, meaning it is not triggered by the same brain mechanisms. Therefore, NREM and REM sleep may have different initiating and controlling mechanisms, which may depend in part on the previous waking experience.

There are multiple excellent reviews describing in great detail a dozen sleep regulation theories and their experimental basis[1,2,8–12]. There is currently no consensus or generally accepted theory explaining sleep–wake cycle regulation, but all researchers agree on the fact that sleeping and waking are intimately united. You cannot understand sleep without understanding wakefulness and its mechanisms, and vice versa. Deep mechanisms of waking behavior are connected with mechanisms of sleep.

DETERMINANTS OF DAYTIME SLEEPINESS

Not all daytime sleepiness is a result of inadequate amounts of total sleep time. The human sleep–wake cycle is regulated by two primary processes, process S and process C[13]. Process S is the homeostatic drive to sleep. This drive increases during wakefulness and decreases during sleep. If a sufficient amount of sleep is not achieved, either through decreased total sleep time (sleep quantity) or sleep fragmentation (sleep quality), our homeostatic drive for sleep increases and results in daytime sleepiness. The amount of slow-wave sleep (stage 3 and 4) achieved is primarily linked to process S and the duration of prior wakefulness[14]. Process C is the circadian drive for sleep, which acts independently of sleeping and waking. This drive increases sleepiness and alertness during different parts of the subjective day. Process C also controls our drive for REM sleep. REM sleep propensity is circadian phase dependent and not altered by an increasing homeostatic drive for sleep[14,15].

Other factors in addition to homeostatic and circadian influences may affect an individual's drive for sleep or wakefulness.

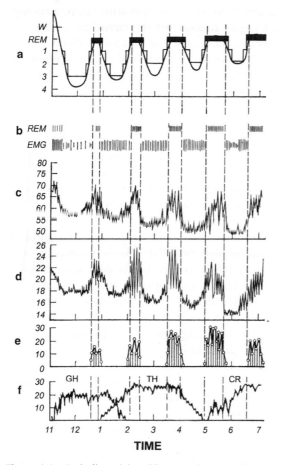

Figure 1.1 Periodic activity of functional systems during a night of sleep. (a) Sleep stages; (b) REM (rapid eye movements), EMG (electromyogram); (c) Pulse rate (per minute); (d) Respiration rate (per minute); (e) Nocturnal penile tumescence (erection); (f) Hormonal release of growth hormone (GH), thyroid hormone (TH) and cortisol (CR). W, wakefulness. Based on materials from Jovanovic, 1972, Shepovalnikov, 1981 and others

Certain etiologies of hypersomnia, such as narcolepsy and central nervous system (CNS) hypersomnia, appear to be regulated by other CNS processes which are not well understood. Several medications may enhance or reverse the effects of daytime sleepiness. Finally, it should be remembered that many of the above factors may act together to produce an additive effect.

Homeostatic factors

Sleep quantity

The degree of daytime sleepiness is directly proportional to the amount of sleep achieved during the prior night[16]. The total amount of nocturnal sleep that an individual requires to alleviate daytime sleepiness is unknown, and is likely to vary on an individual basis. It is believed that healthy young adults require between 8 and 8.5 h of sleep per night[6]. A recent epidemiological study of young adults has suggested that this group suffers from chronic partial sleep deprivation, as their average length of nocturnal sleep achieved on weekdays was only 6.7 h[17]. Total or partial sleep deprivation will result in daytime sleepiness even after only 1 evening of sleep loss. Data indicate that nocturnal sleep periods reduced by as little as 1.3 h for 1 night result in a 32% reduction of daytime alertness, as measured by the multiple sleep latency test (MSLT)[18].

Conversely, lengthening the nocturnal sleep period beyond 8 h results in significantly increased alertness and improved reaction times[19,20]. Moreover, studies assessing the effects of late afternoon naps and sleep extension (increasing total sleep time beyond baseline normal levels) have demonstrated significant decreases in the homeostatic drive for sleep[21–23]. Daytime naps have also been shown to improve daytime sleepiness after acute sleep deprivation. Notably, although sleep extension results in statistically significant improvements in performance and decreased deep stages (SWS), some authors debate the clinical significance of these improvements[24], especially in individuals without previous complaints of sleepiness.

Sleep quality

The degree of daytime sleepiness is also regulated by sleep continuity. The sleep continuity theory states that consolidation of sleep is as important as total sleep time. In general, the degree of daytime sleepiness is directly proportional to the degree of sleep fragmentation[25].

Neurocognitive performance deficits are common in individuals experiencing sleep fragmentation[25–27]. Studies of nocturnal sleep fragmentation demonstrate that daytime sleepiness increases and neurocognitive performance decreases even after one night of sleep fragmentation[25–27]. The number of shifts from other sleep stages to stage 1 sleeping or waking, and the percentage of stage 1 sleep correlates with excessive daytime sleepiness in various patient groups[28]. It appears that the total number of sleep fragmenting events is as important as their distribution over the night. Similar numbers of sleep fragmenting events result in similar deficits in daytime function whether the events are evenly spaced or clustered[29].

In clinical practice, sleep fragmentation may result from primary sleep disorders including obstructive sleep apnea and periodic limb movement syndrome. Several medical disorders are also associated with sleep fragmentation including chronic obstructive pulmonary disease (COPD) and congestive heart failure (secondary to Cheyne–Stokes respirations in stage 1 and 2 sleep)[30]. Chronic pain syndromes, including fibromyalgia, are linked to an alpha-delta sleep pattern which is associated with non-restorative sleep[31]. Finally, frequent awakenings due to nocturnal urination are common in older males and individuals using diuretics.

Circadian factors

The circadian system is the internal pacemaker, or time clock, of the human body. The human sleep–wake cycle, as well as several other neuro-hormonal cycles, are synchronized to the day–night cycle through the circadian system. The human sleep–wake cycle demonstrates a strong relationship to the deep circadian pacemaker, as it has strong influences on both the timing and the duration of sleep in normal individuals[32].

There is a biphasic pattern of objective sleepiness, demonstrated by multiple sleep latency testing in normal young adults and elderly subjects over a 24 h period[33]. When using core body temperature (CBT) as the surrogate marker for the circadian pacemaker, sleep onset is closely linked to the downslope of the CBT curve[15,32]. Two peaks in sleep tendency and troughs in alertness are evident in humans. The major peak in sleep tendency occurs between the hours of 2 a.m. and 6 a.m. and is linked to the nadir and rising limb of the CBT curve. A second, weaker increase in sleep tendency and decrease in alertness occurs between the daytime hours of 2 p.m. and 6 p.m.[33].

Conversely, there is also a biphasic pattern to objective alertness. The two peaks in alertness occur at opposite ends of the clock, around 9 a.m. and 9 p.m. This biphasic pattern also correlates with increasing and peak CBT, respectively[33,34]. The main troughs in alertness correspond to those times of increased sleep tendency as mentioned above.

Owing to the biphasic shifts in sleepiness and alertness throughout the 24 h day, the major determinant of duration of sleep is the phase of the endogenous pacemaker rather than the duration of prior wakefulness[32]. For these reasons, when normal individuals are placed into an environment free of time cues, they demonstrate a shorter sleep duration when a chosen bedtime is near the temperature cycle minimum and a longer sleep duration when sleep is initiated near the temperature cycle maximum. As stated above, these patterns persist regardless of the prior length of wakefulness[32].

The differential diagnoses of sleepiness related to circadian disturbances include primary and secondary disorders. Primary circadian disturbances that may result in daytime sleepiness are caused by the patient's internal clock being constantly out of phase, or unsynchronized, with the external environment. These disorders include:

(1) Delayed sleep phase syndrome;

(2) Advanced sleep phase syndrome;

(3) Non-24 h/irregular sleep–wake syndrome.

Secondary circadian related sleep disorders occur when:

(1) The external stimuli that normally entrain the internal clock change abruptly such as in jet lag or rapidly changing shift work;

(2) Individuals are required to work at times of the day/night when sleep tendencies are the greatest, e.g. shift workers who work the night shift routinely.

Central factors

Several syndromes that result in daytime hypersomnia are caused by CNS processes which, for the most part, have poorly understood mechanisms of disease. The most recognized syndromes in this category include narcolepsy, idiopathic central nervous system hypersomnia[35,36] and Kleine–Levin syndrome.

Although the underlying mechanisms responsible for narcolepsy still remain unclear, several hypotheses have been put forth. Currently, no structural abnormalities of the brain have been consistently identified in patients with narcolepsy. Genetics are likely to play a role, with the most probable scenario that of multiple genes being influenced by environmental factors. A strong association has been demonstrated between two human leukocyte antigen (HLA) haplotypes on human chromosome 6: HLA DQB1*0602 and DQA1*0102 which are found in 85% to 95% of narcoleptics as compared to 12% to 38% of the general American population[27,28], with the HLA DQB1*0602 haplotype being more closely associated with cataplexy[37,38].

Several recent findings have identified a potential biochemical basis for narcolepsy in dogs, mice and humans[39–42]. In the canine model of narcolepsy, a genetic defect in the hypocretin receptor 2 (Hcrtr2) gene results in a non-functional hypocretin receptor 2[40]. A human study has also demonstrated that hypocretin neurotransmission was deficient in 7 of 9 narcoleptic patients[42]. These data suggest that hypocretins (orexins) may be the major neurotransmitters responsible for narcolepsy (see Chapter 9).

BIOCHEMICAL REGULATION OF SLEEP–WAKE BIORHYTHM

Several neurotransmitters are involved directly and indirectly in the initiation and maintenance of sleep and wake states. Several of these same neurotransmitters have been linked to the development of psychiatric disorders, thus providing the link between sleep (and its disorder) and mental functions (and their disorders). This section will present a brief overview of how many of the currently defined neurotransmitters are involved in the control and regulation of sleeping and waking states as well as how they may be involved in sleep-related psychiatric diseases.

The catecholaminergic system

The existence of catecholaminergic neurons was discovered about 25 years ago in the rat brain by Swedish investigators and in 1983 in humans. Originally Jouvet[3] collected evidence that the majority of these neurons were situated in the locus ceruleus with widespread connectors and are critically involved in wakefulness and paradoxical sleep (REM). Later it was demonstrated that dopamine plays an important role in the maintenance of wakefulness as well as the maintenance of paradoxical sleep. Later studies have suggested that the involvement of norepinephrine in waking and its involvement in paradoxical sleep are in opposition to each other: during waking there is activity of norepinephrine neurons, whereas REM activity is decreased or prevented but does not play an essential role in the maintenance of waking[44]. REM sleep is a much more vulnerable state; basically α_1 and α_2 agonists as well as β_1 antagonists decrease REM, whereas α_1 and α_2 antagonists and β_1 agonists increase it.

The serotoninergic system

The serotoninergic system plays a key role in both sleep–wake and behavior regulation; any disruption of serotoninergic function induces modification of sleep and waking behavior[45]. The brain serotonin system arises from neurons in the midbrain (dorsal raphe nucleus (DRN)) with widespread projections. Under normal physiological conditions, the activity of the serotoninergic neurons is at a maximum during wakefulness, reduced during NREM sleep and almost totally abolished during REM sleep. Serotonin is no longer considered a 'sleep promoting neurotransmitter', or 'antiwaking' agent, but as a modulator with a very complex role: during wakefulness the activated serotoninergic system (in the hypothalamus) prepares and later promotes sleep occurrence; during sleep, the deactivated serotoninergic system controls the production of the REM stage.

Impairment of serotonin metabolism has specific effects on the states of vigilance. Using serotoninergic precursors results in a reduction of the waking state. Conversely, serotonin reuptake inhibitors suppress REM. The prevention of serotonin synthesis in the CNS induces severe insomnia. Low serotonin level in the CNS is a common finding in a variety of behavior and emotional disorders. (Sometimes REMs in NREM sleep could be related to the selective serotonin reuptake inhibitors.)

Histaminergic system

Histamine was synthesized by Winders and Vogt in 1907[46] but its physiological activity was only recently recognized. First it was shown to stimulate smooth muscle and was isolated from the liver and the lungs; later it was found in the hypothalamus[46]. In 1958 it was discovered that administration of histamine causes desynchronization of cortical EEG. Since histamine does not cross the blood–brain barrier, the waking effect could be related to a reflex activation of the reticulocortical projectors through a nociceptive or chemoceptive afferent system[46]. Current data support the hypothesis that histamine has a physiological function in modulating arousal mediated by H_1 receptors.

Cholinergic system

As long ago as 1931, Hess's experiments[47] indicated that the cholinergic or parasympathetic system was involved in sleep promotion. Since then, new evidence (see Tononi and Pompeono[48]) demonstrated more specifically that the cholinergic system serves two functions:

(1) An involvement in thalamic, cortical and hippocampal activation;

(2) A central role in the generation of REM sleep.

Release of acetylcholine (ACh) is associated with hippocampal rhythmic slow activity called theta rhythm. As we now know, theta rhythm appears during the different states of vigilance such as SWS, it episodically appears in REM and as 'superfocused attention' during high levels of athletic performance. ACh has been the first neurotransmitter implicated by Jouvet in 1962 as a regulator of wakefulness and a REM sleep generator[49].

ACh receptors are involved both in tonic as well as in phasic PGO components of REM. Additional evidence for the involvment of the cholinergic system in sleep–wakefulness comes from the study of sleep and psychiatric pathology. In patients with depression, for example, sleep abnormality such as short REM latency, increased REM percentage and reduction of NREM, particularly SWS, seem to be associated (at least in part) with an alteration in the cholinergic system with possible up-regulation of muscarinic receptors. Drugs with cholinominetic or antiaminergic properties produce depression-like symptoms. Sleep disorders, such as narcolepsy associated with cataplexy (a sudden loss of muscle tone during active waking, a sort of 'atonia without REM sleep'), are most clearly related to cholinergic mechanisms. Thus, the cholinergic system is closely involved in orchestrating wakefulness, REM sleep, altered states of consciousness, body postures and vestibular reflexes, as well as in mood and sleep disorders.

GABA-ergic/benzodiazepine system, sleep and mood

Although γ-aminobutyric acid (GABA) was discovered as recently as 1950, there is clear evidence that GABA is the most important inhibitory neurotransmitter of the mammalian CNS (see Müller[50]). Activation of central GABA-ergic inhibitory receptors represents the mechanism of action of the benzodiazepine class and of the newer compounds: zopiclone and zolpidem, as well as other hypnotics such as the barbiturates etomidate and methaqualone. GABA-ergic interneurons inhibit most neuronal systems determining the sleep–wake cycle, such as monoaminergic structures of the brainstem and the hypnogenic structures in the lower brainstem. Impairment of the GABA-ergic system is associated with both insomnia and anxiety disorders.

CNS peptides and sleep

The discovery of endogenous sleep promoting substances by Ishimori in 1909[51] and Legenore and Pierson in 1913[51] was appreciated only in the 1980s when a large number of endogenous substances were described as sleep modulators, i.e. sleep peptides (see Inouë[51]). Among them, the most studied were delta sleep inducing peptides (DSIPs). DSIPs are intrinsically involved in the circadian sleep–wake rhythm programming along with growth hormone releasing hormone, a melanophore-stimulating hormone and others. It is also important to note that DSIPs are involved in the neuroendocrine regulation of reproduction and antistress by the changes in the state of vigilance[51].

Another well-studied CNS peptide is glutathione (found in astrocytes, but not in neurons), which enhances NREM sleep, and is involved in brain temperature regulation. Concentration of glutathione is decreased in the substantia nigra of patients with Parkinson's disease. Muramyl peptides and cytokines were found to be directly connected sleep regulators with bacterial and viral immunomodulations. It was also reported that murine macrophages produce and release somnogenic and pyrogenic muramyl peptides through phagocytic digestion of bacteria[51]. This means that sleep may serve as a host defense response[51]. Interleukin-1, tumor necrosis factor (TNF) and interferon promote NREM, suppress REM and never occur during the normal daily vigilance[51]. However, corticotropic releasing hormone (CRH) and another CNS peptide, thyrotropin releasing factor (TRF), are known to be sleep-suppressive peptides[51]. Cytokines are also linked with neuroendocrine activity of the hypothalamic and pituitary hormones such as growth hormone releasing hormone (GRH), growth hormone (GH), adrenocorticotropic hormone (ACTH), thyrotropin releasing hormone (TRH), thyroid stimulating hormone (TSH) and prolactin which non-specifically but correlatively modulate sleep and wakefulness, serving as possible neuroendocrine transducers. Satiety-related factors such as cholecystokinin (CCK), bombesin and acidic fibroblast growth factor (aFGF) increase sleep shortly after eating[51].

Acidic fibroblast growth factor

Acidic fibroblast growth factor (aFGF) is the most potent satiety-inducing substance yet found. Administration of aFGF causes a dramatic increase in NREM sleep but not in REM sleep.

Vasoactive intestinal polypeptide and nonapeptide vasopressin

These peptides serve as REM sleep factors[51]. Further investigations of CNS peptides may bring new evidence of direct interactions between sleep, immune defense and states of vigilance in normalcy and pathology.

Adenosine

Recently, adenosine has received much attention from sleep researchers. Extensive experimental data by Radulovacki[5] placed adenosine

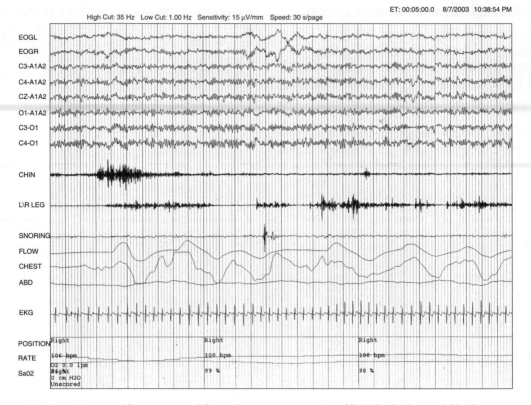

Figure 1.2 Stage 1 non-rapid eye movement sleep (slow eye movements), stable alpha rhythm, variable electromyogram

as one of the cornerstones of sleep–wake metabolism. Adenosine is a nucleoside, consisting of the purine base adenine linked to ribose, and acts as a neurotransmitter in the CNS. Adenosine A_1 receptors are located in many areas of the brain (with high affinity for adenosine) whereas A_2 receptors (low affinity for adenosine) are presented only in the striatum and nucleus accumbens. Adenosine and its analogs produce a strong hypnotic effect (through stimulation of A_2 receptors and inhibiting release of activated neurotransmitters). They increase both SWS and REM sleep. Benzodiazepines affect the CNS at least partially through adenosine A receptors[1]. Prolonged deprivation of REM sleep increases the number of adenosine receptors in a similar way to that of long-term use of caffeine. This suggests that the stimulating effects of caffeine and other methylxanthines are due to the blockade of central adenosine receptors[52],

which in turn suggests the existence of 'endocaffeine'.

HORMONES AND SLEEP

Human sleep is unique because of its consolidation in a single 6 to 8 h period, whereas fragmentation of the sleep period is typical for other mammals. Humans are also unique in their capacity to ignore circadian signals, and to maintain wakefulness despite an increased pressure to go to sleep. Also now humans typically live for long periods of time in an artificial environment (i.e. lights on during the night). In experimental situations, the results with human subjects are different from those in animal studies.

Sleep and circadian rhythmicity are controlled by the CNS and are both closely associated with the timing of hormonal release. The

Epoch: 136/983 Stage: 2 Body Position: Supine

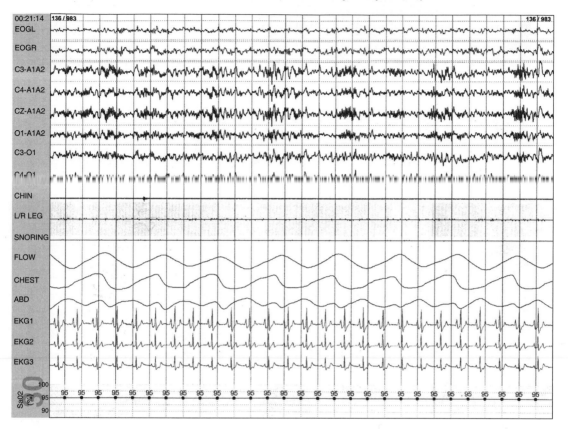

Figure 1.3 Stage 2 non-rapid eye movement sleep (spindles) and K complexes – high-amplitude theta waves followed by a spindle

timing, duration and characteristics of sleep are partially controlled by circadian rhythmicity. Current evidence does not support the notion that some hormones are entirely 'sleep related' such as 24 h rhythm of GH and prolactin without any input from the circadian system. Other hormones with 24 h profiles, such as cortisol, are entirely circadian dependent and are not influenced by the sleep–wake condition. It is accepted now that there are both circadian and sleep–wake inputs in the 24 h profiles of all pituitary-dependent hormones. New evidence suggests that hormones that are not directly controlled by the hypothalamic–pituitary axis, such as insulin and the hormones regulating water balance, also change during wakefulness and sleep[53].

The effect of sleep on endocrine secretion may be stimulatory or inhibitory. Sleep stimulates the secretion of GH and prolactin and increases plasma renin activity. Sleep inhibits the secretion of cortisol and interrupts the elevation of TSH, which is normally initiated during the early evening[53]. On the other hand, sleep deprivation leads to an approximately two-fold increase in nighttime TSH levels. As for the reproductive axis, the effects of sleep vary according to the stage of sexual maturation. In pubertal children, sleep enhances the release of gonadotropins; in adults, men are mostly unchanged, but in women the pulsatile release of the gonadotropins is inhibited during the follicular phase of the menstrual cycle but not during the luteal phase[53].

Epoch: 223 / 1099 Stage: 4 Body Position: NA

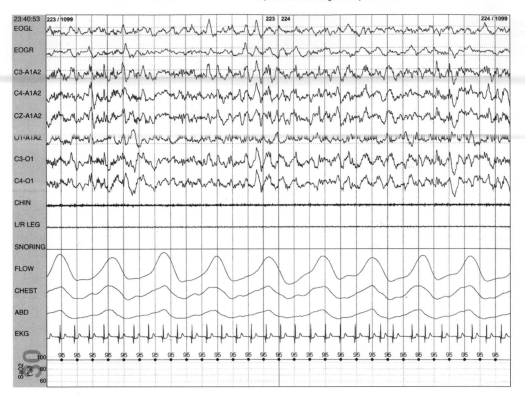

Figure 1.4 Stage 3 and 4 non-rapid eye movement sleep (delta sleep)

Glucose tolerance is decreased during sleep (because of a reduction in glucose utilization by the brain). Chronic partial sleep deprivation has also been associated with reduced glucose tolerance[43]. In short, the effects of sleep on hormones and the effect of hormones on sleep are of great functional significance.

The nocturnal rise of TSH, when cortisol secretion is quiescent, ends with the beginning of sleep. In the early morning period GH, TSH and prolactin concentrations are low, but cortisol level is high. Thus the release of all four pituitary hormones follows a highly co-ordinated program. With prolonged sleep deprivation and frequent awakenings, cortisol secretion is less pronounced and occurs earlier than in normal sleep, thus decreasing the efficient stress response.

Growth hormone and prolactin rise at the beginning of sleep. GH is released in pulses.

The most significant and sometimes the only burst of GH secretion occurs shortly after sleep onset during the first cycle of NREM[54]. The longer the first cycle of NREM, the more GH is secreted. In one study, whenever sleep was interrupted by a spontaneous awakening, the ongoing GH secretion was abruptly suppressed[55]. A detailed study by Van Coevorden and co-workers[56] showed that, in healthy elderly men (aged 67–89 years) the total amount of GH secreted over the 24 h span averaged one-third of the 24 h GH secretion of a young man, and that the amount of SWS in the elderly was also reduced three-fold.

The notion that sleep is a time of reparation is true for normal SWS with sufficient release of GH. In the elderly and especially in growing youngsters, SWS deprivation and disruption of GH may induce orofacial abnormality and other soft neurological signs[57]. Prolonged awakenings and frequent sleep

Epoch: 565 / 913 Stage: R Body Position: Supine

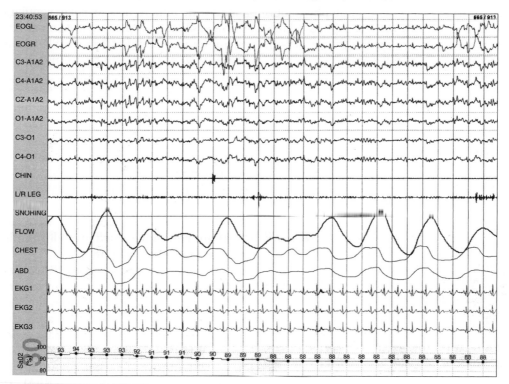

Figure 1.5 REM sleep (rapid eye movement, sawtooth waves, phasic EMG, irregular heart rate and breathing)

interruptions in young men are consistently associated with decreasing prolactin concentration, and with associated emotional and behavioral lability typical for the elderly[53]. The treatment with GH for children with GH deficiency shows a positive effect on sleep EEG[58].

Plasma renin activity is increased at the beginning of REM episodes[59]. In patients with obstructive sleep apnea who have increased urine and sodium excretion and decreased activity of the renin–angiotensin system, treatment with continuous nasal positive airway pressure (CPAP) induced REM rebound and restored plasma renin activity, which in turn contributed to the normalization of urine and sodium outputs[59].

Administration of the pineal hormone melatonin is capable of re-synchronizing the sleep–wake cycle in a variety of conditions, including real or simulated jet lag, or delayed sleep phase syndrome[53]. In elderly subjects,

there are significant correlations between daily endogenous melatonin production, total REM sleep and REM latency[60].

PHYSIOLOGICAL CHANGES IN SLEEP

The review of physiological changes in sleep is important for those interested in sleep psychiatry for two reasons:

(1) To verify how each state of vigilance – NREM, REM, quiet wakefulness, athletic or intellectual performance – are different in their physiological foundations (Figures 1.1–1.5);

(2) Sleep disorders as well as disordered daytime emotions or behaviors are, in essence, heightened displays of underlying normal physiological and psychosomatic signs.

Almost every system in the body undergoes changes during sleep. The pathophysiological changes associated with many medical disorders may be associated with changes in both sleeping and waking states.

Autonomic changes during sleep (Table 1.1)

There are extensive reviews of physiological changes in sleep[9,69]. In a nutshell, the most important of the autonomic changes during sleep involve the heart, circulation, respiration, and thermal, pupillary and erection regulation. The basic autonomic changes during sleep include increased parasympathetic tone and decreased sympathetic activity during NREM sleep. In REM sleep there is further increase of parasympathetic activity, and further decrease of sympathetic activity with short spikes of increased sympathetic activity during REMs, arousals or K complexes in NREM sleep[2]. The implications of physiological changes during sleep are profound. Dysfunction and abnormal changes in the autonomic nervous system during human sleep may be seen in disorders such as: multiple system atrophy; secondary autonomic posture; obstructive sleep apnea; cluster headaches; sleep terrors; REM-related sinus arrest; and painful penile erections, to name a few.

Respiratory function in sleep

Most normal individuals demonstrate circadian changes in their pulmonary function, with peak function occurring in the late afternoon and a nadir in function occurring in early morning hours[61,62]. Changes in pulmonary function are more specifically associated with changes in the CBT curve, with the nadir in function linked to the nadir in the CBT curve. The amplitude between peak and nadir flow and spirometric values in normal individuals is between 5% and 8%[63].

In normal people, during both REM and NREM sleep, cyclic changes are noted in tidal volume and respiratory rate with resultant changes in minute and alveolar ventilation[63]. During NREM sleep, minute ventilation falls by approximately 0.1–1.5 l/min. Sleep onset is characterized by periodic breathing, with regular increases and decreases in the amplitude of the individual's tidal volumes. This pattern may last from minutes up to an hour after sleep onset. As sleep progresses further into NREM sleep, breathing becomes more regular. Minute ventilation becomes reduced, probably due to a combination of reduced respiratory rate and tidal volumes. As a result of the fall of alveolar ventilation, blood gases are also altered: PCO_2 rises by 7–8 mmHg; PO_2 decreases by 3–10 mmHg, with a resultant reduction in the oxygen saturation by up to 2%[62].

In contrast to NREM sleep, REM sleep is marked by an irregular pattern of respiratory frequency and amplitude. Respiratory muscle tone is markedly reduced. There are clear discrepancies with regard to the changes in respiratory rate and minute ventilation in REM sleep, with little overall changes in these parameters when compared to NREM sleep. Reduction in oxygen saturation in relation to hypoventilation may be more pronounced during REM sleep[62].

Heart rate and circulation during sleep

Circulatory changes in sleep are well described in the literature[2,61,64]. Physiological changes in the heart during sleep include heart rate and cardiac output variations. Changes in circulation are reflected by blood pressure swings, changes in peripheral vascular resistance, and blood flow. Heart rate decreases during NREM sleep and is unstable during REM sleep. Heart rate changes are due to the predominance of parasympathetic activity during sleep and additional decrease of sympathetic activity during phasic REM[2]. Cardiac output falls progressively during sleep, particularly during the last REM cycle early in the morning[2]. This is a possible explanation of why predisposed

Table 1.1 Physiological variability between non-rapid eye movement (NREM) and rapid eye movement (REM) sleep

Function	NREM	REM
Electroencephalogram	Slow waves (theta and delta)	Low amplitude; tooth waves
Evoked potentials	None	Decreased amplitude
Eye movements (electro-olfactogram)	Slow, pendulum-like	Rapid eye movements
Chin electromyogram	Normal	Significant decrease or absence
Mono-synaptic reflex	Normal	Weak
Pupils	Normal	Myopic
Babinski symptoms	Apneas	Disappear
Intra-cerebral pressure	Decreases	Increases
Body movements	Typical	Absent
Brief finger movement	Not typical	Typical
Arousal threshold	Increases	Decreases
Type of thinking	Realistic thoughts	Emotional images
Dreams	Rare	Frequent
Sleep talking	Understandable; long, frequent	Not understandable, brief, rare
Blood pressure	Increased, lowest during stages 3 and 4; reduced variability	Short increases possible (40 mmHg); magnitude of change greater in hypertensive patients
Heart rate	Decreased; breathing variablity	Increased variability; bursts of eye movements accompanied by brief tachycardias, followed by bradycardia
Cardiac activity	Reduced cardiac output; vasodilatation	Transient vasoconstrictions in skeletal muscle circulation; cardiac arrest (during sleep) more frequent during this stage
Cerebral blood flow	Twenty-five per cent reduction of flow to brainstem; 20% reduction to cerebral cortex	Significantly increased blood flow, especially to cochlear nuclei
Temperature	Decreased brain and body temperature (rectal)	Increased brain temperature; absence of thermoregulation
Perspiration (except palms)	Maximal	Fluctuates by waves
Fever	Increased	Decreased
Palms perspiration	Decreased	Increases during REM bursts
Skin galvanic response (SGR)	Increases with body movements	Decreased
Seizure activity	Increased	Suppressed
Respiration	Respiratory rate decreased; upper-airway muscles may be hypotonic, obstructing oxygen flow in patients with sleep apnea	Breathing rapid and may be irregular
Oxygen metabolism	Decreased	Significantly increased
Blood CO_2 consumption	Maximal	Lowest
Endocrine functions	Growth hormone and prolactin secretion increased	ACTH–cortisol rhythm increased (in the morning)
Renal function	Decreased urine volume, excretion of sodium, potassium, chloride and calcium	Variable
Pain	Decreased receptor activity to noxious tactile stimuli	Decreased pain at level of tooth pulp
Sexuality	n/a	Nocturnal penile tumescence: increased

Data derived from Kales[1], Chokroverty[2], Kryger et al.[12]

15

people are most likely to have heart attacks during their sleep early in the morning[65]. Systemic arterial blood pressure falls by about 5–16% during NREM and significantly fluctuates in REM sleep. Cutaneous, muscular and mesenteric blood flow show little change during NREM but have profound vasodilatation in REM sleep. Cerebral blood flow and cerebral metabolic rate for glucose and oxygen decrease by 5–23% in NREM but increase by up to 41% above waking levels during REM sleep[2,61,64,65].

Neuromuscular changes in sleep

Somatic, cranial and respiratory muscle tones are maximal during wakefulness, slightly decreased in NREM and almost absent in REM sleep. For limb muscle atonia in REM sleep, the dorsal pontine tegmentum appears to be the central postsynaptic inhibitor of the motor neurons responsible for atonia of the somotic muscles. Upper airway muscles, such as the genioglossus, levator veli palatini and palatoglossus show phasic inspiratory and tonic expiratory activities. During sleep their muscle tones decrease, causing increased upper airway resistance and decreased airway space[66]. Selective reduction of genioglossal or hypoglossal nerve activity by alcohol and diazepam is worth emphasizing as well as the fact that protriptyline and strychnine each selectively increase such activity and might be used in some cases of increased upper airway resistance[2]. Masseter contraction causes bruxism and jaw clenching in sleep. Masseter electromyogram (EMG) decreases immediately before the apnea is present and increases again at the end of the apnea episode[67]. It may be caused by hyperoxic hypercapnia and inspiratory resistance.

Three types of REM sleep-related changes in respiratory muscle activity have been described[68]:

(1) Atonia of EMG during REM period;

(2) Rhythmic activity of diaphragm persists in REM but certain diaphragmatic motor units fail to fire. Kline and colleagues[2] described intermittent decrements of diaphragmatic activity during single breaths;

(3) Fractionations of diaphragmatic activity (clusters of pauses 40–80 ms correlated with PGO waves during REM).

The mechanism of muscle atonia in upper airway muscles during REM is believed to be related to glycine-mediated postsynaptic inhibition of the trigeminal, but not the hypoglossal motor neurons[2]. The roles of GABA and the serotonin system are also postulated.

Gastrointestinal physiology in sleep

Gastrointestinal physiology in sleep is a relatively new field, owing to difficulties in recording techniques. Extensive clinical and experimental work by Orr[69] and others shed some light on the importance of gastrointestinal changes in sleep.

In terms of gastric secretions, Orr[69] found no relationship between acid secretions in REM vs. NREM sleep. The most striking finding was failure of inhibition of acid secretion during the first 2 h of sleep. Overall gastric motility decreased in sleep.

Esophageal function (swallowing) is suppressed during sleep, specifically in stages 3–4 (delta sleep)[70], resulting in prolonged mucosal contact with refluxed acid which causes nocturnal gastroesophageal reflux (GER). Salivation in normal individuals decreases in sleep. Orr and co-workers[69,70] showed that arousals associated with swallowing prevented acid clearance and GER during sleep.

Intestinal motility in sleep is not well studied as yet, although a special pattern of intestinal motility, called migrating motor complex, was discovered, and consists of recurring motility every 90 min in the stomach and small intestine[71]; no clear differences of intestinal motility between REM and NREM sleep were found.

Temperature regulation in sleep

Body temperature follows a circadian rhythm independent of the sleep–wake rhythm[2]. During REM sleep thermoregulation seems to switch to poikilothermia. Body and brain temperature increases and sweating stops in REM sleep and shortly after this animals and humans become poikilothermic. NREM sleep is associated with a reduction of body temperature of 1–2 °C, due to vasodilatation; with the lowest temperature during the third sleep cycle[72] and increased sweating. The mechanism is probably related to the reduced activity of the preoptic nucleus of the hypothalamus[73]. MacFadyen and Oswald[74] observed increased SWS after 2–3 days of fasting. They believe that the purpose of this is conservation of energy. Increased body temperature and hypothalamic heating are associated with increased SWS.

Several clinical conditions are connected to thermoregulation problems. Jet lag and shift work may disrupt the linkage of temperature with SWS[2]. Menopausal hot flushes are considered a disorder of thermoregulation[75]. Hot flushes are associated with increased delta sleep. Some have also suggested a role of hyperthermia in sudden infant death syndrome[76].

CONCLUSION

Variation of physiological functions in normal sleep may be exaggerated in cases of sleep disorders to a degree that sets a condition for development of emotional, behavior and cognitive pathology, such as depression, confusion, or impulsive behavior. On the other hand, psychiatric problems further desychronize circadian rhythms. Anxiety, mood disorders, impulse control problems and other psychiatric pathology share neurophysiological processes with sleep and its disorders. Psychotropic medications may also play a major part in the physiological changes of sleep.

Neurophysiological changes in sleep are under the control of the same mechanisms that are responsible for control of wakefulness, levels of alertness, cognitive and motor activity and mood. Sleep–wake cycles are intimately connected states of vigilance. Disorders of sleep could lead to disorders of alertness during wakefulness, including psychiatric problems.

Further study of the role of neurophysiological mechanisms of sleep in the development of psychiatric pathology has tremendous potential.

References

1. Drucker CR, Merchant NH. Evolution of concepts of mechanisms of sleep. In Kales A, ed. *The Pharmacology of Sleep*. Berlin, New York: Springer-Verlag, 1995:1–21
2. Chokroverty S. Physiological changes in sleep. In Chokroverty S, ed. *Sleep Disorders Medicine*, 2nd edn. Boston: Butterworth/Heinemann, 1999:95–126
3. Jouvet M. The role of monoamines and acetylcholine containing neurons in the regulation of the sleep–wake cycle. Ergeb Physiol 1972; 64:166
4. Hernandez-Peon R. A cholinergic hypnogenic limbic forebrain hindbrain circuit. In Jouvet M, ed. *Aspects Anatomo-functionnels de Sumeil*. Paris: Centre National de la Recherche Scientifique, 1965
5. Radulovacki M. Pharmacology of adenosine system. In Kales A, ed. *The Pharmacology of Sleep*. Berlin, New York: Springer-Verlag, 1995:297–322
6. Hobson A, McCarley RW, Wyzinski PW. Sleep cycle oscillation: reciprocal discharge by two brainstem neuronal groups. *Science* 1989;55–8
7. Ambrozini MV, Sadile AG, Carnevaleu G, *et al*. The sequential hypothesis of sleep function. 1. Evidence that the structure of sleep depends on the nature of the previous waking experience. Physiol Behav 1988;43:325–37
8. Berbely A. *Secrets of Sleep*. New York: Basic, 1986
9. Steriade M. Brain electrical activity and sensory processing during waking and sleep states. In Kryger M, Roth T, Dement W, eds. *Principles and Practice of Sleep Medicine*, 3rd edn. Philadelphia: WB Saunders, 2000:93–111

10. Siegel JM. Brainstem mechanisms generating REM sleep. In Kryger M, Roth T, Dement W, eds. *Principles and Practice of Sleep Medicine*, 3rd edn. Philadelphia: WB Saunders, 2000:112–33

11. Jones BE. Basic mechanisms of sleep–wake states. In Kryger M, Roth T, Dement W, eds. *Principles and Practice of Sleep Medicine*, 3rd edn. Philadelphia: WB Saunders, 2000:134–54

12. Pommeggiani PL. Physiological regulation in sleep. In Kryger M, Roth T, Dement W, eds. *Principles and Practice of Sleep Medicine*. Philadelphia: WB Saunders, 2000:179–92

13. Borbely A. A two process model of sleep regulation. *Hum Neurobiol* 1982;1:195–204

14. Dinges D. Differential effects of prior wakefulness and circadian phase on nap sleep. *Electroencephalogr Clin Neurophysiol* 1986;64:224–7

15. Czeiler C, Zimmerman J, Ronda J, et al. Timing of REM sleep coupled to the circadian rhythm of body temperature in man. *Sleep* 1980;2:329–46

16. Carskadon M, Dement W. Normal human sleep: an overview. In Kryger M, Roth T, Dement W, eds. *Principles and Practice of Sleep Medicine*, 3rd edn. Philadelphia: WB Saunders, 2000:15–25

17. Breslau N, Roth T, Rosenthal L, et al. Daytime sleepiness: an epidemiological study of young adults. *Am J Public Health* 1997;87:1649–53

18. Rosenthal L, Roerhs T, Rosen A, et al. Level of sleepiness and total sleep time following various time in bed conditions. *Sleep* 1993;16:226–32

19. Roerhs T, Timms V, Zwyghuizen-Doorenbos A, et al. A two week sleep extension in sleepy normals. *Sleep* 1989;12:449–57

20. Carskadon M, Dement W. Sleepiness during extension of nocturnal sleep. *Sleep Res* 1979;8:147

21. Feinberg I, Fein G, Floyd T. Computer detected patterns of electroencephalographic delta activity during and after extended sleep. *Science* 1982;215:1131–3

22. Feinberg I, March J, Floyd T, et al. Homeostatic changes during post nap sleep maintain baseline levels of delta EEG. *Electroencephalog Clin Neurophysiol* 1985;61:134–47

23. Karacan I, Williams R, Finley W, et al. The effects of naps on nocturnal sleep: influence on the need for stage-1, REM and stage-4 sleep. *Biol Psychiatry* 1970;2:391–9

24. Harrison Y, Horne J. Should we be taking more sleep? *Sleep* 1995;18:901–7

25. Bonnet M. Infrequent periodic sleep disruption: effects on sleep, performance and mood. *Physiol Behav* 1989;45:1049–55

26. Bonnet M. Effect of sleep disruption on sleep, performance and mood. *Sleep* 1985;8:11–19

27. Bonnet M. The effect of sleep fragmentation on sleep and performance in younger and older subjects. *Neurobiol Aging* 1989;10:21–5

28. Stepanski E, Lamphere J, Badia P. Sleep fragmentation and daytime sleepiness. *Sleep* 1984;7:740–3

29. Martin S, Brander P, Deary I, et al. The effect of clustered versus regular sleep fragmentation on daytime function. *J Sleep Res* 1999;8:305–11

30. Fleetham J, West P, Mezon B, et al. Sleep, arousals, and oxygen desaturation in chronic obstructive pulmonary disease. *Am Rev Respir Crit Care Med* 1982;126:429–33

31. Saskin P, Moldofsky H, Lue F. Sleep and post traumatic rheumatic pain modulation disorder (fibrositis syndrome). *Psychosom Med* 1986;48:319–23

32. Czeisler C, Weitzman E, Moore-Ede M. Human sleep: its duration and organization depend on its circadian phase. *Science* 1980;210:1264–7

33. Richardson G, Carskadon M, Orav E, et al. Circadian variation of sleep tendency in elderly and young adult subjects. *Sleep* 1982;5:S82–94

34. Dijk D, Duffy J, Czeisler C. Circadian and sleep–wake dependent aspects of subjective alertness and cognitive performance. *J Sleep Res* 1992;1:112–17

35. Bassetti C, Aldrich M. Idiopathic hypersomnia: a series of 42 patients. *Brain* 1997;120:1423–35

36. Billiard M. Idiopathic hypersomnia. *Neurol Clin* 1996;14:573–82

37. Kadotani H, Faraco J, Mignot E. Genetic studies in the sleep disorder narcolepsy. *Genome Res* 1998;8:427–34

38. Mignot E, Hayduk R, Black J, et al. HLA DQB1*0602 is associated with cataplexy in 509 narcoleptic patients. *Sleep* 1997;20:1012–20

39. Takahashi J. Narcolepsy genes wake up the sleep field. *Science* 1999;285:2076–7

40. Lin L, Faraco J, Li R, et al. The sleep disorder canine narcolepsy is caused by a mutation in the hypocretin (orexin) receptor 2 gene. *Cell* 1999;42:365–76

41. Chemelli R, Willei J, Sinton C, et al. Narcolepsy in orexin knockout mice: molecular genetics of sleep regulation. *Cell* 1999;98:437–51

42. Nishino S, Ripley B, Overeem S, et al. Hypocretin (orexin) deficiency in human narcolepsy. *Lancet* 2000;355:39–40

43. Spiegel K, Leproult R, Van Cauter E. Impact of sleep debt on metabolic and endocrine function. *Lancet* 1999;23:1435–9

44. Wauguier A. Pharmacology of the catecholaminergic system. In Kales A, ed. *The Pharmacology of Sleep*. Berlin, New York: Springer-Verlag, 1995:65–90

45. Adrien J. The serotonin-ergic system and sleep–wakefulness regulation. In Kales A, ed. *The Pharmacology of Sleep*. Berlin, New York: Springer-Verlag, 1995:91–116

46. Monti JM. Pharmacology of the histaminergic system. In Kales A, ed. *The Pharmacology of Sleep*. Berlin, New York: Springer-Verlag, 1995:117–42

47. Hess WR. Le Sommeil. *CR Soc Biol* 1933;107:1333

48. Tononi G, Pompeono O. Pharmacology of the cholinergic system. In Kales A, ed. *The Pharmacology of Sleep*. Berlin, New York: Springer-Verlag, 1995:143–210

49. Jouvet M. Recherches sur les structures et les mechanisms responsibles des differentes phases du sommeil physiologique. *Arch Ital Biol* 1962,100.125

50. Müller WE. Pharmacology of the GABAergic/benzodiazepine system. In Kales A, ed. *The Pharmacology of Sleep*. Berlin, New York: Springer-Verlag, 1995:211–42

51. Inoüe S. Pharmacology of the CNS peptides. In Kales A, ed. *The Pharmacology of Sleep*. Berlin, New York: Springer-Verlag, 1995:243–67

52. Snyder SH, Katims JJ, Annau Z, *et al.* Adenosine receptors and behavioral actions of methylxanthines. *Proc Natl Acad Sci USA* 1981;78:3260–4

53. Van Cauter E. Hormones and sleep. In Kales A, ed. *The Pharmacology of Sleep*. Berlin, New York: Springer-Verlag, 1995:279–306

54. Holl RW, Hartmann ML, Veldhuis JD, Taylor WM, Thorner MO. Thirty-second sampling of plasma growth hormone in man: correlation with sleep stages. *J Clin Endocrinol Metab* 1991;72:854–61

55. Van Cauter E, Kerkhofs M, Caufriez A, *et al.* A quantitative estimation of GH secretion in normal man: reproductivity and relation to sleep and time of day. *J Clin Endocrinol Metab* 1992;74:1441–50

56. Van Coevorden A, Mockel J, Laurent E, et al. Neuroendocrine rhythms and sleep in aging. *Am J Physiol* 1991;260:E651–61

57. Golbin AZ. *The World of Children's Sleep*. Salt Lake City, Utah: Michaelis Publishing Co, 1995

58. Wu RH, Thorpy MJ. Effect of growth hormone treatment on sleep EEGs in growth hormone deficient children. *Sleep* 1988;11:425–9

59. Brandenberger G. Hydromineral hormones during sleep and wakefulness. *Sleep Res* 1991;20A:186

60. Singer CM, Sack RL, Denney D, *et al.* Melatonin production and sleep in the elderly. *Sleep Res* 1988;3:99

61. Orem J. Physiology in sleep. In Kryger M, Roth T, Dement W, eds. *Principles and Practice of Sleep Medicine*, 3rd edn. Philadelphia: WB Saunders, 2000:169–318

62. Krieger J. Respiratory physiology: breathing in normal subjects. In Kryger M, Roth T, Dement W, eds. *Principles and Practice of Sleep Medicine*. Philadelphia: WB Saunders, 2000:229–41

63. Hettzel MR, Clark TJH. Comparison of normal and asthmatic circadian rhythm in peak expiratory flow rate. *Thorax* 1980;35:732

64. Parmegiani PL, Morrisson AR. Alteration of autonomic functions during sleep. In Leucey AD, Spyer KM, eds. *Central Regulation of Autonomic Functions*. New York: Oxford University Press, 1990.367

65. Verrier RL, Muller JE, Hobson JA. Sleep, dreams, and sudden death: the case for sleep as an autonomic stress test for the heart. *Cardiovasc Res* 1996;31:181–211

66. Tangel DJ, Mezzanotte WS, Sanberg EJ, *et al.* Influences of sleep on tensor palatini EMG and upper airway resistance in normal man. *J Appl Physiol* 1991;70:2574

67. Suratt PM, Hollowell DE. Inspiratory activation of the masseter. In Issa FG, Surratt PM, Remmers JE, eds. *Sleep and Respiration*. New York: Wiley, 1990:109

68. Pack AL, Kline LR, Hendricks JE, *et al.* Neural mechanisms in the genesis of sleep apnea. In Issa FG, Surratt PM, Remmers JE, eds. *Sleep and Respiration*. New York: Wiley, 1990:177

69. Orr WC. Gastrointestinal physiology. In Kryger M, Roth T, Dement W, eds. *Principles and Practice of Sleep Medicine*, 3rd edn. Philadelphia: WB Saunders, 2000:279–88

70. Orr WC, Robinson M, Johnson L. Acid clearance during sleep in the pathogenesis of reflux esophagitis. *Dig Dis Sci* 1981;26:423

71. Guyton AC, Hall JE. *Textbook of Medical Physiology*. Philadelphia: WB Saunders, 1996:810

72. Henane R, Buguet A, Roussel B, *et al.* Variations in evaporation and body temperatures during sleep in man. *J Appl Physiol* 1977;42:50–5

73. Berger RJ, Phillips MH. Comparative physiology of sleep. Thermoregulation and metabolism from the perspective of energy metabolism. In Issa FG, Surratt PM, Remmers JE, eds. *Sleep and Respiration*. New York: Wiley, 1990;41

74. McFayden H, Oswald SA. Starvation and human slow wave sleep. *J Appl Physiol* 1973;35:391

75. Woodward S, Freedman RR. The thermoregulatory effects of menopausal hot flashes on sleep. *Sleep* 1994;17:497

76. Kimmonth AL. Review of the epidemiology of sudden infant death syndrome and its relationship to temperature regulation. *Br J Gen Pract* 1990;40:161

2

Development of sleep–wake structure in human ontogenesis

Alexander N. Shepovalnikov and Alexander Z. Golbin

In this short period of time researchers have discovered that sleep is a dynamic behavior. Not simply the absence of waking, sleep is a special activity of the brain, controlled by elaborate and precise mechanisms.

J. Allan Hobson, *Sleep*, 1989[34]

INTRODUCTION

The roots of adaptive human behavior are based on productive wakefulness. Productive wakefulness (meaning sustained alertness and focused attention) is an intrinsic part of the sleep–wake cycle. Simply stated, we cannot truly understand wakefulness without understanding sleep. That is why analysis of the ontogenetic longitudinal changes of sleep–wake states and their mechanisms is key to our understanding of sleep as well as daytime behavior and its disorders.

Investigation of human sleep, specifically sleep states in newborns, has a long and fascinating history involving researchers of many nations. The discovery of bioelectrical activity of the brain and the methodology of its registration, by the German physiologist Berger in 1930[2], sparked interest in this new and promising language of the brain. In 1937, separation of sleep into distinct states was first described by Harvey, Loomis and Hobart[3]. After Aserinsky and Kleitman discovered rapid eye movement (REM) sleep in 1953[4], a flood of research into adult sleep followed. A publication in 1968 by Rechtschaffen and Kales, *A Manual of Standardized Terminology, Techniques and Scoring System for Sleep Stages of Human Subjects*[5], gave the research and clinical studies solid ground. Analysis of sleep–wake states in infants, on the other hand, was not easy. Among the significant works in this area was the 1971 publication of '*A Manual of Standardized Terminology, Techniques and Criteria for Scoring of States of Sleep and Wakefulness in Newborn Infants*' by Anders, Emde and Parmelee[6].

Since that time, new and more advanced techniques of electroencephalography (EEG) analysis have been developed and are presented in this chapter. Current knowledge of sleep–wake development in fetuses, premature infants, full-term infants and older children clearly relates the formation of sleep–wake stages to central nervous system (CNS) maturation. At the same time, deviations in the development of sleep–wake states are considered sensitive and specific indicators of CNS problems and provide an insight into prognosis and long-term outcome[7].

One of the reasons for studying the structure of sleep is to gain knowledge into the function of the different stages of sleep. The second reason to study the structure of sleep is to advance techniques in the understanding of the regulation mechanisms on all levels, including the brain as a whole. The third reason is to search for the roots of sleep and daytime pathology for their presentation or treatment[8].

Although the neuronal structures underlying physiological mechanisms producing delta rhythm are in debate, available data have initiated new ideas. Steriade and colleagues[9] have shown that delta waves can be produced by cortical neurons, contrary to the prior belief that delta sleep is the function of deep brain structures. These cortical neurons are the targets of arousal systems that include the reticular activating forebrain, and hypocretin–orexin arousal systems[10]. The most recent discovery by Feinberg and Campbell[11], using advanced statistical techniques, shows that the amount of delta activity generated during waking is the same whether the subject has spent the day studying science or day dreaming. Examination of delta wave kinetics is consistent with the possibility that delta activity is the physiological correlation of the neuronal systems that underlie consciousness. Neither the state of consciousness nor its 'depth' or 'richness' seem to affect the distribution of delta activity, although it diminishes with age. Based on these data, Feinberg and Campbell concluded that NREM delta activity serves as a specific homeostatic function for the neuronal systems that underlie consciousness.

REM sleep plays an important role in memory, emotions, learning, language and other aspects of neuromental development[11-15]. Major evidence demonstrating the importance of REM sleep in facilitating recall was described in 1982 by Scrima[15], who concluded that the active/REM state and quiet alert states are correlated with CNS maturational changes in the infant. This main state of newborn sleep is the primary time for neurons to grow[16].

As for NREM, the major feature of sleep spindles is that they are a ubiquitous phenomenon in sleep, first appearing and developing

rapidly between 1.5 and 3 months of age. It is postulated that sleep spindles reflect growth and maturation of thalamocortical structures, and their function includes promotion of central activations[17]. Sleep spindle development seems to be an accurate reflection of normal maturation in the CNS. Deficiency or hemispheric asymmetry of spindles signifies CNS abnormality[18].

Ontogenetic development of spindles on an EEG follows and replicates the development of muscle activity. Voino-Yacenecky[19], using an original method of isolation of cortical zones by Khananashvili[20], demonstrated on rabbit embryos that body functions developed, not simultaneously, but sequentially (heterochronic). First, muscle activity goes through its four phases of maturity: (1) tonic slow movements; (2) periodic complexes of low amplitude, but high frequency rhythmic movements (the first level); (3) appearance of 'spindle-type' muscle movements with even pauses in between (the second level); and (4) pauses between 'spindles' becoming uneven and organized into 'groups' synchronized with the rhythms of scratching and 'rhythmical walking reflexes'. Hamburger[21] described identical phases in the development of neuronal activity and, later, similar phases were found in the development of the intestinal system.

Thus, ontogenetic neurophysiological data confirmed that delta and spindle activity (major EEG signs of sleep) developed first and alpha rhythm (sign of wakefulness) developed later.

OVERVIEW OF THE DEVELOPMENT OF THE SLEEP–WAKE STRUCTURE

The development of REM-activity structure in the fetus, REM–NREM in children and organization of circadian sleep–wake cycles all follow neuromotor and central nervous system (CNS) maturation. This development can be affected by multiple endogenic, medical and environmental factors. The main state of the fetus, neonate and infant is sleep. The rhythmic cycle of activity in the fetus can be recorded *in utero* by 20 weeks of conceptional age. By 32 weeks of conceptional age, body movements are absent in 53% of fetuses[22–27].

The sleep of a preterm infant is different from that of a full-term healthy infant at matched conceptional age in terms of:

(1) A longer ultradian sleep cycle (70 minutes versus 53 minutes);

(2) More abundant tracé alternant pattern;

(3) Less abundant low voltage irregular active sleep;

(4) Fewer numbers and shorter periods of arousals;

(5) Fewer body and rapid eye movements.

The number of REMs increases with gestational age. In general, ontogenesis of sleep–wake states is comparable in premature and full-term infants.

The full-term infant spends about 70% of its time in sleep. Sustained periods of wakefulness appear by 6 months of age, distributed during late afternoon and early evening hours. The longest period of sleep moves to throughout the night. REM sleep is a disproportionately longer part of sleep. NREM sleep starts to be clearly demarcated from REM and develops an internal structure (delta sleep, spindles). Slowly, REM decreases to be substituted by wakefulness. The critical period of sleep–wake development is at approximately 3 months of age, having a long-term effect on cognitive, emotional and social functioning. After this time, adult-like REM–NREM sleep stages begin to emerge and circadian rhythm is established. Many factors can influence basic rhythms in newborns and infants; specifically significant are feeding, non-nutritive sucking and predominant body position[28,29]. For example, non-nutritive sucking promotes the 'switch' from wakefulness to sleep (see Chapter 15). 'Quiet' sleep no longer exists when the infant is in the 'prone' body position, which is associated statistically with a high risk for sudden infant death syndrome.

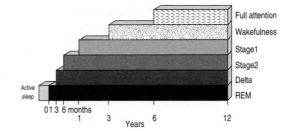

Figure 2.1 Chronology of the development of sleep–wake stages. Sleep stages develop first, wakefulness and attention later. Sleep is a foundation for wakefulness and alertness

There appears to be a relationship between sleep structure maturity at 3 months post-term and 1 to 2 month psychomotor performance[26,27]. Thus, physiological measurements of sleep can be reliable objective indicators and predictors of later psychomotor development. Longitudinally, active sleep transforms into REM, and NREM sleep goes through differentiation of delta sleep, then spindles. Spindle activity is associated with the development of sustained wakefulness and later with alertness and focused attention (Figure 2.1). Maturation of wakefulness, alertness and attention seems to follow the development of the REM–NREM infrastructure.

Between the ages of 9 and 12 months, the REM stage decreases to about 30% and later continues to decrease to adult levels of 20% at about 5–7 years of age. Decreased or REM sleep is eventually substituted by increased daytime wakefulness. Unique characteristics of the physiology of sleep between 1 and 3 years of age include a period of stabilization of sleep stages, although the sleep structure is still different from that in young adults[27]:

(1) A relatively smaller number of state changes occur per hour;

(2) EEG amplitude is significantly higher in all stages;

(3) Slow-wave sleep is considerably longer;

(4) There is a relatively smooth progression of states across the sleep period;

(5) Transition between stages is relatively regular and consistent in comparison with adults who often abruptly cross several stages of sleep at a time.

After 5 years of age, sleep continues to mature, while development of wakefulness, alertness and attention takes the lead. Total sleep time in the middle of childhood is about 2.5 hours longer than in the healthy young adult and is distributed equally throughout all sleep stages. The predominance of sleep during prenatal and early childhood periods signifies its fundamental mental role in both structural 'hardware' and functional 'software' development of body and mind.

DEVELOPMENT OF CNS MECHANISMS OF SLEEP–WAKE CYCLES IN ONTOGENESIS

During evolution, the human brain, especially cortical zones, progressively grew from primate to human and took on more responsibility for bodily functions, including the regulation of circadian rhythms in connection with the environment.

The concept of the 'critical period' should not be forgotten when considering the general principles of longitudinal ontogenetic development[30]. The maturation of the sleep–wake cycles progresses not continuously and smoothly, but in 'spurts' around critical times in CNS development. Such critical periods in the development of bioelectrical activity of the brain are:

(1) At 36–37 weeks of intrauterine life, when EEG passive states vs. active states begin to differentiate;

(2) On the 9th–10th day of postnatal life, when the infant appears to be active after breast feeding, acts of defecation and urination are separated and the phasic activity in sleep becomes significant;

(3) At the end of the first month of postnatal development, when slow waves on the sleep EEG become stable;

(4) At 8–9 weeks of postnatal life, when 'sleep spindles' appear and develop quickly;

(5) In the first month of the third year of life when theta and delta sleep are no longer dominant.

The maturation of active, waking EEG rhythms develops unevenly and not simultaneously (also called heterochronically). First, the mature waking rhythm is observed in the motor zones, as a 'window' with periods of sleep that become stable and consolidated during the day, at about 6 months of age and then, much later, in the occipital areas at about 2 years of age[32,33]. Focused attention appears much later – after 5–6 years of age (Figure 2.1).

What do we know about the sleep–wake regulatory mechanisms? Recent advances in the biochemistry of sleep have increased our understanding of the biochemical mechanisms of sleep and their deviations. Approximately 24 peptides are capable of modulating slow (NREM) and paradoxical (REM) sleep[34]. New data about molecular mechanisms of biological clocks increase our understanding of the functional roles of sleep in the link of biochemical transformations in the brain and body[8]. One of the key questions remains: what is the mechanism of the systemic reorganization of cortical centers in sleep? Also, what is the mechanism of maintenance of individual personality features during the absence of consciousness in deep sleep?

The development of a method to analyze integrative brain activity is the essence of current neurophysiology[3–33,35,36]. One of the productive methodological approaches for analyzing integrative brain activity is the method of evolutionary physiology. Evolutionary physiology is based on the fact that, during various disorders, both brain and body functions are temporarily returned to the previous phase of development. By analysis of these regressive changes, the level of pathological changes can be evaluated. Among the 'key structures' is a net of intercorrelations between different cortical 'centers'. Such intercentral constellations are relatively stable for each stage of sleep and for wakefulness, as well as for different ages of normalcy and some forms of pathology.

It is known that, during phylogenetic development, new rostral formations accept the functions previously belonging to the caudal structures. (For example, the cortical structure in reptiles has functions that belong to the midbrain in fish.) With the development of the frontal brain, the cycles of sleep–wake change: paradoxical sleep (analog of REM in humans) becomes shorter, slow-wave sleep is longer. The period of sleep is also relatively longer[25].

Early human postnatal ontogenesis repeats phylogenesis. The electrographic structure of wakefulness and phases of sleep quickly change (maturing from archetypal to 'human' REM). The cycle of sleep–wake transforms from polyphasic to biphasic. These changes are in agreement with the concept of 'heterochronic' development of the child's brain: the formation of (phylogenetically) older structures is completed sooner than evolutionarily younger structures such as frontal or temporal–parietal cortical zones (Figure 2.2).

In short, mechanisms of sleep develop earlier than mechanisms of alertness and prolonged wakefulness[30]. The electroencephalogram is commonly used for quantitative and qualitative analysis of the levels of sleep and alertness in children and adults. The development of new methods of investigation of the functional states in the brain, such as positron emission tomography (PET) or magnetic resonance imaging (MRI), made visually scored EEG less useful. However, the combination of EEG with other polygraphic parameters (electro-olfactogram, electromyogram, electrocardiogram, skin galvanic response, pneumogram, etc.) and, most importantly, with the new computerized EEG analysis, make EEG once again an indispensable tool for the study of integrative brain activity. The level of correlations between EEG waves from different leads and their changes can be interpreted as a level of functional connections between distant parts of the brain. This ability to provide instant temporal resolution between specific

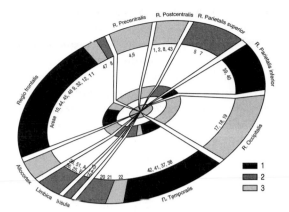

Figure 2.2 The primary system complex of phylogenetically new cortex zones used specifically in human work and speech activities. (1) Cortex zones growing progressively from primate to human; (2) zones that are relatively stable in primate species; and (3) zones that decrease relatively if compared to the overall dimension of the cortex from primate to human (according to Shevchenko, 1972[31])

brain areas is a distinct advantage of EEG even compared to PET.

Registration and analysis of EEG in newborns and infants is accompanied by several methodological difficulties, including quick changes in sizes of cortical zones and their projections on the skull (especially for temporal and frontal parts). For example, motor zones in children in the first few months after birth are projected under the parietal area of the skull, and not under the temporal bone, as is the case in children over 6 years of age. The relative sizes of the frontal lobes in infants are smaller but the occipital ones are larger.

Another obstacle is that impedance between EEG electrodes of newborns and infants is very high, which makes the quality of recording difficult. The most important obstacle is that typical EEG functional tests are impossible to perform in infants as there are multiple biological artifacts, which might be interpreted as slow brain activity due to pulsation of the brain, acts of sucking, tongue movements and jaw tremors, etc. The conceptual difficulty in the interpretation of EEG pathological changes is that some EEG phenomena in newborns and infants might be relatively normal. It is important to remember that the reaction of the immature brain is different to that of the mature brain.

Previously, investigations suggested that the beginning of sleep in newborns is paradoxical sleep similar to REM in adults. However, according to current knowledge of neuro-physiological and biochemical chronobiologi-cal dynamics, the REM stage should follow the slow-wave stage[36,37].

Based on the distribution of correlations between distant cortical zones in REM and NREM sleep, it was possible to conclude that the ontogenetic development of intercortical functional relations typical of paradoxical sleep is formed later than slow-wave sleep. Thus, it is clear that, at the beginning, sleep in a newborn is not REM sleep.

The transition from wakefulness to drowsi-ness and light sleep is difficult to determine visually by EEG. Typically, during light sleep the EEG registers a polymorphic 4–7 Hz, low-amplitude (30 mV) activity. With deepening of sleep, the EEG amplitude is increased and the frequency decreased. Some waves are as high as 180–100 mV of 0.5–1.5 Hz. The frequency of such delta waves is not significant (about 5–8 per 20 s). At the end of the first month, the EEG of slow-wave sleep becomes similar to the pattern of delta sleep (stage 3–4) of adults. The main indication of stage 2 (sigma rhythm or sleep spindles) is not registered until 15 months of age, so the dynamics of transitions from wakefulness to stages 1 to 2 to 3 to 4 is difficult to follow in small children.

As previously mentioned, paradoxical sleep in newborns is a sleep period that follows a slow-wave stage. Newborns' 'paradoxical sleep' differs from the adult REM stage by frequent high-amplitude (50 mV) theta and delta waves. Typically stage 4 (stable delta pattern) is not developed until the end of the second month of life.

Advanced methods of computerized EEG analysis, such as correlation and coherent analysis demonstrate that the levels of inter-cortical EEG wave correlations reflect their functional relationships.

A systematic study of the time–space distribution of biopotentials of the brain

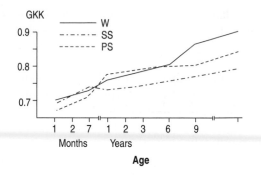

Figure 2.3 Age dynamics of EEG correlations in differ-ent functional states during sleep and wakefulness. W, wakefulness; SS, slow-wave (delta) sleep; PS, paradoxical (REM) sleep; GKK, general correlation coefficient (sum-mary of all coefficients). This indicator allows integration of both parameters of EEG, frequency and amplitude

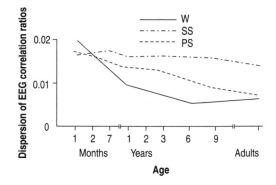

Figure 2.4 Age differences in integrated EEG activity in sleep and wakefulness. W, wakefulness; SS, slow-wave (delta) sleep; PS, paradoxical (REM) sleep

demonstrated that the distribution of inter-central correlations along the sagittal line during waking and sleep in children is significantly different from that in adults. The younger the child, the more notable are the changes (Figures 2.3 and 2.4).

The times of EEG inter-central correlations of bioactivity in occipital areas are brief in duration. In the parietal and frontal zones, on the other hand, the inter-central functional relationships are low and equal. The center of symmetry is in the posterior parietal zone. With age the frontal zones' functional connec-tions grow quickly.

Inter-central (functional) correlations on EEG, during wakefulness and sleep, are simi-lar at first. There are no negative correlations

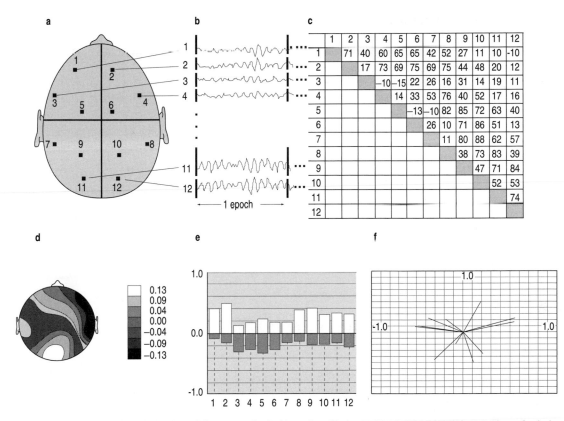

Figure 2.5 Automated analysis of spatial–temporal relations of oscillations of brain biopotentials. (a) Chart depicting the arrangement of electrodes; (b) selecting the standard epoch for EEG analysis; (c) constructing the EEG correlation matrix: in correlation, 0 and point signs are omitted, their values are averaged over 30–40 epochs of analysis; (d) mapping the spatial distribution of the levels of the EEG correlation ratios and their scale; (e), (f) examples of histograms reflecting the changes in the levels of the correlation ratios for corresponding leads (1–12) and an example of the distribution of radial vectors in factorial space

and the level of correlations between electrodes is proportional to the distance, especially in occipital areas.

The level of similarity of electrical cortical activity in different zones during fixed epochs of the EEG reflects systemic integrative brain activity. In other words, this method permits review of how the bioelectrical activity in one zone influences the bioelectrical activity in another zone, and how the EEG from one lead is connected to the EEG from another lead. A graphical representation is shown in Figure 2.5a. The level of similarity is analyzed between each of the two electrodes and then a correlation schema is created automatically

where the level of similarity (Figure 2.5b and 2.5c) between each set of leads of the EEG is between +1 and −1. The full extent of such correlations depends on the quantity of EEG electrodes. If the EEG is registered from eight leads, then for each analyzed epoch (usually 4 s) there will be 28 correlations. If the amount of leads is increased to 20, however, then the number of correlations is increased to 190 (diagonal and symmetrical numbers are not included). To analyze integrative physiological functions, it is not necessary to analyze all spectra of the EEG, but only to analyze the level of statistical similarity in certain levels of frequency waves using so-called coherent

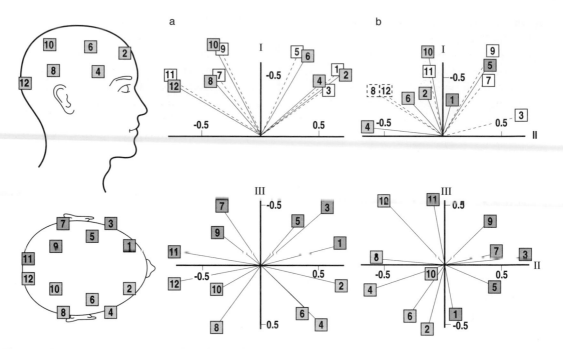

Figure 2.6 Vector representation of results of the multi-parameter analysis of the system organization of brain activity in normal (a) and pathological (b) states. Top panel, projections of electroencephalography (EEG) radial vectors on the plane of factors I–II; bottom panel, on the plane of factors II–III. Numbers of EEG radial vectors (1–12), which correspond to EEG leads as shown on the left. A healthy person in a state of rest has a steady distribution of EEG radial vectors, which reproduce the location of corresponding EEG leads in abstract three-dimensional space. In case of pathology (e.g. a patient with concussion of the brain) this order is disrupted

analysis of the EEG. A detailed theoretical foundation of this method and its reliability and validity are presented in the work of Livanov[35] and Nunez[36]. Currently, correlation and coherent analysis of the EEG are actively used for many conditions including human sleep (Figure 2.6).

The importance of this method is based on the use of a large quantity of numbers. A method of compression of data, which makes them more convenient for visual and express analysis, has been developed and well described[30,32,33,35,36]. The results of EEGs analyzed by this method are presented in a three-dimensional factorial space (Figures 2.5 and 2.6). The key informative parameter reflecting the level of inter-correlations between pairs of electrodes is an angle between radial-vectors (Figure 2.5f). The three-dimensional abstract factorial space is associated with three factors (factors 1, 2 and 3) identical to the actual placement of electrodes on the surface of the skull. Results showed that the EEG organization became more prominent with age. Cerebral pathology leads to different levels of disorganization of this structure. During wakefulness the level of inter-correlation is much higher than during sleep (Figure 2.7). This implies that in sleep the brain works in a less controlled regime than during wakefulness. During wakefulness 'the levels of freedom' in each zone are decreased. Interestingly, with age, the 'order' during wakefulness of the functional relationships between the cortical centers is increased, but their 'level of freedom' during sleep is not changed. It is possible to conclude that the activity of the 'awake brain' in individual ontogenesis progresses more than the activity of the 'sleeping brain'.

The phenomenon of 'emancipation' of the cortical zones in sleep from the hypothetical 'strict central control' systems during wakefulness is in agreement with an interesting and not fully appreciated hypothesis described by Evarts in 1965, a pioneer of microelectrode studies[38]. This hypothesis discusses how different regions of the brain work in sleep versus in wakefulness. It is now known that wakefulness is characterized by the very specific differentiation between groups of cortical neurons (micromodules or neuronal networks) and 'vertical columns' of neuronal circuits. In sleep, especially in delta sleep, many 'micromodules' work in synchrony thus losing their individual specificity. It is probable that this synchronized activity between many distant brain zones is necessary for reparational processes in sleep. In this sense, such 'freedom' from the 'central control' is a preparation for the 'hard-specific job' that is performed during wakefulness. The behavior of an active and alert person demands fast, precise, highly specialized and differentiated reactions with concentrated attention and a variety of modulations. To achieve this, the specialized and differentiated activity of neuronal networks (micromodules) is necessary, in contrast to the synchronized activity which can only produce general responses.

According to Evarts' hypothesis[38], a strict differentiation of neuronal networks is achieved by the central active inhibition system. This system blocks the tendency of neurons for synchronized activity, thus 'forcing' neuronal networks to work in 'individual' patterns. In sleep, the brain is 'free' from these inhibitory 'forces' and neuronal networks switch to the 'relaxed' synchronized patterns. The EEG findings in children are in agreement with the existence of central morphophysiological systems that actively force micromodules to work 'individually' in a different fashion[32,33].

Many peculiarities of a child's EEG can be explained by 'immaturity' of such a 'damping system'. With mild extrapolation of Evarts' hypothesis, it is possible to assume that in small children the system controlling neuronal networks is not developed, a circumstance which makes synchronization easy and differentiated reactions difficult. From an ontogenetic point of view synchronization might have a 'positive' function by providing good conditions for nutritive metabolism. It may be that this is the reason why newborns sleep longer and their behavioral reactions are generalized during short periods of alertness. When a child grows, this 'co-ordinated control damping inhibitory' system develops, providing a neurophysiological basis for specific organized differentiated reactions and activities. Differentiation of micromodules is reflected by differentiation of the EEG and decreased synchronized patterns, allowing EEG contrasts between sleep and wakefulness.

During ontogenetic development of the integrative activity of brain myelinizations, it becomes key to unite distant cerebral structures. The time of myelinization is crucially important for the child's future neuropsychological development. It is interesting that the myelinization of neurons, mostly responsible for the integrative processes in the brain (non-specific thalamocortical paths; reticular formation; corpus collosum; and, especially, inter-cortical associative connections), is completed much later than the myelinization of other brain structures[39]. Integrative processes in the sleeping brain can be visualized by a compressed coherent EEG analysis (Figure 2.7).

Immaturity of structural and functional development of the brain can present in the form of different dysrhythmias, especially paroxysms[25].

How frequent are deviations of sleep and daytime EEGs in newborns? Unfortunately, symptoms of brain dysfunction are frequent, but the traditional methods of EEG analysis do not allow appropriate verification. EEG evaluation (using spectral wave analysis) of newborns in the general population shows that abnormal EEGs might be as frequent as 25%, a number significantly higher than previously thought. These abnormal signs disappear in subsequent days and weeks, but the consequences of ischemia of the basal structures and hippocampal areas may result in neuropsychiatric and autonomic deviations many years later.

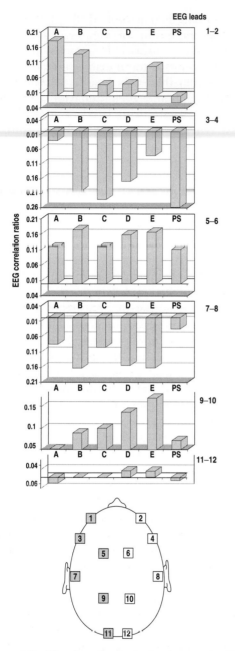

Figure 2.7 The inter-hemispheric changes in EEG during wakefulness (A), different periods of non-REM (B–E) and REM sleep (PS). These data show that bilateral correlations between hemispheres are different and specific in wakefulness as well as in the different stages of sleep. For example, in sleep, especially stages 2 and 4, there is increasing correlation between frontal, central and parietal EEGs, but decreased correlation between frontal temporal and occipital zones. This indicates the special role of temporal zones in the neurophysiological mechanisms of sleep

Stable inter-hemispheric connections, registered from bilateral symmetrical points in the central, posterior temporal and parietal zones, are typical for stage 2; they appear between frontal, anteriotemporal and central regions for stage 3, but are less visible in stage 4. During stage 2 and in the paradoxical stage the most stable correlations are the 'diagonal' distant connections between anterior temporal, posterior temporal and parietal zones.

CLINICAL IMPLICATIONS

Clinicians now appreciate that complications in pregnancy and delivery have a significant impact on the subsequent development of the child's nervous system, which can be diagnosed by changes in the sleep structure of newborns. For example, the length of slow-wave sleep in newborns from mothers who had toxemia late in pregnancy is twice as long as that of newborns from normal pregnancies, but the length of paradoxical sleep is significantly shortened. The proportions of slow-wave sleep and paradoxical sleep in newborns from abnormal pregnancies are about 1:1.4, while in babies from a healthy mother they are 1:34[33], which is significant.

Among other specific phenomena in children born from mothers with late toxemia is a significant, almost two-fold increase in motor activity, especially in the form of paroxysmal focal limb movements. The fast activity on the EEG in these newborns is also significantly increased, which is a sign of increased activation of the CNS. As this increased CNS activation does not change for the next 10 days, these circumstances might have a significant impact on later motor and psychological development[37,38].

Similar EEG changes are characteristic in newborns from mothers who had long and close contact with gasoline inhalation (hazardous professional materials). Professional and industrial hazards are dangerous for pregnant women and for the child in two ways: (1) they slow the processes of pregnancy and weaken delivery; and (2) they have a direct influence on the morphological, physiological and biochemical development of the fetus[40,41].

Difficult delivery by itself negatively affects the newborn's condition, increasing the probability of asphyxia and hypoxic states, changing the brain blood supply and increasing chances of birth trauma. The earlier the abnormal signs of brain trauma are recognized, the more significant the help will be[41,42].

The earliest signs of structural and functional CNS pathology do not appear in focal changes on the EEG, but in the systemic organization of the newborn's states of vigilance, sleep and alertness[39,41].

There are data indicating that perinatal hypoxia induces long-term consequences on brain functions including sleep–wake mechanisms. About 60% of cases with minimal brain damage are connected to perinatal hypoxia[42–44].

Hypoxia causes a significant increase in antistress hormones and peripheral vasoconstriction, which lead to increased anaerobic metabolism. Intrauterine brain hypoxia increases Ca^{++} permeability through the cell wall which causes problems in protein synthesis[44]. Given the fact that somnogenic structures are spread throughout the brain, it is no surprise that hypoxia during pregnancy might have significant negative effects on brain development, such as sleep–wake deviations as physiological foundations for sleep, behavior and mood disorders.

Even prenatal use of alcohol was found to induce abnormal CNS development (probably due to hypoxia) and to modify neonatal sleep–wake organization[45]. Recently, experiments with animal models demonstrated that chronic stress during pregnancy interferes with brain development and induces long-lasting alterations of sleep in offspring[46].

Thus, it is now apparent that, when not recognized and treated in a timely fashion, minimal brain dysfunctions during the newborn period may lead to deviations that will be difficult to correct later.

Inter-hemispheric functional connections are stable but change with age. On the other hand, intra-hemispheric diagonal correlations are not so stable, and are developed later. Using the method of time–space correlations and coherent analysis, it was possible to establish two different systems of inter-cortical connections responsible for two functionally different aspects of cortical activity[32,33]. The first system included long associative connections between frontal and parietal–occipital ends of the brain in each hemisphere and direct commissural connections. This system is responsible for co-ordination of the frontal and posterior sectors of each hemisphere, as well as uniting functional connections between bilateral symmetrical zones of both hemispheres. This system of functional unity of distant zones develops early in ontogenesis. The second system develops later in ontogenesis and consists of short connections between cortical zones within the same hemisphere. These connections are very unstable and are responsible for a separate system of associative connections. Some of these structures are responsible for brain activity as a whole in sleep and wakefulness. They achieve maximal development and some of them are unique, only appearing in humans.

CONCLUSION

The evaluation of sleep–wake structures from an evolutionary standpoint provides a useful model for the interpretation and differentiation of normal development and pathology. The child's developing brain, in sleep and alert stages, has been shown to mirror the ontogenesis of the organ within humans.

Mechanisms responsible for sleep mature earlier in the brain and provide the foundation for future alertness. The wakeful synchronization that follows is predicated upon the scaffold provided by paradoxical periods of unregulated brain activity in sleep.

Computerized EEG analysis provides a new indicator of functional connections between brain systems and their neurophysiological correlates. This methodology can provide clinicians with an insight into the effects of pre-, peri- and postnatal trauma on the infant brain. Specific patterns of impairment, due to hypoxia, toxic exposure and physiological insults, have become more easily recognizable and have led to an increase in our understanding of neural mechanisms.

ACKNOWLEDGEMENT

This presentation is partially supported by Grant RFFI 02-04-49351.

References

1. Hobson J. *Sleep*. New York: Scientific American Library, 1989:1
2. Berger H. Ueber das Elektroenkephalographalogramm des Menchen. *J Psychol Neurol* 1930;40:100–79
3. Harvey EN, Loomis AL, Hobart GA. Cerebral states during sleep as studied by human brain potentials. *Science* 1937;85:443–4
4. Aserinsky E, Kleitman N. Regularly recurring periods of eye motility, and concomitant phenomena, during sleep. *Science* 1953;118:273–4
5. Rechtschaffen A, Kales A. *A Manual of Standardized Terminology, Techniques and Scoring System for Sleep Stages of Human Subjects*. Los Angeles: BIS/BRI;UCLA, 1968
6. Anders T, Emde R, Parmelee AH, eds. *A Manual of Standardized Terminology, Techniques and Criteria for Scoring of States of Sleep and Wakefulness in Newborn Infants*. Los Angeles: UCA Brain Information Service, NINDS Neurological Information Network, 1971
7. Scher MS. A developmental marker of central nervous system maturation. Part II. *Pediatr Neurol* 1988;4:329–36
8. Chase MH. Sleep mechanisms. In Kryger MH, Roth T, Dement WC, eds. *Principles and Practice of Sleep Medicine*, 3rd edn. Philadelphia: WB Saunders, 2000:93–168
9. Steriade M, McCormic DA, Sejnowski TJ. Thalamocortical oscillation in the sleeping and aroused brain. *Science* 1993;262:679–85
10. Moore RY, Abrahamson EA, Van Den Pol A. The hypocretin neuron system: an arousal system in the brain. *Arch Ital Biol* 2001;139:195–205
11. Feinberg I, Campbell I. Kinetics of non-rapid eye movement delta production across sleep and waking in young and elderly normal subjects: theoretical implications. *Sleep* 2003;26:192–200
12. Karni A, Tanne D, Rubenstein BS, *et al*. Dependence on REM sleep of overnight improvement of a perceptual skill. *Science* 1994;265:679–82
13. Wilson MA, McNaughton BL. Reactivation of hippocampal ensemble memories during sleep. *Science* 1994;265:676–9
14. DeKoninck J, Christ G, Hebert G, *et al*. Language learning efficiency, dreams, REM sleep. *Psychiatr J Univ Ottowa* 1990;15:91–2
15. Scrima L. Isolated REM sleep facilitates recall of complex associative information. *Psychophysiology* 1982;19:252
16. Sheldon SH, Spire JP, Levy HB. *Pediatric Sleep Medicine*. Philadelphia: WB Saunders, 1992:14–27
17. Louis J, Zhang JX, Revol M, *et al*. Ontogenesis of nocturnal organization of sleep spindles: a longitudinal study during the first 6 months of life. *Electroencephalogr Clin Neurophysiol* 1992;83:289–96
18. Willis J, Schiffman R, Rosman NP, *et al*. Asymmetries of sleep spindles and beta activity in pediatric EEG. *Electroencephalogr Clin Neurophysiol* 1990;21:48–50
19. Voino-Yacenecky AV. *Primary rhythms of activity in ontogenesis*. Academy of Science, USSR. Leningrad: Nauka, 1974:32–64
20. Khananashvili MM. The operation of isolation of function of brain's hemispheres. *Physiol J USSR* 1961;47:661
21. Hamburger V. Some aspects of the embryology of behavior. *Rev Biol* 1963;38:342
22. Shinozuka N, Okai T, Kuwabara Y, *et al*. The development of sleep–wakefulness cycle, its correlation to other behavior in the human fetus. *Asia Oceania J Obstet Gynaecol* 1989;15:395–402
23. Curzi-Dascaloba L, Peirano P, Morel-Kahn F. Development of sleep states in normal premature, full-term newborns. *Dev Psychobiol* 1988;21:431–44
24. Anders TF, Keener MA, Kraemer H. Sleep–wake organization, neonatal assessment, development in premature infants during the first year of life. II. *Sleep* 1985;8:193–206
25. Scher MS, Steppe DA, Dahl RE, *et al*. Comparison of EEG sleep measures in healthy full-term, preterm infants at matched conceptional ages. *Sleep* 1992;15:442–8
26. Parmelee AH. Neurophysiological, behavioral organization of premature infants in the first months of life. *Biol Psychiatry* 1975;10:500–12

27. Sheldon SH. *Evaluating Sleep in Infants and Children*. Philadelphia: Lippincott-Raven, 1996: 11–20

28. Matsuoka M, Segawa M, Higurashi M. The development of sleep, wakefulness cycles in early infancy, its relationship to feeding habit. *Tohoku J Exp Med* 1991;165:147–54

29. Golbin AZ. *The World of Children's Sleep*. Salt Lake City, Utah: Michaelis Publishing, 1995:244

30. Shepovalnikov AN. *Activity of the Sleeping Brain*. Leningrad: Nauka, 1971:144

31. Shevchenko UG. *Development of the Brain Cortex from the Point of View of Ontophylogenetic Relations*. Moscow: Medicina, 1972

32. Shepovalnikov AN, Tsitseroshin MN. Spatial order of functional organization of the whole brain. Human physiology, September 1988: 371–85 (translation from *Hum Physiol* 1987; 14(6))

33. Shepovalnikov AN, Tsitseroshin MN, Pogosyan AA. The role of different cortical areas and their connections in the postnatal development of the spatial pattern of the field of brain biopotentials. *Hum Physiol* 1997;23:136–46

34. Hobson JA. *Sleep*. New York: Scientific American Library, 1989:35–77

35. Livanov MN. *Space-temporal Organization of Potentials and System Activity of the Brain*. Moscow: Science, 1989:400

36. Nunez PL. *Electric Fields of the Brain: The Neurophysics of EEG*. New York: Oxford University Press, 1981

37. Oniani T, ed. *Neurobiology of the Sleep–Wakefulness Cycle*. Tbilisi: Metsniereba, 1988:519

38. Evarts EV. Neuronal activity in visual and motor cortex during sleep and waking. In *Neurophysiologie des Etats de Someil*. Paris, 1965:189–209

39. Yakovlev PI, Lecours AR. The myelogenetic cycle of regional maturation of the brain. In Minkovski A, ed. *Regional Development of the Brain in Early Life*. Oxford: Blackwell, 1967:3–70

40. Evsjukova II. Features of formation of sleep cycles in newborns, whose mother had late pregnant toxicosis. *Questions of protection of mothers and childhood*. 1972(11):66–72

41. Ratner AU. *Neurology of Newborns*. Kazan University, 1995:368

42. Nordstrom L, Arulkumaran S. Intrapartum fetal hypoxia and biochemical markers: a review. *Obstet Gynecol Surv* 1998;53:645–57

43. Berger R, Garnier Y. Perinatal brain injury. *Perinat Med* 2000;28:261–85

44. Vannucci RC. Hypoxic–ischemic encephalopathy. *Am J Perinatol* 2000;17:113–20

45. Hayes MJ, Sallinen BA, Gilles A, Stoughton J, Zeman J, Brown E. Prenatal alcohol: neonatal sleep organization and spontaneous movements. *Sleep* 2003;26:A148

46. Le Marec N, Bach TM, Godboat R. Sleep in rats born from chronically mild stressed mother. *Sleep* 2003;26:A57

3

The psychophysiology of REM sleep in relation to mechanisms of psychiatric disorders

Vadim S. Rotenberg

A THEORETICAL BACKGROUND – SEARCH ACTIVITY CONCEPT

Numerous investigations on sleep psychophysiology in psychiatry have provided science with interesting empirical data. However, there are many contradictions in these data and the most important and substantial questions are still far from being solved. The only way to overcome these contradictions and to elucidate the role of sleep alteration in the general pathogenesis of mental disorders is to develop an integrative theory of the basic sleep functions, which are equally relevant for humans and animals, for psychology and physiology, for mental health and for psychopathology. Obviously, this is a difficult task. It would be too optimistic to expect that such an integrative theory would appear at once in its final and comprehensive version. Thus, it is worth producing different versions of such a theory for broad discussion, to provide in the future a holistic picture from all of these puzzles. The task of the present chapter is to use one such theory (search activity concept) for the revision of some contradictions and for the discussion of some theoretical assumptions.

The search activity concept[1–5] deals mostly with the function of rapid eye movement (REM) sleep, although the alteration of NREM sleep seems also to be very important for understanding the mechanisms of mental disorders. However, NREM sleep deficiency is an unambiguous and general finding in many psychiatric patients with different diagnoses, while data on REM sleep are much more contradictory. The discussion of the nature of such contradictions may be very productive.

Search activity is defined as activity that is oriented to changing the situation (or at least the subject's attitude to it) in the absence of the precise prediction of the outcome of such activity but taking into consideration the results at each stage of the activity. According to this definition, search activity is a component of many different forms of behavior: self-stimulation in animals, creative behavior in humans, as well as exploratory and active defense (fight/flight) behavior in all species. In all these forms of activity the probability forecast of the outcome is indefinite, but there is a feedback between the behavior and its outcome enabling the subject to correct his behavior according to the outcome.

Many forms of behavior do not include search activity. Renunciation of search is opposite to search activity and encompasses depression and neurotic anxiety in humans, freezing in animals and learned helplessness in both species. Neurotic anxiety, according to psychodynamic conceptions, is a consequence of the repression of an unacceptable motive from consciousness. The repression can be regarded as a purely human variant of renunciation of search, of the modes of realization of the unacceptable motive in behavior, and modes of integration of this motive with other, realized, behavioral orientations. The difference between productive emotional tension (the normal anxiety of a healthy individual in a state of stress), which is instrumental in mobilizing all psychological and physical resources to overcome obstacles, and unproductive emotional tension, which hampers successful activity, is determined by the presence or absence of search activity in the structure of emotional tension[6].

Panic reaction can imitate search activity, but a subject in a state of panic does not consider the real outcome of his behavior and is unable to correct it. The common clinical condition of panic is depression. Stereotyped behavior is based on the precise prediction of the outcome and is not flexible; thus it also does not fit with the idea of search activity.

I have proposed this new classification of behavior because our investigations have shown that search activity has a very important psychobiological meaning[1,6–13]. All forms of behavior that include search activity, but differ in other respects, increase body resistance, while absence of search decreases body resistance and predisposes a person to mental and psychosomatic disorders. Persons with psychosomatic illness have a more pronounced tendency to give up than do healthy subjects, especially in stressful conditions and after facing failure. We concluded that the process of search activity in itself, independent of the pragmatic results of such activity (i.e. whether it is successful or not) and independent of the accompanying emotions, protects persons from somatic disorders.

Herein lies the basic difference between the concept of search activity and the concept of coping behavior[14] that must be successful in order to be protective.

The protection of search behavior reflects a particular self-service and a positive feedback: search activity requires a lot of effort and stimulates a person to enter unpredictable and potentially dangerous situations, and prevents exhaustion in such situations. All details of the investigations performed on animals and humans as well as all aspects of the theoretical discussion can be found in the above-mentioned publications.

The biochemical mechanisms of search activity have been insufficiently studied but it is possible to suggest that the brain's monoamine system is closely connected with search behavior. Learned helplessness accompanied by somatic disturbances emerges when the brain monoamine level drops[15]. An artificial reduction of brain catecholamine levels by tetrabenazine speeds passive behavior whereas the prevention of its depletion by monoamine oxidase (MAO) inhibitors raises stress resistance, restoring the animal's ability for an active reaction to stress[16]. In animals that cannot control the stressful situation the brain level of norepinephrine drops particularly low and they show the greatest distress[17,18]. Finally, the locus ceruleus plays a major role in the organization of various forms of search behavior[19].

On the basis of the preceding facts the following hypothesis has been advanced[3,20]. Search activity can begin in the presence of a certain critical level of the brain monoamines that are utilized in the course of search. Search activity itself, once it starts, stimulates the synthesis of the brain monoamines and ensures that they remain at adequate, or even excessive, levels. The task of such a system with positive feedback (brain monoamines – behavior – brain monoamines) is to support search activity.

At the same time, a stable high level of brain monoamines causes a hyposensitivity of the inhibitory α_2-adrenoreceptors. As a result, in order to switch on the negative feedback that regulates homeostasis of the brain monoamines, its level has to be excessively high.

In a state of renunciation of search the above-mentioned positive feedback between brain monoamines and behavior does not function. Moreover, in this state, which manifests itself in depression and maladaptive emotional tension, the monoamine expenditure climbs. The requirement for brain monoamine production and expenditure decreases because the behavior that requires brain monoamines is absent. At the same time, the low level of brain monoamines by itself does not stimulate its own production. The brain monoamine system is only partly homeostatic. If the appropriate behavior (search activity) is absent, activation of the brain monoamine system is not required. When the level of brain monoamines is constantly low the inhibitory α_2-adrenoreceptors become adapted to it and maintain this low level. If search activity is of such great biological relevance, and the absence of search, and especially renunciation of search in stressful conditions, leads to illness and death, why has the latter regressive behavior survived in the course of evolution and what makes it emerge?

All higher mammals, including humans, at the early stages of ontogenesis inevitably experience helplessness determined by the relatively slow development of the central nervous system and all mechanisms (nervous, hormonal and vegetative) that ensure subsequent search behavior. Naturally, during the early stages of ontogenesis such a state cannot be called renunciation of search. It is normal and inevitable and the only accessible form of a defense reaction for an immature organism. Nevertheless, the organism thus acquires an early experience of passive reaction, an experience of helplessness. Both this experience and the ways to overcome it are of colossal relevance to the individual's entire subsequent life. In the case of the correct attitude of the primary group, above all the mother, this early experience of helplessness can be successfully and painlessly overcome. However, all injuries of early childhood, from physical separation from the mother to insufficient emotional contact with her and the feeling of insufficient protection as a result of strained relations between the parents, can consolidate the experience of primary helplessness and produce a tendency to give up. The imprinting mechanism may lead to the development of a state of renunciation of search in an adult, especially if the emotional problems encountered in some way resemble the conflicts of early childhood. Thus, readiness for the development of mental and psychosomatic illnesses is formed. It is exactly from these general biological positions, the relations between early helplessness and the formation of search activity, that the present author proposes considering the Freudian theory of the role of early psycho-traumatizing situations in the entire subsequent development of the individual. Regressive behavior in the case of neuroses and psychosomatic illnesses, according to Freud, is indeed a regression towards a biologically earlier state of helplessness that assumes a form of renunciation of search.

However, if search activity is so important for survival, and renunciation of search is so destructive and dangerous for health, it would be reasonable to assume a natural brain mechanism that can restore search activity after temporary renunciation of search. I believe that dreams in REM sleep fulfil this function. A covert search activity in dreams compensates for the renunciation of search in previous wakefulness and ensures the resumption of search activity in subsequent wakefulness. I base this claim on the following findings:

(1) Different forms of animal behavior that contain search activity (self-stimulation, fighting) suppress REM sleep in subsequent sleep without a restorative rebound effect[21,22]. This means that less REM sleep is required after such overt behavior.

(2) Renunciation of search produced by the direct stimulation of the hypothalamus causes an increase in REM in subsequent sleep[1]. This corresponds to data[23] that REM sleep increases along with a moderate reduction of norepinephrine system activity, while the excessive decrease or increase of this activity suppresses REM

sleep (see discussion in references 12, 20). This means also that search activity can start in REM sleep with a lower level of brain monoamines than is required in wakefulness. This conclusion corresponds to data[25] that in REM sleep α_2-adrenoreceptors are much more sensitive than in wakefulness; thus the fine regulation of brain monoamines can be performed on their lower level.

(3) If, during REM deprivation, the subject is involved in active behavior (exploration, active defense reaction), the REM rebound effect during subsequent sleep is substantially reduced[20].

(4) Depression, neurotic anxiety and generalized learned helplessness as manifestations of renunciation of search are accompanied by increased REM sleep requirement (REM sleep latency is decreased while the duration of the initial REM episodes is increased)[27–29]. A correlation was detected between learned helplessness and REM sleep percentage[30,31].

(5) Both REM sleep and search activity in wakefulness are characterized by a regular and synchronized hippocampal theta-rhythm. Moreover, the more pronounced the theta-rhythm in wakefulness, the less pronounced it is in subsequent REM sleep[26]. REM sleep in animals regularly contains pontogeniculo-occipital (PGO) spikes, which are electroencephalographic (EEG) signs of neural activation. In wakefulness, PGO correlates with orienting activity[32]. The presence of the PGO spikes in REM sleep may mean that the animal is predisposed to react to novel stimuli, including spontaneous changes of dream content.

(6) When a special part of the nucleus ceruleus (nucleus ceruleus aleph) in the brainstem is artificially destroyed and as a result muscle tone does not drop during REM sleep, animals demonstrate complicated behavior that can be generally described as orienting (or search) activity[33].

(7) The same psychological variables that predispose the subject to renunciation of search – trait anxiety, fixation on obstacles according to Rosenzweig[34], motivation of avoidance of failures – have a tendency to correlate with REM percentage[8].

(8) REM sleep is increased in students who display a stable emotional tension both before and after an examination, even with its positive outcome (when the stress situation no longer exists) as compared with students who display emotional tension only before an examination[2]. It is possible to suggest that this stable emotional tension, which is not compatible with the actual situation, is similar to neurotic anxiety and represents renunciation of search.

(9) Healthy subjects with normal search activity during wakefulness are characterized by active participation in their own dreams. This active participation correlates with heart rate acceleration and eye movement density in REM sleep[35].

(10) The more characters and descriptive elements that appear in the dream, and the more active the characters and the dreamer himself, the larger the decrease in the scale of unhappiness during the night[36]. It can be suggested that the characters' activity represents search activity in dreams. One must stress that, in the case of healthy subjects, the decrease of unhappiness after sleep correlates only with the above-mentioned dream variables, not with the sleep physiology. As I see it, this means that, as long as the dream is functionally effective and is able to restore search activity, REM sleep requirement does not increase. It is increased only when dreams are going to lose their restorative capacity, for instance in clinical or pre-clinical disorders (depression and subsyndromal depression, neurotic anxiety, narcolepsy).

The dreams of healthy subjects represent a very specific kind of search activity, which, however, is compatible with the above-mentioned notion of search activity: the subject is active in his dreams but is unable to make a definite forecast according to the outcome of dream events. The dream does not apparently fit solely those parts of the notion emphasizing the permanent consideration of the behavioral outcome. This is true only if the dream is not self-reflective and does not include self-control, i.e. if activity in the dream is a chaotic activity. However, it was demonstrated[37] that, in the vast majority of spontaneous dreams, the dreamer is moderately self-reflective and effective in dream control.

Dreams provide a good opportunity for search activity after giving up. First, the subject is separated from reality while sleeping, including those aspects of reality that caused renunciation of search. Thus, in dreams a person is free to start from the beginning. Second, within his dream, the dreamer can be very flexible in his behavior: it may be an attempt to solve an actual problem in a metaphoric manner, or it can be an attempt to solve another problem, one that displaces the actual problem[38], since not the topic of search, but the search process itself is the main restorative factor. Moreover, in dreams, one is not restricted by logical and conventional rules while manipulating the problems. One is able to use image thinking, which is polysemantic by nature and as a result much more flexible than logical thinking and, unlike the waking consciousness, can avoid contradictions[5,20,24,39,40]. Image thinking is free from the probability forecast[41,42]. Since we assume that the final aim of the dream work is not the real solution of the actual problem but only the restoration of search activity, all the above features contribute substantially to the restoration.

The proposed explanation of the functional significance of the REM sleep in the restoration of search activity helps us to understand a very well-known phenomenon in human sleep, the 'first-night effect' (FNE). It is an alteration of sleep structure observed on the first night of the multinight sleep study relative to subsequent nights[43,44]. Compared with later nights, the first night in the laboratory is characterized by increased REM sleep latency, combined with a moderate REM sleep reduction, especially in the first part of the night, usually without the subsequent REM sleep rebound. Sleep latency is also often increased and sleep stages shift, while sleep efficiency is decreased. FNE reflects the natural increase of the sleeper's state of vigilance in an unfamiliar sleeping environment as part of the adaptive orientation in the new situation[45], and is much less prominent in healthy subjects sleeping at home where they are reacting only to the monitoring equipment[44,46]. Such adaptive orientation includes search activity (orienting behavior, as I have stressed, is a manifestation of search activity); thus according to the search activity concept, the requirement of REM sleep in the night sleep has to be decreased. That is exactly the case. It means that the FNE can be used for the estimation (even quantitative estimation) of the subject's ability to display search activity.

Another theoretical outcome of the search activity concept is the conclusion that REM sleep may be efficient or inefficient according to its main function – restoration of search activity[5,35]. If dreams do not contain a covert search activity, and moreover, if it is a continuation of the renunciation of search in dreams, it is possible to suggest REM sleep as inefficient. REM sleep inefficiency displays itself not only in the stable feeling of helplessness and giving up in dreams, in the passive position of the dreamer facing the dangerous events in the dream, but also in the decrease of dream reports after awakenings in REM sleep and in the impoverishment of these reports (fewer images and events). Such features characterize, for instance, dreams of depressed patients[38,47,48]. As mentioned before, there are some physiological correlations of the subjects' imaginative activity in their own dreams. Thus, it is possible to use such physiological variables for the estimation of REM sleep functional activity even without awakenings.

In the following sections of this chapter I will discuss alterations of sleep psychophysiology in different mental disorders using the frame of the search theory.

POST-TRAUMATIC STRESS DISORDERS

Complaints about sleep disorders – difficulty falling or staying asleep, increased number of spontaneous awakenings, recurrent distressing dreams (nightmares) – belong to the main diagnostic features of post-traumatic stress disorders (PTSDs). In most cases these complaints are confirmed by polysomnography: the sleep of PTSD patients is characterized by disturbances in sleep continuity, including increased sleep latency, increased number of awakenings, especially awakenings in REM sleep during nightmares, and low sleep efficiency[49–54]. However, data on sleep structure in PTSDs, and especially data on REM sleep variables, are very ambiguous and contradictory.

First, PTSDs are characterized by a high variability of REM sleep latency. In comparison to healthy control subjects, REM latency in PTSD patients has been reported to be either shortened or lengthened[55–60]. Correspondingly, REM sleep time was either increased[61] or decreased[57]. In some investigations, there was no difference in the mean REM time and REM latency between healthy subjects and combat veterans[62].

PTSDs are often accompanied by major depression (MD) or other depressive disorders such as dysthymia[54,63,64]. Thus, it has been reasonable to assume that the difference between PTSD patients in REM sleep variables may be determined by the presence or absence of PTSD co-morbidity with depression[54]. Comparison of PTSD and MD patients has shown that REM sleep time was reduced in PTSDs; however, this reduction was presumably a side-effect of the decreased sleep duration[54]. In contrast to healthy subjects, the decrease of the total sleep time in PTSD patients was not accompanied by a compensatory increase in the percentage of REM and slow-wave sleep (SWS). At the same time, REM latency does not differ significantly between both clinical groups. However, it was difficult to draw a definite conclusion from this study that PTSD patients display REM sleep latency typical for depression. First, depression in the group of MD patients was not severe, and only 47% of these patients had REM latency less than 60 min. On the other hand, 20% of PTSD patients suffered from co-morbid MD, and 40% of these patients had prior depressive episodes. Moreover, within the PTSD group there was no significant trend for REM latency to be reduced in patients with the current co-morbid depression. Thus, the suggestion of depression as a reason for the high variability of REM latency in PTSDs was neither confirmed nor refuted.

The investigation of Woodward and colleagues[65] seems to give a more definite answer to this question. Two groups of PTSD patients – one with and one without co-morbid depression – demonstrated similar mean REM sleep latencies, although the variability of REM latency was higher in patients with a co-morbid depression. Thus it is not depression itself, or at least not only depression, which determines the decrease of REM latency in some PTSD patients and causes heterogeneity of REM latency in all groups of these patients. The authors concluded that 'a (unknown) factor emerges in PTSD which exerts a specific effect upon REM sleep timing and amount. … This factor is related to the apparent increase in both tonic and phasic REM phenomena in sleep of PTSD patients'.

In discussing this topic, it is also worth emphasizing that some core physiological features of PTSD are the converse of those in depression. PTSD patients in comparison to healthy subjects, and contrary to depressed patients, are characterized by the decreased basal cortisol level and by the increased negative feedback regulation of cortisol excretion (see reference 66). Patients with PTSDs demonstrate augmented cortisol suppression in response to dexamethasone, while depressed patients are characterized by non-suppression of cortisol in this test[67,68]. PTSD patients have more, and depressed patients have fewer, type II glucocorticoid receptors in circulating lymphocytes than do normal controls[69,70]. Platelet α_2-adrenergic receptor binding, platelet MAO activity and platelet serotonin uptake are decreased in PTSD patients in comparison to normal subjects[71]. The increased activity and reactivity of the monoamine system in PTSDs is confirmed by increased nocturnal noradrenergic excretion[53]. Thus, it is possible to suggest an exaggeration of the normal adaptive physiological response to stress in PTSD – although without any real stressful condition – and this exaggerated response to stress is the opposite to what may be found in depression. This exaggeration of the normal response is confirmed in the investigation of the FNE[45]. According to the REM sleep variables, and especially to REM latency, PTSD inpatients were bidirectionally sensitive to the degree of familiarity they associated with the sleep laboratory conditions. In comparison to non-ill trauma-free controls, in-patients familiar with the laboratory environment demonstrated reduced FNE (increased extinction of the orienting reaction), while patients unfamiliar with this environment demonstrated enhanced FNE. At the same time MD patients, in contrast to normal subjects, often demonstrate a reduced FNE in the unfamiliar situation (see below). Thus, PTSD symptomatology is very complicated. On the one hand, depression is a common PTSD co-morbidity and there are some factors that make REM sleep variables in isolated PTSD similar to those in depression. However, on the other hand, PTSDs differ from depression according to many physiological variables. We will show that this distinction has real roots in the clinical picture and in the pathogenesis of PTSDs.

The clinical picture of PTSDs includes, on the one hand, a persistent re-experiencing of the past traumatic events manifested as intrusive distressing recollections (images, thoughts, perceptions, dreams, dissociations like illusions, hallucinations and flashback episodes) accompanied by increased physiological reactivity on exposure to internal or external cues that symbolize or resemble an aspect of the traumatic event. It can be assumed that persistent symptoms of increased arousal such as irritability, hypervigilance, exaggerated startle reaction, prominent orienting reaction and FNE, difficulty falling and staying asleep, although they are usually considered separately, belong to the same group of symptoms – group I.

On the other hand, the same patients (and this is worth emphasizing) display persistent avoidance of stimuli associated with the trauma and numbing of general responsiveness (conscious avoidance and repression of thoughts, feelings, memories and activities associated with the trauma; diminished interest in any forms of activity and interpersonal relationships, as in depression; a hopeless view on the future). This group II of symptoms is obviously opposite to group I, and both groups compose a contradictory clinical picture, where symptoms of group I are continuously displaced by symptoms of group II and vice versa, or even partly appear together.

However, it is possible to integrate these different symptoms in one holistic frame. The central point of the PTSD diagnosis is the feeling of helplessness caused by the traumatic event. It is the central feature of the entire clinical picture. Fear of death and fear of ego-destruction produces helplessness because it is a very distressing and disorganizing emotion – there are no clear ways to cope with a fear of death, if the psychological defense mechanisms become insufficient[72]. The feeling of helplessness is very difficult to resist. It is a state of giving up, of renunciation of search, with all negative outcomes on human behavior and health, as shown in the Introduction. By considering helplessness as a corner-stone of PTSDs, it is possible to explain all group I symptoms as attempts to cope with this feeling of helplessness and loss of control which accompanied the traumatic event. Hypervigilance, and exaggerated startle reaction, reflect the mobilization for coping. However, unfortunately, this coping is irrelevant and cannot be successful, because the object of coping is elusive: it is the traumatic event that already happened in the past, and the subject is unable to win back. In principle, the re-experience of trauma may help to re-examine the traumatic event and to include it in a more broad and polydimensional picture of the world where trauma is able to find its definite and restricted place and will no more cause general helplessness. However, for this re-examination, the subject has to be well equipped with skills of the right-hemispheric polysemantic way of thinking[39,73], and exactly these skills are underdeveloped in PTSD patients[74]. In these patients traumatic experiences are fragmental, not integrated in the holistic picture of the world, and reappear in a very rigid form of primitive and frustrating images in wakefulness, in altered states of consciousness and in nightmares. Such coping is stereotypic in its nature; however, it can include a very strong physiological mobilization. The position of the subject in this state of coping can be very active, but the final goal – a freedom from helplessness and from a feeling of being a victim – cannot be achieved. It is like a fight with a shadow where you never can win. Traumatic events, instead of being coped with, restore every time the same distressing frame and do not help to overcome helplessness. It is a key point of this unsuccessful coping.

Group II symptoms reflect an attempt to avoid the negative experience with which the subject is unable to cope. To avoid does not mean to solve, but only to conserve the problem. Trauma after such avoidance remains isolated from the normal integrative function of the brain and from the larger associative network of memory. Actually, these group II symptoms display a giving-up state in front of traumatic experience after the unsuccessful coping. However, giving up only increases helplessness, and it forms a vicious circle. Coping and avoidance work in opposite ways towards the same goals, but both are unsuccessful. The continuous oscillations between unsuccessful attempts to cope and giving up (avoiding) can explain the complicated and contradictory picture of PTSDs and their sleep alterations.

For instance, Woodward and co-workers[45] proposed that helplessness and not clinical depression may be a factor related to increases in both tonic and phasic REM phenomena and reduced REM latency. Conversely, the predominance of group I symptoms (active coping) may be responsible for increased REM latency in some PTSD patients and in the exaggeration of FNE. The same patient may demonstrate different sleep structures at different time points.

By taking into consideration the role of REM sleep and dreams in balancing behavioral attitudes and restoration of search activity, it is reasonable to pay attention to the dream content. In contrast to the increased variability of REM latency and REM sleep time, eye movement (EM) density in REM sleep in PTSD patients seems to be unambiguously increased[54,62,66]. According to the above-mentioned relationships between EM density and dream content[35,75], it is possible to suppose that the increase of EM density in PTSD patients corresponds to their typical complaints of traumatic dreams and nightmares[59,76–79]. However, direct investigation of this topic in the sleep laboratory does not confirm this proposition. According to Greenberg and associates[55], most REM awakenings in Vietnam War veterans with PTSD symptoms led to content-less reports. Kramer and colleagues[81] have also shown a lower than normal (around 50%) dream recall rate after spontaneous awakenings from REM sleep. In the investigation of the Lavie group[49,82] these findings have been substantially enlarged, and they deserve elaboration. The authors systematically collected dreams from REM sleep in well-adjusted and poorly adjusted Holocaust survivors, and compared them to the control group of aged persons without the Holocaust experience. The estimation of the level of adjustment was based on clinical interview regarding all main areas of life: marital and familial problems, problems at work, social relationships, somatic and mental problems, and general satisfaction in life. It is worth stressing that the well-adjusted group presented not only fewer somatic complaints than the poorly adjusted group, but also even fewer complaints than the control group. Members of the well-adjusted group were characterized by stronger ego-forces, in comparison to the poorly adjusted group. Their emotional feelings were positive. Recollection of the Holocaust contents occurred infrequently and was under their control.

The less well-adjusted group was disturbed by their Holocaust experience. According to the clinical picture, the less-adjusted group displayed a moderate PTSD complex, including decreased sleep efficiency in comparison to both other groups. In sleep structure, including REM sleep variables, no differences were found among the groups. (This is not very surprising if we consider the variability of sleep in PTSD patients.) The most prominent differences between groups were in dream reports and in dream content. The control group reported a normal percentage (80%) of dream content when awakened from REM sleep. The percentage of reports in the less well-adjusted group was 50.7% – equal to the percentage reported by the PTSD patients of Kramer and associates[81], and Bleich and co-workers[83]. This percentage is also approximately equal to the percentage of dream recall (54.6%) presented by mentally ill patients (with depression, anxiety, hypochondria and hysterical neurotic disorders[84]). At the same time, the well-adjusted group had the lowest dream rate (33.7%). Moreover, in contrast to both other groups, well-adjusted survivors were unable to realize not only the content of the dream, but also even the fact of dreaming. The survivors' dreams, particularly those of the well-adjusted group, were less complex and salient in comparison to dreams of the control group. The number of anxious dreams was high in both groups of survivors and especially high in the poorly adjusted group. However, only the less well-adjusted survivors experienced nightmares resulting in spontaneous awakenings. In dreams of the less-adjusted group the dreamers were usually the victims, while in the well-adjusted group dreams were characterized by hidden hostility in which survivors were not directly involved. This is a very important point, because according to the search activity concept a feeling of being a victim means the continuation of giving up and the renunciation of search

from wakefulness into dream, and this feeling reflects the functional insufficiency of the dream. Only the well-adjusted survivors demonstrated indifferent responses toward their dream content after awakening, even if the content was stressful. Similar to controls, and in contrast to the less well-adjusted survivors, the well-adjusted subjects dreamed about their present life rather than about the past.

Dreams of both groups of survivors contained more danger to the dreamer, more anxiety and hostility, and more interpersonal conflicts than dreams of the control group, although all these features were more prominent in the less-adjusted group. By taking into consideration this similarity, and the relative similarity in the low number of dream reports, Kaminer and Lavie[49] concluded that both groups, and especially the well-adjusted one, were characterized by the repression of dreams, and the stronger the repression, the better was the psychological adjustment. However, this explanation looks very doubtful. First, it has already been stressed that according to many important features (such as general physical and mental health, sleep efficiency, psychological response to the negative dream content during sleep and after awakening, position in dream – victim versus non-victim) the well-adjusted group of survivors is closer to the healthy control group than to the poorly adjusted group, while according to the number of dream reports it is most different from the control group. Second, it is very difficult to accept the statement that repression is a healthy defense mechanism. As has been shown previously, repression is a very specific human form of renunciation of search, according to the psychodynamic concept of neurotic free-floating anxiety. We have shown[85] that in psychologically maladapted somatic and psychosomatic patients there is a positive correlation between repression (measured according to Plutchik and associates[86]) and the D scale of the Minnesota Multiple Personality Inventory (MMPI), which measures depression and neurotic anxiety. This correlation was absent in psychologically adapted subjects; thus it is possible to suggest that high levels of repression caused increased anxiety. If anxiety required repression for its compensation, such positive correlation would be present in psychologically adapted subjects. In addition, the high strain of repression characterized essential hypertension. This means that repression does not belong to the most adaptive defense mechanisms. Moreover, repression increases together with anxiety after REM/dream deprivation[80,87]. This means that in normal subjects dreams are used for the compensation of repression and for the prevention of anxiety, and it would be very paradoxical to assume that the repression of dreams serves psychological health. It is possible to suggest repression of the functionally insufficient dreams to explain the lack of dream reports in the poorly adjusted group of PTSD patients; however, it looks very doubtful that repression can serve psychological health and is used by well-adjusted survivors.

The search activity concept provides another explanation of the extremely low number of dreams in the well-adjusted group. Members of this group appear to have a very strong search activity. They are usually successful and active business people, with high social achievements[49]; they cope with problematic situations well, perhaps better than people without the Holocaust experience. This resembles hyper-compensatory activity and can explain their normal health as well as a decreased dream requirement. Thus, the number of dream reports is decreased in this group not owing to the dream repression but to the high search activity during wakefulness. However, in the less-adjusted group the low number of dream reports reflects suppression of the functionally insufficient REM dreams[35]. Thus, dreams in PTSDs are either anxious and hostile (coping) or repressed (avoidance of experience).

DEPRESSION

Sleep in depression has been investigated in more detail than sleep in any other psychiatric disorder and there is a general consensus regarding the sleep structure in depression. Slow-wave sleep (SWS) deficiency, especially in adults; decreased sleep duration caused by the increased sleep latency; awakenings during the night sleep and early morning awakenings; decreased REM sleep latency and the redistribution of REM sleep with its concentration in the first half of the night; increased EM density in the first cycle – various combinations of these features characterize the sleep of depressed patients[64,88–91]. However, what these alterations mean and the cause-and-effect relationship between them and other clinical symptoms of depression is still an open question.

There is contradiction in the literature regarding REM sleep variables: they have been claimed to normalize during remission[92,93], but this finding has not been confirmed in other investigations[94,95]. Thus, the alteration in REM sleep variables may be a trait or state marker of psychopathology[96,97]. REM sleep deprivation was used as an effective treatment for depression[98]; thus REM sleep may even play a role in the pathogenesis of depression. Alternatively, REM sleep redistribution may reflect either an altered circadian rhythm[99] or an attempt by the brain to compensate for depression. This latter proposition appears to be more explanatory and ties in with theories concerning the adaptive function of REM sleep in healthy subjects, especially in the domain of mood[28,36,100]. The search activity concept also fits this proposition because depression is a typical state of renunciation of search that requires search activity in dreams for compensation and for the restoration of overt search behavior in the subsequent wakefulness[5]. According to this point of view, the decreased REM latency and increased REM duration and EM density in the first sleep cycle reflects an increased requirement in REM sleep. This increased REM sleep pressure in depression was confirmed in our recent investigation[101]: while in normal subjects and in schizophrenic patients the incorporation of wakefulness in the first sleep cycle increases REM latency in proportion to the incorporated wakefulness, it does not happen in depression. The absence of the FNE, according to REM sleep variables, in many patients with severe depression[102–105] can be considered not only as an outcome of the diminished orienting reaction in depression, but also as a sign of the increased REM pressure. In our investigations[106,107], FNE was present only in 44% of patients with MD. According to our criteria, FNE was present if REM sleep latency on the first night of study was at least 30 min longer than REM sleep latency on the second night. FNE was absent in most patients with mood-congruent psychotic features (delusional depression) highly resistant to the antidepressant drugs and with more previous hospitalizations (as was shown ׳˙·˙˙ ̄ ̄ ̄ ̄ ̄ ̄ ̄ ̄ ̄ ̄ ̄ ̄[111]), and clinical improvement in these patients without FNE was achieved only after electroconvulsive therapy (ECT). Thus, absence of the FNE characterized depressed patients in a more severe clinical state. However, and especially interesting, depressed patients who exhibited FNE also demonstrated increased REM sleep pressure. The delayed first REM sleep period in the first night was increased, in comparison to the first REM sleep period in the subsequent nights of patients with FNE as well as in comparison to the first REM sleep period in all nights of patients without FNE. In depressed patients the first REM sleep period duration is usually increased, in comparison to healthy subjects, but in patients with FNE the first REM sleep period on the first night was especially high and occupied 44% of REM sleep. Moreover, REM sleep latencies on the second and third nights in patients who exhibited FNE were significantly shorter than REM sleep latency of the corresponding nights of the group without FNE. In patients with FNE total REM sleep was increased in the second night compared with the first night. In addition, patients with FNE showed an increased number of short cycles (less than 40 min) in all nights. By taking into consideration all these data, it is possible to suggest that depressed patients who display the FNE are also characterized by the high REM sleep requirement; however, they are more flexible in their physiological responses, in particular in the response of their REM sleep system, in comparison to patients without FNE. Being in an unfamiliar environmental condition, they are able to react to this condition with a FNE, like healthy subjects – by increasing the REM sleep latency. However, presumably due to the high REM sleep requirement, they demonstrate a 'rebound effect' not typical for healthy subjects: a shift of REM sleep to the first cycle and an increase of REM sleep in the subsequent nights. I cannot exclude that they are less resistant to the treatment partly owing to this flexibility of orienting and REM sleep systems.

In parallel with the increased REM sleep requirement, it could be suggested that REM sleep in depression has an adaptive function. This suggestion is partly based on the relationship between REM sleep quality and SWS restoration during night sleep. As was stressed previously, depression in general is characterized by SWS deficiency, and SWS is often restored only after successful treatment[102,108]. Patients who display FNE exhibit more SWS in their night sleep[106]. In addition, SWS in depression is often redistributed compared to healthy subjects: it predominates in the second, and rarely even in the later cycles. We have shown[109] that in REM sleep episodes just before such an 'explosion' of SWS in the third or fourth cycle, EM density is increased in comparison to all previous REM episodes, while such an explosion does not happen in depression with a flattened EM density distribution. Thus, it is possible to speculate that in some particular cases REM sleep, characterized by enhanced EM density, contributes to the improvement of the mental state of depressed patients and determines the psychophysiological condition that allows SWS to appear. This conclusion is in agreement with data of some recent investigations: the increase of the positive dream content from the first to the last REM sleep periods is related to the remission from depression[27]; at the same time the increase of REM density from the first to the last sleep cycle in depressed patients (a relatively rare finding) is accompanied by mood improvement from evening to morning[110].

However, the concept of the restorative and compensatory function of REM sleep at the first glance contradicts some experimental data, and this contradiction requires explanation. First, this concept does not correspond to the beneficial effect of REM sleep deprivation[98]. Second, the duration of the first REM sleep period and its EM density are usually increased in depression[91]; however, this does not contribute to mental health improvement. When EM density is highest in the first cycle, mood does not change from evening to morning, or even becomes worse. While EM density in the fourth cycle correlated positively with mood restoration, REM sleep duration in the first cycle correlated negatively with the same variable[110,118]. Also, the high EM density in the first REM sleep period, even if it exceeds EM density in any other cycle, does not predict or determine the increase of SWS in the second cycle. As stressed above, only in the second part of the night, after the second cycle passed, was any significant increase of SWS preceded by enhanced EM density. Previously, we have shown[2] that not the first, but the second REM sleep period increased in healthy students in the process of adaptation to stress. Thus, it is possible to suggest that the first REM sleep period is functionally different and less efficient in comparison with the subsequent REM sleep periods.

According to Cartwright and colleagues[27,28], it looks as if the first REM period serves as a bridge between the emotional state of the preceding wakefulness and its regulation in the subsequent REM sleep periods. In healthy non-sensitive subjects without strong negative pre-sleep mood dream activity, the first REM period is usually short and less elaborate, and corresponds to the short REM duration and low EM density. A shift toward more intense dreams in the first REM period may represent a response to excessive levels of pre-sleep negative affect, and in such dreams this affect is still not compensated. A normal dynamic in normal subjects with a high pre-sleep negative affect is the change from the initial negative affect in the first dream to increasing positive affect in subsequent dreams. According to Cartwright and Lloyd[111], depressed patients who had an enhanced dream-like quality of mentation during the first REM sleep period showed decreased Beck Depression Inventory scores at follow-up assessment. An enhanced dream-like activity may indicate that the brain starts to deal with negative affect in the first REM period. Such dealing is a necessary but insufficient condition for adaptation and mood regulation. The sufficient condition may be the restoration of search activity in the subsequent dreams. However, when speaking about resistant depression such restoration is usually not available. There are doubts whether the normal adaptive process even starts in the first REM period, in spite of its increased duration and enhanced phasic activity. There are even more doubts about the functional sufficiency of subsequent REM periods characterized by flattened EM density, in contrast to normal subjects who display an increase of EM density from cycle to cycle[91]. In depressed patients the number of dream reports after awakenings in REM sleep during the night is decreased, dreams are shorter and simpler, and contain fewer images than dreams of healthy subjects[112]. We have found that in patients with MD, subjective estimation of sleep latency correlated with EM density in the first REM sleep period and subjective estimation of the number of awakenings correlated with the total EM scores[113]. In healthy subjects, as has been shown previously[35,75], EM density correlates with dream reports. Thus, it is possible to suggest that in depression psychic activity in REM sleep is often not perceived as dream mentation. Dreams may be repressed from the consciousness if they contain failures and feelings of helplessness. As a result, REM sleep is considered subjectively as wakefulness. This may be one of the reasons for the underestimation of sleep duration in depression. However, at the same time it is a sign of the proposed functional insufficiency of REM sleep that it does not provide an opportunity for the restorative search activity in dreams[5,35]. Thus, the increased need for REM sleep in depression is combined with the functional insufficiency of REM sleep.

The insufficient dreams cannot restore search activity; moreover, such dreams may conserve or even increase the renunciation of search. The functional insufficiency of REM sleep and dreams may explain the positive outcome of REM deprivation in depression.

SCHIZOPHRENIA

In patients suffering from schizophrenia, polysomnographic findings are less consistent than in depression. Some authors noted SWS reduction[114]; however, this was not confirmed by other investigators[115,116]. Lauer and associates[117] did not find any significant differences in sleep structure between a paranoid group of schizophrenic patients and a healthy control group, while, according to Mendelson and co-workers[118], REM sleep percentage increases exactly before the exacerbation of psychotic symptoms and tremendously decreases during the exacerbation.

In some studies REM sleep latency was reduced[115,119–121], while in other studies it was normal[122–124]. Some authors[121] suggested that symptoms of depression may be related to the decrease of REM sleep latency in schizophrenia; however, in other investigations[114,125], REM latency was not related to depressive symptoms.

The difference between schizophrenia with the predomination of positive and negative symptoms in numerous clinical and physiological variables allows a prediction that this difference may also influence sleep architecture. Some sleep investigations have been performed using this paradigm directly or indirectly[115,120,122,126]. These investigations concentrated mostly on the relationships between positive versus negative symptoms, SWS and REM sleep latency.

We investigated 34 patients with chronic schizophrenia on stable doses of neuroleptic medication[10,127]. They were divided into two groups according to the positive and negative syndrome score (PANSS) rating[128]. Group I contained seven men and two women (mean

age 40 years) with positive/negative ratio > 1. Group II contained eight men and two women (mean age 41 years) with positive/negative ratio < 0.5. Thus, positive symptoms dominated in group I (28.1 vs. 11.8 in group II) and negative symptoms dominated in group II (30.8 vs. 20.0). The neuroleptic treatment was approximately similar in both groups. Sleep data were collected on two consecutive nights. There were no significant differences between both groups according to most sleep variables except for REM sleep percentage and EM density in REM sleep. In group I the mean REM sleep percentage was significantly lower (20%) than in group II (25%). REM sleep in the first cycle displayed a tendency to be higher in group II, but REM sleep latency was similar in both groups.

We also compared positive and negative symptoms in 11 patients with more than 25% REM sleep (group A) and in 14 patients with less than 20% REM sleep (group B). The mean level of positive symptoms was 15 in group A, and 20 in group B, while the mean level of negative symptoms was 27 and 25, respectively. Negative symptoms were relatively more predominant in group A with the increased REM sleep percentage. REM sleep latency demonstrated a non-significant tendency to be shorter in the group with an increased REM sleep percentage; however, it was in the normal range.

According to these data the ratio between positive and negative symptoms is not the only factor determining the representation of REM sleep. In group I this ratio was > 1; however, the mean REM sleep percentage was 20, while in group B, where REM sleep was less than 20, this ratio was less (0.8). On the other hand, in group II positive/ negative ratio was 0.38 and REM sleep percentage was 25%, while in group A, where REM percentage was more than 25%, this ratio was 0.55. In control healthy subjects matched to patients with schizophrenia according to age, the mean REM sleep percentage was 19%, very similar to patients in group I. These results suggest that a strong predominance of negative symptoms is associated with a relative increase of REM sleep percentage. However, the predominance of positive symptoms is not associated with REM sleep suppression less than the normal level and there is no linear relationship between REM sleep variables and the positive/negative symptom ratio.

Also, we have estimated the relationship between EM density (averaged EM frequency in 1 min of REM sleep) and positive versus negative symptoms. In subgroups with a high (> 6) and low (< 2.5) mean EM density the level of negative symptoms was almost equal (31 and 33), but the level of positive symptoms was significantly higher in the subgroup with low EM (25.2 vs. 12.6). This finding was confirmed in further analysis of the data. In patients with a low score of positive symptoms, mean EM density was significantly higher than in patients with high scores[127]. At the same time in patients with high and low scores of the negative symptoms EM density was similar. In patients with positive/negative symptom ratio < 0.4, EM density achieved maximum values in the first cycle. In other cycles, it was lower and almost equal, thus resembling EM distribution in depressed patients[129]. A significant negative correlation was found between the score of the positive symptoms and EM density in the first and third cycles, −0.45 and −0.50, respectively. These findings are in agreement with Neylan and colleagues[125], who reported an increased severity of psychosis after neuroleptic withdrawal simultaneously with the decrease in EM density. Our results correspond also with those of Tandon and associates[115], who reported that schizophrenic patients who were drug free only for 2–4 weeks (when the effect of neuroleptics is still present) displayed higher EM density in comparison with schizophrenic patients who were drug free for a longer time or drug naive. Tandon and co-workers[115] did not present data on positive symptoms after drug withdrawal. It is, however, not rare that the withdrawal of neuroleptics causes the exacerbation of psychotic (positive) symptoms[125].

Although the relationships between clinical symptoms and both REM sleep variables (REM sleep percentage and EM density) are in the same direction, it is worth mentioning the difference. The increase of REM sleep percentage is determined mainly by the predominance of negative symptoms, while the decrease of EM density is related to the level of positive symptoms. However, this is at least one possible interpretation of both relationships in the frame of the search activity concept. I suggest that the increased REM sleep percentage in group II is caused by the absence of search activity in patients with predominantly negative symptoms. Negative symptoms (apathy, flattened affect, low social activity, inattentiveness, lack of spontaneity in behavior and in mental activity, poverty of speech), like depression, display a lack of search activity that requires REM sleep for its compensation. However, in contrast to depression, negative schizophrenia is not accompanied by the regular decrease of REM sleep latency. It may depend on the different context of the renunciation of search in depression and negative schizophrenia. While in depression, and especially in anxious and agitated depression, renunciation of search is usually combined with increased affective tension, in negative schizophrenia it is usually accompanied by flattened affect. At the same time, any form of schizophrenia may be combined with depressive symptoms, and this can be an additional factor determining the lack of linear relationships between positive/negative symptom ratio and REM sleep.

There is another possible interpretation of the normal REM sleep latency in our patients. It has been shown[121,125] that REM latency correlates with SWS time. The exacerbation of psychosis following acute neuroleptic withdrawal may determine the suppression of SWS and as a result the decrease of REM latency[125]. At the same time, the relapse of psychosis after neuroleptic withdrawal decreases the total REM time. Thus, the relapse of psychosis may cause a paradoxical combination of decreased REM sleep latency, decreased REM time and decreased phasic REM activity, while stable neuroleptic treatment, like in our investigation, causes a combination of increased REM duration and REM activity with normal REM sleep latency. However, the relationships between positive/negative symptoms and sleep structure may be even more complicated and contradictory. Not only may the exacerbation of positive symptoms suppress SWS, Ganguli and associates[122] showed also that SWS and negative symptoms were negatively correlated, which may influence REM latency, especially in non-medicated schizophrenic patients. Positive symptoms represent very particular, misdirected and maladaptive, but at the same time very intense, search activity[20]. Paranoid ideation and hallucinations correspond to the definition of search activity: active overt or covert behavior without definite forecast. Auditory hallucinations are associated with increased metabolic activity in brain centers for inner speech, i.e. that represent active verbalization. A schizophrenic patient cannot be sure about future 'events' in the artificial world he is building for himself, or about outcomes of his interactions with this world. At the same time, the person remains sensitive to all events and outcomes related to this artificial world. The hyperactivity of the brain catecholamine system in positive symptom schizophrenia also corresponds to the notion of search activity[20].

In healthy subjects, EMs in REM correlate with the active participation of the dreamer in dream scenarios and with dream content[35,75]. Active events in dreams represent search activity that has to compensate the renunciation of search in the previous wakefulness[5]. If search activity during wakefulness is already high, there is no need for high EM density in REM sleep. From my point of view, this may explain how neuroleptic withdrawal precipitated a psychotic relapse associated with the decline in REM sleep duration and EM activity[125], and explains why positive symptoms correlated negatively with EM density in our investigation.

The peculiarity of the FNE in schizophrenia also can be explained in the frame of the search activity concept. Neylan and associates[125] did not find FNE in schizophrenic patients on and off haloperidol therapy. In our investigations[10,127], FNE according to our criteria (see above) was present only in 35% of schizophrenic patients, less than in MD. Interestingly, the age of patients who demonstrated FNE was significantly higher than the mean age of patients without FNE. Positive symptoms were higher in patients with FNE while negative symptoms were almost equal in both groups. When the ratio of positive/negative symptoms was > 0.6, FNE was present in 71% of all cases, whereas when this ratio was < 0.4, FNE was present only in 17%. It was difficult to discriminate the influence of age and positive symptoms on the difference between REM sleep latency on the first and the second nights. The ratio of the first REM period to the total amount of REM sleep was not increased in the first night of schizophrenic patients, and in patients with FNE this variable was less than on the second night. In patients with a FNE, sleep efficiency on the first night was lower and the number of awakenings higher than on the first night in the control group of healthy subjects who demonstrated a FNE. Thus, it is possible to suggest that there is an exaggerated FNE in schizophrenic patients with relatively high positive symptoms in comparison to normal subjects.

Although patients with FNE were, in general, older than patients without FNE, it is very unlikely that FNE is directly determined by age. In the investigation of Ganguli and co-workers[122] almost half of the patients suffering from schizophrenia demonstrated FNE although all patients were young. In normal young subjects, FNE is a typical finding[45,130]. There are some reasons to suggest that positive symptoms play a key role in the FNE:

(1) Schizophrenic patients with positive symptoms, like PTSD patients, display an exaggerated orienting reaction[131]. At the same time, patients whose negative symptoms predominate demonstrate a failure to respond to the environment[132].

(2) Schizophrenic patients with positive symptoms display higher reactivity to

sensory and affective stimuli in comparison to patients with negative symptoms[133]. Such sensitivity may increase with age.

(3) A relatively higher response of the brain monoamine system in patients with positive symptoms, in comparison to patients with negative symptoms[134], may also explain the appearance of the FNE as an exaggerated reaction in a new environment.

(4) As we have already shown, positive symptoms decrease REM sleep pressure. As a result, REM sleep pressure does not prevent FNE (the reverse of the situation in depressed patients with high REM sleep pressure and a low REM sleep flexibility).

It is interesting to discuss the difference between schizophrenic patients with positive symptoms and the above-mentioned patients with psychotic depression. The latter do not display FNE. It is possible to speculate that hallucinations and delusions of schizophrenic patients cause an active and outside oriented, although inappropriate and misdirected, search behavior while delusions in depressed patients are often mood-congruent and are related to the feeling of guilt, worthlessness, failure, to ruminative self-blaming and self-annihilation. Such delusions provide a basis for renunciation of search. It was shown[135] that psychotic depressive patients, in comparison to melancholic patients and to those with major depression without psychotic features, were significantly more likely to demonstrate marked psychomotor disturbances, to report feeling sinful and guilty, and to suffer from constipation, terminal insomnia, appetite loss and loss of interest and pleasure.

Our approach to the difference between psychotic mood-congruent depression and schizophrenia is in line with data[136] that cortisol non-suppression on the dexamethasone suppression test is most prominent in depression with mood-congruent delusions, in comparison to both non-psychotic depression and depression with mood-incongruent delusions. Lower rates of non-suppression were also observed in schizophrenia[137].

These data suggest that psychotic features in depression and schizophrenia may have different significance, and this proposition is confirmed by our data derived from sleep investigations.

Our group has shown that melatonin treatment of chronic schizophrenia definitely restored FNE in these patients in comparison to placebo treatment[138]. There are different possibilities to explain these data. It is possible that melatonin enhances the alertness of schizophrenic patients in the unfamiliar situation as an outcome of the improved sleep quality on melatonin treatment during the previous nights[138]. The restoration of FNE may result from the modulation of dopaminergic activity by melatonin in the neuroleptic-treated patients with schizophrenia.

Finally, we have investigated the relationship between objective sleep variables and subjective sleep estimation in schizophrenia[139]. There are no systematic investigations of this topic. Patients with chronic schizophrenia demonstrated a high, and unexpected, ability to estimate correctly the duration of sleep latency. The correlation between objective and subjective sleep latency in patients was higher than in healthy subjects and in depressed patients. In healthy subjects and patients with mood disorders the duration of wakefulness before sleep onset is probably overestimated, owing to emotional tension caused by sleep delay. This emotional tension may interfere with the ability to estimate sleep latency. In chronic schizophrenic patients with a relative predominance of negative symptoms and with blunted affect, alteration of sleep onset does not cause any emotional reaction and its subjective estimation is not distorted.

At the same time, the subjective estimation of the duration of wakefulness in sleep correlated in schizophrenic patients with EM density in REM sleep. The same correlation was found in patients with MD (see above). As stressed previously, in healthy subjects EM density correlates with some features of dream reports. However, in schizophrenic patients we found a negative correlation between EM density and dream reports. It is possible to speculate that schizophrenic patients, as well as patients with MD, perceive mental activity in REM sleep as wakefulness, and it is an important sign of the REM sleep functional insufficiency. According to the search activity concept, such functional insufficiency of REM sleep may play an important role in the pathogenesis of different mental disorders.

ADAPTIVE VS. MALADAPTIVE EMOTIONAL TENSION (ANXIETY) AND SLEEP

It is well known that anxiety is one of the main reasons for sleep disturbances. Anxiety causes prolonged sleep latency, decreased total sleep time, reduced SWS and reduced sleep efficiency partly due to the increased number of awakenings. Beyond the alterations of the objective sleep structure, anxiety may cause a negative subjective estimation of sleep[140]. Sleep latency may be overestimated; awakenings filled with anxious feelings might be more easily fixed in memory than those without and will result in reports of poor sleep. Moreover, awakenings in NREM sleep, especially in the first sleep cycles, may cause the underestimation of the depth and duration of the preceding part of sleep[84].

The alterations of REM sleep variables in anxiety are less definite than alterations of non-REM sleep or of sleep duration. This may relate to the problem of the definition of anxiety.

Emotional tension (anxiety) is not a united psychophysiological state. It can be either maladaptive or adaptive in both nature and outcome. Adaptive emotional tension helps the subject to solve problems and to overcome obstacles, and has no negative outcome on health. Despite the theoretical and practical importance of the distinction between adaptive and maladaptive emotional tension, neither adequate theoretical approaches nor valid methods appear to distinguish between the two in past research. According to general activation theory, an optimal level of emotional tension is adaptive in helping the individual to solve problems and to overcome

obstacles without any negative outcome for the organism. The Yerkes–Dodson law is when the level of tension is extremely low or high, and its outcome is regarded as negative with respect to performance, adaptation and health[141,142]. However, there are many exceptions to the Yerkes–Dodson law. First, pathological emotional tension (neurotic anxiety) is always harmful, with respect not only to health but also to performance, thereby decreasing the effectiveness of the latter in a linear manner[143,144]. Second, even a very high level of emotional tension can promote the activity of the subject (Figure 3.1).

According to Dienstbier[145], naturally evoked peripheral catecholamines never seem to be too high for optimal performance. In addition, when methods of coping were available, even very high arousal levels failed to elicit discomfort and negative emotions[146].

I suggest that the difference between productive emotional tension (the normal anxiety of a healthy individual in a state of stress), instrumental in mobilizing all psychological and physical resources to overcome obstacles, and unproductive emotional tension that hampers successful activity is determined by the presence or absence of search activity in the structure of emotional tension. Until search activity is present, anxiety is adaptive. All forms of maladaptive anxiety (like panic and neurotic anxiety) do not correspond to search activity, both according to the theoretical notion and clinical observations. During panic the results of the activity are not considered at any stage and cannot be used for the correction of behavior. Panic behavior during catastrophic events is usually displaced by or combined with depression[147,148]. Panic may represent an exaggeration of normal anxiety that corresponds to the final point of the curvilinear line displaying relationships between emotional tension and adaptation or performance (see Figure 3.1). In this final point the emotional tension is very high while performance and adaptation are low. This happens, in particular, when vital motivations are increased and fear of the consequences of failure predominates over constructive attempts to find

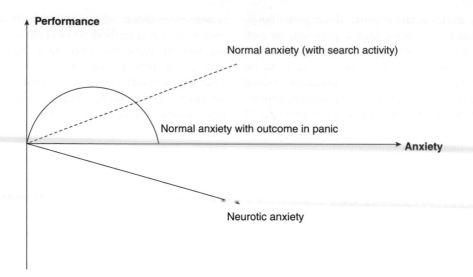

Figure 3.1   The relationships between different types of anxiety and performance

a reasonable solution to the problem; such fear does not allow the subject to follow up, to the end, any way of search and to use the current outcome of his/her own activity in order to correct this way. Finally, such fear deteriorates behavior. In panic, like in other states of emotional tension without search activity, the expenditure of brain monoamines exceeds their synthesis, and eventually there comes a pronounced drop in their levels and a secondary depression.

Neurotic anxiety, according to the psychodynamic concept, is a consequence of the repression of an unacceptable motive from consciousness. The repression can be regarded as a purely human variant of renunciation of search, of the modes of realization, of the unacceptable motive in overt behavior, and modes of integration of it with other realized behavioral orientations. Thus, repression simply represents a state of giving up in front of the inner motivational conflict and its outcome is, speaking metaphorically, a mental 'freezing'. It is the reason why neurotic anxiety caused by repression is maladaptive[85] and does not follow the Yerkes–Dodson law.

Benzodiazepines have different outcomes for adaptive and maladaptive emotional tension. It is well known that benzodiazepines

sometimes enhance and sometimes diminish the behavior (motor) response to threatening signals[149]. In moderate doses, they do not block active avoidance or even increase it, but they usually block freezing as a sign of renunciation of search[150]. Maladaptive anxiety is more sensitive to anxiolytics, and because of the competition between renunciation of search and search behavior, freezing can be replaced by active avoidance.

However, benzodiazepines also block adaptive anxiety containing search activity, by increasing the sensory threshold for any meaningful information that can cause frustration. Imagine, for instance, a lecturer who is worrying about the possible outcome of his lecture. Even if it is a mobilizing and adaptive emotional tension, subjectively it is accepted as an unpleasant anxiety and has a negative connotation for the person: he prefers not to worry. If in order to cope with this anxiety he uses benzodiazepines, the adaptive mobilization is reduced and the lecture will be less successful.

Ledoux and Gorman[151] have recently confirmed our approach to anxiety. They stressed that a shift from passive suffering to active coping is the best way to treat anxiety caused by recent social events.

The search activity concept helps to solve some contradictions related to the dynamic of autonomic patterns in different forms of anxiety. Thus, there is a marked difference between the habituation of orienting reactions in healthy subjects versus subjects with psychopathology. In healthy subjects, the amplitude of the electrodermal reaction (EDR) during the first two orienting reactions is higher and the habituation is faster, while the spontaneous electrodermal activity is lower[152]. If the spontaneous electrodermal activity reflects an inner emotional tension not relevant to the external task, and the evoked EDR reflects the emotional tension during decision making[153], it can be suggested that pathological subjects are overwhelmed by their emotional tension, which causes hyperarousal. This high arousal, however, reflects maladaptive emotional tension, is in competition with search activity and blocks normal forms of behavior requiring search activity, in particular, the orienting reaction. From my point of view, this is a more reasonable explanation than the explanation according to the 'law of initial level'[154]. Wilder proposed that the higher the initial level of activity of the physiological system, the lower the reaction of the system on the relevant task. However, in healthy subjects involved in a meaningful activity and highly motivated, autonomic variables may increase regardless of their initial level[155,156]. Wilder's law seems to be relevant only for pathological anxiety. Thus, the low autonomic reaction in pathologically anxious persons may not relate to the high initial level by itself, but rather to the inability of the subject to accept the challenge of the task that requires search activity.

Sleep structure is also able to separate adaptive and maladaptive anxiety. We analyzed sleep change in 27 healthy students on a post-examination night in comparison to post-holiday nights[2]. Thirty minutes before the examination and 30 min after, we recorded their heart rate frequency, arterial blood pressure and bioelectrical activity of the orbicular muscles of the mouth. The latter, as other autonomic variables, is very sensitive to emotional tension. The control data on these indices were obtained on one of the term days. Before the examination all subjects showed an increase in autonomic variables and muscle tension compared with the control measures. However, after the examination, two groups could be separated. The group I subjects' (16 students) indices dropped to the control level, whereas the indices of subjects in group II remained at a stable high level. Students of group II demonstrated a significant increase in REM sleep percentage on the post-examination night compared with the control night and with the post-examination night of the group I subjects. On the post-examination night, the subjects of group II showed a positive correlation between the total duration of sleep and the proportion of REM sleep (0.74) and a negative correlation (– 0.6) between the duration of REM sleep and that of delta sleep. The subjects of group II showed worse results in resolving logical tasks on the evening after the examination (before sleep) than on the following morning; also, their results were worse than those of group I. They were working relatively faster but they made significantly more mistakes – thus they behaved in a more impulsive way. It is important to note that subjects in both groups did not differ according to the objective outcome of the stressful situation – all students passed the examination. Thus, stable emotional tension was not caused by the negative outcome of the examination.

We have proposed a hypothesis that the subjects of group I exhibited normal emotional tension, which ensured psychophysiological mobilization for overcoming the stressful situation and diminished when the situation passed. The subjects of group II displayed maladaptive emotional tension. It did not diminish after the stressful situation was over and required REM sleep for its disappearance. Additional support for this approach comes from data demonstrating that slow post-stress catecholamine decline is accompanied by poor performance, neuroticism and pathological anxiety[157].

Almost everybody who has ever passed examinations is familiar with such maladaptive tension. It prevents concentration on the particular text the subject is studying because the subject is overwhelmed with fears according to the predicted negative outcome of examinations. Instead of reading the text the subject is continually counting the number of pages he has yet to go. It is possible to suggest that coming examinations, as every stressful condition, provoke in such subjects deep and old neurotic complexes and feelings of inferiority, and this is the reason why the anxiety does not disappear even after the actual stressful situation is over. In order to cope with these activated complexes and feelings that provoke renunciation of search the subject has to go through REM sleep. Maladaptive anxiety determines paradoxical relationships between sleep disturbances and daytime alertness. Recently, we investigated daytime wakefulness/sleepiness and night sleep structure in patients with sleep apnea and in patients with depression/anxiety[158]. We found that in patients with sleep apnea the ability to remain awake during soporific circumstances measured by the maintenance of wakefulness test (MWT) correlated negatively with stage 1 sleep. The latter correlated negatively with the total sleep time and with SWS. It looks very natural – the more disturbed the night's sleep due to sleep apnea, the more difficult it is to maintain daytime alertness. However, in patients with depression/anxiety, MWT scores correlated negatively with total sleep time and SWS (stage 3), while the multiple sleep latency test correlated negatively with total sleep time and sleep efficiency. This means that the more disturbed the night's sleep, the less easily is the subject able to go to sleep during the day. Maladaptive tension disturbs nighttime sleep and at the same time prevents daytime sleep. It determines a very well known paradoxical combination of subjective sleepiness (caused by nighttime sleep disturbance) with high irritation and inability to sleep.

ROLE OF SLEEP IN MEMORY FUNCTION: REM SLEEP, BEHAVIOR AND MEMORY

The outlined ideas concerning the function of REM sleep and dreams presented in part of this chapter can help to solve many debatable problems of sleep psychophysiology. Among such problems, in particular, is the role of sleep in memory and learning. Jenkins and Dallenbach[159] in their classical investigation demonstrated that recall was diminished less by a night of sleep than by an equivalent amount of wake time, and may explain why a person with psychophysiological in somaia (somatized tension anxiety) does not nap either. However, in their theory no active role in memory consolidation and storage was ascribed to sleep; it was considered only as a period free from sensory interference.

The discovery of REM sleep and different NREM sleep stages elicited many modern investigations on the active role of these sleep stages in memory. The recent review by Stickgold[160] summarized data of investigations performed on animals and humans. It was shown that in animals, REM sleep increases after training on very different but complex tasks such as the multiple-goal maze, shuttle avoidance, classical conditioning and operant bar press, mostly after the so-called unprepared learning according to Seligman[161]. This REM sleep increase appeared in special time periods (REM sleep 'windows'[162]), often just before the critical level of success in the learning process was achieved[163] and correlated with the successful learning of new material. REM sleep deprivation performed after the learning process in such critical periods ('windows') disturbs retention. At the same time, performance of simple tasks was not impaired by REM sleep deprivation[164].

Investigations performed on humans have also shown that the relationship between the learning process and sleep depends on the task peculiarity. Tasks related to declarative memory (word recognition, retention of the word list or paired associates) are REM sleep independent and REM deprivation produced no effect on these tasks[165], while tasks related to procedural memory that require the development of new and flexible perceptual or motor skills – like mirror writing, the word fragment completion task or the Tower of Hanoi task[166] – are REM dependent[160].

Declarative memory as opposed to procedural memory depends on SWS[167–169].

According to the above-mentioned data, many authors[160,162,164,170,171] suggest that REM sleep *per se* plays an important role in the consolidation of unusual and emotionally significant information, but not in the retention of ordinary information. However, it was shown that the creative (unusual) task, in most cases, is not solved in REM sleep *per se*, although after a dream with an active position of the dreaming subject the creative task in subsequent wakefulness is solved more successfully[172]. On the other hand, REM sleep deprivation does not influence the learning process, if the learning prior to the deprivation was performed with intensity and success, and the task was realized during wakefulness[170]. This means that REM sleep is not obligatory for the retention of information even if the task by itself is complex. There are some additional arguments against the idea of the direct participation of REM sleep in consolidation mechanisms:

(1) During the active search behavior in the stressful situation, consolidation of the new experience is essential for survival, but under these conditions REM sleep does not increase, and even decreases.

(2) The REM sleep percentage increase under neuroleptic treatment[118] has no beneficial effect on memory.

(3) Activating drugs, like amphetamine, have a tendency to suppress REM sleep but, at least, do not disturb memory[173].

(4) Despite marked suppression of REM sleep, antidepressants on the whole do not disrupt learning/memory[174].

As already mentioned, REM sleep becomes longer at certain stages during the solution of emotionally significant complex problems, which the animal or human subject is originally unprepared to handle[170]. There is evidence suggesting that the greatest increase of REM sleep occurs during the 24 h before the critical level of success in the learning process[175,176]. REM sleep deprivation carried out directly in this period impedes it. It is possible to suggest that REM sleep is particularly important for the animal during the critical period of an acute conversion from the previous stereotypical behavior to the new and flexible style of behavior.

It might be a sign that REM sleep plays only an indirect role in the process of retention by carrying out its main function – compensation of renunciation of search and restoration of search activity[4]. A complex problem that the subject is not ready to solve, a difficult task that requires unprepared learning, may cause renunciation of search with much greater probability than a simple one, especially at the early stages of the solution when failures prevail over successes. In experiments on animals 'the learning situation imposed is undoubtedly the most important and traumatic event in the life of the organism'[171], and such an event has a significant chance of producing a giving-up reaction (renunciation of search). Actually, the non-learning rats (rats that remain below the learning criteria) displayed a considerable majority of freezing responses during training and thereby received the highest number of electric shocks[177]. If search activity in REM sleep is unavailable (due to REM deprivation) and, consequently, does not overcome the state of renunciation of search, the latter itself will make it impossible to find the right solution or keep it in memory. REM deprivation after training leaves memory in a labile form and delays the process of consolidation[178], presumably due to the predominance of the maladaptive state of renunciation. Therefore, the lengthening of REM sleep exactly before the critical point in the learning, after which the animal fully develops the habit, is not surprising.

However, in some cases the lengthening of REM sleep may be insufficient to compensate for the very prominent state of renunciation of search. In such cases, REM sleep may increase precisely in those animals that are the least successful in forming the new habit[179], resembling the increase of REM sleep in depression. It is possible to suggest that in non-learning rats the compensatory REM sleep system is usually weak and functionally insufficient. This hypothesis corresponds to data[177] that the average duration of REM sleep episodes of baseline sleep of non-learning rats is significantly shorter in comparison to learning rats. These episodes may be less stable. In such cases stressful conditions of training may cause a relative increase of REM sleep that is nevertheless insufficient for compensation.

The peculiarity of neuronal activity in different functional states also does not confirm the theory of REM sleep's direct participation in memory consolidation. According to the dynamic of neuronal activity, in quiet rest and in SWS, information flows from hippocampus to neocortex, while in REM sleep and during active exploration in wakefulness[160,180], information flows in the opposite direction – from neocortex to hippocampus. Thus according to this variable, as well as according to the hippocampal theta-rhythm, active exploration in wakefulness and REM sleep are very similar to each other and opposite to SWS.

This confirms our conclusion about active exploration (search activity) in functionally sufficient REM sleep. However, it shows also that it is not necessary to ascribe memory consolidation by itself to REM sleep. The above-mentioned explanation of the indirect contribution of REM sleep in memory function is here more relevant. Renunciation of search makes any functions in wakefulness and sleep, including memory, less efficient, and if REM sleep overcomes renunciation of search and restores search activity it has also a positive outcome on memory. Furthermore, this approach provides an explanation for data being difficult to explain by the concept of memory consolidation in REM sleep. For instance, what is the functional meaning of the REM sleep increase after immobilization stress or learned helplessness? What sort of information is it so necessary to consolidate by means of REM sleep after such an experience? The subject needs only to overcome the unproductive state of renunciation of search elicited by these conditions. This means that the concept of the indirect positive role of REM sleep in memory functions seems to be more comprehensive and broad.

This concept also allows explanation of some data showing that REM sleep has a double effect on retention: facilitative and inhibitory[169]. Latash and Manov[167] have performed an investigation on the task of declarative memory. Human subjects were awakened in the first or second cycle in delta sleep close to REM sleep or after the first or second episode of REM sleep. Every subject passed all four experimental conditions, but every night each subject had only one awakening, during which he was tested for the amount of retention of material he had learned before going to sleep. The authors found that retention after the second REM sleep episode was lower than immediately before this episode. The addition of a short period of time that corresponds to the second REM sleep period had an unexpected inhibitory influence on the declarative memory retention. At the same time, REM sleep facilitated the positive effect of SWS on retention. From my point of view, this facilitative effect was indirect and can be explained as an outcome of the general positive effect of REM sleep on mental state due to the restoration of search activity. A direct negative effect of REM sleep on retention may be due to the interference between dream images and learned material. This double effect of REM sleep may explain the different outcomes of REM sleep deprivation in different conditions. If the learning process *per se* causes renunciation of search, the requirement in REM sleep has to be particularly high and REM deprivation will inhibit retention. If the learning process stimulates search activity, REM sleep deprivation may sometimes even facilitate retention.

In addition, by accepting this concept, some other contradictions are avoided. As mentioned above, there are data that declarative memory tasks depend on SWS while procedural memory tasks depend on REM sleep. Of course, there are differences between some substantial aspects of declarative and procedural memory tasks – for instance, procedural tasks are more complex and the subject is less prepared for such tasks and this can cause giving up (renunciation of search) during training. However, it is difficult to imagine that these two sorts of task are even opposite according to the essential process of information retention and memory consolidation and that they are related to the opposite directions of flow of information.

It was shown recently[181] that several brain areas activated during the execution of a serial reaction time task during wakefulness were significantly more active during REM sleep in subjects previously intensively trained on the task than in non-trained subjects. In addition, this task was performed better after sleep than before sleep. According to the authors, these results support the hypothesis that memory traces are processed during REM sleep in humans. However, the same brain structures may be involved in search activity during training in wakefulness as well as in REM sleep, and these data can be explained without ascribing to REM sleep a direct participation in memory function. On the other hand, it was shown[182] that dreams may represent, in a very direct way, the previous waking experience and problems the subject was preoccupied with in previous wakefulness. If subjects have been involved in task performance (and even periodically failed in this performance) they can imagine this task in dreams and the relevant brain area may be activated during such imagination, as happens during the imagination in wakefulness. Does it really mean that such imagination contributes to memory consolidation? It seems to be very doubtful because usually people do not see in their dreams any elements of information they have to consolidate in their memory.

The outcome of REM sleep deprivation before training on memory function deserves a short special discussion. A long REM sleep deprivation on the wooden platform before learning destroys simple active avoidance[183], while a short REM deprivation can even stimulate active avoidance[26]. If REM deprivation is short, then search activity is frustrated, but brain monoamines and physiological mechanisms responsible for search activity are not yet exhausted. The change from the frustrating conditions on the wooden platform to the conditions of learning and testing may cause a rebound of motor activity and search activity[4]. Such new conditions can even promote some forms of learning, for instance, active avoidance. Conversely, if REM deprivation is prolonged, a renunciation of search activity appears, and the whole process of learning is destroyed. Memory traces then become more sensitive to disturbing influences. Thus, REM sleep deprivation before learning creates distress that can interfere with memory.

References

1. Rotenberg VS, Arshavsky VV. Search activity and its impact on experimental and clinical pathology. *Act Nerv Super (Praha)* 1979;21:105–15
2. Rotenberg VS, Arshavsky VV. REM sleep, stress and search activity. *Waking Sleeping* 1979;3:235–44
3. Rotenberg VS. Search activity in the context of psychosomatic disturbances, of brain monoamines and REM sleep function. *Pavlov J Biol Sci* 1984;19:1–15
4. Rotenberg VS. Sleep and memory I. The influence of different sleep stages on memory. *Neurosci Biobehav Rev* 1992;16:497–502
5. Rotenberg VS. REM sleep and dreams as mechanisms of the recovery of search activity. In Moffitt A, Kramer M, Hoffmann R, eds. *The Functions of Dreaming*. Albany, NY: State University of New York Press, 1993;261–92
6. Rotenberg VS, Boucsein W. Adaptive vs. maladaptive emotional tension. *Genet Soc Gen Psychol Monog* 1993;119:207–32
7. Rotenberg VS, Schattenstein AA. Neurotic and psychosomatic disorders: interdependence in terms of search activity concept. *Pavlov J Biol Sci* 1990;25:43–7
8. Rotenberg VS, Korosteleva IS. Psychological aspects of the search activity and learned helplessness in psychosomatic patients and healthy testees. *Dynamische Psychiatrie Dynamic Psychiatry* 1990;120:1–13
9. Rotenberg VS, Sirota P, Elizur A. Psychoneuroimmunology: searching for the main deteriorating psychobehavioral factor. *Genet Soc Gen Psychol Monogr* 1996;122:329–46
10. Rotenberg VS, Hadjez J, Martin T, *et al*. First night effect in different forms of schizophrenia (pilot investigation). *Dynamische Psychiatrie Dynamic Psychiatry* 1998;172/173:421–30
11. Rotenberg VS. Sleep after immobilization stress and sleep deprivation: common features

and theoretical integration. *Crit Rev Neurobiol* 2000;14:225–31

12. Rotenberg VS. The revised monoamine hypothesis: mechanism of antidepressant treatment in the context of behavior. *Int Physiol Behav Sci* 1994;29:182–8

13. Rotenberg VS. Anorexia nervosa: old contradictions and a new theoretical approach. *Int J Psychiatry Clin Pract* 2000;4:89–92

14. Coyne J, Lazarus R. Cognitive style, stress perception and coping. In Kutash I, Schlezinger L, eds. *Handbook on Stress and Anxiety: Contemporary Knowledge, Theory and Treatment*. San Francisco: Jossey-Bass, 1980:57–79

15. Seligman M. *Helplessness. On Depression, Development and Death*. San Francisco: W.H. Greeman, 1975

16. Katz R, Roth K, Carrol B. Acute and chronic stress effects on open field activity in the rat: implication for a model of depression. *Neurosci Biobehav Rev* 1981;5:247–51

17. Lehnert H, Reinstein D, Strowbridge B, Wurtman R. Neurochemical and behavioral consequences of acute uncontrollable stress: effect of dietary tyrosine. *Brain Res* 1984;303:215–23

18. Kohno Y, Hoaki Y, Glavin G, *et al*. Regional rat brain NA turnover in response to restraint stress. *Pharmacol Biochem Behav* 1983;19:287–90

19. Paul A, van Dongen G. The human locus coeruleus in neurology and psychiatry. *Prog Neurobiol* 1981;17:97–139

20. Rotenberg VS. An integrative psychophysiological approach to brain hemisphere functions in schizophrenia. *Neurosci Biobehav Rev* 1994;18:487–95

21. Cohen H, Edelman A, Bower R, Delmont W. Sleep and self-stimulation in the rat. Presented at the *Eleventh Annual Meeting of the Associated Professional Sleep Societies (APSS)*, New York, 1975:abstr 75

22. Putkonen P, Putkonen A. Suppression of paradoxical sleep following hypothalamic defense reactions in cats during normal conditions and recovery from PS deprivation. *Brain Res* 1971;26:334–47

23. Kafi S, Bouras C, Constantinidis J, Gaillard J-M. Paradoxical sleep and brain catecholamines in the rat after single and repeated administration of alpha-methyl-parathyrosine. *Brain Res* 1977;135:123–34

24. Rotenberg VS. Richness against freedom: two hemisphere functions and the problem of creativity. *Eur J High Ability*, 1993;4:11–19

25. Gaillard J. Involvement of noradrenaline in wakefulness and paradoxical sleep. In Wauquier A, Gaillard JM, Monti JM, Radulovacki M, eds. *Sleep: Neurotransmitters and Neuromodulators*. New York: Raven Press, 1985:57–67

26. Oniani TN, Lortkipanidze ND. Effect of paradoxical sleep deprivation on the learning and memory. In Oniani TN, ed. *Neurophysiology of Motivation, Memory and Sleep–Wakefulness Cycle*. Tbilisi, Georgia: Metsniereba, 1985;4:214–34

27. Cartwright R, Luten A, Young M, Mercer P, Bears M. Role of REM sleep and dream affect in overnight mood regulation: a study of normal volunteers. *Psychiatry Res* 1998;81:1–8

28. Cartwright R, Young MA, Mercer P, Bears M. Role of REM sleep and dream variables in the prediction of remission from depression. *Psychiatry Res* 1998;80:249–55

29. Kupfer DJ. REM latency – a psychobiological marker for primary depressive disease. *Biol Psychiatry* 1976;11:159–74

30. Adrien J, Dugovic C, Martin P. Sleep–wakefulness patterns in the helpless rat. *Physiol Behav* 1991;49.257–62

31. Rotenberg VS. Learned helplessness and sleep: discussion of contradictions. *Homeostasis* 1996;37:89–92

32. Kuiken D, Sikora S. The impact of dreams on waking thoughts and feelings. In Moffitt A, Kramer M, Hoffmann R, eds. *The Functions of Dreaming*. Albany: State University of New York Press, 1993;419–76

33. Morrison A. Central activity states: overview. In Beckman AL, ed. *The Neural Basis of Behavior*. New York: Spectrum, 1982:3–17

34. Rosenzweig S. A test for types of reaction to frustration. *Am J Orthopsychiatry* 1935;5:395–403

35. Rotenberg VS. Functional deficiency of REM sleep and its role in the pathogenesis of neurotic and psychosomatic disturbances. *Pavlov J Biol Sci* 1988;23:1–3

36. Kramer M. The selective mood regulatory function of dreaming: an update and revision. In Moffitt A, Kramer M, Hoffmann R, eds. *The Functions of Dreaming* Albany, NY: State University of New York Press, 1993:139–96

37. Purcell S, Moffitt A, Hoffmann R. Waking, dreaming and self-regulation. In Moffitt A, Kramer M, Hoffmann R, eds. *The Functions of Dreaming*. Albany, NY: State University of New York Press, 1993:197–260

38. Greenberg R, Pearlman C. The private language of the dream. In Natterson J, ed. *The Dream in Clinical Practice*. New York: Aronson, 1980:85–96

39. Rotenberg VS. Word and image: the problem of context. *Dynamische Psychiatrie Dynamic Psychiatry* 1979;59:494–8

40. Rotenberg VS. Sleep dreams, cerebral dominance and creation. *Pavlov J Biol Sci* 1985;20:53–8

41. Rotenberg VS, Arshavsky VV. Psychophysiology of hemispheric asymmetry: the 'entropy' of

right hemisphere activity. *Integr Physiol Behav Sci* 1991;26:183–8

42. Rotenberg VS, Arshavsky VV. Right and left brain hemisphere activation in the representatives of two different cultures. *Homeostasis* 1997;38:49–57

43. Agnew H, Webb W, Williams R. The first night effect: an EEG study of sleep. Psychophysiology 1966;2:263–6

44. Sharpley A, Solomon R, Cowen P. Evaluation of first night effect using ambulatory monitoring and automatic sleep stages analysis. *Sleep* 1988;11:274–6

45. Woodward SH, Bliwise DL, Friedman MJ, Gusman FD. First night effects in post-traumatic stress disorder inpatients. *Sleep* 1996; 19:312–17

46. Coates T, George J, Killen J, Marchini E, Hamilton S. Thorensen C. First night effect in good sleepers and sleep maintenance insomniacs when recorded at home. *Sleep* 1981;4:293–8

47. Riemann D, Low H, Shredil M, Wiegand M, Dippel B, Berger M. Investigation of morning and laboratory dream recall and content in depressive treatment with trimipramine. *Psychiatr J Univ Ott* 1990;15:93–9

48. Armitage R, Rochlen A, Fitch Th, Madhukar T, Rush AJ. Dream recall and major depression: a preliminary report. *Dreaming* 1995;5:189–98

49. Kaminer H, Lavie P. Sleep and dreams in well-adjusted and less adjusted Holocaust survivors. In Stroebe MS, Stroebe W, Hansson RO, eds. *Handbook of Bereavement*. USA: Cambridge University Press, 1993:331–4

50. Ross RJ, Ball WA, Sullivan KA, Caroff SN. Sleep disturbance as the hallmark of post-traumatic stress disorder. *Am J Psychiatry* 1989;146:697–707

51. Inman DJ, Silver SM, Doghramji K. Sleep disturbance in post-traumatic stress disorder: a comparison with non-PTSD insomnia. *J Traum Stress* 1990;3:429–37

52. Rosen J, Reynolds CF, Yeaer AL, Houck PR, Hurwitz LF. Sleep disturbances in survivors of the Nazi holocaust. *Am J Psychiatry* 1991;148:62–6

53. Mellman ThA, Kumar A, Kulick-Bell R, Kumar M, Nolan B. Nocturnal/daytime urine noradrenergic measures and sleep in combat-related PTSD. *Biol Psychiatry* 1995;38:174–9

54. Mellman ThA, Nolan B, Hebding J, Kulick-Bell R, Dominguez R. A polysomnographic comparison of veterans with combat-related PTSD, depressed men, and non-ill controls. *Sleep* 1997;20:46–51

55. Greenberg R, Pearlman C, Campel D. War neuroses and the adaptive function of REM sleep. *Br J Med Psychol* 1972;45:27–33

56. Kauffmann CD, Reist C, Djenderedjian A, Nelson JN, Haier RJ. Biological markers of affective disorders and post-traumatic stress disorder: a pilot study with desipramine. *J Clin Psychiatry* 1987;48:366–7

57. Schlosberg A, Benjamin M. Sleep patterns in three acute combat fatigue cases. *J Clin Psychiatry* 1978;9:546–9

58. Lavie P, Hefez A, Halperin G, Enoch D. Long-term effects of traumatic war-related events on sleep. *Am J Psychiatry* 1979;136:175–8

59. Hefez A, Metz L, Lavie P. Long-term effects of extreme situational stress on sleep and dreaming. *Am J Psychiatry* 1987;144:344–7

60. Glaubman H, Mikulincer M, Porat A, Wasserman O, Birger M. Sleep of chronic post-traumatic patients. *J Traumat Stress* 1990;3: 255–63

61. Van Kammen WB, Christiansen C, van Kammen DP, Reynolds CF. Sleep and the prisoner-of-war experience – 40 years later. In Giller IR, ed. *Biological Assesment and Treatment of Posttraumatic Stress Disorder*. Washington DC: American Psychiatric Press, 1990:159–72

62. Ross RJ, Ball WA, Dinges DF. Rapid eye movement sleep disturbance in posttraumatic stress disorder. *Biol Psychiatry* 1994;35:195–202

63. Kulka RA, Fairbrank JA, Hough RL, Marmar CR, Weiss DW. *Trauma and the Vietnam Generation: Findings from the National Vietnam Veterans Readjustment Study*. New York: Brunner/Mazel, 1990

64. Benca RM, Obermeyer WH, Thisted RA, Gillin C. Sleep and psychiatric disorders. A meta-analysis. *Arch Gen Psychiatry* 1992;49: 651–68

65. Woodward SH, Friedman MJ, Bliwise DL. Sleep and depression in combat-related PTSD inpatients. *Biol Psychiatry* 1996;39:182–92

66. Emilien G, Penasse C, Charles G, Martin D, Lasseaux L, Waltregny A. Post-traumatic stress disorder: hypothesis from clinical neuropsychology and psychopharmacology research. *Int J Psychiatry Clin Pract* 2000;4:3–18

67. Bauer M, Priebe S, Graf KJ, *et al.* Psychological and endocrine abnormalities in refugees from East Germany. II. Serum levels of cortisol, prolactin, luteinizing hormone, follicle stimulating hormone and testosterone. *Psychiatry Res* 1994;51:75–85

68. Carrol BJ, Feinberg M, Greden JF. *et al.* A specific laboratory test for the diagnosis of melancholia. *Arch Gen Psychiatry* 1981;38:15–22

69. Whalley LJ, Borthwick N, Copolov D, *et al.* Glucocorticoid receptors and depression. *Br Med J* 1986;292:859–61

70. Yehuda R, Boisoneau D, Lowy MT, Giller FL. Dose response changes in plasma cortisol and

lymphocyte glucocorticoid receptors following dexamethasone administration in combat veterans with and without posttraumatic stress disorder. *Arch Gen Psychiatry* 1995;52: 583–93

71. Perry BD, Giller EL, Southwick SM. Altered platelet alpha2-adrenergic binding sites in posttraumatic stress disorder. *Am J Psychiatry* 1987;144:1511–12

72. Gershuni BS. Thayer JF. Relations among psychological trauma, dissociative phenomena, and trauma-related distress: a review and integration. *Clin Psychol Rev* 1999;19:631–57

73. Rotenberg VS. Right hemisphere insufficiency and illness in the context of search activity concept. *Dynamische Psychiatrie Dynamic Psychiatry* 1995;150/151:54–63

74. Schore AN, The effects of early relational trauma on right brain development, affect regulation, and infant mental health. *Infant Ment Health J* 2001;22:201–69

75. Hong Ch Ch-h, Potkin SG, Antrobus JS, Dow BM, Callaghan GM, Gillin JCh. REM sleep eye movement counts correlate with visual imagery in dreaming: a pilot study. *Psychophysiology* 1997;14:377–81

76. Kinzie JD, Fredrickson RH, Ben R, Fleck J, Karls W. Posttraumatic stress disorder among survivors of Cambodian concentration camps. *Am J Psychiatry* 1984;141:645–9

77. Goldstein G, van Kammen W, Shelly C, Miller D, van Kammen D. Survivors of imprisonment in the Pacific Theatre during World War II. *Am J Psychiatry* 1987;144:1210–14

78. Kramer M, Schoen LS, Kinney L. Nightmares in Vietnam veterans. *J Am Acad Psychoanal* 1987;15:67–81

79. Husain AM, Miller PP, Carwile ST. REM sleep behavior disorder: potential relationship to post-traumatic stress disorder. *J Clin Neurophysiol* 2001;18:148–57

80. Greenberg R, Pillard R, Pearlman Ch. The effect of dream (stage REM) deprivation on adaptation to stress. *Psychosom Med* 1972;34: 257–62

81. Kramer M, Schoen LS, Kinney L. The dream experience in dream-disturbed Vietnam veterans. In van den Kolk BA, ed. *Post-traumatic Stress Disorder: Psychological and Biological Sequelae*. Washington DC: American Psychiatric Press, 1984:81–95

82. Lavie P, Kaminer H. Dreams that poison sleep: dreaming in Holocaust survivors. *Dreaming* 1991;1:11–21

83. Bleich A, Attias Y, Dagan Y, Lavie P, Shalev A, Lerrer B. Psycho-neuro-physiologic characteristics of combat veterans with posttraumatic stress disorder. *Clin Neuropharmacol* 1990; 13(Suppl 2):334

84. Rotenberg VS. Sensitivity, neuroticism and sleep disturbances: some controversial problems. *Waking Sleeping* 1980;4:271–9

85. Rotenberg VS, Michailov AN. Characteristics of psychological defense mechanisms in healthy testees and in patients with somatic disorders. *Homeostasis* 1993;34:54–8

86. Plutchik R, Kellerman H, Conte HR. A structural theory of EGO defenses and emotions. In Izard E, ed. *Emotions in Personality and Psychopathology*. New York: Plenum Publishing, 1979:229–57

87. Grieser C, Greenberg R, Harrison R. The adaptive function of sleep: the differential effects of sleep and dreaming on recall. *J Abnormal Psychol* 1972,80.200–6

88. Kupfer DJ, Frank E, Grochocinski VJ, Gregor M, McEacharon AB. Electroencephalographic sleep profiles in recurrent depression. *Arch Gen Psychiatry* 1990;15:678 81

89. Ansseau M, Kupfer DJ, Reynolds CF III. Internight variability of REM latency in major depression: implications for the use of REM latency as a biological correlate. *Biol Psychiatry* 1985;20:489–505

90. Reynolds CF III, Kupfer D. Sleep in depression. In Williams RZ, Karacan I, Moore CA, eds. *Sleep Disorders, Diagnosis and Treatment*. New York: John Wiley, 1988:147–64

91. Benson E, Zarcone VP. Rapid eye movement sleep eye movements in schizophrenia and depression. *Arch Gen Psychiatry* 1993;50:474–82

92. Riemann D, Berger M. EEG sleep in depression and in remission and the REM sleep response to the cholinergic agonist RS 86. *Neuropsychopharmacology* 1989;2:145–52

93. Thase ME, Reynolds CF III, Frank E, *et al*. Polysomnographic studies of unmedicated depressed men before and after cognitive behavior therapy. *Am J Psychiatry* 1994;151: 1615–22

94. Rush AJ, Erman MK, Giles DE, *et al*. Polysomnographic findings in recently drug-free and clinically remitted depressed patients. *Arch Gen Psychiatry* 1986;43:878–84

95. Buysse DJ, Kupfer DJ, Frank E, Monk TH, Ritenour A. Electroencephalographic sleep studies in depressed outpatients treated with interpersonal psychotherapy. II. Longitudinal studies at baseline and recovery. *Psychiatry Res* 1992;40:27–40

96. Kupfer DJ, Ulrich RF, Coble PA, *et al*. The application of automated REM and slow wave sleep analysis (normal and depressives). *Psychiatr Res* 1984;13:325–34

97. Reynols CF, Kupfer DJ. Sleep research in affective illness: state of the art circa 1987. *Sleep* 1987;10:199–215

98. Vogel GW, Vogel F, McAbur RS, Thurmond AJ. Improvement of depression by REM sleep deprivation. *Arch Gen Psychiatry* 1980;37:247–53

99. Wirz-Justice A, Van den Hoofdaker RH. Sleep deprivation in depression: what do we know, where do we go? *Biol Psychiatry* 1999;46: 445–53

100. Greenberg R, Pearlman Ch. Cutting the REM sleep nerve: an approach to the adaptive role of REM sleep. *Perspect Biol Med* 1974;17: 513–21

101. Rotenberg VS, Shamir E, Barak Y, Indursky P, Kayumov L, Mark M. REM sleep latency and wakefulness in the first sleep cycle as markers of major depression. A controlled study vs. schizophrenia and normal controls. *Prog Neuro-Psychopharmacol Biol Psychiatry* 2002;26: 1211–15

102. Kupfer DJ, Frank E, Ehlers CL. EEG sleep in young depressives: first and second nights effects. *Biol Psychiatry* 1989;25:87–97

103. Reynolds CF III, Newton TF, Shaw DM, Coble PA, Kupfer DJ. Electroencephalographic sleep findings in depressed outpatients. *Psychiatry Res* 1982;6:65–72

104. Coble P, Foster C, Kupfer D. Electroencephalographic sleep diagnosis of primary depression. *Arch Gen Psychiatry* 1976;33:1124–7

105. Akiskal HS, Lemmi H, Yerevanian B, King D, Belluomoni J. The utility of the REM latency test in psychiatric diagnosis: a study of 81 depressed outpatients. *Psychiatry Res* 1982;7: 101–10

106. Rotenberg VS, Hadjez J, Kimhi R, *et al*. First night effect in depression: new data and a new approach. *Biol Psychiatry* 1997;42:267–74

107. Rotenberg VS, Kayumov L, Indursky P, *et al*. REM sleep in depressed patients: different attempts to achieve adaptation. *J Psychosom Res* 1997;42:565–75

108. Reynolds CF III, Hoch CC, Buysse DJ, *et al*. Sleep in late-life recurrent depression: changes during early continuation therapy with nortriptyline. *Neuropsychopharmacology* 1991;5: 85–96

109. Rotenberg V, Kayumov L, Indursky P, *et al*. Slow wave sleep redistribution and REM sleep eye movement density in depression: towards the adaptive function of REM sleep. *Homeostasis* 1999;39:81–9

110. Indursky P, Rotenberg VS. Change of mood during sleep and REM sleep variables. *Int J Psychiatry Clin Pract* 1998;2:47–51

111. Cartwright RD, Lloyd SR. Early REM sleep: a compensatory change in depression? *Psychiatry Res* 1994;51:245–52

112. Kramer M, Roth T. A comparison of dream content in dream reports of schizophrenic and depressive patients groups. *Compr Psychiatry* 1973;14:325–9

113. Rotenberg VS, Indursky P, Kayumov L, Sirota P, Melamed Y. The relationship between subjective sleep estimation and objective sleep variables in depressed patients. *Int J Psychophysiol* 2000;37:291–7

114. Keshavan MS, Reynolds GF, Kupfer D. Electroencephalographic sleep in schizophrenia: a critical review. *Compr Psychiatry* 1990;30: 34–47

115. Tandon R, Shirpley JE, Taylor S, *et al*. Electroencephalographic sleep abnormalities in schizophrenia: relations to positive/ negative symptoms, and previous neuroleptic treatment. *Arch Gen Psychiatry* 1992;49: 185–94

116. Hudson JI, Lipinski JP, Keck PE, *et al*. Polysomnographic characteristics of schizophrenia in comparison with mania and depression. *Biol Psychiatry* 1993;34:191–3

117. Lauer TCM, Schreiber W, Pollmacher Th, Holsboer F, Krieg J-Ch. Sleep in schizophrenia: a polysomnographic study of drug-naïve patients. *Neuropsychopharmacology* 1997;16: 51–60

118. Mendelson WB, Gillin JCh, Wyatt RJ. *Human Sleep and its Disorders*. New York: Plenum Press, 1977

119. Hiatt JF, Floyd TC, Katz PH, Feinberg I. Further evidence of abnormal non-rapid-eye-movement sleep in schizophrenia. *Arch Gen Psychiatry* 1985;42:797–802

120. Benson E, Zarcone VP. Low REM latency in schizophrenia. *Sleep Res* 1985;14:124

121. Zarcone VP, Benson KL, Berger PA. Abnormal rapid eye movement latencies in schizophrenia. *Arch Gen Psychiatry* 1987;44:45–8

122. Ganguli R, Reynolds ChF III, Kupfer DJ. Electroencephalographic sleep in young, never-medicated schizophrenics. *Arch Gen Psychiatry* 1987;44:36–44

123. Kempenaers C, Kerkhofs M, Linkowski P, Mendlewicz J. Sleep EEG variables in young schizophrenic and depressive patients. *Biol Psychiatry* 1988;24:833–8

124. Riemann D, Gann H, Fleckenstein P, Hohagen F, Olbrich R, Berger M. Effect of RS86 on REM latency in schizophrenia. *Psychiatry Res* 1991;38.89–92

125. Neylan ThC, van Kammen DP, Kelley ME, Peters JL. Sleep in schizophrenic patients on and off haloperidol therapy. Clinically stable vs. relapsed patients. *Arch Gen Psychiatry* 1992; 49:643–9

126. Kupfer DJ, Wyatt RJ, Scott J, Snyder F. Sleep disturbance in acute schizophrenic patients. *Am J Psychiatry* 1970;126:1213–23

127. Rotenberg VS, Hadjez J, Shamir E, Martin T, Indursky P, Barak Y. Sleep structure as a mirror of the clinical state in schizophrenic patients. *Dynamische Psychiatrie Dynamic Psychiatry*, 1999;176/179:334–40

128. Kay SR, Fiszbein A, Opler LA. The positive and negative syndrome scale (PANSS) for schizophrenia. *Schizophr Bull* 1987;13:261–76

129. Foster FG, Kupfer D, Coble P, McParland RJ. Rapid eye movement sleep density. *Arch Gen Psychiatry* 1976;33:119–23

130. Toussaint M, Luthringer R, Schaltenbrandt N, *et al*. First night effect in normal subjects and psychiatric inpatients. *Sleep* 1995;18:463–9

131. Kim DK, Shin YM, Kim ChE, Cho HS, Kim YS. Electrodermal responsiveness, clinical variables and brain imaging in male chronic schizophrenics. *Biol Psychiatry* 1993;33:786–93

132. Frith CD. *The Cognitive Neuropsychology of Schizophrenia*. Hove, UK: Lawrence Erlbaum, 1992

133. Docherty NM. Affective reactivity of symptoms as a process discriminator in schizophrenia. *J Nerv Ment Dis* 1996;184:535–41

134. Wolkin A, Sanfilipo M, Duncan E, *et al*. Blunted change in cerebral glucose utilization after haloperidol treatment in schizophrenic patients with prominent negative symptoms. *Am J Psychiatry* 1996;153:346–54

135. Parker G, Hedzi-Pavlovik D, Brodati H, *et al*. Sub-typing depression. II. Clinical distinction of psychotic depression and non-psychotic melancholia. *Psychol Med* 1995;25:825–32

136. Ayuso-Gutierrez JL, Almoguera MI, Carcia-Camba E, Frias JQ, Cabranes JA. The dexamethasone suppression test in delusional depression: further findings. *J Affect Disord* 1985;8:147–51

137. Schatzberger AF, Rothshild AJ, Langlais PJ, Bird ED, Cole JO. A corticosteroid/dopamine hypothesis for psychotic depression and related states. *Psychiatr Res* 1985;19:57–64

138. Shamir E, Rotenberg VS, Laudon M, Zisapel N, Elizur A. First-night effect of melatonin treatment in patients with chronic schizophrenia. *J Clin Psychopharmacol* 2000;20:691–4

139. Rotenberg VS, Indursky P, Kimhi R, *et al*. The relationship between objective sleep variables and subjective sleep estimation in schizophrenia. *Int J Psychiatry Clin Pract* 2000;4:63–7

140. Ware JC. Sleep and anxiety. In Williams RL, Karacan I, Moore CA, eds. *Sleep Disorders. Diagnosis and Treatment*. New York: John Wiley & Sons, 1988;189–214

141. Yerkes RM, Dodson JD. The relation of strength of stimulus to rapidity of habit formation. *J Comp Neurol Psychol* 1908;18:459–82

142. Lens W, De Volder M. Achievement motivation and intelligent test scores: a test of the Yerkes-Dodson hypothesis. *Psychol Belg* 1980:49–59

143. Spielberger CD. The effects of manifest anxiety on the academic achievement of college students. *Ment Hyg* 1962;46:420–6

144. Lader M. *The Psychophysiology of Mental Illness*. London: Routledge, 1975

145. Dienstbier RA. Arousal and physiological toughness: implications for mental and physical health. *Psychol Rev* 1989;96:93–104

146. Gal R, Lazarus RS. The role of activity in anticipating and confronting stressful situations. *J Hum Stress* 1975;1:4–20

147. Zuckerman M. Sensation seeking: a comparative approach to human traits. *Behav Brain Sci* 1984;7:413–34

148. Rosenbaum DL, Seligman MEP. *Abnormal Psychology*. New York: Norton, 1989

149. Gray J. *The neuropsychology of anxiety; an inquiry into the functions of septohippocampal system*. Oxford: Oxford University Press, 1982

150. Soubrie P. Inferring anxiety and anti-anxiety effects in animals. *Behav Brain Sci* 1982;5:502–3

151. Ledoux JE, Gorman JM. A call to action: overcoming anxiety through active coping. *Am J Psychiatry* 2001;158:1953–5

152. Lader M. The orienting reflex in anxiety and schizophrenia. In Kimmel HD, van Olst EH, Orlebeke JF, eds. *The Orienting Reflex in Humans*. Hilsdale, NY: Erlbaum, 1979:607–17

153. Rotenberg VS, Vedenyapin AB. GSR as a reflection of decision-making under conditions of delay. *Pavlov J Biol Sci* 1985;20:11–14

154. Wilder L. Das 'Ausgangswert-Gesetz' – ein unbeachtetes biologische Gesetz: Seine Bedeutung fur Forschung und Praxis. *Klin Wiss* 1931;41:1889–93

155. O'Gorman JG, Jamieson RD. Short latency acceleration of human heart rate as a function of stimuli intensity. *Percept Motor Skills* 1977;45:579–83

156. Lovallo WR, Pincomb GA, Wilson MF. Predicting response to a reaction time task. Heart rate reactivity compared with Type A behavior. *Psychophysiology* 1986;23:648–56

157. Lader M. Anxiety and depression. In Gale A, Edwards JA, eds. *Physiological Correlates of Human Behavior. Individual Differences and Psychopathology*. London: Academic Press, 1983;155–67

158. Kayumov L, Rotenberg VS, Buttoo K, Auch Ch, Pandi-Perumal SR, Shapiro CM. Interrelationships between nocturnal sleep, daytime alertness, and sleepiness: two types of alertness proposed. *J Neuropsychiatry Clin Neurosci* 2000;12:86–90

159. Jenkins JG, Dallenbach KM. Obliviscence during sleep and waking. *Am J Psychol* 1924; 35:605–12

160. Stickgold R. Sleep: off-line memory reprocessing. *Trends Cogn Sci* 1998;2:484–92

161. Seligman MEP. On the generality of the laws of learning. *Psychol Rev* 1970;77:406–18

162. Smith C. Sleep states and learning. A review of the animal literature. *Neurosci Biobehav Rev* 1985;9:157–68

163. Smith C, Kitahama K, Valatx JL, Jouvet M. Increases in paradoxical sleep in mice during acquisition of a shock avoidance task. *Brain Res* 1974;77:221–30

164. Pearlman Ch. REM sleep and information processing: evidence from animal studies. *Neurosci Biobehav Rev* 1979;3:57–68

165. Conway J, Smith C. REM sleep and learning in humans: a sensitivity to specific types of learning tasks. Presented at the *12th Congress of the European Sleep Research Society*, Florence, Italy, June 1994

166. Smith C. Sleep states and memory processes. *Behav Brain Res* 1995;69:137–45

167. Latash LP, Manov GA. The relationship between delta-sleep and REM sleep phasic components with the retention and reproduction of the verbal material learned before sleep. *Fiziol Cheloveka* 1975;1:262–70

168. Plihal W, Born J. Effects of early and late nocturnal sleep on declarative and procedural memory. *J Cognit Neurosci* 1997;9:534–47

169. Rotenberg VS. Sleep and memory. II. Investigations on humans. *Neurosci Biobehav Rev* 1992;16:503–5

170. McGrath MJ, Cohen JB. REM sleep facilitation of adaptive making behavior: a review of the literature. *Psychol Bull* 1978;85:24–57

171. Smith C. REM sleep and learning: some recent findings. In Moffitt A, Kramer M, Hoffmann R, eds. *The Functions of Dreaming*. Albany, NY: State University of New York Press, 1993:341–62

172. Montangero J. Dream, problem solving and creativity. In Cavallero C, Foulkes D, eds. *Dreaming as Cognition*. Harvester Wheatsheaf, 1993:93–113

173. Coenen AML, van Luijtelaar FLJM. Effects of benzodiazepines, sleep and sleep deprivation on vigilance and memory. *Acta Neurol Belg* 1997;97:123–9

174. Vertes RP, Eastman KE. The case against memory consolidation in REM sleep. *Behav Brain Sci* 2000;23:867–76

175. Leconte P, Hennevin E, Block V. Analyse des effets d'un apprentisage et de son niveau d'acquisition sur le sommeil paradoxal consecutive. *Brain Res* 1973;49:367–79

176. Pagel I, Pegram V, Vaughan S, Donaldson P, Bridge W. The relationship of REM sleep with learning and memory in mice. *Behav Biol* 1973;9:383–8

177. Giuditta A, Ambrosini MV, Montagnese P, et al. The sequential hypothesis of the function of sleep. *Behav Brain Res* 1995;69:157–66

178. Fishbein W. The case against memory consolidation in REM sleep: Balderdash! *Behav Brain Sci* 2000;23:934–6

179. Fishbein W, Kastaniotis C, Chattman I. Paradoxical sleep: prolonged augmentation following learning. *Brain Res*, 1974;79:61–75

180. Chrobak JJ, Buzsaki G. Selective activation of deep layer (V–VI) retrohippocampal cortical neurons during hippocampal sharp waves in the behaving rat. *J Neurosci* 1994;14:1660–70

181. Maquet P, Laureys S, Peignen Ph, et al. Experience-dependent changes in cerebral activation during human REM sleep. *Nat Neurosci* 2000;3:831–6

182. Greenberg R, Katz H, Schwartz W, Pearlman Ch. A research-based reconsideration of the psychoanalytic theory of dreaming. *J Am Psychoanal Assoc* 1992;40:531–50

183. Stern WC. Acquisition impairments following rapid eye movements sleep deprivation in rats. *Physiol Behav* 1971;7:345–52

4

Gender and sleep

Howard M. Kravitz, Louis G. Keith,
Emma Robinson-Rossi and Alexander Z. Golbin

AGE-RELATED CHANGES AND GENDER DIFFERENCES

Women's and men's sleep differs, behaviorally and physiologically. Their sleep patterns change differently with age, and changes in sleep patterns across the life span can be measured polysomnographically[1]. Some changes in the sleep-wake cycle are non-specific, whereas others have important significance. The mechanism(s) and significance of these differences remains a mystery.

Gender differences in sleep begin in the fetal and neonatal growth periods. Analysis of fetal and neonatal movement patterns shows that fetuses/neonates display decreasing numbers of leg movements per minute during antenatal development (30 to 37 weeks), followed by increasing numbers of leg movements per minute during postnatal development (birth to 6 weeks of age)[2]. According to Almli and co-workers[2], males display greater numbers of leg movements per minute compared with females during both antenatal and postnatal development. At the same time, females display a stronger and different fetal-to-neonatal movement continuity pattern compared with males. These results indicate a differential time course for neurobehavioral development in male and female fetuses/neonates[2].

Postnatal differences were examined in 4- to 14-month old infants by Menna-Barreto and associates[3], who found that girls tended to sleep more than boys after 10 months old. Sloan and Shapiro[1] have summarized gender differences in sleep architecture across the life span, based on the published results of Williams, Karacan and Hursch[4]. These early pioneers in sleep research conducted cross-sectional sleep laboratory studies on males and females ranging in age from 3 years to 79 years[4].

Studies on gender differences in adolescent sleep habits have shown that girls, compared to boys, get less nighttime sleep, complain more of poor sleep quality, and spend more time in bed and get up later on weekends[5-7]. These differences may be related to girls' more advanced pubertal status compared with that of boys of the same chronological age[6].

Lee and colleagues[8] demonstrated gender differences in sleep disturbances in a racially diverse sample of early adolescents aged 11–14 years. They analyzed school night and weekend sleep patterns and daytime sleepiness. Results show that boys consumed significantly more caffeinated beverages than girls did, which was related to self-reported parasomnias. Significant gender differences were present for self-reports of daytime sleepiness. Moreover, weekday wake-up time for boys was significantly later than for girls. Those who reported consuming alcohol during the week were likely to fall asleep in the classroom before lunch. Girls, who awakened earlier than boys on school days, were more likely to report falling asleep on the way home from school[8]. College students displayed a significant positive correlation between increased daytime sleepiness and negative mood states[9]. Specifically, sleepiness may correlate with higher negative moods.

Gender differences in circadian patterns in adults were described by Natale and Danesi[10]. Using the Morningness–Eveningness Questionnaire (MEQ) to measure sleep-wake cycle preferences of 1,319 individuals aged 18–30 years, 240 morning-types, 284 evening-types and 795 intermediate-types were identified. Men had more pronounced eveningness preferences than did women. There was a significant gender-by-circadian typology interaction for wake-up time, meaning evening-type men preferred waking up later than did evening-type women, but morning-type men had a propensity to wake up earlier than did morning-type women. These results suggest that the circadian system may be more flexible in men than in women[10].

In a Japanese study, Park and co-workers[11] looked at the MEQ scores of 2,252 individuals aged between 6 and 89 years and found that gender differences in sleep changed with age and showed sharp changes in young adulthood, i.e., puberty. They analyzed the effects of age and gender on the habitual sleep-wake rhythm in randomly selected subjects living in Shimonoseki, Japan. Study subjects were divided into 21 age groups with a matched number of males and females in each. During the period from primary school to adolescence, bedtime became delayed and sleep length decreased. After that period, with increasing age, bedtime became earlier and sleep length increased. The number of awakenings and the length of daytime naps increased markedly after 50 years of age and 70 years of age, respectively. In this study, gender differences were attributed to the women's social and domestic customs in

Japan. Gau and co-workers[12] found an association between morning/evening type and mood and anxiety symptoms in young Taiwanese adolescents. Evening type was associated with severe mood problems in boys but not in girls.

Spindles, as a specific sleep electroencephalographic (EEG) phenomenon, can be used as a biological marker to differentiate sleep cycles between genders. Huupponen and colleagues[13] examined gender differences in sleep spindle typography in 40 healthy subjects aged 22 to 49 years. Women, compared with men, had a significantly higher percentage of spindles in the left frontal channel. According to the investigators, this difference was gender and not age related[13]. However, interindividual spindle variability was at least as large as that stemming from gender.

Carrier and colleagues[14] assessed the effects of age and gender on sleep EEG power spectral density in a group of 100 health subjects aged 20–60 years who enrolled in the Pittsburgh Study of Normal Sleep. Results of the quantitative EEG analysis suggested that the aging process did not differentially influence men and women. Power density was higher in women than in men within the delta, theta, low alpha, and high spindle frequency ranges. With increasing age, the investigators observed a decrease in power in slow-wave, theta, and sigma activity, and higher power in the beta range. These results suggested that increasing age might be related to an attenuation of homeostatic sleep pressure and an increase in cortical activation during sleep[14].

Armitage and co-workers[15] analyzed slow wave activity (SWA) in non-rapid eye movement (NREM) sleep, and showed that significant differences between patients and controls were restricted to the first NREM period only for 20–30 year olds. Sex differences in the depressed group were twice as large as those seen in the control group. Changes in slow-wave sleep (SWS) presumed to reflect homeostatic sleep regulation of SWA were abnormal only in depressed men. Depressed women showed no evidence of an abnormal SWS time course. In individuals with affective disorders, men but not women showed impaired SWA regulation that was evident from 20–40 years of age[15].

Autonomic regulation (heart rate variability) has clear gender differences[16]. Compared with women, men showed a significantly elevated low frequency (LF) to high frequency (HF) ratio during rapid eye movement (REM) sleep, and a significantly decreased HF band power during waking. It is interesting that there were no significant sleep- or gender-related changes in LF band power. These data suggest that there are gender differences in autonomic functioning during waking and sleep, manifested as decreased vagal tone during waking and increased sympathetic dominance during REM sleep in men.

Men and women have different dream recall[17]. A total of 480 men (mean age 37.7 years) and 242 women (mean age 35.9 years) completed a sleep questionnaire measuring sleep pattern, sleep quality, presleep mood, and dream frequency during the previous 2 weeks. Women, compared with men, tended to rate their sleep quality lower and felt less refreshed in the morning. Women also reported awakening more at night and a lower presleep emotional balance, but no differences in tiredness. Women scored higher on dream recall. Moreover, engagement in dreams, an item in which women also scored markedly higher, nearly completely explained the gender difference concerning dream recall. Such findings suggest that the gender-specific pattern in factors connected with dream recall frequency may be explained by the different levels of dream recall[17].

GENDER, HORMONES, AND SLEEP

Childbearing years

Manber and Armitage[18] extensively reviewed the evidence for the effects of reproductive hormones on sleep, which strongly suggests that endogenous and exogenous sex steroids both can have an impact. Progesterone primarily affects NREM sleep, whereas estrogen primarily affects REM sleep. Gender differences in REM sleep are strongly influenced by androgens, i.e., testosterone. Estrogen and progesterone act on the central nervous system through interaction with intracellular receptors that trigger genomically directed interactions in protein synthesis and through a more rapid nongenomic alteration of neuronal excitability involving binding sites on neurotransmitter-gated ion channels such as the gamma-aminobutyric acid-A receptor complex[18].

Although the literature suggests that there are menstrual phase effects on sleep architecture, these differences across the menstrual cycle may not be significant. This inconsistent picture of menstrual cycle effect on women's sleep may be due to varied research methodologies, including small sample sizes, timing of sleep studies relative to menstrual cycle phase, and substantial interindividual differences such as age of study participants and lack of control for psychological factors (e.g., mood symptoms).

Women with premenstrual syndrome and premenstrual dysphoric disorder, compared with women without these cyclical symptom exacerbations, report more insomnia symptoms, increased difficulty wakening in the morning, heightened mental activity during the night, more frequent and unpleasant dreams, and increased daytime sleepiness[19]. However, published research suggest that compared with controls these women show no remarkable differences in sleep architecture, and there is a disparity between their sleep self-reports and polysomnographic measurements[20].

Pregnancy and the postpartum period are life cycle events that have important effects on women's sleep, both subjectively and polysomnographically. Sleep can be disturbed by physiological changes due to hormonal factors, physical factors due to the growing fetus, and sleep-wake cycle changes associated with the newborn infant's unpredictable sleep-wake schedule[21]. Lee[22] has published a comprehensive review of sleep during the pregnancy and postpartum period. Polysomnography with pregnant women has demonstrated increased awakening and time awake during the night and decreased slow wave sleep[20]. Sleep deprivation, which can be attributed to the disturbed sleep, produces daytime sleepiness and fatigue. To compensate, about 50% of pregnant women nap on average once daily for 30–60 minutes and sleep about 30–60 minutes longer on weekends[20]. The good news is that postpartum sleep tends to improve by 3–5 months, with less time awake and increased sleep efficiency[23].

Mid-life and the menopausal transition

In middle-aged women entering the menopausal transition, self-reported sleep difficulty increases dramatically, with prevalence rates ranging from 28–63% in surveys of peri- and post-menopausal women[24]. Whereas insomnia is uncommon among persons younger than 20 years old, according to data from a representative community survey, 23.6% of women and 14.4% of men between 45–49 years old report sleep difficulties, and 39.7% of women and 15.3% of men report not sleeping well by their early 50s[25]. In a survey of 200,000 men and women aged 30–59 years, Brugge and associates[26] estimated that 44–50% of perimenopausal and postmenopausal women had complaints of insomnia. Studies involving other representative community samples confirm that the female preponderance of sleep problems most often involves women aged 40 years and older[27–30].

In a community survey of 12,603 middle-aged women (40–55 years) of diverse ethnicities, conducted as part of the Study of Women's Health Across the Nation (SWAN), 38% reported sleep difficulties[31]. Prevalence rates differed among ethnic groups: 28% in Japanese women, 32% in Chinese women, 36% in African-American women, 38% in Hispanic women, and 40% in Caucasian women. Menopausal status, but not age *per se*, was significantly associated with sleeping difficulties. Late perimenopausal and both naturally and surgically postmenopausal women had the highest rates in the adjusted analysis, while early perimenopausal women

and postmenopausal women using hormone replacement therapy (HRT) had rates of difficulty sleeping similar to rates reported by the premenopausal group.

Whether the increase in difficulty sleeping in middle-aged women is due to aging, stress, psychosocial and physical problems, or the effects of hormonal changes associated with menopause remains unclear[32–34]. For example, among women 65 years of age and older, difficulty falling asleep and frequent awakenings continue to increase with age[35]. On the other hand, across a woman's life cycle, hormonally related events unique to women, such as menstruation and pregnancy, also are associated with disrupted sleep patterns[36,37]. Disturbed sleep, including trouble falling asleep and frequent nocturnal awakenings, are reported commonly by perimenopausal and postmenopausal women as well as by premenopausal women who have had a bilateral oophorectomy[1,38].

Vasomotor symptoms may be related to hormonal factors as well as to disturbances in thermoregulation[32,34,39,40]. During the perimenopausal years, sleep difficulties increase and tend to be attributed to hot flashes and related perimenopausal symptoms[24]. Shaver and co-workers[37] found that the sleep patterns of healthy perimenopausal and premenopausal women were similar but perimenopausal women experiencing hot flashes compared to those without hot flashes had more sleep instability, as indexed by the sleep efficiency index. Woodward and Freedman[41] studied the thermoregulatory effects of hot flashes on sleep by measuring skin conductance level and confirmed that hot flashes disrupt sleep. Vasomotor symptoms may have more negative effects on sleep in surgically menopausal women who did not use HRT, compared with women who went through the menopausal transition naturally or who used HRT postmenopausally[42]. In addition to alleviating sleep disruption caused by vasomotor symptoms in perimenopausal as well as surgically menopausal women, Moe and co-workers[42] suggested that oral estrogen replacement may decrease sleep disruption in postmenopausal women experiencing sleep disruption from environmental factors. However, HRT has had mixed effects on disturbed sleep[43,44] and may be less effective for women not experiencing vasomotor symptoms[44,45], which further complicates understanding the relationship among vasomotor symptoms, hormones, and sleep.

Young and colleagues[46] used cross-sectional data from the Wisconsin Sleep Cohort Study to show that postmenopausal women slept better than premenopausal women as measured by all-night polysomnography (longer total sleep times, increased delta sleep, less time awake in bed) despite their self-report of more sleep dissatisfaction. More specifically, women who reported less quality during sleep reported more dissatisfaction but did not differ on any objective measure of sleep quality during a single night of polysomnography. These results may reflect postmenopausal women's estrogen deficiency, which leads to more daytime fatigue and a consequent increased drive for sleep[47]. Another consideration is that these statistically significant findings may not be physiologically significant. These interesting findings require confirmation in a longitudinal study of women transitioning to menopause.

Menopause may affect sleep quality in ways other than through effects of vasomotor symptoms. These include increasing the prevalence of breathing-related and periodic limb movement sleep disorders, social changes associated with middle-age such as reentering the work force, stress and psychological distress, and aging *per se*[48]. Polysomnography is required to assess sleep apnea and periodic limb movement disorders. The role of other factors mentioned would be better assessed with longitudinal studies.

SLEEP DISORDERS

Sleep breathing disorders

The prevalence of sleep-disordered breathing (SDB), in particular, obstructive sleep apnea (OSA), increases in the mid-life years, with narrowing the high male-to-female ratio,

from 8–10:1 in younger clinic-based cohorts to 2-4:1 in population-based studies of mid-life adults[49–52]. The prevalence of obstructive sleep apnea also increases with age, with prevalence rates two to three times higher in the 65 years and older group compared with those in middle age, 30–64 years[52]. In a population-based study, Young et al[51] estimated that the prevalence of SDB in middle-aged men and women was 24% and 9%, respectively, and that 2% of middle-aged women and 4% of middle-aged men had sleep apnea syndrome according to the criteria of an apnea-hypopnea index of 5 or higher plus daytime hypersomnolence. Data from the Wisconsin Sleep Cohort Study indicate that gender differences in sleep apnea diagnosis are due to gender bias; women with OSA are less likely than men to be evaluated and diagnosed in clinic settings[53].

Upper airway resistance syndrome (UARS) is part of the spectrum of SDB that may be more prevalent in women, especially premenopausal women, than in men because the female upper airway is less compliant and thus more resistant to collapse. UARS has been diagnosed in nonobese individuals with repetitive increased respiratory effort that is terminated by transient arousals; there is no associated airway collapse, hypoventilation, or oxygen desaturation[54]. UARS may evolve into OSA during the menopause transition due to increased fat deposition in and subsequent narrowing of the upper airway.

Data supporting menopause as a risk factor for SDB and HRT as a protective factor for SDB are few and not definitive[55]. A recent study by Bixler et al[49] examined this association. Defining sleep apnea as 10 or more apneas or hypopneas per hour, plus clinical symptoms such as daytime sleepiness, they found that the prevalence increased from 0.6% in premenopausal women to 2.7% in postmenopausal women who were not on HRT but remained low (0.5%) in postmenopausal women who used HRT[49]. Polo-Kantola and co-workers[56] found that the severity of SDB in postmenopausal women was not related to the severity of vasomotor symptoms or to circulating estradiol levels.

In the past, a substantial proportion (37%) of postmenopausal women in the USA was taking HRT[57]. Now that the findings from the Women's Health Initiative (WHI)[58] are available, questions regarding risk and benefit of HRT for treating postmenopausal SDB are relevant. One survey of HRT users conducted 6 months after publication of the WHI results indicated that 40% had discontinued use[59]. The relevance of this finding is that Bixler et al[49] found that hormone replacement reduced the menopause-associated risk for SDB. Compared with premenopausal women, the adjusted odds ratios for SDB were higher for postmenopausal women not using HRT but not for postmenopausal women who did use HRT. Premenopausal women and postmenopausal women using HRT did not differ on SDB risk. Nevertheless, Young[55] advised a cautious approach to these data, which require further study and replication, and the implication that menopause is an independent risk factor for SDB that can be modified by HRT. In considering the American College of Obstetricians and Gynecologists recommendation for short-term use of combination HRT for relief of menopausal symptoms, it remains important to learn about the impact of HRT on breathing during sleep in postmenopausal women.

Insomnia

Ohayon[60] reviewed more than fifty community studies and found that about one-third of adults reported at least one sleep complaint or problem (e.g., difficulty falling asleep or staying asleep, or early morning awakening). Most studies have shown that the prevalence of sleep problems increases with age and is higher for women than for men. Whereas prevalence estimates of insomnia in childhood and adolescents do not appear to differ between boys and girls, and gender differences are small or nonexistent between persons 20–40 years old, investigations spanning the age range from 18–79 years indicate that women, compared with men, are about 1.3 times more likely to report insomnia-like sleep problems[61].

A recent study of gender-related factors in insomnia among adults 18–65 years old in the Chinese population in Hong Kong showed that women had an estimated 1.6 times higher risk for insomnia than did men[62]. Similar to other studies, reasons suggested for these differences included differences in psychiatric comorbidities, gonadal steroids, sociocultural factors and coping strategies. Studies also show that women are prescribed and use hypnotic medications at rates significantly higher than in men[1].

However, the gender differences may be related more to the self-perception of sleep quality and the propensity for reporting symptoms. A meta-analysis of the prevalence of insomnia conducted by Lack and Thorn[63], based on 61 surveys published from 1962 to 1987, revealed that women reported more general sleep difficulties and difficulty falling asleep but gender differences in self-reported sleep maintenance difficulties and early morning awakening were not as clear-cut. Gender differences in self-reported sleep difficulties may be due at least in part to how survey questions are worded. Ruler and Lack[64] found that women were more likely than men to demonstrate this bias in reporting sleep difficulty when questions were negatively worded; they found no gender difference when specific, neutrally worded questions were used. When polysomnography is used as an objective indicator of sleep disturbance, women tend to sleep at least as well as men do, and in older age groups, men have more sleep disruption and less slow wave sleep than do women[65].

In a cross-sectional survey of 405 long-time married couples (married 35 years or more) participating in the Alameda County Study in 1999, Strawbridge and associates[66] found that spouses' sleep problems negatively impacted their partners' health and well-being. However, no gender differences were found, suggesting that regardless of whether the husbands or the wives have the sleep problems, the resulting relationships with quality of life for their partners appear to be the same.

In an epidemiological survey of cardiovascular risk factors in employed men and women, 19–65 years old, conducted in central Sweden, Akerstedt et al[67] observed that disturbed sleep was predicted by being female and older than 45 years. As in Li et al's[62] study, women had a 1.6 times higher risk than men for reporting disturbed sleep. Sleep difficulties also were strongly linked to stress and the social isolation at work as well as to the inability to stop worrying about work and marital problems.

Kripke and colleagues[68] examined mortality in association with sleep duration and insomnia in more than 1.1 million men and women aged 30–102 years participating in the Cancer Prevention Study II of the American Cancer Society. Data were analyzed separately for men and women. The lowest mortality risk was experienced by persons reporting that their usual sleep was 6.5–7.4 hours per night. Higher risks were found for those sleeping 8 hours or more and for those sleeping 6 hours or less. Increased risk exceeded 15% when reported sleep was more than 8.5 hours or when less than 4.5 hours among men or less than 3.5 hours among women. Interestingly, self-reported "insomnia" was not associated with excess mortality risk for either men or women after controlling for sleeping pill use and other comorbid conditions. In fact, the covariate-adjusted hazard ratios actually were significantly less than the reference (i.e., no self-reported insomnia) for both men and women. On the other hand, self-reported prescription sleeping pill use was associated with increased mortality hazards regardless of whether insomnia was reported.

Patel and associates[69] examined the relationship between sleep duration and mortality in the Nurses' Health Study. Participants were 82,969 women from the original cohort established in 1976, which had included 121,700 married female nurses, aged 30–55 years, who resided in eleven large U.S. states. The sleep duration question was introduced in 1986 and was repeated in 2000. In this predominantly Caucasian female sample, mortality risk was lowest among those sleeping 6 to 7 hours, consistent with findings from the American Cancer Society study[68], which included males, and from the Japanese Collaborative Cohort Study on Evaluation of Cancer Risk[70].

Periodic limb movements and restless legs

Periodic limb movements in sleep (PLMS) and restless legs syndrome (RLS) have been increasingly recognized as causes of disturbed sleep and daytime sleepiness (see Chapter 10). The two can co-occur; approximately 85% of people with RLS experience PLMS. Furthermore, the prevalence of RLS (as well as nocturnal leg cramps) is higher in women, particularly during pregnancy[1]. Symptoms may first develop when a woman is pregnant and prevalence estimates of RLS during pregnancy range between 11–27%[71]. On the other hand, there appears to be no gender difference in PLMS.

Fibromyalgia syndrome

Fibromyalgia syndrome (see Chapter 22) is characterized by chronic diffuse non-articular musculoskeletal aches, pains and stiffness, nonrefreshing and disrupted sleep, fatigue, and multiple localized tender points. Moldofsky et al[72] described a subgroup of patients with sleep-related involuntary leg movements who experienced disturbed sleep and the typical alpha EEG intrusions of fibromyalgia syndrome. These afflicted individuals, mainly women, experienced more pain, morning fatigue, and sleep stage shifts than individuals with sleep-related limb movements and daytime somnolence. However, the prevalence of this sleep-related limb (especially legs) activity (i.e., periodic limb movements in sleep, (PLMS)) in patients with fibromyalgia syndrome is not known, nor is it known whether PLMS reflects a generalized sleep-related increase in muscle activity in persons with fibromyalgia[73,74].

Parasomnias

Some parasomnias are more common in women than in men, whereas others are more common in men or show no gender differences. Parasomnias are reviewed in Chapters 10–15.

CONCLUSION

As noted by Sloan and Shapiro[1], there is a dearth of information about many relevant aspects of gender-related sleep differences. Yet, as described herein, clearly sleep differs in men and women in some important ways.

Hormonal changes and the aging process are just two factors involved in producing these differences. Together with psychosocial and cultural factors they provide a biopsychosocial framework for further study. Understanding gender differences from this perspective may help us to better understand the physiological processes underlying changes in sleep across the life cycle. To the extent that sleep is a manifestation of psychiatric illness and sleep disturbances can contribute to the development of psychiatric disorders, understanding gender differences should facilitate further study of the role of gender in psychopathology.

References

1. Sloan EP, Shapiro CM. Gender differences in sleep disorders. In Seeman MV, ed. *Gender and Psychopathology*. Washington, DC: American Psychiatric Press, 1995:269–85
2. Almli CR, Ball RH, Wheeler ME. Human fetal and neonatal movement patterns: gender differences and fetal-to-neonatal continuity. *Dev Psychobiol* 2001;38:252–73
3. Menna-Barreto L, Montagner H, Soussignan R, *et al*. The sleep/wake cycle in 4- to 14-month children: general aspects and sex differences. *Braz J Med Biol Res* 1989;22:103–6
4. Williams RL, Karacan I, Hursch CJ. *EEG of Human Sleep: Clinical Applications*. New York: John Wiley & Sons, Inc., 1974
5. Gau SF, Soong WT. Sleep problems of junior high school students in Taipei. *Sleep* 1995;18:667–73
6. Laberge L, Petit D, Simard C, *et al*. Development of sleep patterns in early adolescence. *J Sleep Res* 2001;10:59–67
7. Manni R, Ratti MT, Marchioni E, *et al*. Poor sleep in adolescents: a study of 869 17-year-old Italian secondary school students. *J Sleep Res* 1997;6:44–9
8. Lee KA, McEnany G, Weekes D. Gender differences in sleep patterns for early adolescents. *J Adolesc Health* 1999;24:16–20
9. Jean-Louis G, Von Gizycki H, Zizi F, *et al*. Mood states and sleepiness in college students: influences of age, sex, habitual sleep, and substance use. *Percept Motor Skills* 1998;87:507–12
10. Natale V, Danesi E. Gender and circadian typology. *Biol Rhythm Res* 2002;33:261–9
11. Park YM, Matsumoto K, Seo YJ, *et al*. Changes of sleep or waking habits by age and sex in Japanese. *Percept Motor Skills* 2002;94:1199–213
12. Gau SS-F, Soong W-T, Merikangas KR. Correlates of sleep-wake patterns among children and young adolescents in Taiwan. *Sleep* 2004;27:512–9
13. Huupponen E, Himanen S, Vaerri A, *et al*. A study on gender and age differences in sleep spindles. *Neuropsychobiology* 2002;45:99–105
14. Carrier J, Land S, Buysse DJ, *et al*. The effects of age and gender on sleep EEG power spectral density in the middle years of life (ages 20–60 years old). *Psychophysiology* 2001;38:232–42
15. Armitage R, Hoffmann R, Trivedi M, *et al*. Slow-wave activity in NREM sleep: sex and age effects in depressed outpatients and healthy controls. *Psychiatr Res* 2000;95:201–13
16. Elsenbruch S, Harnish MJ, Orr WC. Heart rate variability during waking and sleep in healthy males and females. *Sleep* 1999;22:1067–71
17. Schredl M. Gender differences in dream recall. *J Ment Imagery* 2000;24:169–76
18. Manber R, Armitage R. Sex, steroids, and sleep: a review. *Sleep* 1999;22:540–55 [Errata. *Sleep* 2000;23:145–9]
19. Manber R, Colrain IM, Lee KA. Sleep disorders. In Kornstein SG, Clayton AH, eds. *Women's Mental Health: A Comprehensive Textbook*. New York: The Guilford Press, 2002:274–94
20. Moline ML, Broch L, Zak R. Sleep in women from adulthood through menopause. In Lee-Chiong TL, Sateia MJ, Carskadon MA, eds. *Sleep Medicine*. Philadelphia, PA: Hanley & Belfus, Inc., 2002:105–14

21. Campbell I. Postpartum sleep patterns of mother-baby pairs. *Midwifery* 1986;2:193–201

22. Lee KA. Alterations in sleep during pregnancy and postpartum: a review of 30 years of research. *Sleep Med Rev* 1998;2:231–42

23. Hertz G, Fast V, Feinsilver SH, *et al*. Sleep in normal late pregnancy. *Sleep* 1992;15:246–51

24. Krystal AD, Edinger J, Wohlgemuth W, *et al*. Sleep in perimenopausal and post-menopausal women. *Sleep Med Rev* 1998;2:243–53

25. Cirignotta F, Mondini S, Zucconi M, *et al*. Insomnia: an epidemiological survey. *Clin Neuropharmacol* 1985;8(Suppl 1):S49–54

26. Brugge KL, Kripke DF, Ancoli-Israel S, *et al* The association of menopausal status and age with sleep disorders. *Sleep Res* 1989;18:208

27. Bixler EO, Kales A, Soldatos CR, *et al*. Prevalence of sleep disorders in the Los Angeles metropolitan area. *Am J Psychiatry* 1979;136:1257–62

28. Karacan I, Thornby JI, Anch M, *et al*. Prevalence of sleep disturbance in a primarily urban Florida county. *Soc Sci Med* 1976;10:239–44

29. Quera-Salva MA, Orluc A, Goldenberg F, *et al*. Insomnia and use of hypnotics: study of a French population. *Sleep* 1991;14:386–91

30. Weyerer S, Dilling H. Prevalence and treatment of insomnia in the community: results from the Upper Bavarian Field Study. *Sleep* 1991;14:392–8

31. Kravitz HM, Ganz PA, Bromberger J, *et al*. Sleep difficulty in women at midlife: a community survey of sleep and the menopausal transition. *Menopause: J North Am Menopause Soc* 2003;10:19–28

32. Driver HS. Sleep in women. *J Psychosom Res* 1996;40:227–30

33. Driver HS, Shapiro CM. A longitudinal study of sleep stages in young women during pregnancy and post-partum. *Sleep* 1992;15:449–53

34. Erlik Y, Tataryn IV, Meldrum DR, *et al*. Association of waking episodes with menopausal hot flushes. *J Am Med Assoc* 1981;245:1741–44

35. Newman AB, Enright PL, Manolio TA, *et al*. Sleep disturbance, psychosocial correlates, and cardiovascular disease in 5201 older adults: the Cardiovascular Health Study. *J Am Geriatr Soc* 1997;45:1–7

36. Owens JF, Matthews KA. Sleep disturbances in healthy middle-aged women. *Maturitas* 1998;30:41–50

37. Shaver J, Giblin E, Lentz M, *et al*. Sleep patterns and stability in perimenopausal women. *Sleep* 1988;11:556–61

38. Janowsky DS, Halbreich U, Rausch J. Association among ovarian hormones, other hormones, emotional disorders, and neurotransmitters. In Jensvold MF, Halbreich U, Hamilton JA, eds. *Psychopharmacology and Women: Sex, Gender, and Hormones*. Washington, DC: American Psychiatric Press, 1996:85–106

39. Polo-Kantola P, Erkkola R, Helenius H, *et al*. When does estrogen replacement therapy improve sleep quality? *Am J Obstet Gynecol* 1998;178:1002–9

40. Polo-Kantola P, Erkkola R, Irjala K, *et al*. Climacteric symptoms and sleep quality. *Obstet Gynecol* 1999;94:219–24

41. Woodward S, Freedman RR. The thermoregulatory effects of menopausal hot flashes on sleep. *Sleep* 1994;17:497–501.

42. Moe KE, Larsen LH, Vitiello MV, *et al*. Estrogen replacement therapy moderates the sleep disruption associated with nocturnal blood sampling. *Sleep* 2001;24:886–94.

43. Assmus JD, Kripke DF. Differences in actigraphy and self-reported sleep quality in women on estrogen replacement therapy. *Sleep* 1998;21(Suppl):268

44. Moe KE, Larsen LH, Vitiello MV, *et al*. Objective and subjective sleep of post-menopausal women: effects of long-term estrogen replacement therapy. *Sleep Res* 1997;26:143

45. Thomson JT, Oswald I. Effect of oestrogen on the sleep, mood and anxiety of menopausal women. *Br Med J* 1977;2:1317–9

46. Young T, Rabago D, Zgierska A, *et al*. Objective and subjective sleep quality in premenopausal, perimenopausal, and postmenopausal women in the Wisconsin Sleep Cohort Study. *Sleep* 2003;26:667–72

47. Polo O. Sleep in postmenopausal women: better sleep for less satisfaction. *Sleep* 2003;26:652–3

48. Shaver JLF, Zenk SN. Sleep disturbance in menopause. *J Wom Health Gender Based Med* 2000;9:109–18

49. Bixler EO, Vgontzas AN, Lin H-M, *et al*. Prevalence of sleep-disordered breathing in women: effects of gender. *Am J Respir Crit Care Med* 2001;163:608–13

50. Redline S, Kump K, Tishler PV, *et al*. Gender differences in sleep disordered breathing in a community-based sample. *Am J Respir Crit Care Med* 1994;149:722–6

51. Young T, Palta M, Dempsey J, *et al*. The occurrence of sleep-disordered breathing among middle-aged adults. *N Engl J Med* 1993;328:1230–5

52. Young T, Skatrud J, Peppard PE. Risk factors for obstructive sleep apnea in adults. *J Am Med Assoc* 2004;291:2013–6

53. Young T, Hutton R, Finn L, *et al*. The gender bias in sleep apnea diagnosis: are women

missed because they have different symptoms? *Arch Intern Med* 1996;156:2445–51

54. Guilleminault C, Chowdhuri S. Upper airway resistance syndrome is a distinct syndrome. *Am J Respir Crit Care Med* 2000;161:1412–3.

55. Young T. Menopause, hormone replacement therapy, and sleep-disordered breathing. Are we ready for the heat? *Am J Respir Crit Care Med* 2001;163:597–601

56. Polo-Kantola P, Rauhala E, Saaresranta T, *et al*. Climacteric vasomotor symptoms do not predict nocturnal breathing abnormalities in postmenopausal women. *Maturitas* 2001;39: 29–37

57. Keating NL, Cleary PD, Rossi AS, *et al*. Use of hormone replacement therapy by post-menopausal women in the United States. *Ann Intern Med* 1999;130:545–53

58. Writing Group for the Women's Health Initiative Investigators. Risks and benefits of estrogen plus progestin in healthy post-menopausal women: Principal results from the Women's Health Initiative randomized control trial. *J Am Med Assoc* 2002;288:321–33

59. Lawton B, Rose S, McLeod D, *et al*. Changes in use of hormone replacement therapy after the report from the Women's Health Initiative: cross-sectional survey of users. *Br Med J* 2003; 327:845–6

60. Ohayon NM. Epidemiology of insomnia: what we know and what we still need to learn. *Sleep Med Rev* 2002;6:97–111

61. Zorick FJ, Walsh JK. Evaluation and management of insomnia: an overview. In Kryger MH, Roth T, Dement WC, eds. *Principles and Practice of Sleep Medicine, 3rd edn*. Philadelphia, PA: W.B. Saunders Company, 2000:615–23

62. Li RHY, Wing YK, Ho SC, *et al*. Gender differences in insomnia – a study in the Hong Kong Chinese population. *J Psychosom Res* 2002;53: 601–9

63. Lack LC, Thorn SJ. Sleep disorders: their prevalence and behavioral treatment. In Caddy GR, Byrne DG, eds. *Behavioral Medicine: International Perspectives, Vol 2*. Norwood, NJ: Ablex Publishing Corporation, 1992:347–95

64. Ruler A, Lack L. Gender differences in sleep surveys. *Sleep Res* 1988;17:244

65. Bearpark HM. Insomnia: causes, effects and treatment. In Cooper R, ed. *Sleep*. London, UK: Chapman & Hall Medical, 1994:587–613

66. Strawbridge WJ, Shema SJ, Roberts RE. Impact of spouses' sleep problems on partners. *Sleep* 2004;27:527–31

67. Akerstedt T, Knutsson A, Westerholm P, *et al*. Sleep disturbances, work stress and work hours: a cross-sectional study. *J Psychosom Res* 2002;53:741–8

68. Kripke DF, Garfinkel L, Wingard DL, *et al*. Mortality associated with sleep duration and insomnia. *Arch Gen Psychiatry* 2002;59:131–6

69. Patel SR, Ayas NT, Malhotra MR, *et al*. A prospective study of sleep duration and mortality risk in women. *Sleep* 2004;27:440–4

70. Tamakoshi A, Ohno Y. Self-reported sleep duration as a predictor of all-cause mortality: results from the JACC study, Japan. *Sleep* 2004;27:51–4

71. Manconi M, Ferini-Strambi L. Restless legs syndrome among pregnant women. *Sleep* 2004;27:350

72. Moldofsky, H. Management of sleep disorders in fibromyalgia. *Rheum Dis Clin North Am* 2002;28:353–65

73. Finestone DH, Sawyer BA, Ober SK, *et al*. Periodic leg movements in sleep in patients with fibromyalgia. *Ann Clin Psychiatry* 1991;3: 179–85

74. Kravitz HM, Helmke N, Hansen G, *et al*. Muscle activity and sleep continuity in women with fibromyalgia syndrome. *Sleep Res* 1989; 18:343

Section 2:

The effect of sleep disorders on health and mental function

5

Insomnia: perspectives from sleep medicine and psychiatry

Jamie K. Lilie and Henry W. Lahmeyer

INTRODUCTION

Insomnia can have a serious impact upon one's ability to perform at work and maintain healthy social relationships, and it can be the source of, or contribute to, a variety of psychological disturbances, including major mood and anxiety disorders. Several studies have also indicated that the length and quality of sleep are related to general health and longevity. Given the potential impact insomnia can have on physical and mental health and well-being, it is not surprising that there has been a proliferation of research in the areas of assessment and treatment for this sleep disorder[1-5].

EPIDEMIOLOGY

Despite advances in pharmacological and behavioral treatments, insomnia remains a common problem for both children and adults. Some surveys estimate that in the USA about 75 million people feel their sleep is inadequate[3]. Several large-scale surveys of sleep problems, both in the USA and in Britain, have found that about 30–35% of adults report at least occasional difficulties with falling asleep or staying asleep[3-5]. Furthermore, large-scale studies have consistently found that females report more complaints than males and that the incidence of sleep complaints increases with age[6-8].

DEFINITION OF INSOMNIA

Insomnia is defined as an inability to obtain adequate sleep. This statement is sufficiently broad to permit classification of essential commonalities, which are persistence of the complaint (i.e. more than a transient poor night of sleep), and the subjective element as noted by the word *adequate*. The latter also highlights the fact that individuals vary in their need for sleep.

Insomnia is a complex problem, and it is now widely recognized that there can be multiple causes for sleep disruption, including conditions such as sleep apnea, delayed sleep phase, periodic limb movements (PLMs), gastroesophageal reflux and drug reactions[9,10]. However, clinicians are more likely to treat insomnia that is the result of anxiety, depression, conditioned arousal, stress and sleep–wake cycle disturbances[3,10].

SLEEP LABORATORY STUDIES

Sleep laboratory measurements are essential in diagnosing and treating disorders of excessive somnolence, such as sleep apnea and narcolepsy, but the information garnered from polysomnography is also thought to be necessary to evaluate the insomnias. For example, Reynolds and colleagues[11] demonstrated in 1987 that polysomnography added to, refuted or failed to support the initial clinical impression in nearly 50% of a sample of consecutive cases referred for insomnia. Commonly, four specific parameters of sleep are used to assess insomnia[5].

They are as follows:

(1) Sleep onset latency is simply the length of time it takes for an individual to initiate sleep (abnormal if over 30 minutes).

(2) Wake after sleep onset is the amount of time an individual is awake after sleep onset prior to final awakening. This measure is useful for evaluating the extent of a sleep maintenance problem (abnormal if over 15 minutes, or 30 minutes in the elderly).

(3) Sleep efficiency is the proportion of total sleep time to total time in bed (abnormal if less than about 80–90% in adults).

(4) Total sleep time is the sum of the time spent in sleep throughout a sleep period and is usually measured in minutes (abnormal if less than 360 minutes).

In addition to polysomnography, various self-report measures have been used to study insomnia. Sleep logs are varied in type but essentially ask the patient to systematically record time spent in bed each night and to estimate total sleep obtained, latency to fall asleep, number of awakenings, time of sleep onset and time of final awakening. Another form of sleep log requires a patient to keep a record of all sleep obtained per 24-hour period. This type is especially helpful in documenting a circadian rhythm disturbance such as phase delay insomnia characterized by late sleep onset and late final awakening, or phase advance insomnia usually seen in the elderly where very early sleep onset and final awakening are consistently found[12].

Lacks[4] noted that, although insomniacs usually overestimate sleep latency and underestimate total sleep time, their self-reports are consistent and thus provide a reliable and valid relative measure of insomnia. Sleep logs have also been shown to have high test–retest reliability and to correlate well with both electroencephalogram (EEG)-defined measures of sleep and bed partner reports. In short, the sleep log or diary has become the standard self-report measure of severity and type of insomnia, and its widespread use has permitted cross-study comparisons. Sleep laboratory studies are usually necessary to determine the efficacy of a new hypnotic early in its development, while out-patient sleep-log studies are used to study large numbers of individuals with insomnia to demonstrate efficacy needed for Food and Drug Administration (FDA) approval.

PSYCHIATRIC MANAGEMENT OF SLEEP DISORDERS

Since most insomnias have psychiatric components and many are completely the result of the underlying psychiatric conditions, most psychiatrists should be familiar with the differential diagnosis and treatment of insomnias, and in most cases should attempt management on their own or in some instances collaborate with therapists. If treatment is unsuccessful and/or a primary sleep disorder is suspected, a sleep laboratory referral can be made.

MEASUREMENT OF SLEEP AND AROUSAL

Since many sleep disorders have a psychiatric component[12], a thorough psychiatric history should always be taken before initiating treatment. The major psychiatric conditions associated with disturbances in sleep or wakefulness must be carefully diagnosed. These include: sleep in affective disorders (major depression), dysthymia, mania, dementia, schizophrenia, schizoaffective disorders, anxiety disorders and alcoholism or other drug abuse[5,12].

A comprehensive medical history should be routinely obtained from patients presenting with sleep-related complaints. Attention should be directed to any signs of major systemic illness since sleep disorders may be a sign of disease in liver, heart, brain, kidney, or endocrine systems. Furthermore, sleep may exacerbate pre-existing medical conditions, such as seizure disorders, heart and lung disorders and migraine headaches[5].

A number of standardized measures of mood and psychological functioning are useful in examining the sleep disorder patient. The single most widely used personality inventory is the Minnesota Multiphasic Personality Inventory (MMPI). It has been well established that patients with insomnia differ from normal sleepers and from patients with other types of sleep disorders in their MMPI profile[1,3,4,12]. Since many sleep disorder patients present with symptoms of depression and anxiety, other self-report scales which focus on these symptoms have been employed. These include the Beck Depression Inventory, the State–Trait Anxiety Inventory and the Profile of Mood States[12].

If the patient is felt to have primary insomnia, behavioral treatments are appropriate initial therapy; several useful tests and papers review the details of how to conduct this form of therapy[2,4,12].

Briefly the therapies that are most widely used are as follows:

(1) Sleep restriction reduces the time in bed and results in increased sleep efficiency and reduced sleep fragmentation. This is an effective therapy which depends on patient compliance[2].

(2) In stimulus-control therapy[2] the clinician instructs the patient to get out of bed if unable to sleep for over 20–30 minutes and to do something else. When sleepiness returns they return to bed. The bedroom and patient's bed become associated with sleep rather than wakefulness.

(3) Sleep hygiene[13] is a series of techniques that emanate from knowledge of sleep physiology:

(a) Fixed bedtime and wake-up time are useful because regular sleep patterns, especially wake-up time, entrain circadian rhythms so that maximal sleep drive is at night and maximal alerting brain activity occurs during the day.

(b) Late-night stimulating activities, exercise and alcohol should be avoided, as these behaviors interfere with normal midbrain sleep-inducing neural activity.

(c) Bed should be used only for sleep and not for watching television or doing work. Both these activities create the association of bed = wakefulness.

(d) Excessive daytime napping should be avoided. While a planned late-afternoon nap can be useful for the elderly, unplanned, late or long naps will delay sleep onset significantly in most people.

(e) A late-night light snack may promote sleep by increasing brain serotonin or by stimulating the tractus-solitarius of the vagus nerve.

(f) Hypnotics should be used sparingly as a 'rescue procedure' when anxiety is high or other techniques fail.

AFFECTIVE DISORDERS

Sleep is very disrupted in depression and mania[5,12]. Major depression usually produces initial insomnia and sleep maintenance insomnia including early morning awakening. Patients most often complain of the inability to return to sleep as easily as usual. Individuals with atypical depressions and seasonal affective disorders more often complain of hypersomnolence. A sleep laboratory recording may document specific abnormalities associated with depression. These include early onset of rapid eye movement (REM) sleep, increased number of eye movements, reduction in stage 3 and stage 4 and poor sleep continuity. Several studies have now demonstrated that 1 year of chronic untreated insomnia leads to depression in up to 50% of people.

Adequate treatment with antidepressants and psychotherapy will usually ameliorate the insomnia as the depression improves. Most effective antidepressants significantly suppress REM sleep[14]. Partial sleep deprivation, another effective treatment for depression, reduces REM by keeping the patient awake when REM sleep predominates (3–7 a.m.) Electroconvulsive therapy (ECT) also reduces REM time and normalizes REM– NREM cyclicity[12].

In general, it has been shown that the amount of REM sleep suppression produced by an antidepressant correlates with its efficacy[13]. Reduced REM latency is a consistent biological marker of depression. Patients who have a REM latency less than 60 minutes respond dramatically to fluoxetine, while patients with REM latency longer than 65 minutes respond the same as placebo subjects[14].

ANXIETY DISORDERS

Chronic anxiety usually produces sleep onset insomnia. Panic attacks can occur at the onset of sleep or during stage 2–stage 3 transition. Those occurring during REM sleep are called REM anxiety attacks[15]. The differential diagnosis must include nocturnal seizures and night terrors. Anxiety disorders do not appear to produce the typical abnormalities seen in major depression such as shortened REM latency. In fact, there are no consistent specific differences between the sleep parameters of patients with anxiety disorders[16]. Anxiolytic agents may be needed chronically by some patients and it is best if these are given once daily at bedtime. Short half-life benzodiazepines, such as triazolam or lorazepam, produce 'rebound insomnia' when abruptly discontinued, which frequently leads to continued use of the drug beyond clinical necessity[17]. Sleep is improved and most patients will not develop tolerance if the dosage is fixed and if drugs such as clonazepam with longer half-lives are used[18].

ALCOHOL AND DRUG ABUSE

About 10–15% of patients with chronic insomnia abuse substances, especially alcohol and other sedatives[12,18]. Although alcohol in low to moderate doses initially promotes sleep, it disrupts and fragments sleep later in the night. Alcohol may exacerbate sleep-related breathing disorders in some patients[19]. A persistent sleep disturbance has been demonstrated in chronically abstinent alcoholics[20]. However, it is unwise to treat abstinent alcoholics with benzodiazepines or barbiturates since they are cross-tolerant with alcohol and patients can quickly become addicted to these drugs. People who are alcoholic or addicted to sedative-hypnotics have severe insomnia during acute withdrawal. Hospitalization may be required for such patients for supervised gradual withdrawal. Insomnia may persist for months following withdrawal. Sleep hygiene techniques must be taught and the underlying psychiatric syndromes should be treated[1,2,21].

PHARMACOLOGY OF SLEEP HYPNOTICS (SEE CHAPTER 27)

Despite the recent progress in the use of non-benzodiazepines, physicians remain reluctant to prescribe drugs with sedative properties, i.e. hypnotics, because the risks are perceived to be too high[2]. Many physicians have the impression that onerous side-effects are inevitable. In general, physicians should favor short-acting hypnotics over long-acting drugs in primary insomnia when short-term use is anticipated. Chronic insomnia associated with the anxiety disorders respond better to hypnotics with longer half-lives to reduce daytime anxiety[5].

Benzodiazepine hypnotics

Virtually all hypnotic drugs work by potentiating the inhibitory actions of γ-aminobutyric acid (GABA receptor) within the brain[17]. Benzodiazepine receptors are part of a large complex of proteins at the synapse in the target neuron. When a hypnotic drug molecule binds to this synaptic complex, both GABA-A and GABA-B receptors, chloride channels in the neuronal membrane open, facilitating the inhibitory effects of GABA.

The benzodiazepines increase total sleep time primarily by prolonging stage 2 sleep, rather than extending slow-wave sleep (stages 3 and 4) and REM sleep[22]. Sleep induced by benzodiazepines is therefore considered inferior to natural sleep. In general, while most patients are likely to prefer shorter-acting hypnotics, there are many chronic psychiatric patients with insomnia for whom a longer-acting benzodiazepine will remain the drug of choice. Anxious, depressed, bipolar and schizophrenic patients may benefit from the persisting anxiolytic effects of long-acting benzodiazepines such as flurazepam and clonazepam, for example[23]. Such patients may also benefit from protection from rebound anxiety, which may occur as a short-acting benzodiazepine wears off.

Non-benzodiazepine hypnotics

For many patients with insomnia, newer non-benzodiazepine hypnotics such as zolpidem, zaleplon and zopiclone may prove to be superior alternatives to the benzodiazepines. Zolpidem is a short-acting (half-life 2.5–3 h) rapid-onset imidazopyridine that selectively binds to the GABA-A benzodiazepine receptor[24]. This is in contrast with the benzodiazepines, which bind to GABA-A and -B receptors in the brain. This receptor-binding selectivity is presumed to account for the relatively specific hypnotic action of zolpidem. In doses of 5–10 mg, zolpidem has no antianxiety, anticonvulsant, muscle relaxant properties, while it produces potent effects on sleep by increasing total sleep time, reducing awake time and maintaining normal sleep architecture[25].

Preliminary evidence suggests that tolerance and rebound insomnia do not occur with the extended use of zolpidem as they can with triazolam or other benzodiazepines[26]. Zolpidem may therefore prove to be the drug of choice for the treatment of chronic insomnia. Nevertheless, the efficacy and safety of zolpidem with extended use remain to be formally established.

Precautions with hypnotic therapy

The treatment of transient insomnia is the single most appropriate use of hypnotics. Such patients only require hypnotic support for a night or two. If the circumstances that provoked the transient insomnia are with some certainty likely to recur, the patient may be prescribed medication for use on those nights. The same guidelines apply in the treatment of short-term insomnia[2].

Like all central nervous system depressants, hypnotics interfere with normal control of respiration and must therefore be prescribed cautiously for patients with breathing problems, such as symptomatic sleep apnea[5].

There are numerous contraindications for the use of hypnotics that must be seriously considered. Hypnotics are contraindicated in people with a history of alcoholism or drug abuse and are generally inappropriate for children. Also, people who may need to be alert at a moment's notice, such as firefighters and other emergency workers, should not be given hypnotics of any kind. The safety of hypnotics in pregnant women has not been established. Sedating antidepressants are safer during pregnancy if treatment must be given. Similarly, nursing mothers should not be given hypnotic drugs, as these medications and their active metabolites have been found in breast milk[2,5].

The psychiatrist faced with managing chronic insomnia in a chronically depressed, anxious, psychotic or demented patient should always use the psychotropic drug of choice at adequate dosages for an adequate length of time to ameliorate symptoms. It is nearly axiomatic that a well-treated depression leads to sound sleep[10]. In cases where it does not, the clinician should try changing the time of day that the psychotropic agent is given. Night is usually best, but for fluoxetine and buproprion, the reverse is usually true[12]. Many depressed patients do better if given a hypnotic for the first 1–3 weeks of therapy since the patient feels improved immediately and the antidepressant compliance is significantly improved. For example, patients particularly responsive to fluoxetine can benefit from adjunctive trazadone, a tricyclic antidepressant, or an atypical antipsychotic such as queitiapine or olanzapine given at bedtime. Anxious depressives can benefit also from clonazepam at bedtime, while bipolar disorders can benefit from mood stabilizer or an atypical antipsychotic at bedtime. Post-traumatic stress disorder usually requires polypharmacy that addresses target symptoms – a benzodiazepine or anticonvulsant for nightmares, antidepressants and anti-anxiety agents for the other symptoms[12] (see Chapter 16). Psychiatric patients will usually sleep well if given adequate antipsychotics at bedtime but some also benefit from clonazepam or zolpidem given at night[2].

A major challenge in the pharmacological management of psychiatric patients is finding a drug that improves cognitive function rather than impairs it. Many patients maintained for a few years on tricyclic antidepressants will experience improved energy, memory and concentration when gradually switched to a selective serotonin reuptake inhibitor (SSRI). Likewise, many elderly patients will improve cognitively when switched from a benzodiazepine to zolpidem or zaleplon, a very low dose of an atypical antipsychotic given at night.

It must be kept in mind that many psychotropic drugs are usually sleep promoting in low doses but less so as the dosage is increased. Examples include trazadone, quetiapine, paroxetine, etc.

Another common problem is drug-induced insomnia. As hypnotic drugs are increased in dosage, sleep will eventually deteriorate into a fragmented, light sleep with often severe daytime impairment[10].

Daytime functioning is usually impaired by insomnia[6,7,14]. This consists of increased anxiety, dysphoria, and memory and concentration deficiency[6,7]. Behavioral treatment of insomnia, when it works, produces improvement in daytime functioning[9,10]. Zolpidem may improve daytime cognitive alertness with short-term use. Psychotropics may improve mood and anxiety, while drugs like trazadone, the tricyclics and the benzodiazepines may actually decrease daytime alertness, memory and concentration. The wise assessment of these trade-offs constitutes the art of clinical psychiatry.

References

1. Bootzin RR, Engle-Friedman M. The assessment of insomnia. *Behav Assess* 1981;3:107–26
2. Bootzin RR, Nicassio PM. Behavioral treatments for insomnia. In Hersen M, Eisler R, Miller P, eds. *Progress in Behavioral Modification*. New York: Academic Press, 1978;6:1–45
3. Kales A, Kales JD. *Evaluation and Treatment of Insomnia*. New York: Oxford Press, 1984
4. Lacks P. *Behavioral Treatment of Persistent Insomnia*. New York: Pergamon, 1987
5. Martin-Gonzalez D, Obermeyer W, Benca R. Comorbidity of insomnia with medical and psychiatric disorders. *Prim Psychiatr* 2002;9:37–49
6. Gallup Organization. 1991
7. Gallup Organization. 1994
8. Lichstein K, Morin C, eds. *Treatment of Late Life Insomnia*. London: Sage Publications, 2000
9. Lilie JK, Rosenberg R. Behavioral treatment of insomnia. In Hersen M, Eisler R, Miller P, eds. *Progress in Behavioral Modification*. New York: Academic Press, 1978:25
10. Lilie JK, Lahmeyer H. Psychiatric management of sleep disorder. *Psychiatr Med* 1991;9:245–60
11. Reynolds CF, *et al.* Is polysomnography useful in the evaluation of chronic insomnia? *Sleep Res* 1987;16:416
12. Ford DE, Kamerow DB. Epidemiologic study of sleep disturbances and psychiatric disorders. An opportunity for prevention? *J Am Med Assoc* 1989;262:1479–84
13. Hauri DJ, Esther MS. Insomnia. *Mayo Clin Proc* 1990;5:869–82
14. Heiligenstein JH, Faries DE, Rush AJ, *et al.* Latency to rapid eye movement sleep as a

predictor of treatment response to fluoxetine and placebo in nonpsychotic depressed outpatients. *Psychiatry Res* 1994;52:327–39

15. Balfer MB, Uhlenhuth EH. The beneficial and adverse effects of hypnotics. *J Clin Psychiatry* 1991;52:16–23

16. Speilman AJ, Saskia P, Thorpy MJ. Sleep restriction: a new treatment of insomnia. *Sleep Res* 1983;12:286

17. Bonnet MH. Effects of sleep disruption on sleep, performance, and mood. *Sleep* 1985;8:11–19

18. Bootz RR, Lahmeyer HW, Lilie JK. *Integrated Approach to Sleep Management*. Belle Meade, NJ: Cahner's Healthcare Communications, 1994:1–32.

19. Ware JC. The symptoms of insomnia. Causes and cures. *Psychiatr Ann* 1979;9:27–499

20. Lahmeyer HW. Hypnotics: a powerful tool for a serious problem. *Pharm Therapeut* 1995;438–55

21. Coats TJ, Thorensen CE. Treating sleep disorders: a few answers, some suggestions and many questions. In Turner SM, Calhoun KS, Adams HE, eds. *Handbook of Clinical Behavior Therapy*. New York: John Wiley, 1981:24240–89

22. Kupfer DJ, Hanson I, Spiker D, *et al.* Amitriptyline plasma levels and clinical response in primary depression II. *Commun Psychopharmacol* 1978;2:441–50

23. Vogel GW. A review of REM sleep deprivation. *Arch Gen Psychiatry* 1975;32:749–61

6

The sleep apnea–hypopnea syndrome and sleep-related consequences of other chronic respiratory disorders: associations with neurocognitive dysfunction, mood and quality of life

Neil S. Freedman

This chapter will review the relationships between sleep-related chronic respiratory disorders and neurocognitive dysfunction, mood disorders with an emphasis on depression, and quality of life. The majority of the chapter will focus on the sleep apnea–hypopnea syndrome (SAHS), as there is an abundance of evidence-based data concerning its epidemiology, underlying mechanisms of disease and response to treatment.

THE SLEEP APNEA–HYPOPNEA SYNDROME

The SAHS, often referred to as obstructive sleep apnea (OSA) is not rare. One large epidemiological study of middle-aged adult Americans estimates that the condition affects 4% of men and 2% of women[1]. SAHS is most commonly associated with symptoms and consequences of increased daytime sleepiness and is a factor that places patients at increased risk for cardiovascular disease[2]. Although somewhat less publicized, SAHS is associated with neurocognitive dysfunction, alterations

in mood and reduced quality of life. This portion of the chapter reviews the relationships between SAHS, neurocognitive dysfunction and mood disorders with an emphasis on depression and quality of life. Evidence-based data are reviewed concerning the epidemiology, the underlying mechanisms of disease and responses to treatment.

Definitions

To understand SAHS better, several definitions will be reviewed initially. SAHS is defined as repeated episodes of obstructive apnea (complete upper airway obstruction) and hypopnea (partial upper airway obstruction) during sleep, together with symptoms of daytime sleepiness and/or altered cardiopulmonary function. It is currently standard in both clinical practice and epidemiological studies to assess the severity of sleep-disordered breathing by combining the number of apneic and hypopneic episodes per hour of sleep into an index called the apnea–hypopnea index (AHI), otherwise known as the respiratory disturbance index (RDI)[3]. Obstructive sleep apnea is defined by an RDI of more than five events per hour of sleep. Increasing severity of disease is typically defined by a higher RDI with or without oxygen desaturations.

Unfortunately, a standard definition of the RDI to quantify disease severity is lacking in much of the literature concerning the relationships between OSA and neuropsychological dysfunction and morbidity. An obstructive apnea is characterized by complete upper airway obstruction causing a cessation of airflow for 10 s or more. Although this definition is universally accepted, until recently the definition of a hypopnea episode was inconsistent. Whereas the duration of reduced airflow secondary to partial upper airway obstruction was well defined at 10 or more seconds, the degree of reduced airflow association with or without electroencephalographic (EEG) arousals and/or oxygen desaturations was inconsistent[4,5]. The most recent definition of hypopnea clearly associates the degree of airflow reduction with at least a 4% oxygen desaturation[3]. Using this definition of hypopnea, the RDI has clearly been associated with a wide range of cardiovascular disease[2]. For the sake of consistency throughout this chapter, the RDI 4% will refer to the newly recognized definition of the RDI requiring a 4% oxygen desaturation[3]. In other instances where a clear definition of hypopnea is not available, the RDI alone will be used. Also, to simplify matters, obstructive sleep apnea (OSA), the sleep apnea–hypopnea syndrome (SAHS) and sleep-disordered breathing (SDB) will be used interchangeably.

SAHS and neurocognitive/psychological functioning

Numerous studies have assessed the effects of sleep disordered breathing on neurocognitive/psychological functioning[6–17]. Altered memory, concentration and reaction times may occur, but the levels of cognitive dysfunction vary over a wide range of performance areas in patients with different degrees of OSA.

The mechanisms responsible for varying degrees of cognitive dysfunction are unclear. Most of the literature focuses on the impact of disease severity, as assessed by the RDI and hypoxemia, on levels of cognitive impairment[11,14,15,18]. For example, Greenberg and colleagues[11] performed neuropsychological testing on 14 OSA patients, a control group of ten patients with other disorders of excessive somnolence and a second control group of 14 healthy volunteers. The sleep disorder groups were matched on two measures of sleepiness. The OSA patients performed significantly worse than both groups of controls on seven of 14 neuropsychological measures and on a rating of global neuropsychological impairment. However, the overall level of performance reflected only moderate impairment. Within the sleep apnea group, hypoxemia severity was significantly correlated with deficits on measures of motor and perceptual–organizational ability. In a larger study by Kingshott and associates[19], few significant relationships were demonstrated between polysomnographic factors and subsequent cognitive performance in 150 patients with OSA and no other co-existing illnesses. These investigators found that intellectual ability weakly correlated with the RDI ($r = -0.14$) and oxygen desaturation ($r = 0.15$). These findings suggest a statistically significant, yet weak, association between the RDI and degree of hypoxemia with decrements in cognitive performance.

The degree of daytime sleepiness that results from SDB may be a better indicator of cognitive performance deficits than the RDI or degree of hypoxemia. This may be related to the fact that the RDI does not necessarily reflect the true degree of sleep fragmentation. Although obstructive apneas typically terminate with an arousal during sleep, hypopneas by definition do not necessarily cause arousals. Hence, it is possible that a patient with predominantly hypopnea-related OSA could have a high RDI with relatively little sleep disruption. In a randomized cross-over study by Martin and colleagues[20], normal subjects exposed to experimentally induced sleep fragmentation, similar to patients with moderate OSA (mean arousal index 34 ± 5 events/h of sleep), demonstrated significant deterioration in their cognitive scores for Trailmaking B and PASAT tests. Although total sleep time was not significantly different between nights, these cognitive deficits were thought to be secondary to an increased homeostatic drive for sleep as demonstrated by increased objective sleepiness on both the multiple sleep latency test (MSLT) and maintenance of wakefulness test (MWT). These results are in agreement with other studies demonstrating that neurocognitive performance deficits are common in individuals experiencing sleep fragmentation[10,11]. Studies of nocturnal sleep fragmentation demonstrate that daytime sleepiness increases and neurocognitive performance decreases even after one night of sleep fragmentation[21-23].

Few studies on the effect of treatment for OSA on neurocognitive function are robust. One small prospective study evaluating the effects of continuous positive airway pressure (CPAP) therapy on 20 patients with severe OSA (mean RDI 67 ± 16) found that most patients demonstrated a significant improvement in cognitive function at 3 months and 12 months after CPAP therapy was instituted[16]. Treatment with CPAP demonstrated significant improvements in concentration, and recent verbal, visual and spatial memory. Munoz and associates[24] prospectively studied 80 patients with severe OSA (mean RDI of 60 ± 21 events/h) and compared them to 80 control patients matched for age and gender. Baseline data demonstrated that the OSA patients were significantly more somnolent ($p < 0.001$), and had longer reaction times ($p < 0.05$) and poorer vigilance ($p < 0.01$) than control subjects. After 12 months of therapeutic nasal CPAP treatment, significant improvements occurred in levels of daytime somnolence ($p < 0.0002$) and vigilance ($p < 0.01$), whereas changes in reaction times were relatively minor.

Several randomized placebo-controlled trials have evaluated the effect of CPAP therapy on the reversibility of neurocognitive deficits in patients with OSA[6,8-10]. A total of 98 patients were evaluated in these trials, with 50 of the 98 patients having relatively mild OSA with an RDI 4% between 5 and 15 events/h of sleep (mean RDI 4% of 26 ± 28 events/h). All patients had an RDI 4% of five or more events, two or more symptoms related to OSA and absence of coexisting illnesses or sleep disorders. Patients were treated with 1 month of CPAP treatment and 1 month of oral placebo treatment. Compared to the placebo arm of the study, all cognitive performance scores demonstrated either trends or significant improvements with CPAP. Significant improvements ($p < 0.05$) with CPAP therapy versus placebo were seen in the Trailmaking B test, WAIS-R Digit Symbol Substitution test, the Performance IQ Decrement test and the PASAT 2s test. Trends toward significant improvement with CPAP therapy were seen with the WAIS-R Block Design subtest and the SteerClear test. Although there were several statistically significant improvements with CPAP therapy, the effective size of these changes was relatively small.

This last finding, concerning the relatively small effect, may be secondary to a significant proportion of the study patients having relatively mild sleep apnea. Another possible explanation could be that 1 month of CPAP therapy may be insufficient to reverse changes that have accumulated over long periods of time (months to years). Also, the mean nocturnal CPAP usage was only 3.3 h/night, which is well below the typical average of 4.5 h/night. Finally, it is possible that some of the cognitive deficits seen in OSA patients are irreversible, possibly related to repeated episodes of nocturnal hypoxemia[19].

Further research is required for better definition of the mechanisms responsible for the neurocognitve deficits observed in some patients with SAHS and to clarify the potential reversibility of the deficits. In addition, larger, more long-term studies will be required to address these questions with patients with varying degrees of OSA severity.

SAHS and mood

The relationship of SAHS with psychiatric disease is unclear and controversial. Several studies link obstructive sleep apnea with major depression and subclinical depressive symptoms[25-30]. Currently, however, no large-scale prospective data accurately estimate the prevalence of depression and other mood symptoms and disorders in these patients. Although the actual prevalence of depression and other mood disorders is unknown, they are estimated to occur in up to 20% of all patients with OSA[25,26,30]. For example, Minnesota Multiphasic Personality Inventory (MMPI) depression scale scores are elevated in 32–49% of patients with varying degrees of OSA[28,31]. The 5-year prevalence of major depressive disorder is estimated to be 58%[30], a figure three times higher than depression prevalence rates in the general population[32]. Eleven per cent of patients with OSA report prior treatment for depression[27]. Finally, although higher rates of depressive symptoms are present in patients with OSA, patients with major depression do not demonstrate an increased incidence of OSA[33].

Several small studies link depressive symptoms to OSA. Ramos-Platon and Espinar-Sierra[34] studied 23 patients with OSA, demonstrating that these patients exceeded scores on five MMPI scales compared to normal controls. Highest scores were seen on scales related to depression, schizophrenia and hypochondriasis. Beutler and colleagues[35] studied 20 OSA patients and compared them to patients with narcolepsy and normal controls. In general, patients with OSA and narcoleptics both demonstrated greater overall psychiatric disturbances compared to normal subjects. Compared to patients with narcolepsy, the OSA patients demonstrated significantly more denial, hypochondriasis and hysteria and less anxiety and social introversion. Borak and associates[16] found that untreated patients with severe OSA demonstrated increased levels of mental stress, depression and anxiety on psychological testing. Both anxiety ($r = 0.68$) and mental stress ($r = 0.56$) correlated with the baseline RDI. Mental stress also correlated with a deficiency of stage 2 non-rapid eye movement (non-REM) sleep ($r = -0.55$).

Aikens and colleagues evaluated 178 OSA patients retrospectively who had been drawn from a university-based sleep disorders center[28]. OSA was diagnosed if the RDI 4% was at least five or more events per hour of sleep. The study population was characterized by a mean age of 48.3 ± 11.1; 87% were male and most were obese (mean body mass index of 39). Each subject completed the MMPI prior to an overnight polysomnography. At least one MMPI elevation was present in 58% of subjects, with depression elevated for 32%, hypochondriasis for 30% and hysteria for 21%. Thirty-eight per cent demonstrated two or more elevations. Interestingly, depression scores were not correlated with any polysomnographic parameters. Aikens and co-workers concluded that OSA patients with core depressive symptoms without other significant psychological symptoms tended to have less severe OSA, and OSA patients with a diverse set of psychological symptoms overshadowing depressive symptoms tended to have more severe OSA as defined by higher RDI 4% and lower oxygen saturations (< 92%). In fact, MMPI elevations (except depression) were more reliably associated with levels of oxygen desaturation than sleep disruption as defined by the RDI 4%. The association of oxygen desaturation with elevated MMPI scores was also demonstrated by Aikens and Mendelson when evaluating changes in the MMPI between patients with primary snoring and OSA[31]. Caution should be used when interpreting these results, because of their retrospective nature and the lack of a control group.

Pillar and Lavie presented data to the contrary[36]. They studied 2271 predominantly male patients (males = 1977) referred to an Israeli sleep laboratory with suspected OSA. All patients completed the SCL-90 Symptom Self-Report Inventory prior to overnight polysomnography. Among men with OSA, no significant complaints of anxiety, depression or any SCL-90 dimension were present regardless of the RDI, body mass index, or age. Depression and anxiety scores were significantly higher in women than in men for all age groups and all levels of RDI. Depression scores were higher in women with more severe OSA compared to women with mild OSA. Pillar and Lavie concluded that neither the existence nor the severity of OSA was associated with depression or anxiety in their largely male sample. Women with more severe OSA tended to have higher levels of perceived depression than women with milder OSA. These data suggest that gender may influence mood independently of, or in conjunction with, OSA.

Bardwell and colleagues[37] propose that psychological symptoms in patients with OSA are related to non-sleep-related variables rather than to OSA itself. They studied 72 patients with mild OSA (mean RDI of 15 events/h of sleep) and compared them to 40 controls without OSA. On initial evaluation, mood symptoms such as depression, anger and total mood disturbance positively correlated with amount of stages 3–4 sleep, REM sleep and/or degree of hypoxemia. When they controlled for age, body mass index and hypertension, however, depression and total mood disturbance no longer correlated with sleep variables, suggesting that many mood symptoms in patients with OSA are related to other non-sleep-related variables.

Several possible explanations exist for the controversial results set forth by the studies of Pillar and Lavie[36] and of Bardwell and co-workers[37]. These studies clearly emphasize the importance of adequate sample size and gender distribution as well as the need to control for underlying co-morbid conditions. Most of the previously mentioned studies were of relatively small sample size (largest 178 patients)[29] and based on predominantly male subjects, making sampling bias a real possibility. Also, the methods used to determine the underlying psychiatric symptoms are of critical importance. In clinical practice, several of the questionnaires used in the studies cited above are only used to help clinicians make a psychiatric diagnosis. Many were developed as screening instruments for patients with known psychiatric disorders and not necessarily validated for the normal population. The previously mentioned studies used several different, although reliable and validated, questionnaires to arrive at their conclusions. Future prospective studies using larger sample sizes, with more equitable gender distribution, using a variety of well-validated questionnaires in addition to psychiatric interviews, may better be able to answer the questions regarding the relationships of psychiatric morbidity to OSA.

Only one relatively large-scale study exists evaluating psychopathology in patients with primary snoring. Aikens and Mendelson[31] compared 49 patients with primary snoring to 49 age- and gender-matched patients with varying degrees of OSA (mean RDI 8% of 55.2 ± 37.2). All subjects completed the MMPI and underwent an overnight polysomnography and MSLT. Compared to patients with primary snoring, OSA patients had more intense depressive symptoms and somatic concerns. As shown in other studies, patients with OSA had higher scores on both depression and hypochondriasis scales. Interestingly, patients with primary snoring demonstrated psychological maladjustment that was qualitatively similar, although quantitatively less severe, than patients with OSA.

The mechanisms responsible for these changes in patients with primary snoring are unclear. Studies evaluating neurocognitive deficits in patients with primary snoring demonstrated deficits in focused attention[38,39], fine motor controls[39] and possibly an increased incidence of nightmares[40,41]. It is possible that some patients with more severe degrees of snoring may suffer cognitive and mood deficits from sleep fragmentation due to microarousals not recognized by the current scoring system[42]. Further research in larger patient populations will be required to define the cognitive and mood deficits seen in some patients with primary snoring.

Assuming that OSA adversely affects mood parameters, data concerning treatment are also variable. Borak and colleagues showed that, although significant early improvements were seen in cognitive function, no significant improvements were seen in any emotional status parameters after 3 months and 12 months of CPAP therapy in 20 patients with severe OSA[16]. Ramos-Platon and Espinar-Sierra[34] prospectively followed 23 patients with severe OSA before, during and after 1 year of CPAP therapy. They found a progressive reduction of psychopathological signs along with a generalized improvement in psychosocial adaptation. The most significant changes were seen for depression ($p < 0.01$) and total adjustment degree ($p < 0.01$) after 1 year of treatment, suggesting that improvements in psychosocial function may gradually take place with proper therapy.

As noted previously, Munoz and co-workers[24] prospectively studied 80 patients with severe OSA (mean RDI of 60 ± 21 events/h sleep) and 80 control patients matched for age and gender. OSA patients were significantly more somnolent ($p < 0.001$), anxious ($p < 0.01$) and depressed ($p < 0.001$) than control subjects at baseline. After 12 months of therapeutic nasal CPAP treatment, significant improvements were seen in levels of daytime somnolence ($p < 0.0002$) and vigilance ($p < 0.01$), but no significant changes were demonstrated in levels of anxiety or depression.

Yu and colleagues[43] studied mood changes in 24 patients with OSA using the Profile of Mood States (POMS) questionnaire. Patients were randomized to treatment with therapeutic CPAP or placebo CPAP for 1 week. After treatment, both groups showed significant improvement in mood states. The authors concluded that the effect of CPAP therapy on mood symptoms could represent a placebo effect. They also concluded that CPAP treatment may be an effective treatment for improving mood states, but only in those patients with severe depressive symptoms secondary to sleep apnea.

Few data are available on the effects of surgical therapy for OSA on mood parameters. Nambu and associates[44] studied psycho-intellectual function in 20 patients with mild to moderate OSA (mean RDI of 19.0 ± 15.6) before and 4 weeks after mandibular advancement surgery. The RDI was significantly decreased to 2.4 ± 1.9 events/h of sleep 4 weeks after surgery. Compared to pre-procedure values, the authors noted significant improvements in state anxiety, trait anxiety and depression scale scores during the postoperative evaluation. They also noted that the patients became less neurotic and less eccentric after treatment as assessed by the Cornell Medical Index and Yatabe–Guilford tests.

The relationship between psychiatric disease and OSA is also variable. In addition to depressive symptoms being common in some patients with OSA, a diversity of other psychological and behavioral problems may also be present. Depressive symptoms may occur in patients with all degrees of severity of OSA, even in those with normal oxygen saturations and less severe OSA. The mechanisms underlying changes in mood and personality in patients with OSA are unclear, but are likely to be related to a combination of factors including chronic partial sleep deprivation induced by sleep fragmentation, chronic nocturnal hypoxemia and other factors yet to be defined. Further research is required to identify the mechanisms and risk factors underlying psychiatric disease that are related to OSA.

SAHS and quality of life

Although currently no gold standard exists for measuring health-related quality of life (HRQL), several tools have been developed to assess this in patients with OSA[45]. Disease-specific tools include the Calgary Sleep Apnea Quality of Life Index (SAQLI)[46] and the Functional Outcomes of Sleep Questionnaire (FOSQ)[47]. The Calgary SAQLI was designed as a disease-specific quality of life measure that would be sensitive in detecting change in the quality of life of people with sleep apnea who have undergone some type of treatment intervention[45,46]. The SAQLI can also be used to measure a patient's baseline quality of life.

This tool has shown a very good test–retest reliability and high face validity[45,46]. The FOSQ, although initially developed to assess the impact of disorders of excessive sleepiness on multiple activities of everyday living, was in part validated using two groups of patients with OSA $(n = 75)$[47]. The FOSQ has been shown to be a valid and reliable measure of quality of life in patients with sleep apnea. Patients with sleep apnea have lower FOSQ scores (poorer quality of life) than patients without sleep disorders[47].

The largest study to date assessing quality of life in patients with OSA involves patients from the Sleep Heart Health Study (SHHS)[39]. The SHHS is a multicenter study involving 6440 men and women over the age of 40[48]. The study's primary goal is to determine the role of sleep-disordered breathing in the development of cardiovascular disease. The investigators recently published results assessing the extent to which sleep-disordered breathing, difficulty initiating and maintaining sleep and excessive daytime sleepiness were associated with impairment of quality of life[39]. HRQL was assessed via the Medical Outcomes Survey SF-36, the most widely used generic health status questionnaire[49]. This tool is sensitive to change in patients with OSA treated with nasal CPAP[50]. The SF-36 has the ability to discriminate between patients with and without chronic diseases and has excellent reliability and validity[51–53]. This instrument is a self-administered survey that measures eight dimensions of health including: physical activity (PF); social activities (SF); physical health problems (RP); bodily pain (BP); general mental health (MH); emotional problems (RE); vitality (VT); and general health perceptions (GH). Scores for each category range from 1 to 100, with higher scores representing better quality of life.

The SHHS data[39] related to quality of life measurements evaluated 5816 participants (52.5% female; mean age of 63.2 ± 11 years). Vitality was the only SF-36 scale to demonstrate a linear association with the clinical categories of SDB (mild SDB (RDI 4% of 4–< 15 events/h), moderate SDB (RDI 4% of 15–< 30 events/h) and severe SDB (RDI 4% of ≥ 30 events/h)). Participants with mild, moderate and severe SDB were 1.20, 1.41 and 1.77 times more likely to have reported poor quality of life for the vitality scale, respectively. Severe SDB was significantly and negatively associated with general health perceptions (odds ratio (OR) 1.56; 95% confidence interval (95% CI) 1.17–2.07), physical functioning (OR 1.54; 95% CI 1.15–2.06), social functioning (OR 1.47; 95% CI 1.11–1.94) and vitality scales (OR 1.53; 95% CI 1.15–2.02). Severe SDB showed no significant association with bodily pain, mental health, or physical health problems scales. Mild and moderate SDB demonstrated no significant associations with any of the SF-36 scales. No significant gender differences were seen for any these associations.

Results were also compared to normative data obtained from 2474 controls from the general US population. Compared to controls, patients with severe SDB reported significantly poorer quality of life on the physical function, physical health problems, bodily pain, general health perceptions and vitality scales. Finally, when the results were compared to normative data from selected disease groups (hypertension, diabetes and clinical depression)[54], patients with severe SDB demonstrated similar numerical profiles to those of patients with hypertension and type II diabetes. Patients with severe SDB also demonstrated poorer scores on bodily pain and physical health problems scales compared to patients with hypertension. Physical function scores were comparable between patients with severe SDB and patients with depression. Mean scores for patients with clinical depression were generally poorer than those of patients with severe SDB, hypertension and diabetes.

The results from the SHHS[39] differ somewhat from an earlier smaller study involving subjects from the Wisconsin Sleep Cohort (WSC)[55]. The WSC study evaluated 737 individuals (mean age 48.4 ± 7.7 years; 43%

female) with OSA. The WSC results suggest that significant linear relationships exist between OSA and mental health, vitality, physical functioning, social functioning, physical health problems and general health SF-36 scales. The SHHS study data demonstrated a significant association only between degrees of OSA and the vitality scale. The reasons for the discrepancies between study results are not totally clear. First, the study groups were not identical, with the WSC group being younger, having fewer females and being significantly smaller. Also, differences in methods of analysis may play a role[39]. Despite disagreement in results, both studies agree that the vitality scale of the SF-36 is negatively associated with OSA.

A third smaller study by Stepnowsky and colleagues[56] studied a sample of 70 African Americans over the age of 65 years. Those subjects with moderate to severe OSA had significantly lower physical component summary scores. After controlling for medical conditions, OSA was significantly related to both general physical functioning and general mental health functioning in individuals with relatively mild OSA (RDI between 5 and 15). Quality of well-being scale scores in the group studied were similar to scores found in patients with depression and chronic obstructive pulmonary disease (COPD). These data, although based on a small sample size, also indicate that varying degrees of OSA may adversely affect daily living and health to similar degrees to those of other chronic medical conditions.

Insufficient data exist to state accurately whether the changes related to quality of life in patients with OSA are partially or totally reversible with adequate therapy. Data obtained from several randomized placebo-controlled trials by Engleman's group[6,8–10] which primarily evaluated the affect of CPAP therapy on neurocognitive function, demonstrated significant improvements in many aspects of quality of life as assessed by the SF-36 questionnaire and the Nottingham Health Profile Part 2 evaluation. These data should be interpreted cautiously, however, as the total sample size was small ($n = 98$ patients) and many of the patients had relatively mild OSA. In a randomized parallel controlled trial of 101 male patients with OSA, Stradling and Davies[57,58] demonstrated that the vitality and energy scale the SF-36 significantly ($p < 0.0001$) improved after 1 month of nasal CPAP treatment at therapeutic levels when compared to controls using CPAP at sub-therapeutic levels. A follow-up study by Jenkinson and colleagues[59], on this same group of patients, demonstrated that these improvements in quality of life measures were sustained after 5 months of therapy. Also, those patients who had initially been randomized to the sub therapeutic arm of the study demonstrated scores similar to those of the active group after being placed on therapeutic CPAP therapy during the following 4-month period.

Conclusions

The sleep apnea–hypopnea syndrome has variable effects on neurocognitive dysfunction, mood and quality of life. The discrepancies between study results are probably related to multiple factors including relatively small sample sizes, short-term follow-up and lack of uniformity between outcome measures. Aside from quality of life measures, which appear to be reduced in patients with severe obstructive sleep apnea, severity of disease has an unclear relationship to neurocognitive dysfunction and mood alterations. It also appears that there are other, as yet unmeasured or undefined, factors that make certain individuals more susceptible than others to these adverse outcomes. Finally, in those patients who are susceptible, it is uncertain whether treatment is totally able to reverse these adverse consequences. Clearly, larger, more long-term studies will need to be performed to help us understand the mechanisms underlying the neurocognitive dysfunction, mood alterations and reduced quality of life in certain subpopulations of patients with sleep disordered breathing.

PSYCHOLOGICAL AND NEUROCOGNITIVE OUTCOMES RELATED TO NOCTURNAL AND SLEEP-RELATED CONSEQUENCES OF OTHER CHRONIC RESPIRATORY DISORDERS

Asthma

Asthma is a chronic respiratory disease characterized by reversible bronchial airways obstruction. It is as common as the sleep apnea–hypopnea syndrome, with a prevalence of 4% of the adult population. Airways obstruction is caused by bronchial smooth muscle constriction and inflammation of the bronchial mucosa and submucosa. Most normal individuals demonstrate circadian changes in their pulmonary function, with peak function occurring in the late afternoon and a nadir in function occurring in the early morning hours. Changes in pulmonary function are more specifically associated with changes in the core body temperature curve, with the nadir in function linked to the nadir in core body temperature curve. The amplitude between peak and nadir flow and spirometric values in normal individuals is between 5 and 8%. Many asthmatics demonstrate greater variations between peak and nadir pulmonary function, with the amplitude of peak flow changes as great as 50%[60]. Increased nocturnal bronchoconstriction during sleep is primarily related to impaired mucociliary clearance and increased parasympathetic nervous system tone. The nocturnal role of changes in inflammatory mediators such as histamine is less clear.

In many asthmatic patients, nocturnal bronchoconstriction may cause sleep disturbances characterized by fragmented sleep and, in some, daytime sleepiness and impaired daytime cognition. Other social implications include more missed days of school and poorer school performance in children with symptomatic nocturnal asthma and more missed days of work for their parents[61].

In spite of frequent reports that symptomatic nocturnal asthma results in fatigue and impaired neuropsychological function, there exist few objective data to support these claims[62]. Compared to non-asthmatic controls, some children with symptomatic nocturnal asthma have demonstrated more psychological problems along with impaired memory and concentration[63]. Improvement in nocturnal asthma symptoms through medication changes was associated with improved psychological and neurocognitive deficits. Other studies in adults with nocturnal asthma symptoms have shown less consistent improvements in neuropsychological outcomes after changing the patient's treatment regimen[62].

Chronic obstructive pulmonary disease

Chronic obstructive pulmonary disease (COPD) refers to a spectrum of lung diseases characterized by fixed or only partially reversible airways obstruction. They encompass the smoking-related chronic obstructive diseases of emphysema and chronic bronchitis as well as the non-smoking-related disease processes related to long-standing under-treated asthma and bronchiectasis.

Patients with COPD may demonstrate accentuation of the normal reduction in oxygen saturation during sleep, with the most severe reductions in oxygen saturation occurring during REM sleep[64,65]. Reductions in oxygen saturation are related to many factors that occur during sleep including hypoventilation, decrease in functional residual capacity and ventilation–perfusion mismatching.

Many patients with COPD demonstrate poorer subjective and objective sleep quality[66]. More than 50% of patients complain of various sleep-related problems including sleep-onset insomnia, sleep-maintenance insomnia and/or frequent awakenings. Sleep disruption is related to many factors including nocturnal hypoxemia, loss of accessory muscle use during REM sleep, increase in airways obstruction and reduced clearance of secretions leading to nocturnal coughing. Sleep disruption appears to be similar in patients with or without nocturnal hypoxemia[67]. Objective studies of daytime sleepiness do not demonstrate evidence of daytime sleepiness as measured by the multiple sleep latency test (MSLT)[68].

Patients with COPD are at higher risk for depression, anxiety and poorer quality of life[69,70]. The risks of psychological dysfunction increase as the severity of the underlying lung disease progresses. No studies have objectively or subjectively evaluated the relationships between sleep-related respiratory dysfunction in patients with COPD and neurocognitive or psychological outcomes.

Conclusions

Unlike the quantity of literature related to psychological and neurocognitive dysfunction and the sleep apnea–hypopnea syndrome, there is a paucity of literature specifically related to sleep-related symptoms and other chronic respiratory diseases. Clearly, future research will need to focus on whether or not nocturnal/sleep-related problems associated with chronic respiratory disorders are associated with neurocognitive dysfunction, mood alterations or reduced quality of life.

References

1. Young T, Palta M, Dempsey J, et al. The occurrence of sleep-disordered breathing among middle-aged adults. N Engl J Med 1993; 328:1230–5
2. Nieto F, Young T, Lind B, et al. Association of sleep-disordered breathing, sleep apnea and hypertension in a large community based study. J Am Med Assoc 2000;283:1829–36
3. Committee Clinical Practice Review. Hypopnea in sleep-disordered breathing in adults. Sleep 2001;24:469–70
4. Redline S, Sanders M. Hypopnea, a floating metric: implications for prevalence, morbidity estimates and case finding. Sleep 1997;20:1209–17
5. Moser N, Phillips B, Berry D, et al. What is hypopnea anyway? Chest 1994;105:426–8
6. Engleman H, Martin S, Kingshott R, et al. Randomized, placebo-controlled trial of daytime function after continuous positive airway pressure therapy for the sleep apnoea/hypopnoea syndrome. Thorax 1998;53:341–5
7. Engleman H, Kingshott R, Martin S, et al. Cognitive function in the sleep apnea/hypopnea syndrome (SAHS). Sleep 2000;23:S102–8
8. Engleman H, Kingshott R, Wraith P, et al. Randomized placebo-controlled crossover trial of CPAP for mild sleep apnea/hypopnea syndrome. Am J Respir Crit Care Med 1999; 159:461–7
9. Engleman H, Martin S, Deary I, et al. The effect of continuous positive airway pressure therapy on daytime function in the sleep apnoea/hyponoea syndrome. Lancet 1994;343:572–5
10. Engleman H, Martin S, Deary I, et al. Effect of CPAP therapy on daytime function in patients with mild sleep apnoea/hypopnoea syndrome. Thorax 1997;52:114–19
11. Greenberg G, Watson R, Deptula D. Neuropsychological dysfunction in sleep apnea. Sleep 1987;10:254–62
12. Redline S, Strauss M, Adams N, et al. Neuropsychological function in mild sleep-disordered breathing. Sleep 1997;20:160–7
13. Kim H, Young T, Matthews C, et al. Sleep-disordered breathing and neuropsychological deficits: a population based study. Am J Respir Crit Care Med 1997;156:1813–19
14. Bedard M, Montplaisir J, Richer F, Rouleau I, Malo J. Obstructive sleep apnea syndrome: pathogenesis of neuropsychological deficits. J Clin Exp Neuropsychol 1991;13:950–64
15. Naegele B, Thouvard V, Pepin J, et al. Deficits of cognitive executive functions in patients with sleep apnea syndrome. Sleep 1995;18:43–52
16. Borak J, Cieslicki J, Koziej M, et al. Effects of CPAP treatment on psychological status in patients with severe obstructive sleep apnea. J Sleep Res 1996;5:123–7
17. Kribbs N, Pack A, Kline L, et al. Effects of one night without nasal CPAP treatment on sleep and sleepiness in patients with obstructive sleep apnea. Am J Respir Crit Care Med 1993;147:1162–8
18. Cheshire K, Engleman H, Deary I, et al. Factors impairing daytime performance in patients with sleep/apnea hypopnea syndrome. Arch Intern Med 1992;152:538–41

19. Kingshott R, Engleman H, Deary I, *et al*. Does arousal frequency predict daytime function. *Eur Respir J* 1998;12:1264–70

20. Martin S, Engleman H, Deary I, *et al*. The effect of sleep fragmentation on daytime function. *Am J Respir Crit Care Med* 1996;153:1328–32

21. Bonnet M. The effect of sleep fragmentation on sleep and performance in younger and older subjects. *Neurobiol Aging* 1989;10:21–5

22. Stepanski E, Lamphere J, Badia P. Sleep fragmentation and daytime sleepiness. *Sleep* 1984;7:18–26

23. Bonnet M. Effect of sleep disruption on sleep, performance and mood. *Sleep* 1985;8:11–19

24. Munoz A, Mayoralas L, Barbe F, *et al*. Long-term effects of CPAP on daytime functioning in patients with sleep apnoea syndrome. *Eur Respir J* 2000;15:676–81

25. Reynolds C, Kupfer D, McEachran A, *et al*. Depressive psychopathology in male sleep apneics. *J Clin Psychiatr* 1984;45:287–90

26. Millman R, Fogel B, Mcnamara M, *et al*. Depression as a manifestation of obstructive sleep apnea: reversal with nasal continuous positive airway pressure. *J Clin Psychiatry* 1989;50:348–51

27. Mendelson W. Depression in sleep apnea patients. *Sleep Res* 1992;21:230

28. Aikens J, Caruana-Montaldo B, Vanable P, *et al*. MMPI correlates of sleep and respiratory disturbance in obstructive sleep apnea. *Sleep* 1999;22:362–9

29. Aikens J, Caruana-Montaldo B, Vanable P, *et al*. Depression and general psychopathology in obstructive sleep apnea. *Sleep* 1998; 21(Suppl):71

30. Mosko S, Zetin M, Glen S, *et al*. Self-reported depressive symptomatology, mood ratings and treatment outcome in sleep disorders. *J Clin Psychol* 1989;45:51–60

31. Aikens J, Mendelson W. A matched comparison of MMPI responses in patients with primary snoring or obstructive sleep apnea. *Sleep* 1999;22:355–61

32. American Psychiatric Association. *Diagnostic and Statistical Manual of Mental Disorders*, 4th edn. Washington, DC: American Psychiatric Association, 1994

33. Reynolds C. Sleep and affective disorders: a minireview. *Psychiatr Clin North Am* 1987; 10:583–91

34. Ramos-Platon M, Espinar-Sierra J. Changes in psychopathological symptoms in sleep apnea patients after treatment with nasal continuous airway pressure. *Int J Neurosci* 1992; 62(3–4):173–95

35. Beutler L, Ware J, Karacan I, *et al*. Differentiating psychopathological characteristics of patients with sleep apnea and narcolepsy. *Sleep* 1981; 4:39–47

36. Pillar G, Lavie P. Psychiatric symptoms in sleep apnea syndrome: effects of gender and respiratory disturbance index. *Chest* 1998;114:697–703

37. Bardwell W, Berry C, Ancoli-Israel S, *et al*. Psychological correlates of sleep apnea. *J Psychosom Res* 1999;47:583–96

38. Verstraeten E, Cluysdts R, Verbraecken J, *et al*. Psychomotor and cognitive performance in nonapneic snorers: Preliminary findings. *Percep Motor Skills* 1997;84:1211–22

39. Baldwin C, Griffith K, Nieto F, *et al*. The association of sleep-disordered breathing and sleep symptoms with quality of life in the sleep heart health study. *Sleep* 2001;24:96–105

40. Thorman F. Snoring, nightmares, and morning headaches in elderly women: a preliminary study. *Biol Psychiatry* 1997;46:275–84

41. deGroen J, Op den Velde W, Hovens J, *et al*. Snoring and anxiety dreams. *Sleep* 1993; 16:35–6

42. Rechtschaffen A, Kales A. *A Manual of Standardized Terminology: Techniques and Scoring System for Sleep Stages of Human Subjects*. Los Angeles: Brain Info. Serv./Brain Res. Int., UCLA (NIH Publ. 2040, 1968)

43. Yu B, Ancoli-Israel S, Dimsdale J. Effect of CPAP treatment on mood states in patients with sleep apnea. *J Psychiatr Res* 1999;33: 427–32

44. Nambu Y, Nagasaka Y, Fujita E, *et al*. Effect of mandibular advancement splint on psycho-intellectual derangements in patients with sleep apnea syndrome. *Tohoku J Exp Med* 1999;188:119–32

45. Flemons W. Measuring health related quality of life in sleep apnea. *Sleep* 2000;23:s109–14

46. Flemons W, Reimer M. Development of a disease specific quality of life questionnaire for sleep apnea. *Am J Resp Crit Care Med* 1998; 158:494–503

47. Weaver T, Laizner A, Evans L, *et al*. An instrument to measure functional status outcomes for disorders of excessive sleepiness. *Sleep* 1997;20:835–43

48. Quan S, Howard B, Iber C, *et al*. The sleep heart health study: design, rationale, and methods. *Sleep* 1997;20:1077–85

49. McDowell I, Newell C. *Measuring Health: A Guide to Rating Scales and Questionnaires*. New York: Oxford University Press, 1996

50. Jenkinson C, Stradling J, Petersen S. Comparison of three measures of quality of life outcome in obstructive sleep apnoea. *J Sleep Res* 1997;6:199–204

51. Stewart A, Hays R, Ware J. The MOS short-form general health survey: reliability and

validity in a patient population. *Med Care* 1988;26:724–35

52. Stewart A, Greenfield S, Hays R, *et al*. Functional status and well-being of patients with chronic conditions: results from the medical outcomes study. *J Am Med Assoc* 1989;262:907–13

53. Ware J, Sherbourne C. The MOS 36-item short-form health survey (SF-36): Conceptual framework and item selection. *Med Care* 1992; 30:473–83

54. Ware J. *SF-36 Health Survey: Manual and Interpretation Guide*. Boston, MA: The Health Institute, New England Medical Center, 1993

55. Finn L, Young T, Palta M, *et al*. Sleep-disordered breathing and self-reported general health status in the Wisconsin Sleep Cohort. *Sleep* 1998;21:701–6

56. Stepnowsky C, Johnson S, Dimsdale J, *et al*. Sleep apnea and health-related quality of life in African American elderly. *Ann Behav Med* 2000;22:116–20

57. Jenkinson C, Davies R, Mullins R, *et al*. Comparison of therapeutic and subtherapeutic nasal continuous airway pressure for obstructive sleep apnea: a randomized prospective parallel trial. *Lancet* 1999;353: 2100–5

58. Stradling J, Davies R. Is more NCPAP better? *Sleep* 2000;23:S150–3

59. Jenkinson C, Davies R, Mullins R, *et al*. Long-term benefit in self-reported health status of nasal continuous airway pressure therapy for obstructive sleep apnoea. *Q J Med* 2001;94: 95–9

60. Hetzel M, Clark T. Comparison of normal and asthmatic circadian rhythms in peak expiratory flow rate. *Thorax* 1980;35:732–8

61. Diette G, Markson L, Skinner E, *et al*. Nocturnal asthma in children affects school attendance, school performance and parents' work attendance. *Arch Pediatr Adolesc Med* 2000;154:923–8

62. Bender B, Annett R. Neuropsychological outcomes of nocturnal asthma. *Chronobiol Int* 1999;16:695–710

63. Stores G, Ellis A, Wiggs L, *et al*. Sleep and psychological disturbance in nocturnal asthma. *Arch Dis Child* 1998;78:413–19

64. Coccagna G, Lugaresi E. Arterial blood gases and pulmonary and systemic arterial pressure during sleep in patients with chronic obstructive pulmonary disease. *Sleep* 1978;1:117–24

65. George C, West P, Kryger M. Oxygenation and breathing pattern during phasic and tonic REM in patients with chronic obstructive pulmonary disease. *Sleep* 1987;10:234–43

66. Cormick W, Olson L, Hensley M, *et al*. Nocturnal hypoxemia and quality of sleep in patients with chronic obstructive lung disease. *Thorax* 1986;41:846–54

67. Brezinova V, Catterall J, Douglas N, *et al*. Night sleep of patients with chronic ventilatory failure and age-matched controls: number and duration of ECG episodes of intervening wakefulness and drowsiness. *Sleep* 1982;5:123–30

68. Orr W, Shamma-Othman Z, Levin D, *et al*. Persistent hypoxemia and excessive daytime sleepiness in chronic obstructive pulmonary disease. *Chest* 1990;97:583–5

69. van Manen J, Bindels P, Dekker F, *et al*. Risk of depression in patients with chronic obstructive pulmonary disease and its determinants. *Thorax* 2002;57:412–16

70. McSweeny A, Grant I, Heaton R, *et al*. Life quality of patients with chronic obstructive pulmonary disease. *Arch Intern Med* 1982;142: 473–8

7

Shift work and circadian rhythm disorders

Jamie K. Lilie

INTRODUCTION

Circadian rhythms, those that recur in every 24-h period, are present in most organisms. In humans, these natural patterns are disturbed by extreme pressures from continuous work and leisure-related activities. The modern, post-industrial society has evolved into a 24-h day with constant opportunities for work, play and global communication. Indeed, when the stock market opens in Tokyo, traders must be sufficiently awake to respond in London, Paris and New York.

Despite the seductive attraction of the 24-h day, humans have not lost the need for a basic rest–activity cycle. Economic and societal demands for increased productivity in a global economy have resulted in the scheduling of round-the-clock shifts in many occupations, including jobs which require high levels of skill and attentiveness (e.g. medical personnel in hospitals, airline pilots and flight crews, police and firefighters, and industrial and military personnel). The deleterious effects of prolonged shift work on health, alertness and decision-making capacity, as well as on the quality of family life, are well documented[1].

NORMAL HUMAN SLEEP AND CHRONOBIOLOGY

Circadian rhythms are inherent to most living systems, from unicellular organisms to man.

The advent of a modern technological society with a 24-h workplace puts increasing demands on biological systems which maintain healthy sleep and alertness. Normal adult sleep follows a typical pattern (called sleep architecture) across the night (or sleep period). In healthy adults, with a consistent sleep pattern, early sleep is characterized by a brief transition through light non-rapid eye movement (NREM) sleep (stages 1, 2) into deeper NREM sleep (delta, stages 3, 4)[2]. The very important dreaming state (rapid eye movement or REM) occurs at approximately 90–100-min intervals throughout the night with progressively longer and more intense dreaming occurring toward morning. Whereas the percentage of REM sleep remains relatively constant across the life span, the percentage of delta sleep declines with age. Both older and more recent research has documented the vital importance of intact REM sleep in maintaining a healthy waking mood and in facilitating learning and memory[3,4].

Sleep and wakefulness are largely regulated by two endogenous processes: (1) an endogenous biological clock, which drives the circadian rhythm, the propensity for sleep and the characteristics of sleep across a 24-h period; and (2) a homeostatic process that increases sleep propensity with longer prior period of wakefulness. Indeed, the duration of

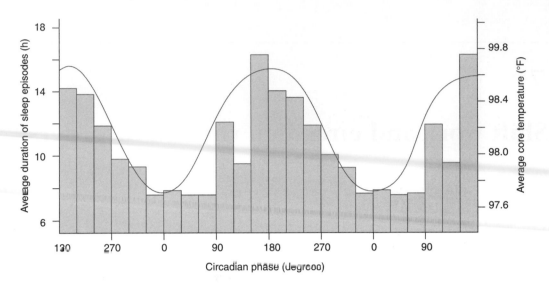

Figure 7.1 The close association between sleep length and the point on the temperature rhythm at which sleep begins, taken from the 'time-free' isolation experiment of Czeisler and co-workers[6]. The circadian cycle is shown in degrees (360° per day), and the columns show sleep lengths. Sleep onset at the time of the temperature trough led to a short sleep of about 8 h, while sleep beginning at the temperature peak led to a long sleep of around 14 h. Reproduced with permission of the American Association for the Advancement of Science

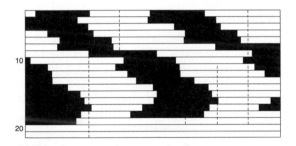

Figure 7.2 Although beyond the scope of this chapter, it is noteworthy that in the free-running condition, CBT and sleep undergo internal phase drift. Adapted from Moore-Ede *et al.*, *The Clocks that Time Us*, by permission of Harvard University Press, 1982[10]

wakefulness prior to sleep onset is directly related to the amount of delta activity during NREM recovery sleep[5]. At the same time, sleep onset at the time of a core body temperature (CBT) trough predicts a short sleep bout while sleep onset at the CBT peak leads to a longer sleep episode[6] (Figure 7.1).

Numerous studies indicate that sleep deprivation in humans, chronic or partial, results in increased daytime sleepiness, decreased subjective alertness and decreased psychomotor performance on a variety of tasks[7,8]. In animals, however, prolonged total sleep deprivation results in death, a fact which clearly emphasizes the fundamental and basic functional nature of sleep as a survival mechanism[9].

Circadian rhythms are biological processes which encompass a period of about 24 h. These rhythms affect sleep, CBT, cognitive performance, blood pressure and endocrine secretions, among other things. The circadian rhythm of sleep is coupled to the rhythm of CBT, is sensitive to ambient light and covers a free-running period of about 25 h in healthy young adults[10] (Figure 7.2).

By measuring the daily rhythm of CBT, sleep and REM, sleep propensity can be predicted. Sleep onset is associated with falling CBT, REM propensity with the nadir of CBT and awakening with a rise in CBT[11] (Figure 7.3).

Humans appear to have two peaks of daytime sleepiness. The first is at night, the second is in mid-afternoon. The 24-h sleep–wake rhythm is driven by the suprachiasmatic nucleus (SCN) synchronized to an environmental light–dark cycle. These rhythms are

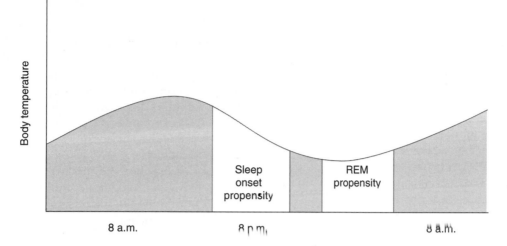

Figure 7.3   Phase of CBT predicts sleep and REM onset and awakening. From Orr WC[11], reproduced with permission

entrained or modified by 'zeitgebers' (time givers) or external cues. Although the major circadian pacemaker in animals is the SCN, a second circadian center may be located in the retina. Cultured retinal cells exhibit a circadian 24-h rhythm of melatonin synthesis. Melatonin is synthesized during the dark phase of the photoperiod in the retina and the pineal gland. It is an immediate precursor to serotonin and has been used as a mild hypnotic by older adults and shift workers. The rhythm of melatonin production by retinal cells and the period of the circadian rhythm based on retinal cultures appear to be genetic. This accounts for a free-running circadian rhythm, which in humans may vary from about 24 to 26 h. It is hypothesized that people with longer pacemakers (toward the 26-h range) tend to be phase-delayed and have difficulty entraining to a normal 24-h day. Those with a shorter period, as seen in some elderly people, tend to have difficulty maintaining sleep, wake up too early and often go to bed earlier than normal.

The universal mammalian zeitgeber is sunlight. Delicate adjustments of circadian rhythms occur in response to changes in available daylight. These processes permit seasonal adjustments to the photoperiod and suggest treatments for circadian rhythm disorders by the application of artificial bright lights[12].

CIRCADIAN RHYTHM DISORDERS

The DSM-IV[13] establishes the following general diagnostic criteria and lists the following four criteria for diagnosing circadian rhythm disorders:

(1) A persistent or recurrent pattern of sleep disruption occurs which leads to insomnia and/or excessive daytime sleepiness secondary to a mismatch between the environment and the individual's circadian sleep–wake pattern.

(2) The sleep–wake disturbance causes clinically significant distress or impairment in social, occupational or other important areas of functioning.

(3) The disturbance does not occur exclusively during the course of another sleep disorder or mental disorder.

(4) The disturbance is not due to the direct physiological effects of a drug of abuse, medication or other general medical condition.

The four following types of disorder are specified and are the most commonly seen in a clinical setting.

Advanced sleep phase syndrome

Individuals are usually drowsy in the evening and awaken too early in the morning. This type sometimes is seen among the elderly, who may experience sufficient lifestyle impairment to warrant treatment. However, people with a strong 'morning' tendency may be called 'larks' and not all present with a phase advanced sleep–wake rhythm which interferes with daily life.

Delayed sleep phase syndrome

These individuals are more alert in the evening and night, tend to stay up much later than usual, and have difficulty awakening in the morning. This is often seen in adolescents and young adults, sometimes referred to as 'owls'. If the desynchrony between internal sleep–wake rhythms and external demands of daily living is severe enough, a diagnosis of phase delayed syndrome is made.

Jet lag

This is sleepiness and alertness experienced at an inappropriate time of day relative to local time, occurring after travel across more than one time zone. Because of the slightly longer than 24-h period for most people, westbound travel, requiring a progressive phase delay, is somewhat easier than eastbound, which requires a phase advance of internal rhythms relative to the new environment.

Shift work

Insomnia may occur during the major sleep period and excessive sleepiness during the major awake period. It is associated with night shift work or frequently changing shifts.

Disorders and symptoms associated with shift work

A variety of factors affect the tolerability of shift work. These include the fit between an individual's assignment and his best time of day, the direction of rotation and the speed of rotation. Figure 7.4 shows that a counter-clockwise rotating shift incurs significant disruption of sleep and necessitates compensatory sleep on days off and vacations.

As society has become more industrialized, an increasing number of individuals are required to undertake shift work, estimates of the number of people thus engaged ranging from 20 to 25% of the work force[14]. Many shift workers are chronically sleep deprived and therefore suffer both sleep onset and maintenance insomnia. During the major waking period, such individuals may suffer fatigue and reduced alertness. Poor mood (irritable, depressed or anxious) may also result from sleep loss. Of perhaps greatest importance is the fact that night shift workers are at increased risk of falling asleep between about 3 and 5 a.m. when the CBT is at its nadir and sleep tendency is greatest. Not surprisingly, many large-scale industrial accidents (e.g. Three Mile Island, Chernobyl and the Union Carbide factory in Bhopal, India) and traffic fatalities occurred in the early morning hours[8,15].

In general, shift workers obtain about 2 h less sleep per day than non-shift workers, because if one is working nights, the physical and social environment makes it more difficult to obtain good quality sleep during daylight hours. Furthermore, the ascending body temperature curve makes morning sleep onset less likely. Under these circumstances, circadian factors exert greater influence on the ability to sleep than do the homeostatic factors (prior sleep loss).

Adaptability to night shift work can be enhanced by the speed and direction of the rotation. Slower rotation used in the United States permit a worker to gradually adjust his circadian rhythms over a period of 2 to 4 weeks. Faster rotas (shifting every 3–5 days), popular in Japan and Europe, assume that

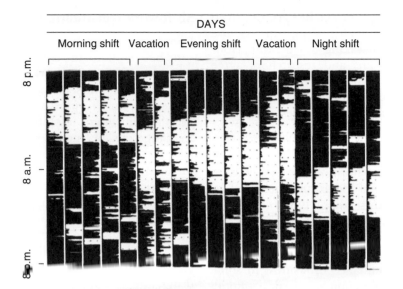

Figure 7.4 Shift worker's sleep–wakefulness cycle when shift rotates: night, evening, morning. From Lavie P[8], reproduced with permission

workers will maintain constant circadian rhythms in co-ordination with the environment. Some authorities believe that this method reduces long-term damage to workers' health[8].

Many hidden costs occur when shift work is assigned without regard for a worker's health, safety or family concerns. For example, in addition to disrupted sleep and compromised alertness, shift workers may have higher job dissatisfaction, greater absenteeism, significant marital and family problems and considerable medical morbidity[14]. Shift workers in particular appear more prone to digestive ailments, including ulcers, constipation and obesity[1]. This is probably due, in part, to poor eating habits, excess intake of caffeine and junk food and too little exercise. Improved health of shift workers may be obtained by modifying diet (e.g. switch to low fat, high fiber) and exercise routines. Of additional concern is the fact that most shift workers revert to the conventional sleep–wake times on days off but often have long periods of compensatory sleep. Thus, social and family obligations may be neglected during time off work.

TREATMENTS

Bright lights

The application of bright, full-spectrum lights with an intensity of at least 2500 lux can efficiently and safely shift biological rhythms[16]. This treatment relieves symptoms of various circadian sleep disorders and can assist in shift work adjustment. The individual is exposed to bright lights, which move sleep–wake rhythms in the following manner. To advance sleep phase (make earlier by a few hours), individuals should be exposed to bright light during the morning. To delay sleep phase (make later), they should be exposed to bright light during the evening. During summer months, exposure to sunlight is most effective. For other seasons or times of day artificial bright lights are used.

Pharmacotherapy

Hypnotics such as benzodiazepines, triazolam, or sedating antidepressants may be used occasionally to initiate sleep. Some central nervous system (CNS) stimulants play a limited role in promoting alertness in sleep-deprived individuals. Also, many shift workers use caffeine to bolster waking functioning. However, most clinicians and researchers agree that reliance on drugs to promote sleep or wakefulness to override the ravages of shift work is not in the individual's best interest.

Melatonin

This endogenous hormone is secreted at night by the pineal gland and mediated by retinal cells, but its secretion is decreased during the day. However, bright lights applied at night can suppress melatonin and increase alertness. Conversely, though, exogenous melatonin may enhance drowsiness in some people and thus function as a weak hypnotic.

Chronotherapy

Progressive delaying of bed/wake times may be applied to individuals with delayed sleep phase syndrome (or others) who cannot fall asleep or awaken at the desired hour. Once established, the schedule must be strictly followed in order to sustain benefits. This method has been quite successful, as it capitalizes on the tendency of the biological clock to have a period slightly longer than 24 h.

Shift-work consultation/planning

Knowledge about human chronophysiology can be applied in selection of suitable individuals for shift work and in rational scheduling of shifts. Most consultants agree that safety on the job as well as a durable, healthy adjustment to shift work is desirable. In dangerous or monotonous jobs, consultants may suggest exercise breaks and planned naps to refresh workers. Finally, counseling workers and family members can do much to protect the shift worker's sleep by providing a quiet, dark environment. Workers themselves must pay close attention to following a healthy diet, obtaining regular exercise and minimizing the use of caffeine or other drugs.

CONCLUSION

Like all living organisms, humans display inherent biological rhythms of many physiological and behavioral systems. Environmental demands produce disorders and symptoms associated with violation of the basic rest–activity cycle, but there are various treatments, including scheduling, drug therapy, bright light therapy and exogenous melatonin, briefly discussed above.

References

1. Moore-Ede M. *Shiftwork and your Health*. Circadian Technologies, Inc, 1986
2. Carskadon M, Dement W. Normal human sleep, an overview. In Kryger MH, Roth T, Dement WC, eds. *Principles and Practice of Sleep Medicine*. Philadelphia: Saunders, 1989: 3–13
3. Crick F, Mitchison G. The function of dream sleep. *Nature* 1983;304:111–14
4. Thase M, Howland R. Biological processes in depression: an updated review and integration. In Backham E, Leber W, eds. *Handbook of Depression*. New York: Guilford, 1995
5. Carskadon M, Dement W. Cumulative effects of sleep restriction on daytime sleepiness. *Psychophysiology* 1981;18:107–13
6. Czeisler C, Moore-Ede M, Coleman R. Rotating shift work schedules that disrupt sleep are improved by applying circadian principles. *Science* 1982;217
7. Horne J. *Why we Sleep: The Functions of Sleep in Humans and Other Mammals*. Oxford: Oxford University Press, 1988
8. Lavie P. *The Enchanted World of Sleep*. New Haven: Yale University Press, 1996
9. Rechtschaffen A. *Perspect Biol Med* 1998;41: 359–90
10. Moore-Ede MC, Sulzman FM, Fuller CA. *The Clocks that Time Us: Physiology of the Circadian Timing System*. Cambridge: Harvard University Press, 1982

11. Orr W. Overview of sleep and circadian rhythms. Presented at *Northside Hospital*, Atlanta GA, 1999

12. Eastman CI, Martin SK. How to use light and dark to produce circadian adaptation to night shift work. *Ann Med* 1999;31:87–98

13. Task Force on DSM-IV, American Psychiatric Association. *Diagnostic and Statistical Manual of Mental Disorders DSM-IV*. Washington, DC: American Psychiatric Association, 1994

14. Dotto L. *The Impact of Sleep on Work: Asleep in the Fast Lane*. Toronto: Stoddart, 1990

15. National Transportation Safety Board. *Fatigue, Alcohol, other Drugs and Medical Factors in Fatal-to-the-Driver Heavy Truck Crashes*. National Transportation Safety Board, 1990

16. Terman M, ed. Task force report on light treatment for sleep disorders. *J Biol Rhythms* 1995; 10:99–176

8

Normal and abnormal dreams

Alexander Z. Golbin and Vadim S. Rotenberg

INTRODUCTION

Dreams, defined as active mental activity in sleep, moved from the domain of folklore and material for an abstract psychoanalytic construction to one of the major topics of sleep research. Dreams are deeply connected with the clinical aspects of medicine, including cardiovascular and psychiatric disorders. The riddle of dreams is finally getting proper attention.

It is now common knowledge that dreams are associated with a stormy turbulence in the brain and the body involving mechanisms of memory, neuro-, endocrinological and biochemistry dynamics. These nighttime dynamics are also intimately related to daytime alertness, attention, mood, judgement and performance. For a long time we were caught in the quagmire of the activation–synthesis hypothesis, which taught us that dreams were nothing but cortical froth or a byproduct, generated by chaotic signals from the subcortical pons. Although this theory could explain why dreams are bizarre, it could not explain the intensity of emotions in the dreams and their frequent incongruence with the subject matter. The content of the dream may or may not be relevant, but emotions and physiological (and pathophysiological) changes are very real and sometimes have dramatic consequences.

Dreams are obvious and common to everyone, yet they are still an elusive phenomenon, which natural science is trying to catch. The question of which dreams to call 'abnormal' is still obscure. Are dreams of mental patients, even during relapses, always abnormal? Could 'crazy' dreams of otherwise healthy persons be considered as 'normal'? In addition, when and how do dreams reflect and affect the body and mind? When and how might they be compensatory and healing or when and how could they trigger sickness and even death? When and how is it possible to use the healing power of dreams and control their destructive force? These questions remain uncertain.

Keeping in mind the clinical orientation of this book, two issues are addressed in this chapter:

(1) Overview of current concepts regarding the physiology of dreams;

(2) The relationship between mental and physical health.

TYPES OF DREAM

Dreams can save lives and dreams can kill. How true is this? Let us judge for ourselves.

Here is an example from a World War II experience:

He was sound asleep. After many hours of trudging through the forest in the German rear, the group of soldiers he was with found what looked like a safe place, and they went to sleep.

Suddenly, he saw his mother in his dreams. She was talking to him and agitatedly pointing to something. He was too exhausted to move. His mother came closer. She shook him, screamed at him, and ordered him to wake up. The soldier woke up, bewildered and angry. He looked around and noticed the Nazis crawling towards them. He was able to alert his companions, and they organized a successful defense.

This dream saved the soldier's life during World War II. A prominent sleep physiology professor, V. N. Kasatkin, in his paper *The Atlas of Dreams*, described it together with 16 000 other carefully selected dreams[1]. N. Y. Grott, in his book *Dreams as a Subject of Science*[2], described many examples of warning signals coming to a dreamer during life-threatening situations, for example: earthquakes, floods, wars, etc. Grott cited a life-saving dream of one respected man who, in his sleep, saw his beloved girlfriend begging him to leave the room immediately. He woke up, frightened and surprised, and left the room. Just a few seconds later, the ceiling collapsed right onto the bed where he had been sleeping. Grott wondered if it were not the barely audible sounds of the ceiling cracking during the earthquake that reached the sleeping semi-conscious brain and gave the most powerful signal[2].

Serious and skeptical scientists accumulated a large number of believable facts about the existence of so-called predictive dreams. They are facts, not fiction. How can they be explained? There is what is known as the statistical theory. According to this theory, your specific worries produce specific images, and you see the same dreams many times. If the subject of your worry really occurs, you remember only this coincidence with the latest dream, forgetting that you saw the same dream many times. A. Shepovalnikov, in his book *How to Order Dreams*[3], offers many examples confirming this theory. A woman who had a dream that her son got killed in the war received a notice the next day informing her of her son's death. One explanation is that she saw the same dream over and over again but remembered only the latest one. Another explanation is that dreams are our connection to the 'collective unconscious'.

A 48-year-old experienced fireman kept a diary of his dreams for several years. He described fires that confirmed his dreams in previous nights. He wrote, 'If I see a fire in my sleep, the very next day, there will be a fire'. He was asked to continue writing his diary for 1–2 months, providing the exact dates of his dreams and dates of fires in his area. After a month and a half he sent this diary back to the sleep center. He had described 17 fire dreams, but there were no real fires during that time.

Does this signify the end of the mystery of predictive dreams? Are all the breath-taking stories just a statistical trick? Let us not rush to conclusions. There is another theory, another group of predictive dreams, which are based on extra sensitivity in sleep. They confirm that there might be truth in predictive dreams. A patient asked me one day to decipher his dream: 'During his service on a submarine, he fell into the cold water and tried to climb back to the platform. A heavy metal part pushed his chest down, preventing him from getting on-board. He tried to scream, but the sound did not come out. He woke up in a cold sweat, frightened to death.' He saw this dream repeatedly, every night, for a few weeks with increasing intensity. He felt normal during the day, working as a truck driver. Our team immediately performed an electrocardiogram, and discovered a heart attack.

Shepovalnikov[3] reported the following examples:

(1) An old man died from a stroke. His only symptom was having repetitive dreams about being scalped by Indians;

(2) A child told his mother that he had a dream about his friend hitting him in the right ear. A few days later, he was diagnosed with right otitis media (ear infection).

If dreams are very concrete, focused around a specific body part, and repetitive, they could be of important diagnostic value. We call them diagnostic dreams. Sub-sensory stimuli are intensified in sleep and reach the central nervous system to produce specific images.

Another medically and socially important type of dream is the suggestive dream. These dreams are fascinating and have a specific meaning for us. They influence our mood and force changes in our daytime behavior. Sometimes those dream images result in death: 'The grandmother called her family in the morning and said calmly, "my children. It's time for me to say goodbye. I saw your father in my dream. He told me to come and join him." The next morning the old woman did not wake up.' Have you heard this type of story? I heard these same words from my grandfather, and this is exactly how he died. What is this? Superstition, super sensitivity or a hidden death wish? Or the power of self-suggestion, which might turn our life off? Animals clearly have the gift to sense their own deaths. Elephants, for example, start the long trip to their place of final rest shortly before they die.

Kasatkin[1] described a young patient who told the doctor that in his dream a relative came and awakened him with the words 'Be awake, son. Be awake. You will die on the 19th'. Two months later, exactly on the 19th, the patient had a cardiorespiratory arrest in his sleep. We should not underestimate the power of self-suggestion. During sleep or in an altered state of consciousness, our hidden worries magnify significant emotional images to the level of post-hypnotic suggestions, exerting a powerful influence on our body, mind and behavior. An example of the power of self-suggestion is the 'anniversary phenomenon', when a person is afraid that he will die, say at age 47, on his birthday, just like his father, and

this person actually dies on that exact day! There is also the 'positive anniversary phenomenon'. My terminally ill grandfather told me that he would not die until he had finished the book of his life. He lived for more years than expected, surprising all of his doctors, and died a few days after he had finished his work.

Sometimes, a coincidence supports public belief in the power of dreams. A young man from Florence saw one day in his dream that he was maimed and killed by a monument of a lion in front of the nearby church. In the morning he told his dream to his friends, and all of them decided that it was ridiculous to believe in it. To prove that he was not afraid, the young man put his hand into the lion's mouth in front of an assembled crowd and…screamed with pain. A scorpion had bitten him. The young man died. This tragic coincidence stunned people. The story became a legend and was used by the church to confirm the power of God.

There are many other instances where the impact of dreams on behavior may be less dramatic but equally tragic. Shepovalnikov[3] cited a number of cases where emotionally unstable adolescents acted upon their dreams. For example, a teenager saw in his dreams that he killed his teacher. He became obsessed with this idea, but did not carry out his plan, only because of timely hospitalization. The suggestive effect of dreams is much more common in children who sometimes may not be able to distinguish between dreams and reality.

There are four factors indicating the suggestive effect of dreams:

(1) The suggestive effect of dreams comes from their unclear images;

(2) We always believe in the situation in sleep. During sleep, everything is real. What would be absurd for the awakened mind seems real and logical to us when we are sleeping;

(3) Sensations in sleep coming from our body, our skin, our nose, our mouth and inner organs make strong 'suggestions' in sleep;

(4) A long-term memory can be revived in sleep.

Altogether these factors produce the extremely believable effect of dreams and influence the person's behavior.

We may also know some interesting and convincing examples of how things escape from our wakened attention and come to us as images in dreams. What we failed to pay attention to during the day may suddenly become highlighted in our dreams. One funny example is described by Grott[2]: the French scientist Delagua had a dream one day that, instead of the broken old lamp outside his apartment, there was an elegant copper lamp. He told his family at breakfast about this strange dream. It turned out, to his embarrassment, that the new lamp had been at the door for the past week. He just had not paid any attention to it.

This specific phenomenon of memory being revived in sleep is probably the basis for the secrets of so-called discovery and creative dreams. Grott told this story as an example: one man was in a financial crisis after the death of his father, and he lost several vitally important documents. In his dream, his father came back and clearly indicated the location of the papers[3].

You might know or have experienced some interesting examples of how problems of real life are solved in sleep. The Russian chemist Mendeleev, author of the famous periodic system of chemical elements, first saw his periodic table in his dreams. He woke up and put his dreams together on paper.

The German chemist, Friedrich Kekule, visualized his famous formula of the benzene ring as a dance of six mice. Grott emphasized the amazing ability of dreams to be a source of creative ideas. As a striking example, he cited 300 poems written by the poet Kollezidger in his sleep[3].

Problem solving in sleep is a common experience. Promising techniques now exist to develop such skills. The present advances in sleep research demonstrate that dreams can be predictive, diagnostic and creative. Dreams may also be emotionally exciting. In sleep, our emotions are not restricted. We feel blissfully happy or endlessly depressed. We are ecstatic or terrified. In sleep we experience flying and falling, moving and spinning. Scientists have yet much to learn before they can fully understand the mechanism of how this happens, the reasons why our bodies and minds have these feelings, and how they can be used to our benefit.

In crisis dreaming according to Cartwright, important thoughts, ideas and problems that people are currently facing invade their dreams and alter them[67]. Often, the themes of the dreams are immediately related to the issue at hand. No matter how many dreams the person has during the night, they all seem to be connected in some way. Since the themes in these dreams happen to be identical to those weighing heavily on the dreamer's mind, they can be referred to as crisis dreams. There can be many advantages to having such dreams. Dreams involving problems and situations that require people to make decisions can prove to be helpful. They may help a person understand his or her own inner fears and feelings about a particular decision. They may also be important in identifying mental obstacles that may stand in the way of some accomplishment.

In other cases, crisis dreams reflect the recurrence of traumatic events. Examples of these would be kidnapping, rape or certain military experiences. Thinking about these occurrences can create feelings of guilt and blame, leading to recurring dreams that focus on the experience itself and the events leading up to it or following it. However, if the dreams are analyzed and the problems therein are recognized and properly addressed, these dreams can be a great help in treatment, and assist the person in recovering from a traumatic experience.

Lucid dreaming, discovered by Stephen LaBerge[4], opens up a whole new world to the human experience. Lucid dreaming occurs when you are conscious and aware of being in a dream state. You are then able to manipulate the content of the dream and its influence upon the body. Often this occurs when, during a dream, something unusual happens that normally would not have taken place in real life, revealing that you are dreaming. This unusual event is called a dream sign. After realizing that you are dreaming, you will have remarkable control of the dream world and your experiences in it. Realization is accompanied by a heightening of the senses observing brighter colors, hearing more sounds, etc. These pleasurable sensations are accompanied by the ability to do anything you want to, literally manipulating the dream world.

One benefit of lucid dreaming is to rehearse a task you are about to perform. For example, if you are eager to succeed in a basketball game that you have the next day, you can practice all of your moves the night before. When you actually play the next day, you will be surprised to find that you feel comfortable with your game plan and know exactly what you are doing. This usage of mental practice to improve physical skills is currently being researched, and new evidence points to the success of this technique.

Through this dream technique, self-confidence can be gained. An example would be a speech that is to be performed soon. The speaker can rehearse a speech and imagine a large crowd, thus practicing the speech and getting used to the crowd at the same time. In some cases, healing oneself may be accomplished by willingly being able to control certain body functions. Finally, fears and lack of self-confidence can be fought, as one can fight and conquer any force that threatens one's peace of mind.

There are some dreams that seriously threaten peace of mind; among them are nightmares. According to Calvin Hall's[5] research into 10 000 'normal' dreams, two-thirds of them were negative, with feelings such as anger, confusion, betrayal and fear being prevalent. Such dreams deserve separate analysis and will be dealt with in detail. Other types of dreams, among them wet dreams, are usually associated with a certain age range.

PSYCHOPHYSIOLOGY OF DREAMS

Early enthusiasm regarding the remarkable correlation between the rapid eye movement (REM) stage of sleep and high physiological activations and reports of vivid dreaming, found by Aserinsky and Kleitman in 1953[6], indicated a belief that the physiological substrate of dreaming was finally discovered.

Similarity between dream images and hallucinations suggested that if we discover the nature of dreams we will understand the physiology of hallucinations and, ultimately, the nature of psychoses. This theory was a logical and very attractive illusion and became one of the beautiful tales of the 20th century. Psychophysiological study of sleep and dreaming was also attractive because it opened new avenues for determining mind–body interactions that are not present during wakefulness[7].

The methodology of the psychophysiological study of sleep includes polysomnography tests and multiple rating scales. Episodes of activations in sleep give good time points of measurement and associations between mentation and physiological parameters. A study showed that dreaming in the non-rapid eye movement (NREM) stage is possible but not frequent (8%) compared to 80% of dream reports from the REM stage. In 1967, Foulkes summarized the argument for the validity of NREM dreams[8]. It was the end of a convenient illusion about REM as a unique dream state. Weak attempts to save the REM tale of changes in semantic definition of dreams as 'coherent and detailed descriptions of dream content' vs. 'vague fragmentary impressions' in NREM did not help.

In some dreams the dreamer passively accepts pictures and discontinuity between objects and events, but there are other types of mentation even in REM:

(1) REM and narcoleptic vivid dreams;

(2) Nightmares where the dreamer may accept some control over dream mentation, or real somatic activation appropriate to a dream might be elicited.

In fact, dreaming may have NREM onset, if it occurs in sleep-like states: meditation, daydreaming, etc. Deprivation of REM does not lead to psychosis. Paradoxically REM deprivation may lead to clinical improvement in some cases of depression, but long morning REM might increase the intensity of negative dreaming. REM and NREM states are different in their mentation. REM is characterized by a greater representation of sensory and motor dimensions, whereas NREM reports show a greater attachment to waking life and are characterized as 'thinking'. Mental activity in stage 1 is similar to REM in terms of hallucinatory perceptual and emotional qualities, but is not organized and real, as in REM, according to Dement and Kleitman[9].

There is some evidence of state-dependent cognitive processes specific to NREM, REM and wakefulness. Is there one single system responsible for dreams with changes in intensity in different states, as each state has it own different system creating unique mentation?

Foulkes brought a new dimension to the psychopathology of dreams in his longitudinal study of dreams in children[10]. A major conclusion from this longitudinal sleep laboratory study on children aged 3–15 years was that 'the development of REM dreaming follows a course parallel to the better documented and well known stages of waking cognitive maturation'. Dreaming is a maturational cognitive process developing from infancy to adulthood.

The absence of relationships between physiological activation and mental activity is especially puzzling. Why, for example, are penile erection and clitoral enlargement in REM not associated with sexual dreams at all? Also, why is the highest electrodermal activity in REM (which is a hallmark of high emotional tension) not correlated to vague, unemotional thought processes?

A variety of electroencephalogram (EEG) features such as the K complex (high amplitude theta or delta wave followed by spindle), sleep spindles, theta or delta bursts and REM 'sawtooth' waves drew attention to the study of sleep mentation. The summary of the study is disappointing: no dreams, but non-intellectualized visual images were found during awakenings for theta bursts and 'sawtooth' waves.

Another type of EEG oscillatory activity has drawn the attention of psychophysiologists. This 20–40-Hz high-frequency rhythm has been noted in animals during wakefulness and sleep but not in NREM sleep. It was assumed that this activity provides a mechanism for integrating multisensory information and mechanism of cognition. However, this study has only just started and the concept is largely speculative.

When researchers turned to the study of motor activity, specifically discrete muscle activity (eye movements) and dream content, this brought more interesting data. The more eye movements, the more vivid are the dreams and the more activity in the dream. The 'scanning hypothesis' proposed that eye movements during REM scan visual images in dreams in the same way as during wakefulness. During lucid dreaming the scanning hypothesis was not valid – eye movements did not reflect any specific images and were not associated with reports. The study of ponto-geniculo-occipital (PGO) spikes responsible for eye bursts did not solve the problem.

The psychophysiological basis of dreams remains a mystery. New findings have brought more questions than answers but the main promise is still held to be true: dreams are essential parts of our sleep life. They were with us from the dawn of civilization and will be with us for good or bad in the future.

THEORIES OF DREAMING

Dreams have existed since ancient time, and so have dream theories. Dream meanings, their nature, origin and causes, and their function and dysfunction, were at the heart of art, culture, religion, science and daily decision making in all times and all cultures. Theories of the spirit world were replaced with the rational concept of Aristotle, then the unconscious drive-related ideas of Plato, expanded later by Freud[11].

Discovery of the association between dreaming and the REM sleep stage by Aserinsky and Kleitman in 1953[6] brought a new tool for dream study and it was felt that the secret of dreams was on the horizon. Well, the horizon is the line that is never reached. An assumption that psychophysiological changes of human emotions are the same in sleep and waking turned out to be false. Electrodermal activity, a hallmark of daytime emotions, is high in delta sleep where there are no emotions and the EEG in REM sleep is very similar to the one in waking.

Twenty years later Hobson and McCarley's[12] research on animals produced the activation–synthesis hypothesis of the dream process, placing emphasis on subcortical levels. Ellman and colleagues[13] showed later how Olds' subcortical reward system[14] might be involved in a motivational aspect of dreams. An excellent review of theories of dreaming is provided by Pivik[7] and Antrobus[15,60].

Theories of dream formation

The neurobiological mechanisms of dreams as a mental state have been intensively investigated by physiologists and psychophysiologists. One of the most popular concepts of dream formation is the activation–synthesis model of Hobson and McCarley[12]. This model in its original form proposed that formal aspects of dream mentation reflect the outcome of attempts by sensorimotor and limbic regions of the forebrain to produce a coherent experience from the incomplete and chaotic inputs received from the brainstem. This theory considered the probable consequences of a shift in visual system input source from the formed visual images on the retina in waking to the chaotic brainstem stimulation of different forebrain areas in REM sleep. These chaotically generated phasic signals arising in the pontine brain lead directly to visual (and not only visual) hallucinations, emotions and distinctively bizarre cognition that characterizes dream mentation. Thus, dreams are considered as a random outcome of an initial chaotic, bottom-up activation process in combination with its resultant secondary semi-coherent, top-down synthetic process based on the interpretation by the cortex of this originally senseless chaotic information.

Sensory information processing in dreaming is related to the activation of the visual and paralimbic cortex and the deactivation of primary visual and dorsolateral prefrontal cortices. The latter is selectively activated during human reasoning tasks, episodic and working memory tasks in wakefulness and is specialized for the central executive function of working memory[16,17]. Its deactivation may be responsible for the illogical explanation of bizarre occurrences in dreams, for the mnemonic deficits and for disorientation in the strange virtual reality of dreams.

This initial activation–synthesis model has recently evolved in the three dimensional framework of the so-called AIM model[18]. High level of cortical activation (A) is a correlate of the mind's ability to access and manipulate significant amounts of stored information from the brain during dream synthesis. (I) is the internal sources – the blockade of external sensory input and its functional replacement by internally generated REM sleep events such as PGO waves, providing the specific activation of sensory and affective centers that prime the cortex for dream construction. According to Braun and co-workers[19] REM sleep is characterized by selective activation of extrastriate visual cortices and attenuation of activity in the primary visual cortex. REM sleep may represent a state with the selective activation of the interoceptive network, which is dissociated from primary sensory and heteromodal association areas at either end of the visual hierarchy that mediates interactions with the external world. (M) is the shift of the brain from aminergic to cholinergic neuromodulation, which alters the mnemonic capacity of the brain–mind and reduces the reliability of cortical circuits, thus increasing the likelihood of bizarre temporal sequences and associations which are uncritically accepted as reality.

According to Hobson and colleagues[18] factors (A) and (I) are similar to factors that characterize sensory deprivation in wakefulness[15]. Factor (I) includes a proprioceptive feedback. Internally generated pseudosensory data can be produced by brainstem mechanisms (via PGO stimulation of the visual cortex), can be recalled from memory or can be intentionally created by directed mental imagery. As proposed by Hobson and co-workers[18], eye movement density in REM provides an estimate of the amount of internally generated pseudo-sensory data and reflects PGO and motor pattern generator activity.

During waking, internal inputs are used mainly in the service of the ongoing sensorimotor integration of external signals. If internal signals become unusually strong they could dominate, resulting in hallucinations.

Hobson's model proposes the following details of dream machinery:

(1) The intense and vivid visual hallucinosis is due to auto-activation of the visual brain by pontine activation processes impinging, initially, at the level of the unimodal visual association cortex and heteromodal parietal areas subserving spatial cognition.

(2) The intense emotions are due to activation of the amygdala and medial limbic structure.

(3) The delusional belief that we are awake, the lack of directed thought, the loss of self-reflective awareness and the lack of insight about illogical and impossible dream experience, results in aminergic demodulation and the selective inactivation of the dorsolateral prefrontal cortex.

(4) The bizarre cognition of dreaming is due to an orientational instability caused by the chaotic nature of the pontine auto-activation process, the absence of frontal cortical monitoring and episodic memory deficits due to failure of aminergic neuromodulation[18].

Thus, according to Hobson's initial and modified models, in dreams senseless experience caused by the chaotic brain activation during REM sleep is secondarily re-interpreted by the associative cortex in the condition of its modulated activity. REM sleep (or a similar state of chaotic brain activation) is an obligate condition for dreams to appear.

However, it is in contradiction with data (see Solms[20]) that dreaming and REM sleep are controlled by different brain mechanisms – dreaming by forebrain mechanisms, REM sleep by brainstem mechanisms. Cholinergic brainstem mechanisms that control REM sleep can only generate the psychological phenomena of dreaming through the mediation of second (dopaminergic) forebrain mechanisms. Dreaming involves concerted activity in a highly specific group of forebrain structures (anterior and lateral hypothalamus areas; amygdala; striatal areas; infralimbic; prelimbic; orbitofrontal anterior cingulate; entorhinal; insular; occipitotemporal cortical areas). At the same time dreams can occur in the absence of REM sleep, in subjects with pontine brainstem lesions.

Antrobus and colleagues[21] also argued that rapid eye movements (the main phasic feature of REM sleep) are not under strict brainstem cholinergic control, but come increasingly under the control of the frontal eye fields as general cortical activation increases. From our point of view it means that the content of dreams can secondarily influence the rapid eye movement activity instead of being totally dependent on its random or stereotyped activity. In the Hobson model there is no place for the initial, purposeful meaning of dreams, or of their special psychological functions. They are in contradiction with many theories of dream functions.

Theories of dream functions

Almost all theories of dream function, starting with Freud[11], emphasized the adaptive functions of dreams for psychological well-being. According to Freud[11], dreams are instigated by unconscious (repressed) wishes and represent their discharge in a modified form into consciousness. According to the psychoanalytic theory, dream experience reflects a compromise between unconscious drives and wishes on the one hand, and censorship that protects consciousness against inappropriate motives and behavioral attitudes on the other.

It is important that, according to the psychoanalytic theory, dreams do not only represent the suppressed wishes that are inappropriate for consciousness. Even some basic needs, such as thirst, that are not in conflict with social motivations and conscious behavioral attitudes could be found in dream content, in a very open form. Because body muscles are paralyzed in the dream state, Freud postulated that the consummatory path in the mental apparatus must flow in a reversed direction from that in a waking state – toward the sensory end rather than the motor end producing the hallucinatory fulfillment of the wish to drink or to eat or to urinate. For instance, thirsty dreamers dream of going to get a glass of water and drinking it instead of waking up and doing the same in wakefulness, and the same happens with other basal needs[11]. It seems unlikely that a random excitation of the forebrain structures[18] could enable the dreamer to hallucinate the whole consequence of behavioral acts in order to satisfy his thirst in his dream.

At the same time, such dreams show that some wishes can appear in dreams without censorship. Possibly this can also happen in dreams dealing with true motivational conflicts. According to the classical psychoanalytic theory, the censorship creates a situation where only the latent content of dreams has a psychological sense relevant for deep interpretation while manifest content uses only day residues to mask an essential latent content. However, Greenberg and Pearlman[22] have shown that manifest content often deals with problems important for the dreamer in his waking life and thus is not opposite to latent content. Sixty per cent of dream reports contained overt emotional problems, most of them connected with actual problems discovered during the waking analysis[22]. According to Cohen and Cox[23], subjects who were confronted by a stressful waking situation and subsequently dreamed about it felt better in the morning than did subjects who had not dreamed about their problems. This corresponds to the recent data of Kahan and LaBerge[24] that cognition sampled from REM sleep was highly similar to waking cognition. When the dream included a tendency to resolve a problem in an open or metaphorical way, the psychological defense in the subsequent wakefulness became more effective and the ability to deal with the problems was enhanced.

It is in agreement with the general concept of the above-mentioned authors that dreams are responsible for adaptation of recent information to stable personal psychological attitudes, especially regarding information which is not relevant to the previous experience. In the process of such adaptation the familiar defense mechanisms are used, and specific and actual emotional problems may be displaced by other situations not necessarily connected with the actual problem. But they can also be presented as they are. The emotional problem by itself is less important than the used and trained defensive mechanisms. Resolving the real or masked problem in a dream may help to confront the actual problem in the subsequent wakefulness.

This explanation is already very close to those proposed by the search activity concept mentioned in Chapter 3. If the main function of the dream is the restoration of search activity to be used in the subsequent wakefulness, then the subject is very free and flexible in his dream. The subject can try to solve his current actual problem in the metaphoric manner, or he can try to solve another problem, one that displaces the actual problem, since the search process itself is the main restorative factor and the content of the search is much less important. Reiser[25] has mentioned that statements of the search activity concept related to dream function are confirmed by data[19,26] and that the 'curiosity–interest–expectancy' command system identified by Panksepp[27] lies in the area of greater activity during REM sleep. It is the same fiber tract that was interrupted by leukotomy in schizophrenic patients, causing lack of initiative and disappearance of dream reports[20].

According to Kramer[28] dreams serve as selective affective regulators, changing the subject's mood in a positive direction. The dream mechanism is especially effective in the relief of a state of subjective unhappiness. According to Kramer, this integrative capacity of dreaming is not solely related to the content of dreams[28]. For instance, manifest dream content may differ both during the same night and from night to night, while the dream's positive influence on mood in healthy subjects is still apparent. Although dream content differs in men and women, the positive change in mood is independent of gender. Moreover, it is independent even of the mood in the dream itself. Dreams often deal with personal preoccupations that exist during wakefulness and such are usually unpleasant and confusing; recurrent dreams especially usually have a threatening content[29]. Nielsen and co-workers[30] even suggested that there is a special process which inhibits positive emotions and facilitates fearful emotions while dreaming. From our point of view, dreaming does not need to include such a process to contain negative emotional features. If the appearance of the dream is stimulated by the renunciation of search in the previous wakefulness, the dream does not reflect the full spectrum of daily emotions but has to deal with this very negative state, especially in the first dream episodes when this state still dominates.

Cartwright and Lloyd[31] and Cartwright and colleagues[32] have shown that depressed patients who had an enhanced dream-like quality of mentation during the first REM sleep period and who displayed the positive dynamic of dream mood from the first to the last REM sleep periods were more likely to be in remission from depression 1 year later. Those with fewer negative dreams at the beginning and more at the end of the night were less likely to be in remission. In healthy subjects a pre-sleep level of the depression scale, being in normal limits, correlated with the affect in the first REM report. Low scorers on this scale (people who are far from the renunciation of search in their waking behavior) displayed a flat distribution of positive and negative affect in dreams. Those with some pre-sleep depressed moods showed a pattern of decreasing negative and increasing positive affect in dreams, reported from successive REM periods[33]. This is a sign that dreams have an adaptive function and contribute to the restoration of normal mood.

The restoration of the normal mood after sleep is relatively independent of mood in dream content. In healthy subjects mood after all REM sleep awakenings was mostly good or neutral regardless of the dream content or phasic/tonic REM sleep features[34]. We suggest that it is possible to explain this by taking into consideration that even dreamers with recurrent dreams and threatening content often participate actively in the course of threatening events and present a fight or flight response[29], which contains search activity elements.

Another theory of the adaptive dream function was proposed by Hartmann[35]. He emphasized that dreaming makes connections between imagined objects and it does this extremely broadly, more broadly and widely than waking in the nets of the mind. In this sense dreaming can be considered 'hyper-connective'. The signal-to-noise ratio is very low in dreaming. It was proposed 30 years ago[36] that dreaming represents the functioning of the cortex without the influence of norepinephrine; this seems to be true[37]. Hartmann[35] also suggests that the dominant emotion of the dreamer is the force which drives or guides the connecting process and determines which of the countless possible connections are actualized at a particular time. This suggestion makes a bridge between the concept of Hartmann and the above-mentioned concepts of Kramer, Greenberg and Cartwright[22,28,31,32,35]. Hartmann has shown that the process of psychological recovery after psychological trauma (a positive outcome) includes a process of connecting the trauma with other emotionally related material from the dreamer's life[35]. It is the process of integration of the traumatic event that prevents the post-traumatic stress disorder (PSTD). What is important is that dreaming allows the making of such connections in a safe place (in the domain of the dream). Hartmann stressed that a similarity between dreaming and the process of psychotherapy is displayed; both first provide a safe place for work to be done.

Hartmann also stressed that people with thin boundaries (open to experience) have more dream recalls and their dreams are more vivid, emotional and bizarre, and have more interaction between characters in comparison to dreams of those with thick boundaries. These thin boundaries between the subject and the polydimensional world also characterize people with a dominant right hemisphere.

Hartmann's approach to the process of psychological recovery after trauma is very close to the approach that was expressed by Rotenberg (see Chapter 3). Rotenberg also suggested that the integration of the traumatic events in the broader picture of the world is the best way for psychological adaptation. However, in addition to this, Rotenberg included the notion of the right hemisphere activity that allows such integration by creating, out of numerous connections between objects and events, a polysemantic context[38–40]. Dreams of normal subjects display a typical example of such context; however, this context is not restricted only to dreams and can also be created in wakefulness. It depends only on the right hemisphere skills which differ in different persons[40]. Recent investigations[41] have confirmed that the same cortical areas (right frontal eye field and dorsolateral prefrontal cortex) are involved in eye movements both in REM sleep and in wakefulness. They suggest that REM sleep eye movements are saccadic scans of targets in the dream scene under right hemisphere control. The main problem of patients suffering from PTSD is their inability to build the polysemantic context in dreaming as well as in wakefulness and consequently to perform search activity in the frame of this broad and powerful context.

The domination of the right hemisphere in human dreams allows us to solve another problem related to the role of dreams in creativity. There are a few very well known stories about the creative acts in dreams, like the discovery of the benzene ring, which Kekule saw in his dream as the image of dancing mice.

However, serious studies devoted to the influence of REM sleep and dreams on creative processes are relatively scarce. Domino[42] and Sladeczek and Domino[43] showed that highly creative subjects have dreams with more primary processes. Individuals with divergent thinking are more creative and produce more dream recall than individuals with convergent thinking. Lewin and Glaubman[44] showed that REM deprivation impaired the carrying out of creative tasks and lowered creativity, whereas it did not impair memory function. These data seem to support the hypothesis[45] that creative acts take place in dreams themselves and even that creativity is one of the tasks of dreaming.

However, first of all, there is a surprisingly small ratio between the insignificant number of discoveries performed in dreams (which is why they are so impressive and fixed in the collective memory) and the huge number of dreams that each individual in the world in each generation experiences from four to five times each night during their life. For the psychobiological system predisposed to discoveries it seems a very low efficiency. Second, if non-conventional tasks which require a creative approach, and are so important for adaptation, are solved in dreams, how is it possible to explain the high variability of REM sleep in the human population? Is it possible that short sleepers with very little REM sleep and a low number of dreams are unable to carry out creative tasks? Moreover, this suggestion is in contradiction with the well known fact that creative people in a state of high creative activity (creative ecstasy) often become short sleepers with a sharp drop in REM sleep percentage in night dreams. It seems a paradox – the creative solution of the problem requires dreams while in the process of the most creative activity dreams disappear.

Finally, it was shown that, although REM sleep and dreams play an important role in the creative solution of complicated problems, the problem itself is not solved in dreams. No precise relationship was found between the presence or absence in dreams of the signs such a problem presented prior to sleep and the subsequent success in solving that problem[46]. When the creative task was successfully carried out the following morning, it was related mostly to the active position of the dreamer as a successful problem solver who is solving not precisely the given task but any task in the dream. The process of the successful solving of any problem unrelated to the actual problem may help the subject to solve the actual problem in the subsequent wakefulness, by restoring search activity which is so important for creative behavior. This approach makes a bridge between the role of dreaming in creative task solution and the general role of dreaming in adaptation to stressful situations and inner motivational conflicts, the latter being a particular form of creative task.

Nevertheless, creative problems are sometimes really solved in dreams, although it is not the precise task of dreams. This happens because the right hemisphere is overactive during dreams and free from conscious (left hemisphere) control. This freedom and the reliance on the flexible polysemantic context helps the subject to restore search activity in a situation when during wakefulness he had already given up. Metaphoric, imaginative thinking is used in dreams to produce artificial problems and to solve them, to perceive oneself as a successful conqueror able to overcome obstacles. At the same time, on occasion, due to the same features of dream mentation, the subject can suddenly find a solution to the concrete problem he was confronted with, especially if he was continuously trying to solve this problem in wakefulness (as occurred with Kekule).

Theories of the role of dreaming in memory function will not be discussed in this chapter, as the possible role of REM sleep (and dreams) in memory was discussed in Chapter 3.

Theories of dreaming (including theories of dream interpretations and theories of brain processes creating dreams)

Theories of dream interpretations assume that dream subjects and events are associated with subjects and events in the dreamer's waking life, and that dreams are created in response to high-order drives and conflicts. Although Freud's[11] assumptions about psychological urges and dreams were not supported in Foulkes' extensive studies of dreams[8,10,47,48], the interaction of dreams and our daily life seems to be utterly intrinsic. It looks as if our daily and nightly lives are mainly independent but have many brief interconnections that may be meaningful or crucial for survival. When and how is still a question.

Studies on pre-sleep situations or traumas show that the stimuli could be included in the mosaic content of dreams. What is important is that stimuli from a 'sick' organ could also be included in a dream. In this sense, interpretations of dreams, although regarded with skepticism, make reasonable sense.

The question of how dreams are produced is still debated. Knowing multiple details about creation is still not the same as knowing the whole picture. Stimulus studies were started by Dement and co-workers[49], who reported that spraying water at the dreamer in REM stage produced dreams that he was sprayed with water by children. The integration of the stimulus in the dream showed that the sleeping brain should be in the active state for this task.

Hobson and McCarley's[12] experiments on positive and cortical stimulation of the cat during waking, NREM and REM provided concrete evidence that REM is a very active state in which the cerebral cortex receives widespread activation from reticular formation. The difference between REM and the waking state is that incoming afferent and outgoing efferent information is strongly inhibited in REM sleep. This means that almost all stimuli the brain is receiving are from inside the body, while the motor response to 'run' or 'fight' is blocked.

During polysomnogram recording the REM stage is recognized by high rapid eye movements (REM bursts). Hobson and McCarley's[12] studies strongly correlated REM bursts with PGO neuronal spikes. They stated that PGO activity is not controlled by the cortex; random dreams are free from cognitive control. Later detailed reviews of Pivik[7] and Antrobus[21] showed that this is not exactly true. Dreams could be elicited between REM bursts, so PGO is not the only information for dreams. Antrobus and colleagues[21] argued that in REM sleep the frontal eye fields are under cortex control. They proposed that saccadic eye movements in REM could not actually contour the object because there is no feedback between the internal object and the retina. In the absence of the visual feedback, the calcarine region to the frontal cortex, the oculomotor system, 'stutters' by repeating its command to the pons resulting in larger PGO. Positron emission tomography (PET) studies[41] supported the concept but showed that the frontal eye field region was indeed activated during REM.

According to Antrobus and colleagues the REM bursts associated with PGO bursts are the sequence of feedback[21]. 'Failure' and the PGO non-random occurrence mean that the theories of dreaming, Hobson and McCarley's[12] and Crick and Mitchison's[50], based on the randomness of PGO lose their basis.

Hobson and McCarley's[12] theory is that the dream is a subcortical process based on the random PGO and not related to cognition. Crick and Mitchison[50] have proposed a theory that dreams are a memory clearing or resetting process and base their assumption on PGO randomness.

Antrobus' 'failure' theory is based on computational models developed in 1986. The basic idea is that there are small units of neural networks that could identify 'microfeatures' which unite into increasingly complex units until they can recognize, locate or name an object or event and give it some meaning. The external stimulus in REM could be recognized by the brain, although the whole object is not based on computational neural networks; activation of just a few units in the cluster is enough to activate the entire cluster, similarly to wakefulness. To recognize one's mother it is enough to hear just a fragment of her voice. Combinations of the smallest unit might lead to imaginary novel pictures from the originals.

It is interesting that novelty in dream pictures is bizarre, as there may be some constraints. Noses are not inverted on faces and planes do not fly in reverse. Those constraints, according to Antrobus' theory, are due to previous intercluster connections. Hinton and associates[51] constructed the top-down model in which there are different levels of neuronal network clusters taking input from bottom to top and controlling from top to bottom. These directional and dynamic processes of dreaming are very promising but detailed research is needed. New developments in physics, such as the Chaos Theory, brought a new direction into the study of brain processes, specifically dreams.

From the Chaos Theory viewpoint, the cluster in any region represents a large number of potential attractor sites with their local input. Attractor sites vary in their strength (based on the frequency with which they have been activated in the past). They compete with each other often and the neural activity is a random, dynamic chaos of attractors producing patterns. It was shown[21] that any random input has some similarity to a previously learned pattern and sequences of images are based on anticipation as a fundamental characteristic of waking perception.

This model also accepts the premise that REM is not the only state that produces dreams. Dreams are also found to be different depending on the time of night. Early night REM dreams are brief and less bizarre. Long, dramatic, bizarre dreams are typical for late-night REM, especially times beyond the usual waking hour. Those dreams are frequently lucid. Mild stressors might have an effect similar to late-sleep REM or NREM as long as afferent input to the cortex is inhibited. The idea of a connection of REM activation with the time of night is so important that Broughton and co-workers[52] suggested studying PET at night. They showed that the occipital cortex is more active in REM-reduced activation of the dorsolateral, prefrontal and lateral orbital cortical areas in sleep and is in agreement with the sleeper's inability to create the visual images in REM that are fully consonant with their larger content. That is why in the waking stage we know that what we saw was only a dream.

Current understanding of dream function

Dreams have belonged to the domain of psychology for a long time. Psychological constructions were difficult to prove or disprove. When REM was discovered in 1953, and later when the connections between REM and vivid dreaming had been established, it was a 'honeymoon' period in dream research. The neurophysiological basis of dreams was thought to have been discovered, the similarity of dreams to hallucinations seemed obvious and expectations of upcoming discovery of the nature of psychotic behavior (and its cure) were high. The 1970s will be remembered as a period of disappointment. The study of dreams faced serious methodological difficulties, samples were small and generally represented healthy young students self-selected on the ability to describe dreams[53]. Besides methodological difficulties another problem emerged that confused what used to be so clear: the dream = REM. Dreams were discovered in all stages of NREM including sleep onset (although dreams in this stage were not as vivid and coherent as REM dreams, but more anxious and unhappy[54,55]). All of this led to the conclusion that NREM dreams are not an epiphenomenon of REM, but an independent continuous mental activity that surfaces during cerebral arousal[53].

According to Hobson and McCarley's 'activation–synthesis hypothesis, dreams are byproducts of the phasic–tonic nature of REM sleep and its underlying neurophysiology. The sensory component of dreams is triggered by the phasic bursts of spikes from the pons before and during the REM phase, which stimulate the production of random images. When these images reach the higher cortex, interpretation (meaning) is added. The interpretation of these ambiguous stimuli is influenced by our past experience, present needs and ongoing interests. As Cartwright put it 'the meaning of dreams is in the mind of the beholder'[53]. The function of dreams, if any, is not clear from this concept; the activation–synthesis hypothesis does not deny the possibility of such functions.

The search for the function of dreams was revived not when the methodology of dream research was standardized but more from the demand of clinical practice, when patients with nightmares, or disturbing cases of acting out dreams with disastrous consequences, etc., were coming to numerous sleep clinics for help.

A psychological model was developed to address the issues of dreams and of affect changes in psychiatric pathology. It started when Snyder[56] reported dreams from 635 REM awakenings over 250 nights from 56 subjects. His conclusion was unexpected: the typical dream is a 'clear, coherent and detailed account of a realistic situation involving the dreamer and other people caught up in very ordinary activities and preoccupations, and usually talking about them'. Another of his stunning suggestions was that emotionally disturbed dreams are coming from emotionally disturbed people, because the dreams reflect this disturbance.

Although these conclusions seem to contradict a common experience, they found support in the dream research of children. Foulkes concluded[10,47] that children's dreams developed in parallel with the child's psychomotor development, meaning that they get more realistic with age.

Dement believed that we need to dream, because of the rebound of REM after REM deprivation[57], but REM deprivation is not always equal to dream deprivation and does not produce hallucinations and other psychotic behavior. In fact, it is the other way around – REM deprivation sometimes improves mental and physical performance.

Psychologists emphasized the notion that dreams have something to do with emotions. Unpleasant dreams are more frequent then pleasant ones. Breger and colleagues[58] studied dreams before and after elective surgery. Their conclusion was that dreams have an information processing function, which is free from a waking logic. The dream function is the attempt at emotional problem solving in sleep. This concept is very close to Rotenberg's 'search activity' concept (see Chapter 3). Kramer[28] confirmed that dreams could improve the person's waking emotional state, specifically from more to less unhappiness. Kramer sums up the function of dreams as 'selective mood regulation'. Cartwright added to this model that the degree and kind of pre-sleep waking affect determines the form of the dream and the functionality of the dream[53]. If the pre-sleep affect is highly negative, the dream might be repetitive with poor quality of 'dream work', and the morning mood will be unchanged. Cartwright suggested that the content of dreams stored in the emotional memory network related to previous experience. Hartmann[59] introduced additional psychological variables such as 'thick' and 'thin' boundaries.

To summarize, the current understanding of the function of dreams is their possible role in searching for solutions and problem solving in normal mental activity and producing maladaptive or even deviated affects in cases of mental pathology.

DREAMS AND PSYCHOPATHOLOGY

Common sense is that dreams reflect mental disorder. 'Crazy' people are supposed to have 'crazy' dreams. The assumption was that if we uncover the secrets of dreams we will find out about insanity. After the discovery of the REM stage, the assumption was that hallucinations and psychosis are REM sleep spilled over into daytime.

Detailed investigations demonstrated that this is not true and these logical theories became a history of beautiful fairytales. Another misconception was based on the confusion between the psychopathology of dreams (meaning abnormal content or nightmares) vs. dreams of patients in psychopathological states (meaning dreams of patients with a mental disorder).

It is now widely accepted that the bizarreness of dream content is a common feature of a perfectly normal person, and a patient with a mental disorder could have a perfectly realistic dream. It is not the dream content but the attitude and interpretations of it by the dreamer that might indicate the presence of psychosis[60]. Kramer, in his review[28], presented descriptions of peculiarities of dreams in different mental disorders. In schizophrenia, for example, dreams were reported to be more primitive; more alienated; less complex; more direct; more sexual, anxious and hostile; and more bizarre and implausible, with the same degree of hallucinations and paranoia as in an awake state (contrary to Freud's compensatory view[11]). The most frequent personage in dreams was a stranger. Schizophrenics were less interested in dream reporting and the interpretation of their significance.

Dream content in depression was studied most intensively because of a natural expectation to find clear connections between dreams and the clinical picture. In approximately 20 studies, the conclusion was that a depressed person dreamed as frequently as a non-depressed person, but the dreams were shorter and had a paucity of traumatic depressive content even after depression was lifted. When hostility was present, it could be directed at or away from the dreamer. In schizophrenia it was directed only at the dreamer. Depressed people, as expected, have more dreams of failure and misfortune. Unexpectedly depressed people have less dream recall both in and out of the laboratory, contrary to previous beliefs[24]. Low dream recall was found to be associated with mania. Dreams of unipolar depressed in-patients were described as mundane and dreams of depressed hospitalized patients were described as trivial. Bipolar patients, before their shift to mania, recalled dreams with bizarre themes related to death and injury. It is interesting that masochism in dreams of depressed divorced women was associated with poor treatment outcome but aggressive dreams coincided with good outcome. This was first noted by Beck in the 1960s[61] and then confirmed in later studies[67,68]. Depressed people in their dreams were predominantly past oriented, but patients with PTSD were past and present focused.

The most important implications of findings about dreams in depressed and anxious patients were that the content of the dream might have prognostic implications.

The more masochistic, past directed, anxious and disorganized the dream, the poorer the expected outcome. The more active, aggressive, hostile – in short, the more increased affect – the better the dreamer's coping capacity, and the better the chances for recovery.

These data confirm Kramer's hypothesis of 'the selective mood regulatory function of dreaming' and Rotenberg's 'search–activity' concept[28]. In approximately 63 studies of dreams in PTSD patients (military and civilian traumas) dreaming was usually disturbed by daytime 'flashbacks'. Ross and co-workers[62] believed that the dreams in PTSD were vivid, emotional, stereotyped and almost specific to PTSD. They also believed that PTSD was a disorder of REM mechanisms[62]. Kramer states that in PTSD dreams are disturbed more than sleep architecture. Disturbed dreams usually occur early at night but it was later suggested that dreams in PTSD are not stage bound and might occur in REM and NREM. The hallmark of dreams in PTSD is that they occur early at night, accompanied by somatic responses such as sweating, arousals and an increased startle response.

Another important feature of the dreams in PTSD is that they are not as disturbing as has been assumed. Taub and colleagues[63] pointed out that REM nightmares are not as intense as night terrors, although anxiety is often present in poorly adjusted survivors. There is extensive literature on types of dreams including re-enactment dreams and meaningless dreams with terror (similar to night terrors). Siegel[64] described 'miracle dreams' in the Holocaust survivors in which a dead relative told them not to give up while in the death camp. Again, focus on the past, anxiety and disorganized dreams with terror were associated with poor adjustment while active and aggressive dreams coincided with better adjustment.

Dream research in PTSD continues to exist but is far from conclusive. The fact that the hallmark of PTSD is a disturbance in the early night points out the involvement of slow-wave sleep (NREM) mechanisms possibly even more than REM sleep. It reminds us of the importance of NREM mechanisms in survival just as the REM stage does.

In Kramer's review of dreams and pathology[28], he stated that dreams might be used in the psychotherapy of many psychiatric disorders including PTSD, depression, alcoholism, eating disorders, organic brain syndromes and even mental retardation.

Sleep, dreams and sudden death

The tranquility of slow-wave sleep is abruptly disrupted several times a night by major changes in brain physiology that cause REM sleep and dreaming (REM stage). In cardiovascular disease, serious consequences may be precipitated by the intense alterations in autonomic activity which accompany dreaming, especially in the late REM stage.

Sudden cardiac death, defined as unexpected death within 1 h of onset of symptoms, occurs during the nocturnal period at an annual rate of 36 000 people in the USA. The impact of sleep may be underestimated by these statistics, since the final early morning bout of intensely phasic REM sleep could initiate coronary plaque disruption, with death delayed until wakefulness.

Clinical reports have provided evidence that REM sleep and dreams play an even greater role in precipitating myocardial infarction and sudden death in patients already afflicted with coronary disease, myocardial infarction or heart failure, and in patients with respiratory disorders ranging from snoring to central and obstructive sleep apnea. This is also true in patients with the pause-dependent long QT syndrome or at risk for sudden infant death as well as in Southeast Asians ('sudden unexpected death').

In regard to physiological and pathophysiological mechanisms responsible for cardiac death in sleep and especially during REM-related dreaming we could summarize as follows:

(1) Central and peripheral autonomic nervous systems have significant influences on cardiac electrical stability in sleep;

(2) Sleep states could induce ventricular arrhythmias;

(3) Patients with nocturnal ischemia and angina: recent studies indicate that mental arousal is a common trigger mechanism of transient myocardial ischemia. It is also widely acknowledged that there is a significant frequency of spontaneous ischemia and angina during the nocturnal period. It has been estimated that 8% to 10% of ischemic attacks and angina occur during sleep. The REM phase of sleep is particularly vulnerable to angina and ST-segment abnormalities. This stage is characterized by increased heart rate and blood pressure, sympathetic nervous system activity and plasma catecholamines.

Dreams could induce sudden death

The belief that dreams can cause sudden cardiac demise is imbedded in folklore and medical history. The experience of being awakened by vivid, frightening dreams, with racing pulse, cold sweat and other physiological responses associated with intense distress, is common. There are documented 'extensive rises in blood pressure during sleep, increased heart action, changes in respiration, and various reflex effects' which exhibit a 'suddenness of development'[65]. These pioneering studies have been substantiated by evidence of heightened autonomic activity associated with dreams.

The impact of dreaming on the heart is most dramatic during night terrors and nightmares. In the former case, there is a partial arousal in panic from stages 3 and 4 of slow-wave sleep, with marked tachycardia and tachypnea without recall dreaming. Nightmares can be precipitated during slow-wave sleep, when they are characterized by pure fear without visual hallucination, or in REM sleep, when vivid and frightening dreams have been reported.

The most striking association between dreaming and sudden death has been observed in Southeast Asians, in whom there is high incidence of sudden, unexplained nocturnal deaths in young (aged 25–44 years), apparently healthy males. Sudden arousal from sleep could be a trigger for life-threatening arrhythmias[66].

CONCLUSION

Dreams have become an important field of science and medicine. Current advances in monitoring and analytical technology help to gain insights about intimate mechanisms of sleep, dreams and body changes in the norm and in disorders. This knowledge could bring new hopes in treatments and prevention of life-threatening diseases.

References

1. Kasatkin VN. *Theory of Dreams*. Leningrad: Nauka, 1983 [Russian]
2. Grott NY. Cited in Shepovalikov AN. *Activity of the Sleeping Brain*. Leningrad: Nauka, 1971:173 [Russian]
3. Shepovalnikov AN. *How to Order Dreams*. St Petersburg: Lenistat, 1987:151
4. LaBerge S. Dreaming and consciousness. In Hameroff SR, Kaszniak AW, Scott AC, eds. *Toward a Science of Consciousness II*. Cambridge, MA: MIT Press, 1998
5. Hall C. Do we dream during sleep? Evidence for the goblet hypothesis. *Percept Mot Skills* 1981;53:239–46

6. Aserinsky E, Kleitman N. Regularly occurring periods of eye motility and concomitant phenomena during sleep. *Science* 1953;118:273–4

7. Pivik RT. Sleep physiology and psychophysiology. In Coles MGH, Donchin E, Porger SW, eds. *Psychophysiology: Systems, Processes and Applications*. New York: Guilford Press, 2000

8. Foulkes D. Nonrapid eye movement mentation. *Exp Neurol* 1967;19(Suppl 4):28–38

9. Dement W, Kleitman N. The relation of eye movements during sleep to dream: an objective method for the study of dreaming. *J Exp Psychol* 1957;53:339

10. Foulkes D. *Children's Dreams*. New York: Wiley, 1982;275

11. Freud S. *The Interpretation of Dreams*. New York: Basic Books, 1955 (original date 1900)

12. Hobson A, McCarley R. The brain as a dream state generator: an activation synthesis hypothesis of the dream process. *Am J Psychiatry* 1977;134:1335–48

13. Ellman SJ, Spielman AJ, Luck D, et al. REM deprivation: a review. In Ellman SJ, Antrobus JS, eds. *The Mind in Sleep*. Erlbaum edition, 1978; John Wiley, 1991

14. Olds J. Hypothalamic substrates of reward. *Physiol Rev* 1962;42:554–604

15. Antrobus JS. Dreaming: cognitive processes during cortical activation and high afferent thresholds. *Psychol Rev* 1991;98:96–121

16. Goel V, Gold B, Kapur S, et al. Neuroanatomical correlates of human reasoning. *J Cognitive Neurosci* 1998;10:293–302

17. Baddely A. Recent developments in working memory. *Curr Opin Neurobiol* 1998;8:234–8

18. Hobson JA, Pace-Schott EF, Stickgold R. Dreaming and the brain: toward a cognitive neuroscience of conscious states. *Behav Brain Sci* 2000;23:793–842

19. Braun AR, Balkin TJ, Wesenten FG, et al. Dissociated patterns of activity in visual cortices and their projections during human rapid eye movement sleep. *Science* 1998;279:91–5

20. Solms M. Dreaming and REM sleep are controlled by different brain mechanisms. *Behav Brain Sci* 2000;23:843–50

21. Antrobus JS, Kondo T, Reinsel R, et al. Dreaming in the late morning: summation of REM and diurnal cortical activation. *Consciousness Cogn* 1995;4:275–99

22. Greenberg R, Pearlman Ch. An integrated approach to dream theory: contributions from sleep research and clinical practice. In Moffitt A, Kramer M, Hoffmann R, eds. *The Function of Dreaming*. Albany, NY: State University of New York Press, 1993:363–80

23. Cohen DB, Cox C. Neuroticism in the sleep laboratory: implications for representational and adaptive properties of dreaming. *J Abnorm Psychol* 1975;84:91–108

24. Kahan TL, LaBerge S. Cognitive, affective, and sensory characteristics of events sampled from REM sleep, NREM sleep, and waking. *Sleep* 2003;26:A89

25. Reiser MF. The dream in contemporary psychiatry. *Am J Psychiatry* 2001;158:351–9

26. Nofzinger EA, Mintun MA, Wiseman MB, et al. Forebrain activation in REM sleep: an FDG PET study. *Brain Res* 1997;770:192–201

27. Panksepp J. *Affective Neuroscience: The Foundations of Human and Animal Emotions*. New York: Oxford University Press, 1998

28. Kramer M. The selective mood regulatory function of dreaming: an update and revision. In Moffitt A, Kramer M, Hoffmann R, eds. *The Function of Dreaming*. Albany, NY: State University of New York Press, 1993;139–96

29. Desjardins S, Marcotte E, Zadra A. Threat simulation in recurrent dreams. *Sleep* 2003;26:A90

30. Nielsen TA, Deslauriers D, Baylor GW. Emotions in dream and waking event reports. *Dreaming* 1991;1:287–300

31. Cartwright R, Lloyd S. Early REM sleep: a compensatory change in depression? *Psychiatry Res* 1994;51:245–52

32. Cartwright R, Young MA, Mercer P, et al. Role of REM sleep and dream variables in the prediction of remission from depression. *Psychiatry Res* 1998;80:249–55

33. Cartwright R, Luten A, Young M, et al. Role of REM sleep and dream affect in overnight mood regulation: a study of normal volunteers. *Psychiatry Res* 1998;81:1–8

34. Hodoba DD, Hrabrik K, Krmpotic P, et al. Dream recall after night awakenings from tonic/phasic REM sleep. *Sleep* 2003;26:A88

35. Hartmann E. Outline for a theory on the nature and functions of dreaming. *Dreaming* 1996;6:147–70

36. Hartmann E. *The Functions of Sleep*. New Haven, CT: Yale University Press, 1973

37. Gottesmann C. The neurochemistry of waking and sleeping mental activity: the disinhibition–dopamine hypothesis. *Psychiatry Clin Neurosci* 2002;56:345–54

38. Rotenberg VS. Word and image: the problem of context. *Dinamische Psychiatrie/Dynamic Psychiatry* 1979;59:494–8

39. Rotenberg VS. Sleep dreams, cerebral dominance and creation. A new approach to the problem. *Pavlov J Biol Sci* 1985;20:53–8

40. Rotenberg VS, Arshavsky VV. Psychophysiology of hemispheric asymmetry: the 'entropy' of right hemisphere activity. *Integrative Physiological Behav Sci* 1991;26:183–8

41. Hong Ch, Gillin JCh, Dow BM, *et al*. Localized and lateralized cerebral glucose metabolism associated with eye movements during REM sleep and wakefulness: a positron emission tomography (PET) study. *Sleep* 1995;18:570–80

42. Domino G. Process of thinking in dream reports as related to creative achievements. *J Consult Clin Psychol* 1976;44:929–32

43. Sladeczek L, Domino G. Creativity, sleep and primary process thinking in dreams. *J Creative Behav* 1985;19:38–46

44. Lewin F, Glaubmann H. The effects of REM deprivation: is it detrimental, beneficial or neutral? *Psychophysiology* 1975;12:349–53

45. French T, Fromm E. *Dream Interpretation: A New Approach*. New York: Basic Books, 1964

46. Montangero J. Dream, problem solving and creativity. In Cavallero C, Foulkes D, eds. *Dreaming in Cognition*. London: Harvester Wheatsheaf, 1993:93–113

47. Foulkes D. Dream research 1953–1993. *Sleep* 1996;19:609

48. Foulkes D, Vogel G. Mental activity at sleep onset. *J Abnorm Psychol* 1965;70:231

49. Dement W, Kahn E, Roffwarg H. The influence of the laboratory situation on the dreams of the experimental subject. *J Nerv Ment Dis* 1965;140:119

50. Crick F, Mitchison G. The function of dream sleep. *Nature* 1983;304:111–14

51. Hinton GE, Dayan R, Frey BJ, *et al*. The wake–sleep algorhythm for unsupervised neural networks. *Science* 1955;268:1158–61

52. Broughton RJ. NREM arousal parasomnias. In Kryger MH, Roth T, Dement WC, eds. *Principles and Practice of Sleep Medicine*, 3rd edn. Philadelphia: WB Saunders, 2000:693–706

53. Cartwright R. Dreaming in sleep disordered patients. In Chokroverty S. *Sleep Disorders Medicine*, 2nd edn. Boston: Butterworth/Heineman, 1999:127–34

54. Rechtschaffen A, Verdone P, Wheaton J. Reports of mental activity during sleep. *Can Psychiatr Assoc J* 1963;8:409

55. Brown J, Cartwright R. Locating NREM dreaming through instrumental responses. *Psychophysiology* 1978;15:35

56. Snyder F. The phenomenology of dreaming. In Madow L, Snow L, eds. *The Psychodynamic Implications of the Physiological Studies of Dreams*. Springfield, IL: Thomas, 1970:124

57. Dement W. The effect of dream deprivation. *Science* 1960;131:1705

58. Breger L, Hunter I, Lane R. The effect of stress on dreams. *Psychol Issues Monogr* 1971;7:27

59. Hartmann E. *Boundaries of the Mind: A New Psychology of Personality*. New York: Basic Books, 1991

60. Antrobus J. Theories of dreaming. In Kryger MH, Roth T, Dement WC, eds. *Principles and Practice of Sleep Medicine*, 3rd edn. Philadelphia: WB Saunders, 2000:472–81

61. Beck A. *Depression*. New York: Harper & Row, 1967:333

62. Ross R, Ball W, Sullivan K, *et al*. Sleep disturbance as the hallmark of posttraumatic stress disorder. *Am J Psychiatry* 1989;146:697

63. Taub J, Kramer M, Arand D, *et al*. Nightmare dreams and nightmare confabulations. *Compr Psychiatry* 1978;19:285–91

64. Siegel JN. Brainstem mechanism generating REM sleep. In Kryger MH, Roth T, Dement WC, eds. *Principles and Practice of Sleep Medicine*, 3rd edn. Philadelphia: WB Saunders, 2000:112–33

65. Verrier RL, Muller JE, Hobson JA. Sleep, dreams and sudden death: the case for sleep as an autonomic stress test for the heart. *Cardiovasc Res* 1996;31:181–211

66. Kirsconer RH, Eckner FAO, Baron RC. The cardiac pathology in sudden unexplained nocturnal death in Southeast Asian refugees. *J Am Med Assoc* 1986;256:2700–5

67. Cartwright R, Lamberg L. *Crisis Dreaming*. New York: Harper Perennial, 1993

68. Cartwright R, Kravitz AH, Eastman C, *et al*. REM latency and recovery from depression; getting over divorce. *Am J Psychiatry* 1991;148:1530

9

Narcolepsy and daytime sleepiness – the impact on daily life

Sharon L. Merritt

Narcolepsy is a chronic neurological disorder that is characterized by instability in the sleep–wake cycle. People with this disorder experience difficulties in maintaining the usual boundaries of sleep and waking states. Regulation of arousal, non-rapid eye movement (NREM) and rapid eye movement (REM) sleep are all affected[1].

Narcolepsy, the most common neurological cause of excessive daytime sleepiness (EDS), is also manifested by REM sleep phenomena, including cataplexy (weakness or sudden loss of voluntary muscle tone brought on by emotions such as laughter or anger), sleep paralysis (an inability to move while falling asleep or waking up) and hypnagogic/hynopompic hallucinations (vivid sensory hallucinations while falling asleep or waking up that are often terrifying)[2,3]. Besides irresistible sleep attacks (involuntary naps usually lasting less than 30 min) at inappropriate times during waking hours, i.e. while eating, talking on the phone or driving, people with this disorder often experience disrupted nighttime sleep with frequent awakenings. In contrast to people who experience physiological sleepiness during waking hours due to insufficient sleep, the EDS of narcolepsy is only transiently relieved by napping. While people with this disorder awaken feeling refreshed following a nap, within 1–2 h the feeling of irresistible sleepiness returns[2].

The symptom burden of narcolepsy can be very disabling with up to one-half of people with this disorder reporting they experienced difficulties at school, work and/or in their social lives, even when under treatment[4]. In studies using the 36-item Short Form Health Survey, narcoleptic patients reported more difficulty with physical and social functioning and experienced less vitality when scores were compared to normative scores for the general population[5] or healthy controls[6]. Compared to other populations, such as epilepsy and Parkinson's patients, those with narcolepsy experience a symptom burden that is similar to, or worse than, these groups[5].

EPIDEMIOLOGY

The prevalence of narcolepsy is 0.02–0.05% in the USA[7], and is more common than multiple sclerosis[8] and nearly as common as Parkinson's disease[9]. Typically, the symptoms arise in mid-adolescence or young adulthood (although they can emerge in childhood) with EDS usually the first symptom to emerge[10]. In one study of 85 consecutive patients, 59% reported experiencing the symptoms of narcolepsy between the ages of 5 and 15[11]. Cataplexy and the other REM-related symptoms can take months or even years to develop[10]. In the experience of this author, when cataplexy develops quickly following EDS, the individual is likely to have a severe case of narcolepsy that can be more difficult to treat pharmacologically. In children, the presenting symptoms are similar to those in adults[2].

Narcolepsy is an underdiagnosed sleep disorder[12] probably because there is no definitive, unequivocal objective means for confirming the presence of the disorder and, therefore, a positive diagnosis is dependent upon the clinical judgement of the clinician. Many people with this disorder report seeing up to five health-care providers over a span of 12–15 years before receiving the appropriate diagnosis. For example, the disorder can be confused with a psychiatric condition or epilepsy, probably owing to the variability with which presenting symptoms may arise. For example, one young man well known to the Center for Narcolepsy Research was hospitalized in a psychiatric ward because of the frequency and intensity with which he experienced frightening hallucinations concurrent with daily sleep attacks. Another young narcoleptic woman, now in her mid-twenties, was treated with anti-epileptic medication from the age of 9 years until she was appropriately diagnosed at the age of 19 years. When untreated, she experienced frequent daily sleep and cataplexy attacks that probably were misconstrued as a seizure disorder.

GENETICS AND NARCOLEPSY

People with a first-degree relative with narcolepsy have a 1–2% chance of developing this disorder. Even though the risk is low, it is still 20 to 40 times higher than the risk to people in the general population[13]. While familial clustering has been observed, narcolepsy is primarily a sporadically occurring neurological disorder. This information can be somewhat reassuring to young adults with narcolepsy who are considering starting a family.

In 1983 narcolepsy was observed to be associated with the human leukocyte antigen (HLA) DR2[14], a finding that was confirmed in subsequent studies in Europe and North America. While no autoimmune pathological changes associated with the presence of this

antigen were subsequently found, these findings did not rule out the possibility that an autoimmune mechanism existed. Using molecular typing at the DNA level instead of serological antibody testing, Mignot determined that narcolepsy with definitive cataplexy is tightly associated with HLA DQB1 *0602 across ethnic groups, with this allele being the better marker for narcolepsy compared to DR2[15].

However, the use of HLA typing to diagnose this disorder is not recommended, for several reasons. While more than 90% of narcoleptics with definitive cataplexy (episodes of muscle weakness triggered by laughter or anger) are positive, narcolepsy patients without cataplexy or with inconclusive cataplexy (e.g. muscle weakness triggered by excitement) are positive for HLA DQB1*0602 only 40 to 60% of the time. Furthermore, up to one-third of control subjects without narcolepsy are also positive for this marker, and a few narcolepsy patients with clear-cut cataplexy do not have this HLA marker[15]. These findings suggest that narcolepsy is more genetically complex than initially thought and that, in addition to a genetic susceptibility, the disorder probably develops in response to some as yet undetermined environmental trigger(s).

NEUROTRANSMITTER/ RECEPTOR SYSTEMS, HYPOCRETIN AND HUMAN NARCOLEPSY

While the exact pathophysiological mechanisms underlying narcolepsy are still unclear, recent findings are beginning to shed new light on this disorder. EDS and cataplexy have been extensively studied in narcoleptic dogs. EDS may be associated with abnormalities in the mesocorticolimbic dopaminergic systems, particularly dopamine and norephinephrine hypoactivity[16]. Cataplexy and the other REM systems may be explained by a cholinoceptive hypersensitivity in the basal forebrain and brainstem. Both systems are known to participate in REM sleep and have connections to the limbic system, possibly explaining why cataplexy is produced by emotions.

Almost simultaneously, canine narcolepsy, phenotypically similar to human narcolepsy, was reported to be caused by a mutation of the hypocretin-2 receptor in narcoleptic dogs[17], and preprohypocretin (the precursor of the hypocretins) knockout mice were found to display behavioral and sleep EEG characteristics similar to narcolepsy[18]. The hypocretins (hypocretin-1 and hypocretin-2, also referred to as orexins) are neuropeptides secreted by cells located in the lateral and perifornical hypothalamus with widespread projections throughout the brain. Recent animal studies suggested that the hypocretins promote wakefulness and inhibit REM sleep[19].

Hypocretin-1 has been reported to be absent in the spinal fluid of most narcoleptic patients with definitive cataplexy, although this protein was also found to be deficient in some people with other neurological disorders; not all narcoleptics with definitive cataplexy have been found to be deficient in this sleep-modulating neurotransmitter[20]. In postmortem studies Thannickal and coworkers found an 85–95% reduction in the number of hypocretin neurons present in the brains of human narcoleptics, with the presence of gliosis in the hypocretin cell region suggesting that a degenerative process contributed to the cell loss[21]. These findings have created a great deal of interest in neuroscience, with emphasis being placed on the study of normal hypocretin physiological function and how malfunction in this system may lead to abnormal sleep–wake function in narcolepsy and a variety of other conditions[22].

As the science associated with the hypocretin system accumulates, new diagnostic and treatment approaches for narcolepsy may emerge. Currently, a less invasive test to measure the amount of hypocretin-1 that is active in the nervous system is needed to avoid the use of a spinal tap, presently the only way that this measurement can be done accurately. A way to supplement hypocretin-1 deficiency with agonists that can centrally penetrate the nervous system is also needed.

CLINICAL PRESENTATION

The classic symptom tetrad of narcolepsy includes EDS, cataplexy, hypnagogic hallucinations and sleep paralysis, although only about 15% of people with this disorder experience all four symptoms[23]. Because the complaint of disturbed nighttime sleep is so common in people with this disorder, some feel that it should be added to the symptom complex. Generally, EDS is the first symptom to appear, often in combination with hypnagogic hallucinations or sleep paralysis. Symptoms usually develop gradually and it may take several years for other symptoms to develop that were not present initially. While some believe there are only minor fluctuations in the severity of the symptoms once they appear, in the clinical experience of the author they can become more intense in times of anxiety and stress.

Excessive daytime sleepiness

EDS is the main symptom of this disorder and is always present at the time of diagnosis. People may use terms such as feeling 'tired' or 'fatigued' to describe their sleepiness. In general medical literature these terms have been used imprecisely, and have been identified and treated in a small proportion of those affected[24]. Generally, the sleepiness associated with narcolepsy is best characterized by a constant subjective feeling of sleepiness that may fluctuate somewhat during the day, and a tendency to fall asleep periodically during the day even in active situations[25]. However, narcoleptics are especially prone to EDS in more passive situations, e.g. while riding in a car or watching the television. For some, reading a book or the newspaper is all but impossible, owing to involuntary sleep attacks. Consequently, maintaining attention and concentration presents particular difficulties with narcoleptics who often complain that they have memory problems. Additionally, automatic behavior, semipurposeful activity for which the individual is amnesic, can occur during the drowsiness that often precedes a sleep attack.

Because of decreased vigilance, individuals may find they have completed some non-sensical task, such as writing something that is illogical or placing salt in the refrigerator[2]. People with this disorder do not sleep more over a 24 h period but experience more frequent bouts of drowsiness and subsequent sleep periods that usually last less than 30 min and from which they can be awakened[25].

Because of difficulties associated with effective treatment, people with narcolepsy report experiencing stigma and intolerance as a result of their sleepiness. They may be labeled as being lazy and become the brunt of family jokes. They often are advised to 'just get more sleep' or are wrongly accused of not trying to control their sleepiness when neither of these measures would be effective in dealing with this neurological disorder.

Cataplexy

Cataplexy, the loss of voluntary muscle control in response to emotion while the person is conscious, is unique to narcolepsy. It occurs in about 70% of people with this disorder[2] and may be partial or complete. In a partial attack, the muscles of the face and neck are more often affected. During complete attacks, loss of muscle tone in the limbs occurs, and the person may drop to the ground and be unable to move for up to several minutes. Key features of a cataplectic attack are that (1) people are aware of their surroundings during an attack and (2) it is triggered by emotion, with laughter being the most common trigger, although people report that a variety of other emotions bring on cataplexy such as anger, excitement and being startled. Partial attacks may be very subtle and difficult to recognize even by the person who is experiencing them.

A neurological examination conducted during an attack typically shows muscle atonia and a loss of tendon reflexes[25]. However, cataplexy usually cannot be provoked in clinical situations. Some people with narcolepsy learn to recognize emotional circumstances that trigger attacks and report being labeled by others as stoic or withdrawn because they avoid these situations. A very graphic film clip illustrating a cataplexy attack can be viewed at the Stanford University Center for Narcolepsy website (http://www.med.stanford.edu/school/Psychiatry/narcolepsy/cataplexy.html).

Hypnagogic hallucinations

These vivid, dream-like sensory experiences occur during the transition from wakefulness to sleep in about two-thirds of narcoleptics[2] and are often described as scary experiences that seem very real and bizarre to the people who experience them. Visual images predominate although auditory and tactile components have been described[25]. When the hallucinations occur as people are waking up, they are referred to as hypnopompic hallucinations. People can report feeling like they are going crazy and may not admit to these experiences unless they are specifically asked about this symptom. When the probable origin of hypnagogic hallucinations, i.e. the intrusion of REM physiology into wakefulness, is explained to the person who is experiencing them, the individual is often quite relieved to know they are associated with this disorder and early REM sleep onset. Over time some people report being able to recognize when the hallucinations are occurring and find them to be less frightening, even when the content has not changed.

Sleep paralysis

Sleep paralysis is a feeling of being unable to move while falling asleep or waking up that can last for as long as 10 min[25]. About 60% of narcoleptics report experiencing this symptom[2]. Sleep paralysis is often accompanied by hallucinatory experiences. People report feeling like they have to struggle to move and are often quite frightened by the experience, especially by the initial attacks. Since hypnagogic hallucinations may be confused with the nightmares experienced by normal individuals, and sleep paralysis has been found to occur in up to 50% of the general population[26], neither of these symptoms are considered diagnostic of narcolepsy.

Disturbed nighttime sleep

People with narcolepsy often have a short latency to sleep onset but many also report waking up frequently during the night. Disturbed nighttime sleep is a complaint of about 75% of people with narcolepsy[2]. The awakenings are usually of short duration but some people report being awake for hours[25]. The relationship of the awakenings to EDS has not been established, nor has how frequently the awakenings occur in narcolepsy compared to the general population. Interestingly, Rogers and Dreher claimed that none of the usual sleep hygiene measures recommended to treat psychophysiological insomnia are effective in narcoleptics who experience nocturnal sleep disruptions[4].

EVALUATING EXCESSIVE DAYTIME SLEEPINESS

Unrecognized or underestimated EDS is a significant public health problem that compromises public safety and quality of life[27]. The EDS associated with narcolepsy places these people at particular risk for workplace and driving accidents when they remain undiagnosed or improperly treated. Narcoleptics report falling asleep while driving and report a 1.5- to 4-fold higher increase in sleep-related automobile accidents[28,29]. While the costs of sleepiness-related automobile and employment-related accidents in the USA are difficult to estimate, conservative estimates are in the range of billions of dollars per year[30,31]. In addition to public health issues, EDS has a significant impact on the personal quality of life of people with narcolepsy and their families, and includes adverse effects on school and work performance, social relations and mood. Complaints of difficulties with maintaining attention, short-term memory, thinking and learning are common[32–35]. Since success in school or work situations is often dependent on cognitive ability, performance

deficits in academic endeavors and decreased productivity in the workplace can result in school dismissal or loss of employment. The most frequent reasons people report contacting the Center for Narcolepsy Research staff for assistance in obtaining a diagnosis and treatment are near-miss or actual crashes while driving, or the threat of job loss or academic failure due to EDS.

Complaints of EDS are frequently not evaluated by health-care professionals in clinical situations because there have been few tools available to measure or confirm pathological sleepiness[36]. Sleepiness is usually evaluated with objective physiological measurements in conjunction with subjective (introspective) assessments made by the individual in order to fully illustrate the problems with sleepiness. However, the association between objective and subjective sleepiness measures is usually low, or moderate at best, even when statistically significant, possibly because the subjective measure may not adequately reflect the individual's propensity to fall asleep or the sleepiness is being underreported[37]. Nevertheless, subjective measures are used to capture dimensions that cannot be illustrated by objective measures.

Objective sleepiness measures

In addition to a complete history and physical examination, the objective polygraphic measures used to diagnose sleep disorders, including narcolepsy, are nocturnal polysomnography (PSG) and the Multiple Sleep Latency Test (MSLT). The PSG provides information about the quality and quantity of sleep, and is used with suspected narcoleptics to rule out the presence of another concurrent sleep disorder that may be contributing to EDS, such as sleep disordered breathing or periodic leg movement. In narcoleptics the PSG usually demonstrates a short latency to sleep onset (< 10 min), a short REM latency (< 20 min) and a poor sleep efficiency with sleep fragmentation and increased stage 1 sleep[2,25,38].

The MSLT is used to aid in determining the cause and extent of EDS when narcolepsy is suspected. Within the past 15 years, the accepted 'gold' standard for the measurement of sleepiness has been the MSLT[39-41]. The MSLT measures physiological sleep tendencies in the absence of alerting stimuli. The person lies down during the day in a quiet, darkened room for four or five nap opportunities scheduled at 2-h intervals from 10:00 a.m. to 6:00 p.m. and is instructed to try to go to sleep. For each nap the latency (time) to sleep onset is evaluated. Additionally, the presence or absence of a REM sleep period within 15 min of sleep onset is also noted. Mean sleep latency scores of 10 min or more are considered to be normal; mean scores of 5 min or less are considered to be in the pathological range and scores of 5–10 min are considered to be abnormal or borderline[39]. Sleep latency measures indicate the severity of the physiological tendency to fall asleep; the underlying cause of the sleepiness may be due to any of several sleep disorders or due to sleep deprivation. However, the presence of two or more sleep-onset REM periods are considered diagnostic of narcolepsy when accompanied by a mean sleep latency from the naps of 5–8 min[26,42].

The Maintenance of Wakefulness Test (MWT) is another polygraphically based objective sleepiness measure that is conducted in a manner similar to the MSLT except that individuals are seated during testing and instructed to try to stay awake[43]. The MWT cannot be used to diagnose narcolepsy since sleep-onset REM periods are much less likely to occur in the sitting position. Recent norms suggested that a mean sleep latency of < 11 min is considered abnormal[44]. Results comparing the individual's ability to go to sleep versus staying awake on these two tests have proved to be discordant[45]. Some experts consider the MWT to be a more ecologically sound test, especially when one is interested in documenting response to treatment, in that it more closely mirrors the sedentary real-life situations in which people are required to maintain wakefulness as well as the outcome of interest – the ability to stay awake. However, like the MSLT, it is expensive to administer,

since a nocturnal PSG is required the evening before testing, inconvenient for the patient, technically demanding and often not covered by health insurers.

Subjective sleepiness measures

In clinical practice, level of alertness is often measured with a visual analog scale (VAS)[46], the Stanford Sleepiness Scale (SSS)[47] or the Epworth Sleepiness Scale (ESS)[48], even though their association with objective measures is likely to be low to moderate. With the VAS, subjects are asked to quantify their current feelings of sleepiness or alertness on a 10-cm line with the low end of the scale being very sleepy and the high end being very alert. The SSS consists of seven items spanning gradations in feelings of alertness from 'wide awake' to 'cannot stay awake'. Responses to these items were validated against objective performance measures in a sleep deprivation experiment. The ESS is a widely used, self-administered inventory on which subjects rate how likely they were to fall asleep (0 = never to 3 = high) in recent times under eight different common life experiences, e.g. while reading or watching television (Table 9.1)[48]. Scores are obtained by summing the rating assigned to each item. Scores can range from 0 to 24 with a score of > 10 indicating moderate sleepiness and ≥ 15 indicating severe sleepiness. The experiences offered are those cited often by persons with confirmed pathological sleepiness as sleep-inducing ones[49]. The observations of a significant other regarding the sleepiness exhibited by a particular patient can also be recorded on the ESS, and may be helpful in situations where the extent of sleepiness is not clearly recognized by the individual being examined. Decreases in ESS sleepiness ratings following treatment have been demonstrated in patients with narcolepsy[50].

The usefulness of these subjective measures has been limited chiefly to describing the subjective perceptions of sleepiness rather than diagnosing and managing sleep disorders. Although the VAS and the SSS may give an

Table 9.1 Epworth Sleepiness Scale (ESS)[48]

Directions: How likely are you to doze off or fall asleep in the following situations, in contrast to feeling just tired? This refers to your usual way of life in recent times. Even if you have not done some of these things recently, try to work out how they would have affected you. Use the following scale to rate your chance of dozing in each situation. *Circle* the correct number to indicate your chance of dozing for each item below.

0 = would never doze
1 = slight chance of dozing
2 = moderate chance of dozing
3 = high chance of dozing

		Circle below:		
1. Sitting and reading	0	1	2	3
2. Watching television	0	1	2	3
3. Sitting, inactive in a public place (e.g. a theater or a meeting)	0	1	2	3
4. As a passenger in a car for an hour without a break	0	1	2	3
5. Lying down to rest in the afternoon when circumstances permit	0	1	2	3
6. Sitting and talking to someone	0	1	2	3
7. Sitting quietly after a lunch without alcohol	0	1	2	3
8. In a car, while stopped for a few minutes in the traffic	0	1	2	3

Reproduced with permission from Johns MW. A new method for measuring daytime sleepiness: the Epworth Sleepiness Scale. *Sleep* 1991;14:540–5

indication of the immediate feeling of sleepiness and can be used to assess sleepiness repeatedly during a short time frame, their reliability in chronically sleepy patients has been questioned[51]. One concern is that the reference points of 'very sleepy' or 'very alert' may be totally different for persons who have experienced EDS for some time, especially when compared to individuals with no sleep deprivation or those who are experiencing an acute, short-term episode. The validity of the SSS has been questioned in view of reports that behaviorally sleepy individuals often evaluate themselves as highly alert[52]. Compared to the VAS and the SSS, the ESS assesses chronic sleepiness but fails to provide a specific timeframe in which the respondents are to rate their propensity to fall asleep (e.g. the last week or the last month) making comparisons between subjects difficult. Additionally, the ESS cannot be used repeatedly during the day, or in the presence of an acute sleep loss that might stimulate a short-term propensity for sleepiness[53].

DIAGNOSING NARCOLEPSY

The current, widely accepted diagnostic criteria for narcolepsy are listed in Table 9.2[26] and are considered a sufficient guide for prescribing medication treatment[25]. The diagnosis is based primarily on the symptoms presented during a thorough clinical interview that includes a comprehensive sleep–wake history and a physical examination with polysomnographic testing used to confirm the clinical diagnostic impression and rule out the presence of another intrinsic sleep disorder[54]. When cataplexy is clearly present, the diagnosis is less complex since this symptom is specific for narcolepsy. However, excessive daytime sleepiness with sleep attacks alone is not specific since these symptoms can be present for a wide variety of sleep disorders,

Table 9.2 International Classification of Sleep Disorders diagnostic criteria for narcolepsy[26]

Symptoms
(1) A complaint of excessive sleepiness or muscle weakness.
(2) Almost daily recurring naps or lapses into sleep for at least the past 3 months.
(3) Sudden bilateral loss of postural muscle tone that occurs with intense emotion (cataplexy).
(4) Associated features including:
    (a) Sleep paralysis
    (b) Hypnagogic hallucinations
    (c) Automatic behavior
    (d) Disrupted consolidated sleep

NPSG and the MSLT
(5) Polysomnographic findings include one or more of the following:
    (a) NPSG sleep latency of < 10 min
    (b) NPSG REM sleep latency of < 20 min
    (c) A mean sleep latency on the 4–5 MSLT naps of < 5 min
    (d) Two or more sleep-onset REM sleep periods

Other criteria
(6) Positive on (HLA) typing for DQB1*0602 or DR2.
(7) No other medical or mental disorder accounts for the symptoms.
(8) Other sleep disorders may be present but do not constitute the primary reason for the symptoms.

Minimum criteria: 2 plus 3, or 1 plus 4 plus 5 plus 7

NPSG, nocturnal polysomnography; MSLT, Multiple Sleep Latency Test; REM, rapid eye movement; HLA, human leukocyte antigen. Data derived from American Sleep Disorders Association. *International Classification of Sleep Disorders, Revised: Diagnostic and Coding Manual*. Rochester, MN, 1997, see page 29

and accompany other medical problems. Some advocate, even when cataplexy is present, that people must demonstrate a pathological sleep latency on the MSLT and the presence of ≥ 2 sleep-onset REM periods for the diagnosis of narcolepsy to be made[3]. However, this is controversial since studies have demonstrated that only 84% of patients with EDS and cataplexy met the ≥ 2 sleep-onset REM period criterion[55]. Likewise, only 84% of narcolepsy subjects with EDS, definitive cataplexy and no detectable hypocretin-1 in their spinal fluid meet this criterion[20]. Additionally, some clinicians consider the early appearance of REM on a nocturnal PSG as meeting the requirement for one of the sleep-onset REM periods[26], while others believe that both REM sleep periods must occur during MSLT testing.

Narcolepsy is probably a more heterogeneous disorder than it was once considered to be. The variability in symptoms with which patients can present may represent a disorder that is in different stages of evolving, or a disorder that is more appropriately described along a continuum of symptoms. Since the International Classification of Sleep Disorders is currently under revision by experts in the discipline of sleep, it will be interesting to see how the current diagnostic criteria for narcolepsy are applied, or whether they are changed, in the next sleep disorder classification.

PHARMACOLOGICAL TREATMENT

Narcolepsy is treated symptomatically with central nervous systems (CNS) stimulants to control EDS, and antidepressants to control cataplexy and the other REM-related symptoms as needed. Many patients experience only mild-to-moderate REM symptoms or experience them infrequently so that antidepressant therapy may not be necessary. The brain mechanisms hypothesized to generate REM sleep and cataplexy, and promote wakefulness, form the basis for the selection of these compounds (Figure 9.1)[15].

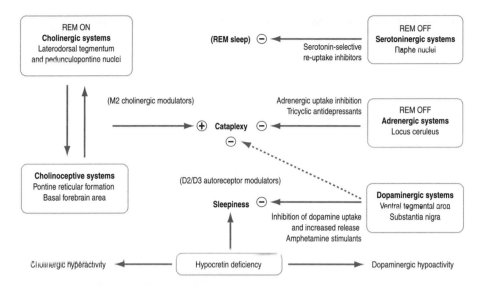

Figure 9.1 Hypothesized neuropharmacological and neurochemical model of cataplexy and excessive daytime sleepiness. Reproduced with permission from Mignot E. Pathophysiology of narcolepsy. In Kryger MH, Roth T, Dement WC, eds. *Principles and Practice of Sleep Medicine*, 3rd edn. Philadelphia: WB Saunders, 2000:663–75

Stimulants

Wake-promoting medications (stimulants and related compounds) are the usual treatment for controlling EDS in narcolepsy. Standards of practice for the use of stimulants as well as other sources cite those listed in Table 9.3 as effective in improving alertness in narcolepsy, although the effects in individual patients can be unpredictable[4,56–59] (Table 9.3). Besides dosage ranges and side-effects, use in pregnancy is included, since this is a frequent concern of young women with narcolepsy who desire to start a family. The goal of therapy is to alleviate sleepiness and allow return of the patient to the fullest possible normal function without the development of significant side-effects.

Modafinil is a novel wake-promoting agent developed in France and approved for use in the USA in 1998 to treat the sleepiness associated with narcolepsy. This compound is chemically distinct from the traditional CNS stimulants; in animals, wakefulness is promoted without the concomitant increase in locomotor activity seen in stimulants[50,58]. While the exact mechanism of action is unknown, it requires an intact α_1-adrenergic system and

has a highly selective activity in the CNS compared to the classic stimulants[50,58]. Modafinil appears to be the first drug of choice in newly diagnosed narcoleptics possibly because of its lower side-effect profile. On average modafinil has slightly fewer alerting effects than the classic stimulants and can be somewhat difficult to use with people who have been on these latter medications. When switched from traditional stimulants to this compound, people need to be informed that (1) modafinil has a more gradual onset of action so they are less likely to experience the burst of wakefulness seen with traditional stimulants; and (2) it is also longer acting so they are less likely to experience the 'sudden crashes' common with the other stimulant medications. The most common side-effect is headache that seems to dissipate with use and can be ameliorated by a gradual initiation of this compound, i.e. administration of 100 mg per day for several days before a gradual titration upwards.

Owing to a potential for causing liver damage, pemoline currently seems to be used as the last option when other compounds have not been effective or tolerated. When prescribed, frequent monitoring of liver function is required[57].

133

Table 9.3 Pharmacological therapy for sleepiness

Medication (Trade name, DEA class)	Usual adult daily dose range; maximum (mg)	Common side-effects	Pregnancy category*
Modafinil (Provigil®, IV)	100–400; 800	Headache, nausea, diarrhea, dry mouth, anorexia	C
Pemoline (Cylert®, IV)	37.5–75; 150	Hepatotoxicity, insomnia, hallucinations, anorexia, weight loss	B
Methylphenidate (Ritalin®, Ritalin SR®, Concerta SR®, II)	30–60; 100	Nervousness, insomnia, anorexia, nausea, dizziness, hypertension, hypotension, tachycardia, headache	Not established
D-amphetamine (Dexedrine®, Dexedrine SR®, Dextrostat®, II)	30–60; 100	Insomnia, restlessness, tachycardia, dizziness, diarrhea, constipation, hypertension, impotence	C
L/D Amphetamine (Adderall®, II)	30–60; 100	Same as D-amphetamine	C
Methamphetamine (Desoxyn®, II)	40; 80	Same as D-amphetamine	C

SR, sustained release. *Pregnancy categories: A, controlled human studies have shown no risk to the human fetus in the first trimester and the possibility of fetal harm is remote; B, no fetal risk in animal studies and no controlled human studies; C, teratogenic or embryocidal effects in animal studies and no controlled human studies; D, evidence of risk to human fetuses but possible benefits may make risks acceptable; X, animal or human studies demonstrate fetal abnormalities and risks outweigh benefits

Methylphenidate may be the most frequently prescribed stimulant for narcoleptics. Studies of narcoleptics using stimulants found that about 50% of the samples were using this compound[60,61]. Methylphenidate is an indirectly acting sympathomimetic that increases the amount of monoamine available within the synaptic cleft of monoamine synapses in the CNS, and blocks the reuptake and enhances the release of norepinephrine, dopamine and serotonin[62]. Common side-effects associated with this compound that can be intolerable to some patients include headache, irritability, anorexia, gastrointestinal complaints, palpitations and disturbed sleep.

The amphetamine compounds inhibit the storage of dopamine and to a lesser extent that of norephinephrine and serotonin, and increase the synaptic release of these mono-amines, but they have little inhibiting effect on dopamine reuptake[59]. Consequently, non-vesicated dopamine is available at the synaptic cleft producing a strong initial effect after administration, but presynaptically dopamine is depleted. Rebound hypersomnolence may result as the compounds are depleted because the dopamine required for wakefulness needs to be resynthesized. Narcoleptics may value the burst of wakefulness they experience after ingesting these compounds, but some are unable to tolerate the nervousness and irritability they can induce, and find the rebound hypersomnolence and crashing effect as the effects wear off to be particularly troubling.

Treatment of EDS usually starts with a low dose of medication that is titrated upward if adequate relief of this symptom is not achieved. Combination therapy is increasingly being tried with a longer acting preparation being used in combination with one that has a shorter half-life, e.g. modafinil with a shorter acting stimulant, or a sustained-release preparation with a regular acting one. Supplementation is not unusual with people on longer acting preparations using a lower dose of a shorter acting one in mid-afternoon if they have an activity planned for later in the day that requires their alertness to be maintained for a longer period. Tolerance to a particular dose or medication can develop over time, requiring an increase in dose or a change in medication.

The objective of treatment is the adequate relief of EDS allowing narcoleptics to return to normal function at work, school and home. However, the relative effectiveness of these compounds in individual patients can be variable. Using published polygraphic data on normal individuals as well as polygraphic studies of the effectiveness of stimulant treatment in narcolepsy, one group of investigators concluded that there is clinical improvement in narcoleptics' sleepiness with these compounds[63]. However, the narcoleptic subjects achieved an average alertness level of only between 50 and 70% of normal controls on the MSLT or MWT: 60 mg methyphenidate, 70% of the alertness level of normals[64]; 40–60 mg methamphetamine, 68%[65]; 60 mg dextroamphetamine, 65%[64]; 200 mg modafinil, 50%[50]; and 112.5 mg pemoline, about 50%[64]. While less sleepy, the narcoleptics were not improved by stimulant treatment to alertness levels comparable to normal control subjects[66,67]. Currently, the undertreatment of EDS in narcolepsy may relate to a reliance on self-reported improvement in EDS to determine the effectiveness of treatment, and concerns that tolerance and drug dependency will develop unless the use of stimulants is limited[68]. Narcoleptics who have been chronically pathologically sleepy may feel subjectively alert when stimulants are prescribed because their frame of reference is a very drowsy state that may have persisted for years[65]. In a large national survey of treated and untreated narcoleptics who were randomly selected from the membership rolls of the American Narcolepsy Association, no significant differences were found between these two groups in the frequency with which the somnolent symptoms were perceived to be experienced. At least 50% of both groups felt that the EDS of narcolepsy moderately or severely interfered with their ability to carry out their activities of daily living[60].

Antidepressants

In contrast to the somnolent symptoms, cataplexy and the other REM symptoms are usually effectively treated with antidepressants because of their REM-suppressing effects (Table 9.4)[4,56-59,69]. These agents vary in the primary neurochemical system affected, with some acting primarily on norepinephrine and others on serotonin[59]. Venlafaxine is an andrenergic/serotonergic re-uptake inhibitor that is available as an extended release or regular acting preparation and appears to have good treatment success. The tricyclic antidepressants commonly used include clomipramine, imipramine and protriptyline, and may be effective in controlling the REM symptoms in lower doses than those used to treat depression. Recently, because of the tricyclic side-effects, particularly sedation, sexual dysfunction and delayed ejaculation and impotence in men, the selective serotonin reuptake inhibitors such as viloxazine hydrochloride and fluoxetine are being used even though they may be less effective than the tricyclic agents and venlafaxine[70].

People on antidepressants need to be warned that rebound cataplexy can occur if these medications are reduced or discontinued. Since the side-effect profile varies somewhat between the compounds, another agent should be tried rather than continuing with one that has very unpleasant side-effects.

Sodium oxybate, often referred to as γ-hydroxybutyrate (GHB), is an old compound that was originally used for its hypnotic properties, and was approved for use in the USA in July 2002 for its effectiveness in reducing cataplexy attacks by a median of 80–90%[71]. This very short acting compound comes in liquid form with the initial dose taken at bedtime and a second dose in the middle of the night. While improvement is seen in 1–2 weeks, several months of treatment may be needed for its full effects to be reached[59]. The exact mechanism of action is unknown. GHB has been shown to be effective in reducing disturbed nighttime sleep and increasing slow-wave sleep. The ESS

Table 9.4 Pharmacological therapy for cataplexy and the other REM dissociation symptoms[4,56–59, 69]

Medication (Trade name, DEA class)	Usual adult daily dose range	Common side-effects	Pregnancy category*
Venlafaxine, adrenergic/ serotonergic re-uptake inhibitor (Effexor®, Effexor SR®)	75–225 mg	Asthenia, sweating, dizziness, insomnia, somnolence, nervousness, dry mouth, anorexia, nausea, constipation, abnormal ejaculation/ impotence	C
Protriptyline – non-sedating TCA (Vivactil®)	10–60 mg	Anticholinergic effects (dry mouth, blurred vision, constipation at high doses), agitation, anxiety, tachycardia, hypotension, weight gain, sexual dysfunction	Not established
Clomipramine, TCA (Anafranil®)	25–150 mg	Same as protriptyline	C
Imipramine, TCA (Tofranil®)	25–150 mg	Same as protriptyline	Not established
Fluoxetine, SSRI (Prozac®)	20–60 mg	Asthenia, nausea, diarrhea, anorexia, insomnia, anxiety, nervousness, somnolence	C
Paroxetine, SSRI (Paxil®)	20–60 mg	Asthenia, sweating, nausea, somnolence, dizziness, insomnia, tremor, abnormal ejaculation	C
Sodium oxybate, hypnotic (Xyrem®, III)	3–9 g, divided dose, twice nightly	Dizziness, headache, nausea, somnolence, confusion, enuresis	B

SR, sustained release; TCA, tricyclic antidepressant; SSRI, selective serotonin reuptake inhibitor. *Pregnancy categories: A, controlled human studies show no risk to the human fetus in the first trimester and the possibility of fetal harm is remote; B, no fetal risk in animal studies and no controlled human studies; C, teratogenic or embryocidal effects in animal studies and no controlled human studies; D, evidence of risk to human fetuses but possible benefits may make risks acceptable; X, animal or human studies demonstrate fetal abnormalities, and risks outweigh benefits. Data derived from references 4, 56–59 and 69

scores improved to the normal range for a substantial number of subjects at the 6 g or 9 g dose in the original clinical trial[72]. However, 85% of the subjects remained on their usual stimulant medication in addition to taking sodium oxybate. Another trial is underway to determine the effectiveness of this compound on EDS.

Adherence

In one published study only 39% of the people with narcolepsy who were on dextroamphetamine or methylphenidate took the amount of medication prescribed, while about 88% of those on pemoline correctly took their medication[73]. Adherence was assessed using a screening questionnaire, sleep diaries and medical records. Twenty-two out of the 43 patients reduced their dosage or did not take any stimulant medication in a 24-h period. People who showed better wakefulness on 24-h ambulatory recordings were no more likely to take their prescribed stimulant medication than those who were less responsive and showed more daytime sleepiness. These findings are consistent with data across a variety of conditions showing that prescribed medication non-adherence varies from 15 to 93% with an average rate of 50%[74,75]. The prevalent pattern is underdosing by taking 'drug holidays', or taking less medication than prescribed. Among people with narcolepsy, underdosing may be due to intolerance of the stimulant side-effects or addiction concerns, although the reasons for non-adherence have not been determined. These finding suggest that narcoleptics need to be asked whether they are having any difficulties with their medications, and providers need to be open to working with patients who are having problems by trying a different medication, dose or schedule. People who contact the Center for Narcolepsy Research staff often report doing so because the person supervising their care is unwilling to listen to their difficulties, or unwilling to try other pharmacological approaches. It can take many experiential trials before the person is able to reach the quality of life desired with adequate symptom control and tolerable medication side-effects.

BEHAVIORAL THERAPIES FOR MANAGING NARCOLEPSY SYMPTOMS

Limited scientific evidence is available that people with narcolepsy can control their symptoms by using behavioral strategies. Nevertheless, people with this disorder are often advised to adopt certain practices, some of which apply to the general population and are consistent with promoting a healthy lifestyle for all individuals.

Structured sleep schedules

Practicing good sleep habits is a frequent recommendation. However, evidence is lacking that EDS and the other symptoms of narcolepsy are under better control when people with this disorder follow two recommendations commonly associated with good sleep hygiene, namely (1) sleep at least 8 h a day; and (2) maintain a consistent time for waking up and retiring every day of the week[76].

Combining frequent, short, scheduled naps (up to five 15-min naps throughout the day) may be helpful in relieving the subjective feelings of sleepiness. However, it is unclear that planned napping reduces or eliminates unscheduled napping, or is more effective when combined with stimulants than using stimulants alone[4]. People with more severe symptoms may receive the most benefit from napping[77]. In one study, long naps of 120 min were effective in maintaining alertness for about 3 h[78]. While narcoleptics report feeling refreshed for about an hour even following brief naps, nap therapy alone to control EDS is usually not effective and, depending upon the frequency and length required by the individual, can be unrealistic to follow. Planning school, work or lifestyle schedules around napping can be difficult.

Dietary modifications

People with this disorder often ask if they can improve their symptoms by altering their diet. In a questionnaire study twice as many narcoleptics compared to controls reported eating daytime snacks between meals and at bedtime, craving sweets and feeling sleepy after regular and big meals[79]. People with narcolepsy may be more sensitive to the sleep-inducing effects of large meals rich in carbohydrates[80]. However, no intrinsic eating disorder was found when sleep, eating behavior and subjective alertness of narcoleptics and controls were compared in isolation laboratory conditions[81]. In narcoleptics subjective alertness ratings peaked 90–120 min before meals but rapidly declined to below pre-meal levels after eating. Controls were more alert than narcoleptics before meals, and their alertness level was maintained for a longer period after meals. Anecdotally, people contacting the center sometimes report that their symptoms are better controlled by limiting their daytime food consumption, although no particular pattern of foods to avoid has been consistently reported.

A reduced caloric intake has been found in people with this disorder[82]. However, narcoleptics who are hypocretin-deficient have been found to have an increased body mass index (BMI) independent of whether or not they were on antidepressant medication compared to healthy controls or controls with other neurological symptoms such as headache or pain[83]. When hypocretin is administered centrally to animals, food consumption increases, leading one to expect that people who are deficient in this neuropeptide would reduce their food intake and would have a decrease in body weight. A reduced energy expenditure due to EDS and reduced activity level have been offered as a possible explanation for the elevated BMI in narcoleptics. An alternative explanation may be that reduced hypocretin levels, which regulate sympathetic and neuroendocrine activity besides sleep, also may reduce metabolic rate and result in an elevated body weight in people with this disorder[83].

Many people with this disorder avoid the use of alcohol because of its sedating effects. In contrast, some use caffeine for its alerting effects, although narcoleptics who daily ingested moderate-to-high levels of caffeine (200–500 mg) were objectively more sleepy on the MWT than those who used no-to-low levels (0–200 mg)[84]. Subjectively, the moderate-to-high users may have perceived that they received some benefit from caffeine ingestion. Consequently, the efficacy of caffeine in controlling EDS in narcolepsy is unclear.

Mood

People with narcolepsy often report having difficulty with feelings of depression[33,35]. In a national sample of 700 narcoleptics 49% of the respondents reported high depressive symptoms on the Beck Depression Inventory compared to national prevalence estimates of 9–31% in the general population. Patients who were married had lower depressive symptoms, while those who were younger and had lower levels of education and income had higher symptoms[35].

In addition to narcolepsy, health-care professionals need to screen for symptoms that indicate that a concurrent mood disorder may be present. This can present a challenge because certain features of narcolepsy overlap with those of depression, namely hypoarousal, a shortened latency to REM sleep, increased REM sleep and increased sleep fragmentation. While investigations into the pathophysiology of depression have traditionally focused on the serotoninergic and noradrenergic systems, interest is growing in the role of hypothalamic neuropeptides in this mood disorder[85]. Reduced hypocretin levels may play a role in the symptoms of depression, and could be a factor in why people with narcolepsy complain of high depressive symptomatology.

Supportive care

People with narcolepsy face difficulties in dealing with this disorder within the health-care system as well as in their daily lives. While not rare, primary health-care providers and even neurology specialists may have little experience with this disorder so that narcolepsy may not be suspected and an appropriate referral made for diagnosis. People with narcolepsy report having repeatedly to request a referral to a sleep specialist from their primary care provider. Even when referred, it can take several months to get an appointment at a sleep center, or the insurer may provide inadequate coverage for expensive PSG and MSLT testing as well as ongoing medication treatment.

Providers are also often concerned about prescribing stimulant therapy for an individual and about the potential for increasing the availability of these compounds in the community[86]. A frequent complaint heard by Center for Narcolepsy Research staff is that the provider will not increase the amount of medication prescribed, or try other medications when the person reported that the medication and dose were no longer effective. Another concern is the need expressed by narcoleptics to educate the provider about the disorder. Center for Narcolepsy Research staff often refer people with this complaint to documents available online that can be copied for primary care staff[57,87].

Once diagnosed, narcoleptics are often interested in getting information about the disorder that can be used to educate employers and teachers as well as family members and peers. They frequently report experiencing mistreatment and stigma because people in their social lives do not understand the involuntary nature of their symptoms. The National Sleep Foundation (www.sleepfoundation.org), the National Institutes of Health (www.nhlbi.nih.gov/health/public/sleep/narcolep. htm) and the American Academy of Sleep Medicine (www.aasmnet.org) provide a wide variety of educational materials about sleep and sleep disorders that are oriented towards the consumer.

Attendance at support group meetings can be helpful although some young individuals may feel more comfortable having one-on-one contact with other young narcoleptics rather than attending a 'public' meeting. The Narcolepsy Network (www.narcolepsynetwork.org) maintains a list of support groups operating in the USA. Many groups are coordinated by sleep professionals who are knowledgeable about the disorder. At one recent center support group meeting, a man in his early 60s expressed amazement at how helpful the meeting had been and stated that he had had narcolepsy for over 30 years and this was the first time he had ever talked to another person with the disorder. Online bulletin boards or newsgroups are also available although people may need to be warned about being cautious in using these resources since many are not moderated by a person knowledgeable about sleep.

Driving can be a concern to some people with this disorder. People with narcolepsy are at increased risk for having automobile accidents, especially when in an untreated state[29,32]. In the USA regulations vary from state to state with some requiring that a history of EDS control be demonstrated before the person can obtain a vehicular license. The health-care provider may be required to provide advice to a licensing agency about whether or not the individual can safely operate a vehicle, even though no objective standards have been established to determine which treated patients can do so[86]. In other states or countries, it is the responsibility of the person with narcolepsy to report their EDS and diagnosis to licensing authorities. Our experience is that (1) people who have been diagnosed with narcolepsy are usually very cautious when it comes to operating a motor vehicle; and (2) some health-care professionals require that the person demonstrates a normal ability to stay awake on the MWT before providing professional advice to governmental authorities, especially if the person is employed in an occupation in which others could be endangered if the individual falls asleep.

The 1990 Americans with Disabilities Act (ADA) requires that, unless an undue hardship would be imposed, employers and schools provide reasonable accommodation(s) for qualified people with disabilities who are capable of performing the essential work or academic functions. This act is particularly important for people with this disorder who do not achieve adequate symptom control on medications alone. The health-care provider may be required to document what accommodations are needed, such as frequent breaks when the person is required to perform tedious tasks that require vigilance, or the need for brief 15-min naps. Information about the ADA and state and local services is available at www.usdot.gov/ert/ada/adahom1.htm.

People with narcolepsy symptoms that cannot be controlled and interfere with their ability to work may qualify for disability benefits, although having narcolepsy does not mean the person automatically qualifies for this benefit. Applying for benefits can be frustrating to the individual because it frequently requires a three-step process during which the individual experiences refusal of benefits. The health-care provider may be required to document the extent of impairments on a sleep impairment questionnaire (see www. talkaboutsleep.com/sleepbasics/medicare_disability_questionnaire.htm for a sample form).

Additionally, this website provides extensive information about the Social Security Disability Insurance (SSDI) application process that may be helpful to individuals seeking benefits. Finally, they may need referral to a legal advocate who can help them with documenting and meeting the SSDI requirements. The National Organization of Social Security Claimant Representatives may be able to help the individual find attorneys or non-attorneys who are experts in representing applicants during the SSDI application process as well as assisting with the process of requesting accommodation in employment or school settings (www.nosscr.org).

CONCLUSION

Narcolepsy is a life-long, complex neurological disorder that is manifested by EDS and, often, cataplexy, and may be accompanied by sleep paralysis, hypnagogic hallucinations and disturbed nighttime sleep. The most debilitating symptom is EDS. Knowledge about this disorder among practitioners is limited, with people often remaining undiagnosed or misdiagnosed. The initial diagnosis usually requires sleep center testing by a specialist. However, primary care staff play an important role in early screening for, and managing of, narcolepsy.

People with this disorder require life-long treatment with wake-promoting agents and, often, antidepressant medications. The effectiveness of treatment can be variable between patients with EDS, a symptom that is often not completely controlled. Since the negative psychosocial impact of this disorder is at least comparable to many other chronic neurological disorders, narcoleptics often require supportive care in addition to medications to obtain an acceptable quality of life. Recent discoveries involving the deficiency of hypocretin-1 in narcolepsy holds promise for advancing the diagnosis and treatment of this disorder.

References

1. Bassetti C, Aldrich MS. Narcolepsy. *Neurol Clin* 1996;14:545–71
2. Thorpy M. Current concepts in the etiology, diagnosis and treatment of narcolepsy. *Sleep Med* 2001;2:5–17
3. Robinson A, Guilleminault C. Narcolepsy. In Chokroverty S, ed. *Sleep Disorders Medicine: Basic Science, Technical Considerations and Clinical Aspects*, 2nd edn. Boston: Butterworth-Heinemann, 1999:427–40c
4. Rogers AE, Dreher HM. Narcolepsy. *Nurs Clin North Am* 2002;37:675–92
5. Beusterne KM, Roger AE, Walsleben JA, *et al*. Health-related quality of life effects of modafinil for treatment of narcolepsy. *Sleep* 1999;22:757–64
6. Merritt SL, Berger B, Ponnaaganti V, *et al*. Symptoms and health status of young adults with narcolepsy. *Sleep* 2003;26(Suppl):A278
7. Hublin C. Narcolepsy: current treatment options. *CNS Drugs* 1996;5:426–36
8. National Commission on Sleep Disorders Research. *Report of the National Commission on Sleep Disorders Research*. DHHS Pub No 93. Washington, DC: US Government Printing Office, 1993
9. Passouant P, Billiard M. The evolution of narcolepsy with age. In Guilleminault C, Dement WC, Passouant P, eds. *Narcolepsy: Advances in Sleep Research*, vol. 3. New York: Spectrum Publications, 1976:179–96
10. Okun ML, Ling L, Pelin Z, *et al*. Clinical aspects of narcolepsy–cataplexy across ethnic groups. *Sleep* 2002;25:27–35
11. Yoss RE, Daly DD. Narcolepsy in children. *Pediatrics* 1960;25:1025–33
12. Nishino S, Okura M, Mignot E. Narcolepsy: genetic predisposition and neuropharmacological mechanisms. *Sleep Med Rev* 2000; 4:57–99
13. Hungs M, Mignot M. Hypocretin/orexin, sleep and narcolepsy. *BioEssays* 2001;23:397–408
14. Juji T, Satake M, Honda Y, *et al*. HLA antigens in Japanese patients with narcolepsy: all the patients were DR2 positive. *Tissue Antigens* 1984;24:316–19
15. Mignot E. Pathophysiology of narcolepsy. In Kryger MH, Roth T, Dement WC, eds. *Principles and Practice of Sleep Medicine*, 3rd edn. Philadelphia: WB Saunders, 2000:663–75
16. Stanford University School of Medicine. *Center for Narcolepsy: Basic Mechanisms Involved in the*

Disease (1). Accessed on June 26, 2003 at http://www.med.stanford.edu/school/Psychiatry/narcolepsy/research.html

17. Lin L, Faraco J, Li R, *et al.* The sleep disorder canine narcolepsy is caused by a mutation in the hypocretin (orexin) receptor 2 gene. *Cell* 1999;98:365–76

18. Chemelli RM, Willie JT, Sinton CM, *et al.* Narcolepsy in orexin knockout mice: molecular genetics of sleep regulation. *Cell* 1999;98: 437–51

19. Scammell TE. The neurobiology, diagnosis and treatment of narcolepsy. *Ann Neurol* 2003; 53:154–66

20. Mignot E, Lammers GJ, Ripley B, *et al.* The role of cerebrospinal fluid hypocretin measurement in the dianosis of narcolepsy and other hypersomnias. *Arch Neurol* 2002;59:1553–62

21. Thannickal TC, Moore RY, Nienhuis R, *et al.* Reduced number of hypocretin neurons in human narcolepsy. *Neuron* 2000;27:469–74

22. Brown RE. Involvement of hypocretins/orexins in sleep disorders and narcolepsy. *Drug News Perspect* 2003;16:75–9

23. Parkes D. *Sleep, its disorders.* Philadephia: WB Saunders, 1985

24. Pigeon WR, Sateia MJ, Ferguson RJ. Distinguishing between excessive daytime sleepiness and fatigue: toward improved detection and treatment. *J Psychosom Res* 2003; 54:61–9

25. Overeem S, Mignot E, van Dijk JG, *et al.* Narcolepsy: clinical features, new pathophysiologic insights and future perspectives. *J Clin Neurophysiol* 2001;18:78–105

26. American Sleep Disorders Association. *International Classification of Sleep Disorders, Revised: Diagnostic and Coding Manual.* Rochester, MN: American Sleep Disorders Association, 1997

27. National Sleep Foundation. Sleepiness in America. Washington, DC: National Sleep Foundation, 1997

28. Aldrich MS. Automobile accidents in patients with sleep disorders. *Sleep* 1989;12:487–94

29. Findley L, Unverzagt M, Guchu R, *et al.* Vigilance and automobile accidents in patients with sleep apnea or narcolepsy. *Chest* 1995; 108:619–24

30. Leger D. The cost of sleep-related accidents: a report for the National Commission on Sleep Disorders Research. *Sleep* 1994;17:84–93

31. Webb WB. The cost of sleep-related accidents: a re-analysis. *Sleep* 1995;18:276–80

32. Broughton R, Ghanem Q, Hishikawa Y, *et al.* Life effects of narcolepsy in 180 patients from North America, Asia and Europe compared to match controls. *Can J Neurol Sci* 1981;8: 299–304

33. Kales A, Soldatos CR, Bixler EO, *et al.* Narcolepsy–cataplexy: II. Psychological consequences and associated psychopathology. *Arch Neurol* 1982;39:169–71

34. Merritt SL, Cohen FL, Smith KM. Learning style preferences of persons with narcolepsy. *Loss Grief Care* 1992;5:115–27

35. Merritt SL, Cohen FL, Smith KM. Depressive symptomatology in narcolepsy. *Loss Grief Care* 1992;5:53–9

36. Broughton RJ. Sleep attacks, naps, and sleepiness in medical sleep disorders. In Dinges DJ, Broughton RJ, eds. *Sleep and Alertness Chronobiological, Behavioral, and Medical Aspects of Napping.* New York. Raven Press, 1989:267–98

37. Mysliwiec V, Henderson JH, Strollo PJ Epidemiology, consequences and evaluation of excessive daytime sleepiness. In Lee-Chiong TL, Sateia M, Carskadon MA, eds. *Sleep Medicine.* Philadelphia: Hanley & Belfus, Inc., 2002:187–92

38. Bassetti C, Aldrich MS. Narcolepsy. *Neurol Clin* 1996;14:545–71

39. Carskadon MA, Dement WC, Mitler MM, *et al.* Guidelines for the Multiple Sleep Latency Test (MSLT): a standard measure of sleepiness. *Sleep* 1986;9:519–24

40. Carsakadon MA, Dement WC. Daytime sleepiness: quantification of a behavioral state. *Neurosci Biobehav Rev* 1987;11:307–17

41. Thorpy MJ, *et al.* The clinical use of the Multiple Sleep Latency Test. *Sleep* 1992;15: 268–76

42. Moscovitch A, Partinen M, Guilleminault C. The positive diagnosis of narcolepsy and narcolepsy's borderland. *Neurology* 1993;43:55–60

43. Mittler MM, Gujavarty KS, Browman CP. Maintenance of Wakefulness Test: a polysomnographic technique for evaluating treatment efficacy in patients with excessive somnolence. *Electroenceph Clin Neurophysiol* 1982;658–61

44. Doghramji K, Mitler MM, Sangal RB, *et al.* A normative study of the Maintenance of Wakefulness Test (MWT). *Electroenceph Clin Neurophysiol* 1997;103:554–62

45. Sangal RB, Thomas L, Mitler MM. Maintenance of Wakefulness Test and Multiple Sleep Latency Test: measurement of different abilities in patients with sleep disorders. *Chest* 1992;101:898–902

46. Weaver ME, Lowe NK. A critical review of visual analogue scales in the measurement of clinical phenomena. *Res Nurs Health* 1990;13: 227–36

47. Hoddes E, Zarcone V, Smythe H, *et al.* Quantification of sleepiness: a new approach. *Psychophysiology* 1973;10:431–6

48. Johns MW. A new method for measuring daytime sleepiness: the Epworth Sleepiness Scale. *Sleep* 1991;14:540–45

49. Roth T, Roehrs T, Rosenthal L. Normative and pathological aspects of daytime sleepiness. In Oldham JM, Riba MB, eds. *Review of Psychiatry/XIII*. Washington, DC: American Psychiatric Press, 1994:707–28

50. USA Modafinil in Narcolepsy Multicenter Study Group. Randomized trial of modafinil for the treatment of pathological somnolence in narcolepsy. *Ann Neurol* 1998;43:88–97

51. Guilleminault C. Disorders of excessive sleepiness *Ann Clin Res* 1985;17:209–19

52. Dement WC. Daytime sleepiness and sleep 'attacks'. In Guilleminault C, Dement WC, Passouant P, eds. *Narcolepsy. Proceedings of the First International Symposium on Narcolepsy. Advances in Sleep Research*, Vol 3. New York: Spectrum, 1976:17–42

53. Mitler MM, Miller JC. Methods of testing for sleepiness. *Behav Med* 1996;21:171–83

54. Aldrich MS. *Sleep Medicine*. New York: Oxford University Press, 1999

55. Moscovitch A, Partinen M, Patterson-Rhoads N, *et al*. Cataplexy in differentiation of excessive daytime somnolence. *Sleep Res* 1991; 20:303

56. Brooks SN, Mignot E. Narcolepsy and idiopathic hypersomnia. In Lee-Chiong TL, Sateia M, Carskadon MA, eds. *Sleep Medicine*. Philadelphia: Hanley & Belfus, Inc., 2002: 193–202

57. Littner M, Johnson SF, McCall V, *et al*. Practice parameters for the treatment of narcolepsy: an update for 2000. *Sleep* 2001;24:451–66 (available online at http://www.aasmnet.org, accessed June 19, 2003)

58. USA Modafinil Multicenter Study Group. Randomized trial of modafinil as a treatment for the excessive daytime somnolence of narcolepsy. *Neurology* 2000;54:1166–75

59. Mignot E. *Narcolepsy: a Guide for Understanding, Diagnosing and Treating Narcolepsy*. [CD ROM]. Washington, DC: National Sleep Foundation, 2003

60. Schumacher A, Merritt SL, Cohen FL. The effect of drug therapy on the perceived symptom and ADL experiences of narcoleptics. *J Neurosci Nurs* 1997;29:15–23

61. Rogers AE, Aldrich MS, Caruso CC. Patterns of sleep and wakefulness in treated narcoleptic subjects. *Sleep* 1994;17:590–7

62. Mitler MM, Aldrich MS, Koob GF, Zarcone P. Narcolepsy and its treatment with stimulants. *Sleep* 1994;17:352–71

63. Mitler MM, Hajdukovic R. Relative efficacy of drugs for the treatment of sleepiness in narcolepsy. *Sleep* 1991;14:218–20

64. Mitler MM, Hajdukovic R, Erman M, Koziol JA. Narcolepsy. *J Clin Neurophysiol* 1990;7: 93–118

65. Mitler MM, Erman, M, Hajdukovic R. The treatment of excessive somnolence with stimulant drugs. *Sleep* 1993;16:203–6

66. Mitler MM. Evaluation of treatment with stimulants in narcolepsy. *Sleep* 1994;17:S103–6

67. Mitler MM, Aldrich MS. Koob GF, Zarcone VP. Narcolepsy and its treatment with stimulants. *Sleep* 1994;17:352–71

68. Workshop on the topic of physician reluctance to prescribe CNS active medication for patients with sleep disorders. La Jolla, CA: Scripps Clinical and Research Foundation, 1991 (unpublished)

69. Orphan Medical. Product monograph: Xyrem® (sodium oxybate) oral solution. Minnetonka, MN: Orphan Medical. (full prescribing information available on p. 36 or at http//www.xyrem.info)

70. Guilleminault C. Narcolepsy. In Chokrovery S, ed. *Sleep Disorders Medicine: Basic Science, Technical Considerations and Clinical Aspects*. Boston: Butterworth-Heinemann, 1994:241–54

71. USA Xyrem Multicenter Study Group. A randomized, double-blind, placebo-controlled multicenter trial comparing the effects of three doses of orally administered sodium oxybate with placebo for the treatment of narcolepsy. *Sleep* 2002;25:42–9

72. USA Xyrem Multicenter Study Group. A 12-month, open-label multicenter extension trial of orally administered sodium oxybate for the treatment of narcolepsy. *Sleep* 2003;26:31–5

73. Rogers AE. Compliance with stimulant medications in patients with narcolepsy. *Sleep* 1997; 20:28–33

74. Eraker SA, Kirscht JP, Becker MD. Understanding and improving patient compliance. *Ann Intern Med* 1984;100:258–68

75. Greenberg RN. Overview of patient compliance with medication dosing: a literature review. *Clin Ther* 1984;6:592–9

76. Zarcone VP. Sleep hygiene. In Kryger MH, Roth T, Dement WC, eds. *Principles and Practice of Sleep Medicine*, 3rd edn. Philadelphia: WB Saunders, 2000:657–61

77. Rogers A, Aldrich MS. The effect of regularly scheduled naps on sleep attacks and excessive daytime sleepiness associated with narcolepsy. *Nurs Res* 1993;42:111–17

78. Helmus T, Rosenthal L, Bishop C, *et al*. The alerting effects of short and long naps in narcoleptic, sleep-deprived, and alert individuals. *Sleep* 1999;20:251–7

79. Bell IR, Guilleminault C, Dement WC. Questionnaire survey of eating habits of narcoleptics versus normals. *Sleep Res* 1975;4:208

80. Bruck D, Armstong S, Coleman G. Sleepiness after glucose in narcolepsy. *J Sleep Res* 1994;3: 171–9

81. Pollak CP, Green J. Eating and its relationships with subjective alertness and sleep in narcoleptic subjects living without temporal cues. *Sleep* 1990;13:467–78

82. Lammers GJ, Pijl H, Iestra J, *et al*. Spontaneous food choice in narcolepsy. *Sleep* 1996; 19:75–6

83. Nishino S, Ripley B, Overeem S, *et al*. Low cerebrospinal fluid hypocretin (orexin) and altered energy homeostasis in human narcolepsy. *Ann Neurol* 2001;50:381–8

84. Mitler MM, Walsleben J, Sangal RB, *et al*. Sleep latency on the maintenance of wakefulness test (MWT) for 530 patients with narcolepsy while free of psychoactive drugs. *Electroenceph Clin Neurophysiol* 1998;107:33–8

85. Iaheri S, Hafizi S. The orexin/hypocretins: hypothalamic peptides linked to sleep and appetite. *Psychol Med* 2002;955–8

86. Douglas NJ. The psychosocial aspects of narcolepsy. *Neurology* 1998;50(Suppl.):S27–S30

87. Hayduk R. An overview of the diagnosis and treatment of narcolepsy for primary care physicans. *Sleep Med Alert* Winter 2001;5:1–6 (available online at www.sleepfoundation.org/publications/sma5.1.html, accessed July 6, 2003.)

Section 3:

Developmental parasomnias: nocturnal behavior and physiological disorders

10

Periodic and rhythmic parasomnias

Alexander Z. Golbin

INTRODUCTION: PARADOXES OF PARASOMNIAS

Parasomnias are sleep-related undesirable behavioral, emotional, mental and somatic phenomena[1]. Multiple 'undesirable' phenomena are known, and descriptions of new parasomnias are forthcoming. Given these circumstances, it is reasonable to ask what should *not* be included in parasomnias from the long list of peculiar sleep events. Could it be that indifferent or even 'desirable' phenomena, say, creative writing in sleep, should be characterized as a parasomnia? This is but the first dilemma or paradox in the study of parasomnias.

The second lies in the distinction between the 'correction' or the 'treatment' of parasomnias. If we use the term treatment, then the question is when does a benign, or 'undesirable', phenomenon become a 'disorder' that requires treatment and what are we treating: elimination of the phenomenon or correction of the underlying pathology?

The third paradox appears as puzzling if one attempts to conceptualize the state in which the person is engaging in parasomnia: is it a waking activity while still asleep, or is it a sleep phenomenon during wakefulness?

The fourth paradox presents as a strange resistance of parasomnias to the treatment (meaning an attempt to suppress 'undesirable' events) and spontaneous disappearance of the symptom (self-cure) without any treatment.

Finally, the fifth paradox is a contrast between the widespread, clear and sometimes very dramatic presentation of parasomnias and the vague understanding of their pathophysiology, and the contrast between abundant literature and an absence of unified theory and effective treatment.

Any concept or theory of parasomnias should attempt to solve all or as many as possible of these paradoxes.

Presently the most accepted classification is based on the notion brilliantly and convincingly presented by Broughton in 1968 that parasomnias are disorders of arousal[2]. This classification consists of (a) NREM arousal disorders, (b) sleep–wake transitional disorders, (c) parasomnias usually associated with REM sleep (REM arousal disorders) and (d) other parasomnias – which comprises a list larger then (a), (b) and (c) together.

Recently, attempts have been made to 'reframe' and add into this classification. For example, nocturnal dissociations, alcohol withdrawal syndrome, hallucinations and paroxysmal events in neonates and infants have been included in this category. Periodic

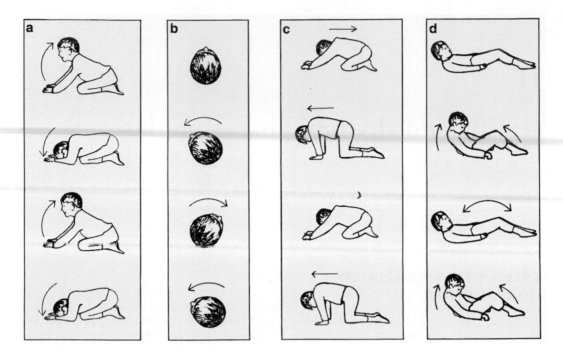

Figure 10.1 Types of rhythmic movements in sleep. (a) Head banging; (b) head and body rocking; (c) shuttling; and (d) folding (see text for explanation)

parasomnias by themselves are a part of the so-called group of periodic disorders.

We propose grouping parasomnias by their clinical presentation and natural course into three categories:

(1)   Periodic or rhythmic phenomena;

(2)   Episodic or paroxysmal parasomnias;

(3)   Static phenomena.

The person with parasomnias usually exhibits one or a small number of phenomena of the same group, and in the course of a lifetime, parasomnias frequently change within the same group (grouping effect).

PERIODIC AND RHYTHMIC PARASOMNIAS

Periodic and rhythmic parasomnias are part of a large group of periodic phenomena, which are common in normalcy and among neurological and psychiatric problems. Sleep-related periodic and rhythmic phenomena range from very mild and benign, such as finger sucking, to bizarre and sometimes injurious disorders, such as violent head banging.

The time and rhythm of periodicity (chronobiological rhythms) is different for each disorder.

SLEEP-RELATED RHYTHMIC MOVEMENT DISORDER

Rhythmic movement disorder (RMD) comprises a group of stereotyped, repetitive movements involving large muscles, including the head and neck[1]. The movements typically occur immediately prior to sleep onset and are sustained during sleep. These movements include head and body rocking, head banging, leg rolling and banging, and many other rhythmic movements (Figure 10.1).

The prevalence of rhythmic movement disorder is surprisingly high[1]. Some form of rhythmic activity is found in two-thirds of all infants at 9 months of age. By 18 months, the frequency declines to less than 50%, and by 4 years it is only 8%[9]. Head and body rocking are more common during the first year of life, but head banging and head rocking continue in older children and adulthood[3-6]. Our oldest patient with severe body rocking was a 63-year-old woman. Stereotyped rhythmic movement disorders are also common in mentally retarded, autistic, brain damaged and socially deprived persons.

Head banging, sleep-related head and body rocking and other similar rhythmic movements are fascinating, puzzling and sometimes frightening phenomena. It is fascinating to the observer, because it presents a very dramatic picture of a child rhythmically banging his/her head against the pillow, his/her fists on the corner of the bed, rocking side-to-side, or otherwise thrashing about for a long period of time. It is puzzling because these phenomena are unusual and contradict the common perception that sleep is a restful state. It is frightening for parents, because they feel helpless against the prolonged and sometimes injurious behavior of their children. Parents often forcibly try to stop these movements. The child stops rocking or banging for a short period of time, only to resume them more intensely. In severe cases, the child can injure him-/herself, resulting in bruises on the face and head. Associated breathing and pulse arrhythmias are common. The family experiences sleepless nights due to loud, annoying and dreadful rhythmical noises from the shaking bed, or may endure complaints about the noise from neighbors or even accusations of child abuse. To further complicate the issue, the child often has difficulty waking up in the morning, and experiences daydreaming, and attention and learning problems at school. Parents may also show a decline in their own performance levels during the day due to sleep deprivation.

Forehead tissue swelling (the 'head banger's tumor') was described in 1982 by Sormann[7] in a 12-year-old Jamaican girl and a 16-year-old West Indian with chronic head banging[7]. Complications are not frequent but might be serious. Cataracts, following chronic head banging, were reported in two institutionalized boys[8].

RMD was frequently observed in deprived children such as infants separated from parents[9,10]. Until the 1980s, rhythmic motor behavior was thought to occur mostly in mentally defective or emotionally disturbed children[9-11]. This view is no longer favored by the majority of clinicians.

Although it is true that brain damaged and severely neglected children are often involved in self-injurious repetitive behavior, in such cases the activities are not always sleep-related and occur in the daytime as self-stimulation or self-soothing activities. Sleep-related rhythmic movement disorders, on the other hand, occur predominantly in intellectually normal or even gifted children who have been raised in caring and loving families[12]. The other misconception is that head rocking and banging, finger sucking and playing with one's hair are generally regarded as 'cute' phenomena of infancy. Unfortunately, it can become an annoying problem that persists through adolescence, young adulthood and into old age.

Rhythmic types of motor activity can be seen in humans and in animals, young and old, in normal and pathological, natural and experimental conditions. To name this distinct clinical entity, the Latin term *jactatio nocturna* serves as an umbrella term, because it reflects movements appearing around the time of sleep in identical cycles with a frequency closely related to the heart rate. It may be rhythmical swinging of the head (*jactatio capitis nocturna*), the body (corpora) or the extremities (arms). The term '*jactatio*' is an abbreviation of the noun *jactation* derived from *jactare*, which literally means 'rhythmical swinging of the body and limbs to and fro'; 'to toss about'; 'to throw back and forth'. Since 1680, French and German literature has commonly used the word jactation to mean rocking. In 1731, in Temple Ess, it was noted that 'Jactation... help or occasion sleep, as we find by cradles or dandling them in their nurses' arms.' In 'Enthus Methodists' (1754) by Levington, there is a chapter entitled 'Various Tumults of Mind and Jactation of Body'. Because of its original meaning of rhythmicity, cyclicity and relation to sleep, the term *'jactatio nocturna'* was formally used in European medical literature from the early 20th century[13].

Clinical forms (subtypes) of *jactatio nocturna*

The clinical and therapeutic differences between patterns of rhythmical movements depend on: the direction (axis) of movement; monotony versus bouts of rhythm; asymmetry; relation to the stage of sleep or level of alertness; age of onset; severity; transformation from one form to another; and progression into adulthood. These parameters seem to be different for each pattern. At least five groups of clinically significant sleep-related rhythmic movement can be identified: 1, head banging; 2, head and body rocking; 3, shuttling; 4, folding; and 5, others (Figure 10.1).

(1) HEAD BANGING (Figure 10.1a) In the prone position, the person repeatedly lifts the head or upper body with outstretched arms and forcibly bangs the forehead or cheeks against the pillow, and fists against the hard edge of the bed. In infants or in mild cases of older children, the child moves only its head. In more severe cases, the whole upper body is involved. The movements are up and down. The force and speed increase on the way down, giving the strong impression of 'beating' the forehead, cheeks or temporal parts against the hard surface. In mild cases or at the beginning, the banging lasts 5–10 minutes without interruptions with a frequency of 60–65 per minute, then increases to 82–89 per minute and appears in clusters. Clusters start and end abruptly as if turned 'on' and 'off'. Several clusters of banging compose an episode, lasting from 1 minute to 2 hours. Episodes may occur through the night and later shift to the day during sleepy or drowsy conditions. External stimuli usually stop movements for a short period of time, but the movements soon resume with greater intensity. Turned to the supine position, the patient either turns back on his stomach or begins to rock his head so vigorously and asymmetrically that it appears as if he is still beating his cheek against the pillow.

(2) HEAD AND BODY ROCKING (Figure 10.1b) In a *mild* form, the patient is usually in the supine position, eyes closed, and performs pendulum-like movements of the head in a sideways fashion. The movements are rhythmic, smooth, stereotyped and with a frequency of 60 to 80 per minute. The length of an episode varies from a single movement to 5–10 minutes. The general pattern of movement (the length and frequency) is individually constant. An episode starts and ends smoothly. The extremities and the whole body are relaxed and immobile, or with some slight movements in the same rhythm as the rocking of the head. Movements occur when falling asleep or waking up. There is no rocking during the daytime. The patient is always aware of the rocking and reports feelings of pleasure and peace from them. In the presence of other people or sounds, these movements stop immediately, but resume shortly thereafter. In the morning, the children have full recollection of the behavior and willingly demonstrate the rocking. In the daytime, such children are cheerful, active and creative. Emotional instability is usually the reason why their parents seek medical help.

In a *moderate* form of rocking, there is greater motor involvement of the extremities and the whole body. An episode occurs with movements that are more intense, and appear in clusters as in banging. The duration of an episode increases, and there is an increase in the number of episodes per night. Movements occur in the daytime when the child becomes excited. The child no longer appears to be relaxed; on the contrary, he is tense while rocking. Sharp movements of the body in the same direction follow sharp movements of the head. An important feature of the moderate form is involvement of the upper extremities and asymmetry of the movements. The arms follow movements of the head, with the elbows bent. The movements are more intense toward one side than to the other. The duration of clusters is greater (up to 30 minutes) with the frequency remaining at 60–90 per minute. The clusters start and end abruptly as if 'plugged in' and then abruptly 'unplugged'. In the presence of another person, the movements stop, but reappear with greater intensity. This is the reason why parents do not try to stop the child. During the daytime, behavior of these children appears to be normal.

In its *severe* form, rocking can be so intense that it looks like a seizure, with sharp throws of the head; the arms and the entire body are flung in a sideways fashion. The arms may be outstretched with fists clenched, or the arms may be bent at the elbows and pressed to the body. The movements are mostly asymmetrical. The asymmetry does not significantly coincide with right- or left-handedness. The duration of a single episode of rocking may be up to several hours, and as many as 2000 movements may be made without stopping. During pauses, electroencephalography (EEG) readings show transitional sleep between stages 2 and 3. In severe rocking, dizziness and vomiting sometimes occur. It is not always possible to forcibly stop the movements, whereas children with mild rocking wake up cheerful, active and showing no signs of sleepiness. However, children with the severe form of rocking frequently have difficulty awakening, are late to school and have learning problems, owing to a shorter attention span and daydreaming. In general, children who rock have a normal IQ and are creative, but may have difficulty in the conformity and discipline required to perform well in school.

(3) SHUTTLING (Figure 10.1c) Shuttling is rhythmic movements of the body at the elbow and knee position, moving forward and backward along the horizontal body line. The term 'shuttling' is readily accepted by patients. Like other non-epileptic forms of movement in sleep, shuttling stops for a short time only to resume with increased intensity. We have observed six children (five males and one female) ages 6–10 years with this problem. Some with shuttling movements were referred to the doctor's office with a chief complaint of masturbation. Video documentation of these children in sleep demonstrated that the movements had nothing to do with masturbation.

The forward component of the shuttling is faster than the backward component. The head is always set against the pillow or the wall. The child actively swivels the head with increased pressure *on the head*. Children do not express pleasure from this activity and only vaguely remember it, and sometimes attempt the activity to get rid of drowsiness, anxiety and unpleasant itching sensations.

(4) FOLDING (Figure 10.1d) A few cases have been described of 'folding up' movements similar to a jack-knife, while in a supine position, with sudden rhythmical movements forward to sit up, back to lie down and then forward to sit up again. The force and speed increases on the way up and forward, possibly causing the child to actually hit his forehead against his knees.

(5) OTHER Rhythmic phenomena may be a part of the above activity as they prelude or else may entail leg or hand waving, kicking, extensive finger or tongue sucking,

151

rhythmic chewing or vocalizations, or rhythmic hair pulling, etc.

The natural course of
jactatio nocturna

Despite many differences between different types of *jactatio nocturna*, common stages or periods in their natural course can be identified.

(1) UNDIFFERENTIATED PERIOD

This is a period of unspecified deviations of the sleep–wake pattern. It reflects instability of the development of the sleep–wake cycles. The child is irritable, is hyperalert, has 'colics', cries at night and is sleepy during the day. This period usually ends with the appearance of *jactatio*.

(2) PERIOD OF 'CRYSTALLIZATION'

This term describes the appearance of rhythmic activity in parallel with 'normalization' (disappearance) of symptoms of instability of sleep. Children sleep better and are more alert during the day. They are normal except for their rhythmical movements. Overall mean onset is 5–6 months of age.

(3) MONOSYMPTOMATIC PERIOD

This term reflects a long period of predominantly one form of *jactatio* in children and adults who are generally normal medically, neurologically and intellectually. This period may last for years and ends by itself (self-cure) or with treatment, or deteriorates.

(4) PERIODS OF SELF-CURE OR DETERIORATION

The term 'deterioration' reflects a period of a dramatic increase in the intensity and amplitude of movements, or the appearance of additional types of movement, medical and psychological symptoms. For example, previous mild head rocking may dramatically increase in amplitude of movements with involvement of the arms

and the entire body. Other parasomnias may appear. This is a period when problems that once occurred only in sleep, and were hidden by the cover of night, begin to appear in the light of day as emotional, learning and behavioral disabilities.

Psychological profiles of children, adolescents and adults with
jactatio nocturna

As was mentioned earlier, the majority of the children, adolescents and adults are intellectually normal with a wide range of intellectual abilities from 'below average' to 'superior'. The general impression is that this is a group of likeable, emotionally warm and active children. Often they are gifted in the humanities and may have difficulty in structural settings and boring tasks. They seem to fancy activities connected with rhythm such as dancing, or music (especially drumming); they like swinging and rotating. Adults also enjoy clear rhythm, as is prominent in jazz music.

These children are generally healthy and without apparent medical problems. However, ear infections, difficult nasal breathing and morning headaches seem to be more commonly encountered than in the general population. Neurological and neurophysiological examinations usually reveal so-called soft neurological signs. These include sensory–motor disintegration; right–left confusion; increased sensitivity to one stimulus and a decreased sensitivity to another; decreased sense of danger and increased anxiety in benign situations.

It is possible to differentiate between 'bangers', 'rockers', etc. Generally, 'head bangers' are more hyperactive during the day, have more problems in early development and have a more turbulent course of the affliction. 'Head bangers' remember their movements less and report more unpleasant sensations, while 'rockers' have a tendency to like the feelings produced by rocking and often perform it voluntarily, which quickly turns *jactatio* into a daytime habit.

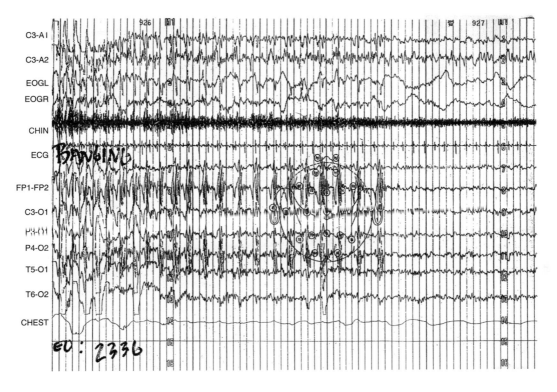

Figure 10.2 Bouts of head banging during transition to sleep

Sleep evaluation of patients with *jactatio nocturna*

Sleep evaluation of patients with *jactatio nocturna* is somewhat difficult because it is unclear what to look for and movements produce artifacts on polysomnogram (Figure 10.2). Examinations of bioelectrical brain activity (EEG) show an increase in maturational deviations compared with age-matched normal controls (especially in head bangers) (Figure 10.3). All changes are soft and diffuse. There are very few cases with epileptic activity.

The most significant findings are shown during all-night recording of sleep using multiple physiological parameters, i.e. polysomnography (EEG, eye movements, heart rate, breathing, muscle activity, etc.). Polysomnograms of patients with a mild-to-moderate degree of rhythmic movements show relatively normal sleep architecture and associations of movements at onset of sleep, in

stages 1 and 2, and rarely at the beginning of stage 3 of non-rapid eye movement (NREM) (Figures 10.3 and 10.4)[14-17].

The case of head banging in REM has been reported[18-21]. Chisholm and Morehouse[21] described a sleep study of two young adults of 19 and 24 years of age, respectively. The older subject was happily married, had two children and a good job. He displayed a typical pattern of head banging with cycles of 10–16 with a short pause in between throughout the night; he was not aware of it. Sleep stage distribution was statistically normal for his age. Head banging was recorded in 14% of all epochs, 54% of stage 1. No respiratory or vascular changes were recorded. The second patient, 19 years old, had poor sleep architecture with REM deficiency. Head banging was not recorded. Both patients had alertness problems during the day and were reportedly helped with clonazepam.

Dyken and co-workers[22] studied RMD with video polysomnography of seven children,

153

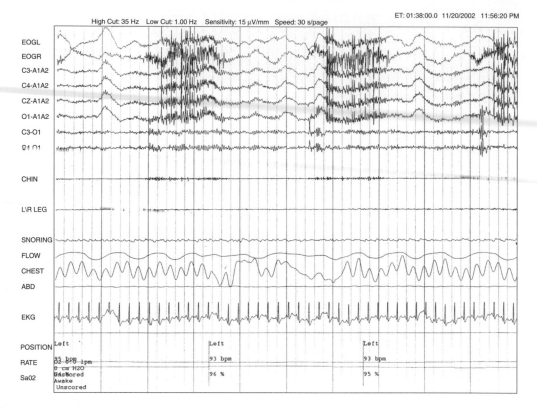

Figure 10.3   Sixty-two-year-old woman with head rolling

from 13 months to 12 years, with a total of 37 episodes of rocking. Two children were normal; one 21-month-old infant was abused and neglected; four teenagers had ADHD and ADD; and one was mentally retarded. Three children (4, 8 and 12 years old) had attention deficit disorder (ADD). The majority of events were recorded in stage 2 (26), nine in stage 1; one episode took place in REM, but was extremely brief. It is interesting that approximately 20 episodes were closely associated with delineated high-amplitude theta and delta paroxysmal discharges.

The sleep architecture of patients with advanced forms of RMD is disorganized. The 'switch' from one state of vigilance to another is difficult, i.e. from restfulness to sleep, from slow sleep to REM, from deep REM sleep to awakening, etc. It is important to mention that episodes of head banging and rocking might occur in any stage of sleep, but predominantly take place between stages. During *jactatio* heart rate, breathing and brainwaves slowly start to be synchronized with the rhythm of the movements. It looks as though stereotyped movements with a rhythm of 0.5–2 per second produce synchronized theta and delta waves on EEG[9]. Movements stop when the child falls asleep. *Jactatio*, in some cases, may serve a function as a 'transmission' or 'pacemaker', switching or stabilizing different states of vigilance. Started as a compensatory phenomenon, rocking and banging may bring many problems later on[5,16].

Several hypotheses have attempted to explain rocking and banging before and during sleep. These include: maternal deprivation, erotic gratification, movement restraint, anxiety relief, disorder of arousal, self-stimulation or perceptual reinforcement, head injury[10,23–29].

It is presently not clear where this natural 'transmission', or switch of states of vigilance is located. It may be a complex of central brain circuits, including the vestibular system. Vestibular tests show that, although the peripheral parts of the vestibular system are

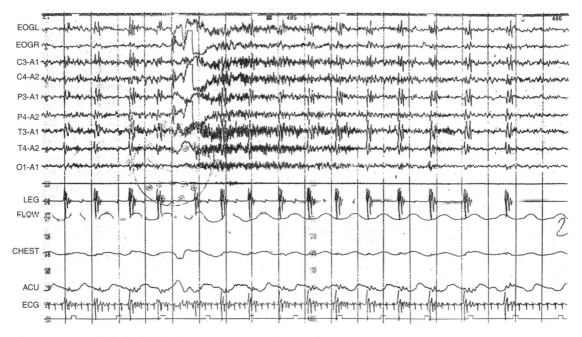

Figure 10.4   Periodic leg kicking in stage 2 NREM with arousal

intact, their central circuits are undeveloped in individuals who exhibit rocking and banging. This is evident by functional asymmetry (superstability of movements in one direction and significant reactions in another direction of movement)[28]. Rhythmic movement disorders can be conceptualized as sensory–motor disintegration. Simply stated, immaturity of the central co-ordinating system might be the basis for self-induced (physiological and pathological) rhythmic movements in specific instances.

PERIODIC LIMB MOVEMENTS AND RESTLESS LEGS SYNDROME

Periodic limb movements disorder (PLMD) and restless legs syndrome (RLS) are well-described in adults[29], but previously were thought to be rare during childhood[16,17]. Symptoms are typically characterized either by a complaint of difficulty initiating and/or maintaining sleep or excessive daytime sleepiness. During the polysomnographic evaluation in a sleep laboratory, periodic episodes of repetitive and highly stereotypical leg movements in sleep are recorded.

Muscle contractions last 0.5–5 s with more than five consecutive movements. The interval between the clusters of such movements ranges from 6 to 90s. Sometimes movements persist during awakenings. Little is known about the character, etiology or clinical significance of these periodic leg cramps. They are different from the slow rhythmic movements of the legs as a part of *jactatio* where the whole limb is involved. In PLMD, only separate groups of muscles are involved in the fast spasm-type of jerk. RLS is seen during the sleep–wake transition. Daytime symptoms of children who have PLMD and RLS range from behavior problems, hyperactivity and school learning difficulties to excessive daytime sleepiness.

BRUXISM

Bruxism is a rhythmic stereotyped grinding or clenching of the teeth which occurs mostly in sleep[30]. The word bruxism is transformed from a Greek work *brychein* (to gnash the teeth) and was coined in 1931 by Frohman to specify sleep-related 'primary' bruxism. Bruxism is observed in about 20% of adults

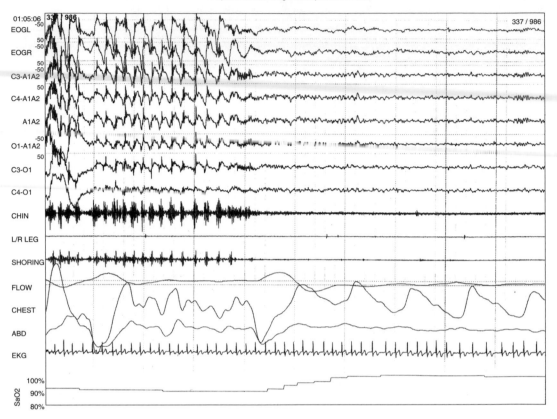

Figure 10.5   Bruxism

and up to 88% of children, occurs in any stage of both NREM and REM sleep and can be very damaging to the teeth[31]. There are multiple causes of bruxism (secondary bruxism), and it can be connected with 'organic' disorders such as orofacial dyskinesia, mandibular distonia, genetic problems, etc.

A current concept of bruxism is that it is a primary disorder of sleep, identified as rhythmic stereotyped parasomnia, and is therefore centrally mediated and, as any centrally mediated phenomenon, may be precipitated or exacerbated by stress[27,32,33].

The study by Vanderas and colleagues[34] of urine catecholamine levels of 314 children with and without emotional stress provides support for the concept that emotional stress is a prominent factor in the development of this parafunction. As with other parasomnias,

precise brain mechanisms of bruxism are unknown. The older the person afflicted with bruxism, the more serious is the pathology associated with it, both medical and psychological. Bruxism appears to be a good biological marker of the levels of consciousness in coma[35,36].

TREATMENT OF SLEEP-RELATED STEREOTYPED RHYTHMIC DISORDERS

The treatment of stereotyped behavior is challenging, to say the least. It is useful to begin the treatment by paying more attention to the child. Special attention before sleep may be particularly helpful for children growing up in unstable families, or having chronic

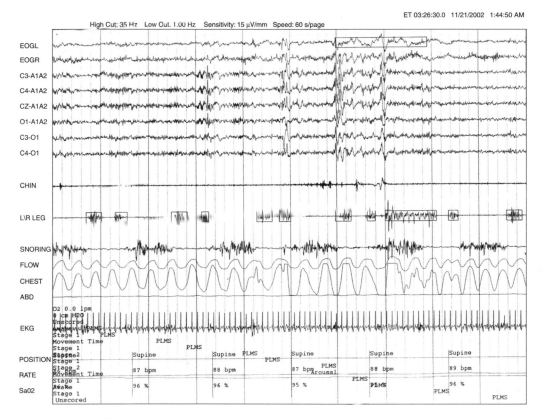

Figure 10.6   Pelvic rolling with loud moaning

illnesses. The value of the attention factor in healing stereotyped movements during sleep, especially in the case of rocking, is shown in the following example.

Jane is 6 years old. When she was 2 months old, she was hospitalized with pneumonia. Shortly after that, the girl was noticed rocking for a long time before falling asleep. She was raised by her grandparents until she was 5 years old. Then she went to live with adoptive parents and soon won their love. In this new family, the rocking symptoms eventually stopped.

Besides attention, such children need physical exercise (skiing, running, jumping rope, etc.).

Rhythm and music therapy occupy an important place among treatment methods. Children often ask to sleep with the sound of music having a clear rhythm, such as a drums or a metronome. Music with a distinct rhythm promotes the process of synchronization in the brain and sleep (for example, a lullaby with rocking). Some families successfully use a metronome. It is known that imagining oneself rocking can cause the same effects of synchronization in the brain as actual rocking. Children with rocking are often distinguished by their vivid imagination. They can easily imagine themselves rocking before sleep. This produces an appearance of EEG waves in the brain, which synchronize in rhythm with such imaginary ramming and rocking. Attempting to stop rhythmic movements in sleep by forcefully waking up the child, or to punish him for 'bad habits', is not recommended because, after a brief pause, the child will resume movements with much greater intensity.

There are anecdotal reports that suggest that rhythmic movement disorders disappear after changing from a conventional bed to a waterbed[23,37], but a significant deterioration of

RMD was observed after a 24-year-old man switched from a conventional bed to a waterbed.

Hypnotherapy was also reported to be[38] a successful technique. Rosenberg described a 26-year-old woman who had been rocking in her bed to fall asleep since her early childhood. The rocking stopped during her adolescent years, but resumed when she got married, which caused family problems. The problem became particularly acute during breastfeeding. Family history, as well as medical examinations, were unremarkable. Hypnosis was used to avoid pharmacological treatment. In the hypnotic state, she was provided an image of watching a television set with a program about her sleeping calmly with her husband. She was trained to produce this image in self-hypnosis at her bedtime. At the time of the 3-month follow-up, only two occurrences of rocking were reported.

Hypnosis has been used successfully for treatment of a variety of sleep disorders, including parasomnias, night terrors in children[38–40] and disorders of arousal in adults, such as sleep terrors and sleepwalking[41]. Rosenberg[38] attributed the efficacy of hypnosis in the disorders of arousal to 'increased control of frenzied and ambulatory behaviors, rather than in the elimination of arousals'.

Moderate or severe cases may require pharmacological treatment. Treatment with benzodiazepines has variable success. Chisholm and Morehouse[21] report a positive effect of clonazepam in two cases of adult head banging. Walsh and colleagues[42] were successful in using oxazepam (10–20 mg nightly) in an 8-year-old girl with head rocking and banging. Freidin and associates[43] had less success with a 27-month-old boy, who had head banging since the age of 10 months to such a severe degree that he broke the headboard and knocked a hole in the wall. Diazepam 2–8 mg at bedtime controlled the symptoms, but for only 4 weeks. Clonazepam received a positive review[44].

Barbiturates are not recommended, because this group of drugs may cause sleep cycle disorganization. Moreover, it slows activities during the day. New anticonvulsants, such as gabapentin, tiagabine and oxcarbazepine, showed promising results. In the most severe cases of stereotyped movements in sleep, use of hydrocarbonate sodium seems to be promising. This method was originally suggested by Hasegawa[28] for patients with vestibular problems, such as Menière's disease.

Antidepressants, including SSRIs, which are so effective for many childhood sleep disorders, such as bedwetting and bedtime fears, do not demonstrate high efficiency for stereotyped activity. Imipramine was better than placebo for head bangers, but less effective than mild tranquilizers, such as clonazepam or alprazolam.

Treatment of periodic limb movements/ restless legs syndrome is based on dopaminergic therapies including both levodopa and dopamine receptor agonists (pergolide, pramipexole, ropinirole)[45] as well as muscle relaxants.

Therapy of bruxism includes a wide range of means such as dental appliances, nonsteroidal and inflammatory agents, muscle relaxants and even suggestive hypnotherapy.

In summary, treatment of periodic and rhythmic parasomnias remains challenging[46]. The search for a better understanding of the nature of these disorders and their successful treatment should be continued.

References

1. *The International Classification of Sleep Disorders. Diagnostic and Coding Manual.* Rochester, MN: American Sleep Disorders Association, 1990: 151–4

2. Broughton J. Sleep disorders – disorders of arousals? *Science* 1968;159:1070–8

3. Happe S, Lüdemann P, Ringelstein EB. Persistence of rhythmic movement disorder

beyond childhood: a videotape demonstration. *Movement Disord* 2000;15:1296–8

4. Alves RS, Aloe F, Silva AB, Tavares SM. Jactatio capitis nocturna with persistence in adulthood. Case report. *Arq Neuropsiquiatr* 1998;56:655–7

5. Thorpy MJ, Spielman AJ. Persistent jactatio nocturna. *Neurology* 1984;34(Suppl 1):208–9 (abstract)

6. Thorpy MJ, Glovinsky PB. Parasomnias. *Psychiatric Clin North Am* 1987;10:623–39

7. Sormann GW. The headbanger's tumour. *Br J Plast Surg* 1982;35:72–4

8. Bemporad JR, Sours JA, Spalter HF. Cataracts following headbanging. a report of two cases. *Am J Psychiatry* 1968;125:245–9

9. Dawson-Butterworth K. Headbanging in young children. *Practitioner (London)* 1979;222:676

10. deLissovoy V. Headbanging in early childhood. *Child Dev* 1962;33:43–56

11. Brody S. Self-rocking in infancy. *J Am Psychoanal Assoc* 1960;8:464–91

12. Golbin AZ. *The World of Children's Sleep*. Michalis Medical Publishing, 1995

13. Zappert J. Über Nachtliche Kopflewegungen der Kindern (jactatio capitis nocturna). *Johnbuch Luer Kinder-Heielkunde* 1905;62:70–83

14. Golbin AZ, Sheldon SH. Parasomnias. In Sheldon SH, Spire JP, Levy HB, eds. *Pediatric Sleep Medicine*. Philadelphia: WB Saunders, 1992:119–35

15. Dyken ME, Rodnitzky RL. Periodic, aperiodic, and rhythmic motor disorders of sleep. *Neurology* 1992;42(Suppl 6):68–74

16. Thorpy MJ. Rhythmic movement disorder. In Thorpy MJ, ed. *Handbook of Sleep Disorders*. New York: Marcel Dekker 1990:119–21

17. Broughton RJ. NREM arousal parasomnias. In Kryger MH, Roth T, Dement WC, eds. *Principles and Practices of Sleep Medicine*, 3rd edn. Philadelphia: WB Saunders, 2000:693–706

18. Gagnon P, De Koninck J. Repetitive head movements during REM sleep. *Biol Psychiatry* 1985;20:187–8

19. Kempenaers C, Bouillon E, Mendlewixz J. A rhythmic movement disorder in REM sleep: a case report. *Sleep* 1994;17:274–9

20. Regestein QR, Hartmann E, Reich P. A single case study: a head movement disorder occurring in dreaming sleep. *J Nerv Ment Dis* 1977; 164:432–5

21. Chisholm T, Morehouse RL. Adult headbanging: sleep studies and treatment. *Sleep* 1996;19: 343–6

22. Dyken ME, Lin-Dyken DC, Yamada T. Diagnosing rhythmic movement disorder with video-polysomnography. *Pediatr Neurol* 1997; 16:37–41

23. Mahowald MW, Thorpy MJ. In Kryger MH, Roth T, Dement WC, eds. *Principles and Practices of Sleep Medicine*, 3rd edn. Philadelphia: WB Saunders, 2000:115–23

24. Greenberg NH. Origins of head-rolling (spasmus nutans) during early infancy. *Psychosom Med* 1964;26:162–71

25. Lourie RS. The role of rhythmic patterns in childhood. *Am J Psychiatry* 1949;105:653–60

26. Fitzherbert J. The origin of headbanging: a suggested explanation with an illustrative case history. *J Ment Sci* 1950;96:793–5

27. Lewis MH, Boumeister AA, Mailman RB. A neurobiological alternative to the perceptual reinforcement hypothesis of stereotyped behavior: a commentary on self stimulating behavior and perceptual reinforcement. *J Appl Behav Anal* 1987;20:253

28. Plepis OY. *Menière's Disease*. Leningrad: Medicina, 1975:270

29. Monplaisir J, Nicolas A, Godbout R, Waltiers A. Restless leg syndrome and periodic limb movement disorder. In Kryger MH, Roth T, Dement WC, eds. *Principles and Practice of Sleep Medicine*, 3rd edn. Philadelphia: WB Saunders, 2000:742–52

30. Lavigne GJ, Manzini L. Bruxism. In Kryger MH, Roth T, Dement WC, eds. *Principles and Practice of Sleep Medicine*, 3rd edn. Philadelphia: WB Saunders, 2000:773–85

31. Attanasio R. Nocturnal bruxism and its clinical management. *Dent Clin North Am* 1991;35:245

32. Mahowald M, Ferber R, Kryger M, eds. *Principles and Practice of Sleep Medicine in the Child. Non-Arousal Parasomnias in the Child*. Philadelphia: WB Saunders, 1995:115–23

33. Satoh T, Harada Y. Tooth grinding during sleep as an arousal reaction. *Experientia* 1971;15:785–7

34. Vanderas PA, Menenakov M, Kouimtzis TH, Paraciannoulis L. Urinary catecholamine levels and bruxism in children. *J Oral Rehabil* 1999;26:103–10

35. Cash RC. Bruxism in children: review of the literature. *J Pedod* 1988;12:107–27

36. Pratap-Chand R, Gourie-Devi M. Bruxism: its significance in coma. *Clin Neurol Neurosurg* 1985;87:113–17

37. Garcia J, Rosen G, Mahowald M. Waterbeds in treatment of rhythmic movement disorders: experience with two cases. *Sleep Res* 1996; 25:243

38. Rosenberg C. Elimination of a rhythmic movement disorder with hypnosis – a case report. *Sleep* 1995;18:608–9

39. Koe GG. Hypnotic treatment of sleep terror disorder: a case report. *Am J Clin Hypnosis* 1989; 32:36–40

40. Kohen DP, Mahowald MW, Rosen GM. Sleep-terror disorder in children: the role of self-hypnosis in management. *Am J Clin Hypnosis* 1992;34:233–44

41. Hurwitz TD, Mahowald MW, Schenck CH, Schutler JL, Bundlie SR. A retrospective outcome study and review of hypnosis as treatment of adults with sleepwalking and sleep terror. *J Nerv Ment Dis* 1991;179:228–33

42. Walsh JK, Kramer M, Skinner JE. A case report of jactatio capitis nocturna. *Am J Psychiatry* 1981;138:524–6

43. Freidin MR, Jankowski JJ, Singer WD. Nocturnal headbanging as a sleep disorder: a case report. *Am J Psychiatry* 1979;136:1469–70

44. Manni R, Tartara A. Clonazepam treatment of rhythmic movement disorders. *Sleep* 1997; 20:812

45. Silber MH, Grish M, Izurieta R. Pramipexole in treatment of restless leg syndrome: an extended study. *Sleep* 2003;26:819–21

46. Clarke JH, Reynolds PJ. Suggestive hypnotherapy for nocturnal bruxism: a pilot study. *Am J Clin Hypnosis* 1991;33:248–50

11

Developmental episodic and paroxysmal sleep events

Alexander Z. Golbin and Leonid Kayumov

Paroxysms, defined as sudden, relatively brief outbursts of autonomic, muscular or behavioral activity, are common events in sleep at all ages, and represent a normal part of the sleep–wake cycle in children and adults. Differentiation of normal from pathological paroxysmal events is both important and challenging.

PAROXYSMAL SLEEP EVENTS IN THE NEONATE AND THE INFANT

Sleep–wake states in neonates and infants are an active and rapidly developing maturational process, associated with multiple paroxysmal events, and are well described[1-3].

Unique sleep state features set the fetus and the neonate apart from the older child and adult[2]. A major sleep reorganization occurs during the first year of life which leads to stable sleep architecture and daytime behavior during childhood. For example, discontinuous electroencephalography (EEG) patterns are noted during quiet sleep in the preterm and full-term neonate, and persist up to 6–8 weeks' post-conceptional age. More arousals and rapid eye movements (REMs) are seen in neonates than during infancy. The percentage of REM sleep drops from 50% to 20% of the total sleep time from birth to 1 year.

Sleep–wake state classifications are similar to behavioral descriptions for neonates. The specific behaviors that define rudimentary REM and non-REM sleep state segments are termed state 1 and 2 in the fetus, or active and non-active sleep states in the neonate. Transitional state 3 suggests a time period during which the cluster of physiological events fails to define wakefulness or sleep (such as a drowsy state in an older person). States 4 and 5 are conventionally defined as quiet–waking and crying–waking states, respectively.

Two unique aspects of neonatal sleep predispose the newborn to paroxysmal events[1,2]. First, 50% of the neonatal sleep cycle consists of active (REM) sleep, during which a greater abundance of motor phenomena, autonomic events and arousals occur. Second, the short neonatal sleep cycle results in rapid transitions between active and quiet sleep segments and wakefulness. Paroxysmal movements in the fetus and neonate include tremulousness or jitteriness, tonic posturing, myoclonus and other state-specific motor activities, which are usually not associated with electroencephalographically proven seizures. Determining whether sleep-related motor phenomena for the fetus or neonate are normal behaviors or are part of an encephalopathic process rests on clinical judgement, supplemented by synchronized video–EEG monitoring.

Tremulousness or jitteriness

The flexion and extension phases of the tremor are equal in amplitude, unlike the unequal phases of clonic movements. Newborns with tremors are generally alert or hyper-alert but can appear somnolent or lethargic. Tremulousness appears with spontaneous or evoked arousals during sleep-to-wake transitions, or within any sleep state. Such movements may follow a brain injury or peripheral neuropathy (e.g. brachial plexus injury), or metabolic or toxin-induced encephalopathy. Tremulousness usually resolves spontaneously over a 6-week period, and in 92% became normal at 3 years of age[4].

Neonatal myoclonus

Clusters of myoclonic activity occur more predominantly during active (REM) sleep, and are more prevalent in the preterm infant[3] and rarely observed in healthy full-term infants. Benign myoclonic movements are not stimulus-sensitive, have no coincident encephalographic seizure correlates and are not associated with EEG background abnormalities. When these movements occur in the healthy full-term neonate, the activity can be suppressed during wakefulness. Benign neonatal sleep myoclonus must be a diagnosis of exclusion, after a careful consideration of pathological diagnoses[5,6].

Infants with severe central nervous system (CNS) dysfunction may also present with non-epileptic spontaneous or stimulus-evoked pathological myoclonus. Encephalopathic neonates may respond to tactile or painful stimulation by isolated focal, segmental or generalized myoclonic movements. Rarely, cortically generated spike or sharp wave discharges as well as seizures may also be noted on the EEG recordings, which is a co-morbid condition with myoclonic movements[7]. Medication-induced myoclonus as well as other movements in sleep, which resolve when the drug is withdrawn, have also been described[8].

A rare familial disorder has been described in the neonatal and early infancy periods, specifically termed *hyperekplexia*[9]. These sleep-related movements usually are misinterpreted as a hyperactive startle reflex, or whole-body myoclonus. Infants are also stiff, with severe hypertonia, which may lead to apnea and bradycardia. EEG background rhythms during myoclonus are generally age-appropriate.

Neonatal dystonia and infants with choreoathetosis

Dystonia and choreoathetosis are not rare paroxysmal movements in infants and are often misclassified as seizures. These non-epileptic movement disorders are associated with either acute or chronic disease states involving basal ganglia structures, or the extrapyramidal pathways that innervate these regions. Antepartum or intrapartum adverse events such as severe asphyxia can damage the basal ganglia (i.e. termed *status mamoratus*[10]).

Specific inherited metabolic diseases[11,12] (e.g. glutaric aciduria) as well as acquired encephalopathies from bilirubin toxicity can cause dystonia. Documentation of electrographic seizures by video–EEG–polygraphic recordings helps avoid misdiagnosis and inappropriate treatment.

Neonatal seizures

Since neonatal and infant seizures are generally brief and subtle in clinical appearance, unusual behaviors are difficult to recognize and classify. The abnormal movements were of non-epileptic origin in 90%[13]. The majority of these non-epileptic events were associated with bicycling, bucco-lingual movements, eye deviation, apnea, autonomic manifestations and irritability noted during sleep or wake–sleep transitions[13]. The diagnosis of suspicious clinical events as seizures, therefore, requires the use of coincident video–EEG recordings to distinguish neonatal clinical 'non-epileptic' seizures from 'epileptic' seizures[14].

The prevalence of paroxysmal events during the first 2 years of life was reported in a Dutch study[15]. One-quarter of the children from the population-based birth cohort of 1854 children had sleep-related paroxysmal episodes.

Benign seizures in infants as parasomnia phenomena

Infantile seizures are subtle and difficult to notice and usually identified by focal appearance[16,17]. Continuous video–EEG monitoring and close observation can help distinguish habitual normal activities of the infant from focal seizures. Guidelines to recognize seizures in infant as well as older children and adults should follow criteria suggested by the International League Against Epilepsy.

Paroxysmal events in sleep and transitional stages include benign as well as epileptic syndromes such as myoclonic epilepsy, Ohtahara syndrome, early myoclonic epileptic encephalopathy, West syndrome or infantile spasms, which are a subset of myoclonic epilepsy that appear during infancy[18]. Clusters of 10–20 contractions in succession may occur during feedings, particularly if the child becomes drowsy. They can occur at the onset of or arousal from sleep. Infantile spasms can be either idiopathic or symptomatic. Idiopathic forms include a small minority of children who are developmentally normal. A classical EEG pattern with the more severe form of infantile spasms includes hypsarrhythmia with asynchronous and random high-amplitude irregular slow waves and intermixed spikes and polyspikes. During sleep this chaotic disorganization of EEG activity can become organized as a suppression burst pattern[19].

Episodic nocturnal movement disorders other than seizures

Episodic nocturnal movement disorders of infancy include events other than epileptic seizures. Their exclusive occurrence during infancy and their functions have not been systematically studied. In particular, **myoclonic, tonic or dystonic movements** may appear after the neonatal period during infancy and reflect epileptic states or non-epileptic movement disorders. These movements may be benign with a high likelihood of resolution, or severe when associated with significant injury. Pathological, non-epileptic myoclonus can be observed in encephalopathic infants and with neonates. **Hyperekplexia** (excessive startle response) may also be misclassified as myoclonus in the infant as with the neonate. **Benign sleep myoclonus** of infancy (as with the neonatal form) consists of focal, multifocal or generalized myoclonic events. Movements occur only during sleep, can be stopped by gentle restraint and are eliminated during arousal. Each jerk lasts only several seconds and tends to recur. EEG demonstrates no change except movement artifact. These infants are typically neurodevelopmentally normal and events usually disappear by 6 months of age, although some persist into childhood. **Shuddering attacks** are unique paroxysmal events of infancy, usually appearing during 4 to 6 months of age[20]. Rarely noted in older children, they may predict essential tremor at older ages[21]. A behavioral arrest may accompany the shuddering attacks without loss of consciousness. These sometimes are noted during the transition from wakefulness to sleep, and EEG activity is generally unremarkable. Despite the appearance of apparent wakefulness with eyes open, some children appear to shudder when hypnagogic hypersynchrony (a pattern of drowsiness) is present on their EEG.

Paroxysmal events in young children

Children with specific medical conditions may experience paroxysmal events in sleep related to a specific organ (for example, GI reflux) at any age.

Gastroesophageal reflux

Both newborns and infants may demonstrate episodic hyperextension and lateral flexion of the head usually with feeding but sometimes spontaneously occurring while asleep or awake. Choking, apnea, laryngospasm and opisthotonus are commonly described[22].

Historically these events were termed 'dystonic dyspepsia' or Sandifer's syndrome, particularly in the preterm infant. The age range for reflux is wide, beginning during the neonatal period and extending into adolescence.

Children with pulmonary diseases including conditions leading to reactive airway disease, specifically bronchial asthma, may experience paroxysmal events with partial arousals or sleep fragmentation. Symptoms of obstructive sleep apnea can also occur from the infancy period, particularly with susceptible individuals with structural abnormalities of the upper airways.

Paroxysmal events occur in children with neurological disease[23]. Developmentally delayed children with diffuse hypotonia due to trisomy 21 or Prader–Willi syndrome may experience multiple movements or cardiorespiratory events during sleep. Neurodegenerative diseases may first present as frequent night awakenings sometimes associated with paroxysmal events. Rett's disorder is accompanied by night awakenings and paroxysmal events, particularly during the first and second years of life. Sleep architecture and continuity may be altered, leading to decreased total sleep time and partial arousals. Other congenital, metabolic or degenerative syndromes are related to disorders of sleep. Hypoventilation can be seen with mitochondrial disease, familial dysautonomia and storage disorders.

Paroxysmal sleep disorders are commonly noted in children with neuromuscular syndromes and structural brain lesions. Myelodysplasia can be associated with apnea, cranial nerve dysfunction including vocal cord paralysis with respiratory stridor and swallowing inco-ordination. Patients with significant myelodysplasia may experience an unusual form of pallid breath-holding spells sometimes commonly referred to as *vagotonia*. These are life-threatening events, which can occur during wakefulness or sleep and can be associated with a sudden bradycardia or asystole. Scher[19] reports that healthy children with migraine variants occasionally present during infancy with cyclic vomiting, partial arousals during sleep and crying from presumed pain.

EPISODIC OR PAROXYSMAL PARASOMNIAS IN OLDER CHILDREN, ADOLESCENTS AND ADULTS

Sleep starts

Sleep starts, or hypnic jerks, are common experiences, usually occurring during the transition between wakefulness and sleep. Most commonly it is a motor sleep start – sudden all-body jerk that may awaken or startle the person or bed partner. Other less common but possibly frightening phenomena are visual (a sudden blinding flash of light), auditory (a loud cracking or snapping noise in the head) or somesthetic (pain or flowing sensations)[24,25]. The mechanism and possible function of sleep starts is unknown. They might represent a sudden intrusion of an isolated REM sleep event into light non-REM[24–27]. However, this suggestion does not explain why, or how, the person can immediately fall asleep after such a dramatic body jerking or sensation. Sleep starts should not be confused with periodic limb movements, considered benign.

Sleepwalking

Sleepwalking is one of the most dramatic and common parasomnias. It is characterized by sudden behavioral events in sleep, which typically occur within the first third of the night during the slow-wave sleep and transitional states. Sleepwalking can occur at any age. As with other parasomnias the pathogenesis of sleepwalking is poorly understood despite obvious dramatic and clear presentation and frequency of the phenomenon.

Sleepwalking has a large spectrum of activity from mild and benign to highly organized and violent (see Chapters 24 and 25). Polysomnographic studies demonstrate that sleepwalking episodes occur within the first few hours of slow-wave sleep. EEG shows sudden rhythmic, high-voltage delta activity that persists during episodes. More commonly, there is a pattern of a low-amplitude mixture of non-REM with non-reactive alpha waves. Sometimes high-amplitude theta and delta outbursts are present in non-REM before the episodes or during the night without sleepwalking.

The treatment of sleepwalking is as unclear as its pathogenesis. Protection, or behavior modification techniques including hypnosis, benzodiazepines and selective serotonin reuptake inhibitors (SSRIs), are the most typical recommendations.

Sleeptalking and groaning

Sleeptalking (somniloquy) is a familiar event, which might range from whispering to very loud speech that can be unclear to prolonged clear conversations even with the awake person. It may arise from non-REM as well as from REM stages. In the latter case it may be associated with recall of a dream[28]. The precise mechanism is not clear and no controlled treatment studies are available.

Sleep-related expiratory groaning might be associated with dyspnea and choking sensations. Etiology, mechanism and treatment are unclear, might be masking and episodes as seizures and other disorders.

Nocturnal headaches

Rare in children and more common in adults, cluster headaches, chronic paroxysmal hemicrania and migraine have been shown, in some cases, associated with REM sleep[29,30]. Obstructive sleep apnea syndrome and carbon monoxide intoxication may cause sleep-related headaches[24].

Nocturnal paroxysmal dystonia and other disorders in older children, adolescents and adults

This condition consists of violent movements of the limbs, associated with spasms that can occur over multiple episodes during the night. No scalp EEG abnormalities are found during the clinical spells, and these events are considered as being partial arousals. Nocturnal paroxysmal disorders might represent epileptic phenomena, which may emanate from the frontal lobe, reminiscent of the nocturnal frontal lobe epilepsies seen in older patients. Seizures must be considered in any sleep-related behavior[24,29]. Nocturnal seizures may be unusual in presentation, and therefore may be underdiagnosed or misdiagnosed in a lack of an absence of scalp EEG abnormalities or unusual clinical manifestations.

Sleep-related seizures

Nocturnal sleep-related seizures should always be ruled out and may take many forms: recurrent dreams; nightmares; sleepwalking or episodic nocturnal wandering; recurrent isolated arousals; unusual autonomic symptoms; nocturnal paroxysmal dystonia; paroxysmal spasms in infants[2].

Rapid eye movement behavior disorder

This interesting condition was described in animals and humans and formally established as a separate parasomnia in 1968 by Schenck and co-workers[30-32], consists of active motor reactions during REM sleep corresponding to dream content. The significance of this disorder is related to paroxysmal (explosive) sudden limb and body movements with potentially traumatic consequences: diving from the bed, or hitting the spouse, walls or furniture. More commonly, the disorder appears as screaming, arm waving or kicking. These episodes appear a few times a week but might be more common. Also, they might appear a few times a night with about a 90-min cycle corresponding to REM phases. It is important to mention that violent and apparently aggressive behavior is discordant to the person's daytime personality. The duration of these episodes is usually a few minutes. Research indicates that one-third of the patients with the disorder have light forms for many years[30,31]. In more than half the patient population the disorder is considered idiopathic, but more typical for patients with CNS pathology such as chronic alcoholism, Parkinson's disease, stroke, etc. The mechanism is due to some sort of lesion or dysfunction of brainstem mechanisms responsible for the suppression of muscle tone in REM.

Polysomnography (PSG) in REM behavior disorder is quite specific, which makes PSG the main diagnostic tool. During REM there are multiple muscle artifacts related to phasic motor activity (eye movements, brief twitching potentials and, unusual for REM, increased background muscle tone). Differential diagnosis is based on exclusion of organic causes, but PSG findings are moderately reliable.

Treatment is mainly medication management, and clonazepam is most commonly used. Tricyclics such as desipramine and SSRIs have been partially helpful. Review of medications to avoid confusion and other complications from drug interactions is necessary and, most importantly, for prevention of injury and treatment of underlying pathology.

Night terrors and nightmares

Night terrors and nightmares are among the most common and most puzzling paroxysmal parasomnias. Their nature and precise physiological mechanisms are yet to be uncovered.

Night terrors and nightmares are frequently described together just to emphasize their differences[32,33] (Table 11.1).

Night terrors are a phenomenon predominantly of NREM, occurring during the first third of the night and presenting essentially paroxysm, a 'storm' in the autonomic nervous system. For carers and observers, night terrors appear as sudden and tremendously intense motor agitation, disoriented behavior, emotional terror and somatic excitement (perfuse perspiration, heart palpitations and tremors).

At the moment of the night terror, the person does not respond to consoling (Figures 11.1

Table 11.1 Differentiation of sleep terrors from nightmares

Characteristic	Sleep terror	Nightmare
Name	pavor nocturnus	anxiety dream
Time of night	first third	last third
Stage of sleep	slow-wave sleep	REM sleep
Movements	somnambulism common	rare
Severity	severe	mild
Vocalizations	common	rare
Autonomic discharge	severe/intense	mild
Recall	fragmented	good
State on waking	confused/disoriented	functions well
Injuries	frequent	rare
Violence	possible	non-violent
Displacement from bed	frequent	none

From Golbin A. *The World of Children's Sleep*. Salt Lake City: Michaelis, 1995, with permission

and 11.2) and cannot be stopped until the episode runs its course and ends by itself.

Surprisingly, afterwards, the 'affected' person does not remember most of it and it does not affect his/her daytime personality and daily life.

In contrast, nightmares are terrifying or otherwise very unpleasant dreams, a part of REM stage disorders (Figure 11.3). The person is actively involved in the content of his/her dreams and the content of the dreams might greatly influence daytime mood, thoughts and behavior.

Paradoxically, despite an intensive emotional content of the dream, autonomic discharges are somewhat weak. Our night 'movies' are significant for us, but their physiological, diagnostic and psychological meaning continues to challenge researchers and clinicians.

The nature, clinical significance and forensic issues of night terrors, dreams and similar phenomena are discussed in detail in Chapters 3, 8, 20 and 25.

Nocturnal panics

Nocturnal sleep-related panic attacks may or may not be associated with daytime panic

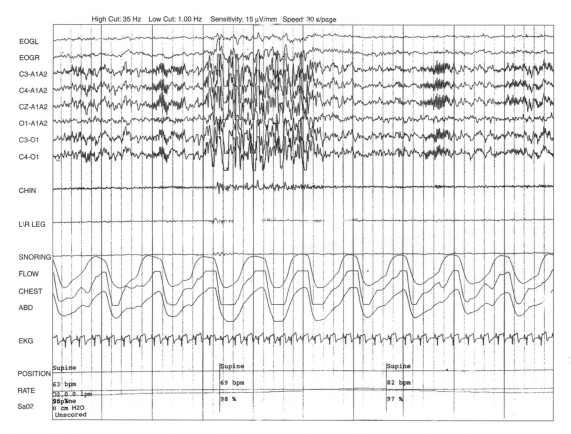

Figure 11.1 Polysomnogram during a brief night terror episode. Diffuse high-amplitude theta and delta waves on EEG

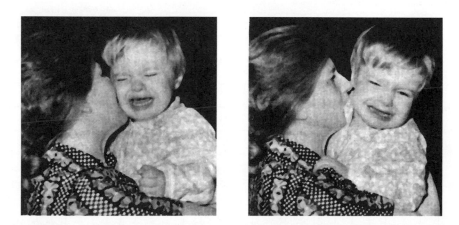

Figure 11.2 Night terrors. The child is confused, screaming loudly and in 'terror'. The mother may desperately try to wake the child, but the child is unresponsive

disorder. Some panic attacks may occur exclusively in sleep during midnight arousals; in other cases, daytime fears may 'spill over' into a sleeping state[24,33].

Nocturnal panic attacks may be a part of other paroxysmal parasomnias such as night terrors, a reaction to forceful awakenings or as a

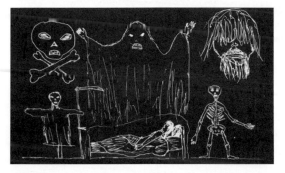

Figure 11.3 A child's interpretive drawings of his nightmare

symptom of multiple sleep disorders and medical problems (Figure 11.4). (For futher details, see Chapter 25.)

CONCLUSION

Paroxysmal events (behavioral, autonomic or electrographic) are extremely common in sleep as well as in transitional stages of vigilance. Some of them are transitory and even a necessary part of ontogenetic development, others are less benign or even pathological and will have significant impact on later development, but all of them signify a level of 'maturity' in sleep–wake regulation. The knowledge of these relationships between paroxysmal events and an underlying CNS mechanism might help in diagnosis and treatment.

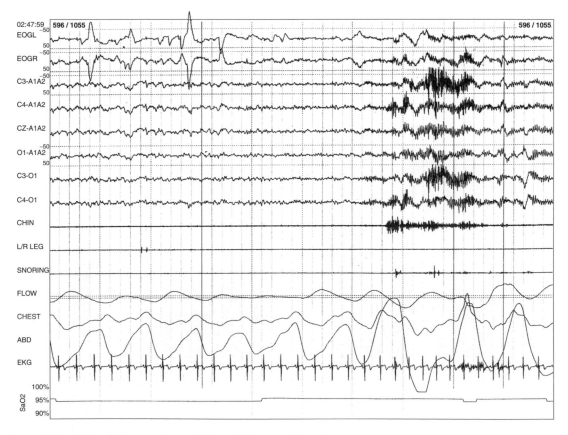

Figure 11.4 Polysomnogram of arousal from REM sleep with panic

References

1. Scher MS. Pediatric sleep assessment by the pediatric neurologist. Understanding sleep ontogeny to assess brain dysfunction in neonates and infants. *J Child Neurol* 1998;13: 467–74

2. Scher MS. Paroxysmal sleep events in the neonate and young infants. In *Recognizing and Treating Pediatric Parasommias*. APSS. 16th Annual Meeting, June 8–13, 2002, Seattle, WA: 1–22

3. Daoust-Roy J, Seshia SS. Benign neonatal sleep myoclonus: a differential diagnosis of neonatal seizures. *Am J Dis Child* 1992;116:1236–41

4. Shupee A, Falzberg J, Weitz R, *et al.* Jitteriness beyond the neonatal period benign pattern of movement in infancy. *J Child Neurol* 1991;6: 243–5

5. Coulter DL, Allen RJ. Benign neonatal sleep myoclonus. *Arch Neurol* 1982;39:191–2

6. Di Capua M, Fusco L, Ricci S, *et al.* Benign neonatal sleep myoclonus: clinical features and video-polygraphic recordings 1993;8: 191–4

7. Scher MS. Pathological myoclonus of the newborn: electrographic and clinical correlations. *Pediatr Neurol* 1985;1:342–8

8. Sexson WR, Thigpen J, Stajich GV. Stereotypic movements after lorazepam administration in premature neonates: a series and review of the literature. *J Perinatol* 1995;15:146–99

9. Brown P, Rothwell JC, Thompson PD, *et al.* The hyperekplexias and their relationship to the normal startle reflex. *Brain* 1991;114:1903–28

10. Volpe JJ. *Neurology of the Newborn*, 4th edn. Philadelphia, PA: WB Saunders, 2001:178–214

11. Barth PJ. Inherited progressive disorders of the fetal brain: a field in need of recognition. In Fukuyama Y, *et al.* eds. *Fetal and Perinatal Neurology*. Basel: Karger 1992:99–313

12. Lyon G, Adams RD, Kolodny EH. *Neurology of Hereditary Metabolic Diseases of Children*, 2nd edn. New York: McGraw-Hill, 1996: 6–44

13. Scher MS, Painter MJ. Electrographic diagnosis of neonatal seizures. Issues of diagnostic accuracy, clinical correlation and survival. In Wasterlain CG, Vert P, eds. *Neonatal Seizures*. New York, NY: Raven Press, 1990

14. Mizrahi EM, Kellaway P. *Diagnosis and Management of Neonatal Seizure*. Philadelphia, PA: Lippincott-Raven, 1998:1–155

15. Klackenberg G. Rhythmic movements in infancy and early childhood. *Acta Paediatr Scand* 1971;224(Suppl):74–83

16. Nordli DR Jr, Kuroda MM, Hirsch U. The ontogeny of partial seizures in infants and young children. *Epilepsia* 2001;42:986–90

17. Nordli DR Jr, Brazil CW, Scheuer ML, *et al.* Recognition and classification of seizures in infants. *Epilepsia* 1997;38:553–60

18. Shupee A, Mimouri M. Problems of differentiation between epilepsy and non-epileptic paroxysmal events in the first year of life. *Arch Dis Child* 1995;73:342–4

19. Scher MS. Neonatal seizures. Seizures in special clinical settings. In Wylie E, ed. *The Treatment of Epilepsy. Principles & Practice*, 3rd edn. Baltimore, MD: Lippincott, Williams & Wilkins, 2001:577–600

20. Holmes GL, Russman BS. Shuddering attacks: Evaluation using electroencephalographic frequency modulation radiotelemetry and videotape monitoring. *Am J Dis Child* 1986; 140:72–3

21. Vanasse M, Bedard P, Andermann F. Shuddering attacks in children: an early clinical manifestation of essential tremor. *Neurology* 1976;26:1027–30

22. Gorrotxategi F, Reguilon J, Arana J, *et al.* Gastroesophageal reflux in association with the Sandifer syndrome. *Eur J Pediatr Surg* 1995; 5:203–5

23. Brown LW, Maistros P, Guilleminault C. Sleep in children with neurologic problems. In Ferber and Kryger, eds. *Principles and Practice of Sleep Medicine in the Child*. Philadelphia, PA: WB Saunders, 1995

24. Mahowald MW, Thorpy MS. Non-arousal parasomnias in the child. In Ferber R, Kryger M, eds. *Principles and Practice of Sleep Medicine in the Child*. Philadelphia: WB Saunders, 1995:115–23

25. Parkes JD. The parasomnias. *Lancet* 1986;851: 10–21

26. Broughton RJ. NREM arousal parasomnias. In Kryger MH, Roth T, Dement WC, eds. *Principles and Practice of Sleep Medicine*, 3rd edn. Philadelphia: WB Saunders, 2000:693–706

27. *The International Classification of Sleep Disorders. Diagnostic and Coding Manual*. Rochester, MN: American Sleep Disorder Association, 1990: 145–7

28. Arkin AM, Toth MF, Baker J, *et al.* The degree of concordance between the content of sleep talking and mentation recalled in wakefulness. *J Nerv Ment Dis* 1970;151:375–80

29. Tinuper P, Cerullo A, Grignota F, *et al.* Nocturnal paroxysmal dystonia with short lasting attacks: three cases with evidence of an

epileptic frontal lobe origin of seizures. *Epilepsia* 1990;31:549

30. Schenck CH, Mahowald MW. REM parasomnias. *Neurol Clin* 1996;14:697–720

31. Mahowald MW, Schenk CH. REM sleep parasomnias. In Kryger MH, Roth T, Dement WC, eds. *Principles and Practice of Sleep Medicine*, 3rd edn. Philadelphia: WB Saunders, 2000: 724–41

32. Nielsen TA, Zodra A. REM sleep disorders. In Kryger MH, Roth T, Dement WC, eds. *Principles and Practice of Sleep Medicine*, 3rd edn. Philadelphia: WB Saunders, 2000:753–72

33. Mellman TA, Uhde TW. Sleep panic attacks: new clinical findings and theoretical implications. *Am J Psychiatry* 1989;146:1204

12

Nocturnal enuresis: a disorder of sleep

Alexander Z. Golbin

Urinating in bed is frequently predisposed by deep sleep: when urine begins to flow, its inner nature and hidden will (resembling the will to breathe) drives urine out before the child awakes.

When children become stronger and more robust, their sleep is lighter and they stop urinating.'

Avicenna (Abu Ali al-Husain ibn Abdallah ibn Sina)[1], *Canon of Medical Science*, AD 1012, Book 3, part 19:338

INTRODUCTION

Nocturnal enuresis (bedwetting) is a 'stumbling block' for theoretical and practical medicine. The literature about enuresis is as large as the population of bedwetters. Nocturnal enuresis is defined as involuntary urination in sleep without urological or neurological causes after the age of 5 at which time bladder control would normally be expected[1,2]. Nocturnal bedwetting in sleep is the most common and least understood parasomnia. The nature of this affliction and its treatment is not simple. Bedwetting becomes clinically significant because of the adverse social and psychological effects on the family structure. Simply stated, no one knows why the child can hold urination all day long, but not during sleep. Often parents ask if the child is aggravating them deliberately. It is difficult to find another disorder in which physical and mental abuse was accepted by society as a formal 'treatment' including such prescriptions as 'wake him up after enuresis and give him hot pepper to punish him'; 'make him sleep with his head down'; 'do not allow him to sleep for a few nights'; etc.[3]

The pervasive influence of psychology in the first half of the 20th century led to the explanation of enuresis as a psychological disorder. Current research into the psychological and social variables linked to primary enuresis yields evidence to support the notion that primary enuresis is a psychological disorder[4]. At the same time individuals tend to develop psychological decrements (i.e. antisocial behavior, low self-esteem, etc.) as a result of their inability to gain urinary control during the night. There are also considerable financial, time and emotional difficulties placed on the guardians and siblings of bedwetters. Children consider their bedwetting as extremely embarrassing and a disaster when discovered by their peers. Even highly educated parents see their children as lazy nuisances[5]. Therefore, children with enuresis may be at significant risk of emotional and physical abuse by society and their own family.

PREVALENCE

According to a questionnaire study involving a sample population of 3344 people from the Shandong Province of China, 7.7% of 2 year olds attained nocturnal urinary control. By the age of 3, this number increased to 53.1%, and by age 5, 93% of children displayed nighttime continence. The overall prevalence of nocturnal enuresis was 1.8%, with a significantly higher rate in boys than in girls. Chinese children attained nocturnal control earlier than children in the Western world[6]. It is often speculated that some of the differences between the reported frequency of enuresis in a given population is related to cultural differences as well as variability in the 'working definition' of enuresis[7]. These numbers seem to be similar throughout all cultures[8,9].

Nocturnal enuresis (NE) is typically divided into primary and secondary forms. Primary nocturnal enuresis (PNE) is urination in sleep since birth. Secondary nocturnal enuresis (SNE) is the re-manifestation of bedwetting after at least 6 months without bedwetting[10].

Monosymptomatic nocturnal enuresis alludes to symptoms of voiding dysfunction in the absence of daytime symptoms. Polysymptomatic nocturnal enuresis is associated with severe urgency, urge incontinence, or a staccato voiding pattern. Approximately 80% of enuretics wet only at night, while 20% also have daytime wetting. The daytime wetters belong to a different category and require an alternative evaluation[2,11,12].

ETIOLOGY

The etiology of PNE is multifactorial and unclear. PNE is a diagnosis of exclusion. All other causes of bedwetting must be ruled out. Skoog[10,13] described monosymptomatic primary nocturnal enuresis as a symptom and not a disease. This symptom has many non-mutually exclusive etiologies that confound any attempt to describe a single pathophysiological mechanism to all individuals with PNE. The major etiological categories are: psychological factors; nocturnal polyuria; developmental delay; urodynamics; genetics; and sleep disorders.

SNE has several causes: idiopathic; urge syndrome/dysfunctional voiding; cystitis; constipation; psychological stress; acquired neurogenic bladder; seizure disorder; obstructive sleep apnea; diabetes mellitus; acquired diabetes insipidus; acquired urethral obstruction; heart block; hyperthyroidism, etc.[11,14].

There is no organ or system that has not been blamed as a cause of enuresis at some time or another.

GENETICS

Formal genetic approaches include family studies, twin studies and segregation analysis[15–17]. Family studies show a 60–80% rate of affected first-degree relatives of enuretic children. There is a 77% recurrence rate if both parents have a history of NE and a recurrence rate of 43–44% if one parent has a history of NE. Family history of enuresis is the most important factor in determining the age of attaining dryness. If two or more first-degree relatives are affected, bladder control is achieved more than 1.5 years later than normal. Monozygotic twins have a concordance rate of 68%, while dizygotic twins display a 36% rate. Segregation analysis shows that the most plausible mode of inheritance was autosomal dominant, with a reduced penetrance of 90% in multigenerational pedigrees. A highly positive linkage between markers D13S291 and D13S263 on the long arm of chromosome 13 (between 13q13 and 13q14.2) was identified by Eiberg[15] in a Danish study of multigenerational families. Two additional markers (D12S260 and D12S43) were found on the long arm of chromosome 12 and on chromosome 8 (D8S260 and D8S257). NE was also mapped to chromosome 22 between the markers D22S446 and D22S343, with a load score of 4.51.

Epidemiological studies have shown NE to be a familial disorder with a high incidence in the parents and siblings of enuretics. Hollmann and co-workers[16,17] noted no statistically significant association between linkage to a chromosome interval and the type of enuresis. There was, however a statistically significant trend towards a high rate of day wetting problems in children with a positive assignment to chromosome 12q. Also there was a high rate of primary NE in children with a positive assignment to chromosome 13q. It is possible that different forms of enuresis coexist in the same family. The author suggests research with larger, multigenerational families in order to determine the association between genotype and the environmental factors that influence phenotype.

By using recombinant DNA technology, a dense map of genetic markers spanning the entire genome has been established. These markers can be used to map a single monogenic trait by linkage analysis. Common traits, such as NE, are heterogenic with either a multifactorial or a polygenic background. Segregation studies have shown that PNE is inherited through several generations as a dominant trait with high penetrance. Von Gontard and co-workers[17], using a total genome scan with more than 800 markers, were able to exclude a locus for PNE from the entire genome except for chromosome 22, between the markers D22S446 and D22S343. Thus, chromosome 22 is the most likely site for PNE.

PSYCHOLOGY/BEHAVIOR

Nocturnal enuresis is rarely caused by psychological factors. A study by Willie and Anveden[4] did not support the theory that PNE is a manifestation of emotional disturbances. These authors found no occurrence of 'symptom substitution' (increase in other neurotic, psychosomatic or emotional symptoms) after treatment. Also, children do not show an increase in behavior or psychological problems, except for their displeasure with bedwetting. Enuresis creates secondary psychological complications that affect

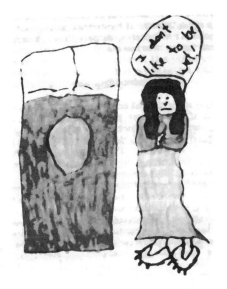

Figure 12.1 Drawing of a 15-year-old girl suffering from bedwetting. She drew similar pictures every night before sleep while praying 'I don't want to be wet'

self-esteem, increase anxiety (Figure 12.1) and create a burden for child and family that often continues into adulthood. The successful treating of PNE contributes to the positive health and development of the patient and the family. Bedwetting after the age of 10 is associated with slight increases in conduct problems, attention-deficit behaviors and anxiety/withdrawal in early adolescence[18]. Byrd and co-workers[8] noted that extreme scores on a 32-item Behavior Problem Index (BPI) were more common among children with frequent or infrequent enuresis opposed to those without enuresis. This particular study did not differentiate between primary versus secondary nocturnal enuresis. Results from a study conducted by Friman suggest that PNE should be considered a common biobehavioral problem, not a psychiatric disorder[7].

Some authors argued that even infrequent episodes of enuresis are associated with significantly higher behavioral problems[3,10,18].

The controversy surrounding the association between bedwetting and behavioral problems is still not solved. It is still unclear whether bedwetting causes behavior problems or vice versa.

Table 12.1 Essential and associated features of noctural enuresis

Essential features
Spontaneous involuntary wetting during sleep
Disturbances of sleep
Changes in levels of wakefulness
Resistance to direct therapeutic intervention and
  spontaneous remission

Associated features
Family pattern of inheritance
Co-existing daytime enuresis
Somatic, endocrinological, neurological and
  urological symptoms

Table 12.2 Disturbances of sleep and alertness in enuretic children

Sleep disturbances in enuresis
Difficulties falling asleep or 'too short' sleep onset
Variation of the sleep depth from too deep
  ('dead') sleep to 'erratic'
Sleep body position changes

Changes of alertness
Agitated or confusional arousals
Sharp variations of daytime motor activity
Significant variations in alertness level and emotional
  lability during the day
Frequent self-stimulating or self-soothing habits

SLEEP AND NOCTURNAL ENURESIS

Nocturnal enuresis (bedwetting) by definition occurs in sleep. Enuresis and sleep seem to be inherently connected. Paradoxically, their connection is not easy to prove and there is no agreement on this subject.

Nocturnal enuresis is not a monosymptomatic condition but a complicated syndrome that consists of a number of essential and associated symptoms (Table 12.1[19,20]).

Significant deviations of sleep and alertness are the essential features of nocturnal enuresis. As seen in Table 12.2, reistance to treatment and spontaneous cure are also related to sleep.

Thus, clinical facts connect enuresis to sleep. It has been reported that enuretics are difficult to arouse from sleep. NE is categorized along with night terrors and sleepwalking as a parasomnia, involving impaired arousal from delta sleep, though a small percentage of enuretic episodes do occur during rapid eye movement (REM) sleep. REM sleep is characterized by increased sympathetic activity while non-REM sleep is characterized by parasympathetic activity. The micturition reflex is initiated by parasympathetic detrusor stimulation and sympathetic inhibition, describing the relationship between non-REM and enuretic episodes. Perhaps the autonomous nervous system is a key link between sleep mechanisms and urodynamics.

Even authors who believe that sleep in enuretic children is polysomnographically normal[31,32,34,41] agree that these children exhibit signs of autonomic arousals associated with acts of urination.

In an attempt to test the hypothesis that enuretic children are difficult to wake, and to find the relationship between bedwetting and other sleep disorders, Neveus and co-workers[21] discovered that enuretics had higher incidents of bruxism and were more often confused when they woke than the controls. The authors showed that enuretics had a higher arousal threshold and occurrence of NE/nocturia in the family. This provides some evidence to speculate that perhaps arousability and nighttime polyuria could be inherited and the combination of these two qualities results in NE.

Interestingly, the majority of enuretic events take place near the onset of sleep. This finding reflects the possiblity of early nocturnal polyuria. Watanabe and Kawauchi[22,23] described the functions of urination and sleep as they develop with age. In infants, the storage and discharge of urine is under the automatic control of the lower urination centrum in the sacral cord. Tension of the bladder wall creates an afferent stimulation from the bladder to the lower centers. The efferent stimulation from the centrum to the bladder could switch the physical condition of the bladder. As an individual develops, the full bladder is sensed consciously in the upper centrum, giving the individual an opportunity to determine whether urination is appropriate or not.

There are data that suggest that acute bladder distension causes the locus ceruleus (LC)

to be activated, resulting in the transition from deep sleep to light sleep. When an individual is in a light sleep (stage 1–2 NREM), bladder distension does not activate the LC. LC activation is effective in switching from deep to light sleep, but in order to fully arouse an individual, further motivation is needed[22].

It is theorized that sleep spindles, generated by the thalamus, prevent arousals and maintain sleep[22,24,25–27]. Classifications have been made by monitoring electroencephalogram (EEG) and cystometry. Roughly 60% of 1252 subjects with PNE belong to type I, 10% belong to type IIa and 30% to type IIb[24].

Type IIb involves the ineffective transmission of urinary sensation to the upper centrum, caused by disturbances in bladder function (latent neurogenic bladder). During sleep, type IIa reflects normal bladder function coupled with a severe disturbance of arousal mechanisms. Because distension of the bladder creates no effect on EEG, it is unknown whether this occurs because of a dysfunction with the arousal systems (namely the LC) or because of an intentional cancellation of activation by an unknown mechanism.

Type I involves a mild disturbance of the arousal systems. Distension of the bladder causes transition from deep to light sleep; however, the transition to full arousal is incomplete. The appearance of sleep spindles increases until the person falls back into deep sleep. Urination occurs during this drowsy or light sleep[23–25].

MECHANISMS OF AROUSAL IN RELATIONSHIP TO BEDWETTING

Using anesthetized rats and cats, Kayama and Koyama[25] were able to determine the key mechanisms of arousal systematically stimulating and recording the activity of brainstem nuclei. The serotonergic projection from the dorsal raphe nucleus is active during waking. Activation of the noradrenergic projection (LC) excites the upper brain sites and activation of the serotonergic projection (dorsal raphe nucleus) depresses upper brain site activity. The cholinergic neurons (laterodorsal tegmental nucleus) constitute a system to induce and maintain REM sleep.

Kawauchi and co-workers[26] and Watanabe and Kawauchi[22] hypothesized that immaturity in the function of the thalamus suppresses the last stage leading to awakening in the type I enuretic. Even though delta waves decrease and sleep spindles increase in response to a full bladder, the thalamus continues to generate sleep spindles. These sleep spindles inhibit the afferent input of internal and external sensory stimuli, thus maintaining sleep. In contrast, type I enuretics who did not wet the bed showed a decrease in the number of delta waves with a corresponding increase in sleep spindles. Eventually both delta waves and sleep spindles appear, leading to arousal and nocturia. Individuals with type IIa enuresis show absolutely no neurological reaction to a full bladder. Delta waves remain high and sleep spindles never appear in the EEG. For this type of enuresis, it is postulated that the arousal mechanisms in the pons or the lower tract may be abnormal or immature.

Watanabe and Kawauchi[22] reviewed physiological mechanisms of arousal. Two independent systems exist in the brain that control arousal and sleep. The 'wet' system involves the sleep-promoting substances that modify sleep according to the circadian rhythms in the body. These substances include amines, cytokines, neuropeptides, nucleosides and prostaglandins as well as other unknown substances. The 'dry' system involves the four neuronal networks projecting to various areas of the brain: norepinephrine (noradrenaline)-activated system from the LC; serotonin from the dorsal raphe nucleus; acetylcholine-activated system from the laterodorsal tegmental nucleus and the pedunculopontine tegmental nucleus; and histamine-activated system from the tuberomammillary nucleus.

The alteration of arousal and sleep is controlled by the harmony among many systems distributed in the brain originating in the LC and projecting to various areas of the brain – thalamus, hypothalamus, cerebral cortex, cerebellum and medulla oblongata. Wolfish[27] studied arousal dysfunction in

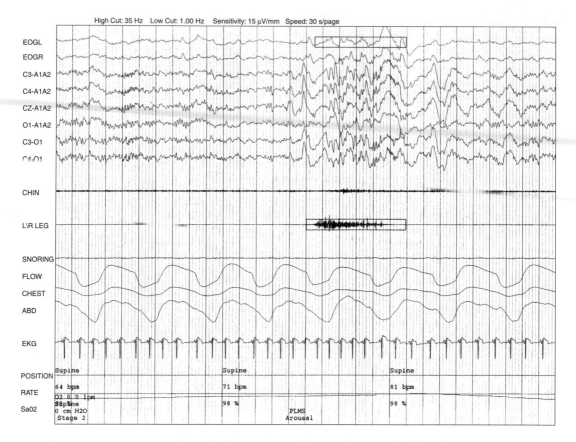

Figure 12.2   Paroxysmal theta or delta wave intrusions with arousals are typical prior to the act of enuresis

enuretics. His research showed that bedwetting events occurred earlier in the night and deceased in frequency as the night progressed. Episodes of brief arousals are typical prior to the act of enuresis (Figure 12.2).

Studies with desmopressin[28–31] also suggest that sleep mechanisms are involved in enuresis as well as bladder dysfunction in some children. Sleep disturbances and bladder dysfunction are common among enuretic children who fail to respond to treatment (desmopressin). Because enuretic events have been stimulated in non-enuretics after fluid loading prior to bedtime, it is speculated that diminished nocturnal bladder capacity is a possible pathological factor in some desmopressin-resistant PNE individuals[12,31,32].

Neveus[29] looked at the sleep records of seven desmopressin responders and 16 non-responders with PNE and found that enuretic events typically took place during non-REM sleep. Desmopressin responders void at the beginning and end of the night, while non-responders void through all parts of the night.

A polygraphy study by Neveus and co-workers[29,30] showed that enuretics displayed a higher proportion of delta sleep during wet nights as opposed to dry nights, which had more superficial sleep. Deep sleep was confirmed using EEG power analysis and the conventional manual polysomnogram description. Computer power analysis showed increased delta power in contrast to the normal manual polysomnographic score. This suggests that enuretics have a greater depth of sleep. Computer power analysis also showed impaired arousals in enuretics. It was

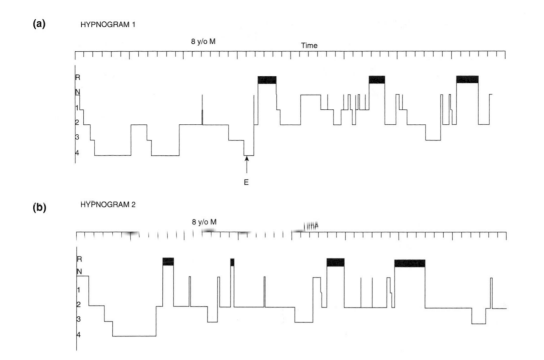

Figure 12.3 Hypnogram of an 8-year-old bedwetter before (a) and after (b) treatment for bedwetting. E, moment of urination. Normalization of sleep architecture after enuresis. After treatment, sleep architecture became age appropriate

concluded that these results pointed to the potential of these sleep components as part of the pathology of NE.

The enuretic event is a non-REM sleep phenomenon that occurs during any part of the night[9,33,34]. It is possible that increased arousability during REM leads to nocturia instead of an enuretic event. We found that paroxysms of delta wave intrusions appear more frequently prior to the act of enuresis (Figure 12.2). The acts of enuresis from stage 3 to 4 are associated with a decrease in heart rate variability. Arousals after the enuretic act are accompanied by tachycardia, body position changes and/or a switch to another sleep stage or awakening (Figure 12.3). Interestingly enough, before the act of enuresis, the first non-REM is prolonged and 'deep' in terms of the very high amplitude of delta waves and low arousability. After the enuretic act, the rhythm of sleep stages seems to 'restore' and 'arousability' increases.

HOW ENURESIS DEVELOPS

The key to the problem of nocturnal enuresis lies in the integration of the known facts regarding this phenomenon. Urination during sleep and the disturbance of the sleep–wake cycle are central features. The question is, which of the two is primary?

The following facts confirm that:

(1) Sleep pattern distortions precede enuresis ontogenically;

(2) During the night, behavioral and EEG distortions precede bedwetting episodes;

(3) Physiological studies demonstrate that arousal or 'switch' stages deviate in primary enuresis;

(4) Following bedwetting, behavioral and EEG patterns normalize;

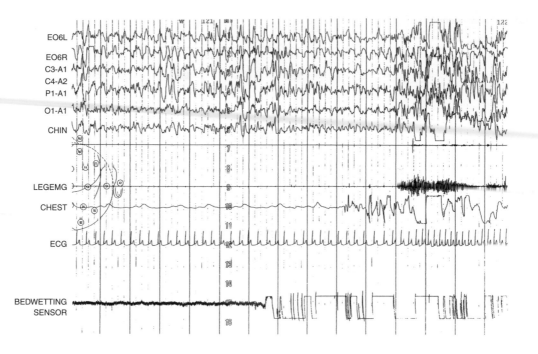

Figure 12.4   Act of bedwetting from stage 3 with subsequent arousal

(5) Clinical experience also suggests that drugs which decrease diuresis (antidiuretic hormone) do not help to restore sleep and produce a short-term effect, followed by deterioration.

Nocturnal enuresis is a sleep disorder

The physiological development of enuresis in sleep can be modeled as follows: the systems of the brain responsible for the smooth transition from wakefulness to sleep, from one stage to another during sleep and from sleep to awakening are often dysfunctional in enuretics. The first non-REM stage is deeper and longer than normal. In this so-called 'dead' sleep, motor activity is absent. A change of stages normally takes place in 60–90 min, but in enuretic children the process of switching from the non-REM to the REM stage in the first cycle is delayed (Figure 12.3a). To compensate and to produce arousal, higher levels of stimulation must occur. This involves increased motor activity; the child becomes episodically restless. It appears that two kinds of motion can activate sleep stage changes: phasic motions (quick, short body jerks), or massive movements (changes in body positions). If such compensatory motor activity does not arise during normal cycles, another paroxysm of urination occurs (Figure 12.4).

The arousal effect appears to apply to enuresis occurring in 'dead' sleep, which is related to deep NREM. Morning cycles may have the same difficulties switching, which end up in morning enuretic episodes.

The compensatory model of enuresis includes the arousal effect as one among many compensatory effects of paroxysmal urination. Different clinical forms of nocturnal enuresis may have different clinicophysiological dynamics and different compensatory mechanisms, which should be investigated in further research (Table 12.3).

Viewing enuresis as a compensatory mechanism of sleep disturbance provides an answer as to why these children should not be

Table 12.3 Explanation of symptoms of nocturnal enuresis (NE) by the compensatory model

Fact	Explanation
The child is capable of holding its urine during the day, but is incontinent during sleep	Because sleep mechanisms are involved, no problem with bladder
Enuretic act in sleep is different from daytime urination	Because different mechanism and different 'purpose' are involved
The forcefully awakened child will urinate again as soon as it falls asleep	Because sleep was disturbed and enuretic act restores normal patterns
Therapeutic resistance	Because NE serves certain physiological function(s)
NE disappears spontaneously when the sleep mechanism matures	Because NE's compensatory function is no longer needed
Enuretics commonly have other parasomnias	Because the latter reflect a hierarchy of compensatory symptoms, which increase in severity if untreated or inappropriately treated

awakened from sleep. This is because a forced awakening will not create a conditioned response, nor will it correct the distortions in the sleep pattern, which are the physiological cause of the enuretic symptom. Moreover, it leads to even greater disorganization of the child's sleep pattern. This is why the awakened child urinates again as soon as he/she falls asleep. Up to a certain age, a child seems to need the enuretic act, and most attempts to eliminate it will fail. As the sleep mechanism matures, enuresis disappears spontaneously since it is no longer needed, and spontaneous recovery ensues. If the sleep mechanism does not mature by a certain period, however, decompensation takes place under the influence of increasing strain on the total organism.

The compensatory model also takes into account the fact that bedwetting tends to normalize the patterns of sleep (Figure 12.3b).

TREATMENT

Because the pathophysiology of enuresis is not completely clear, the therapeutic approach to enuresis is still based on empirical data. Pharmacological therapy is directed at alleviating the symptoms of NE rather than curing the condition[35-37]. Potentially fatal cardiac dysrhythmias have been associated with excessive consumption of imipramine hydrochloride. Imipramine has been associated with a response rate of 20–36%. Desmopressin shows a wide range of efficacy (10–86%). Anticholinergics have been assessed in the treatment of NE. Oxybutynin increases functional bladder capacity; however, in double-blind placebo-controlled studies there was no significant advantage of oxybutynin or placebo in the treatment of primary NE. Oxybutynin may be limited because of its relatively short half-life (< 4 h) and short-term effect on bladder relaxation. Combination therapy with desmopressin and a long-acting anticholinergic agent (hyoscyamine) had a success rate of 60%, which is better than the spontaneous resolution rate[32]. A combination therapy (medications plus behavior modification) has few side-effects and provides symptomatic relief, but is not a cure for enuresis[32].

Biofeedback therapy aims at influencing disco-ordinated patterns of bladder control by helping patients to realize the disco-ordination, allowing cognitive training and cerebral modulation of muscle activity[35,38-41]. With advanced equipment, a flow-triggered training program has been developed to promote ideal striated sphincter relaxation. An immediate success rate of 80% (a long-term effect of over 60%) was found when using biofeedback to treat enuretic children with daytime symptomatology, disco-ordinated voiding (lazy voiding) and urge syndrome. Overall, every therapeutic approach may help to bridge the gap to spontaneous maturation[12].

Behavior training includes bladder training, responsibility reinforcement and classical conditioning therapy using an alarm system.

Alarms wake the child when wetting starts; thus, this is an arduous form of conditioning that may take months.

Current home circumstances must be suitable for the use of an alarm. Dry-bed training refers to regimens that include enuresis alarms, waking routines, positive practice, cleanliness training, bladder training and rewards. From 1998, only 3% of bedwetting children have been prescribed alarms as a primary treatment regimen. Behavior modification requires motivation and positive reinforcement. It may take 2–3 months to see results. Families may lose patience after several months. The combination of work, inconvenience and dedication to the treatment process makes behavior therapy a difficult first choice for families. Because an unstable family environment, family stress, lack of parental concern and multiple bedwetting episodes per night are variables that have a negative response to conditioning therapy, a thorough investigation of the family dynamic is necessary when selecting patients for behavior modification therapy. Motivation is crucial for any form of therapy to be effective. A combination of behavior and medication therapy that improves sleep create an effective treatment.

CONCLUSION

Problems concerning the nature, pathogenesis and treatment of NE remain. Enuresis is a parasomnia that has a complex compensatory and adaptive physiological mechanism. The key to its treatment lies in the means and methods that are used to regulate and normalize sleep. Understanding the nature of nocturnal enuresis might be a gateway to the nature of other parasomnias.

References

1. Avicenna (Abi Ali ibn Sina). *Canon of Medical Science*. UZSSE: Nauka, 1986;Book 3.V.19: 338
2. *Diagnostic and Statistical Manual of Mental Disorders*, 4th edn. DSM-IV. Washington, DC: American Psychiatric Association, 1994
3. Cendron M. Primary nocturnal enuresis: current concepts. *Am Family Physician* 1999; 59:99–111
4. Willie S, Anveden I. Social and behavioural perspectives in enuretics, former enuretics and non-enuretic controls. *Acta Paediatr* 1995;84: 37–40
5. Harari M. Nocturnal enuresis. *Aust Family Physician* 1999;28:113–16
6. Liu X. Attaining nocturnal urinary control, nocturnal enuresis, and behavioral problems in Chinese children aged 6 through 16 years. *J Am Acad Child Adolescent Psychiatry* 2000;39: 1557–62
7. Friman PC. Do children with primary nocturnal enuresis have clinically significant behavior problems? *J Am Med Assoc* 1998;280:2058
8. Byrd RS, Weitzman M, Lanphear NE, *et al*. Bedwetting in US children: epidemiology and related behavior problems. *Am Acad Pediatr* 1996;98:414–19
9. Bader G, Neveus T, Kruse S, Silen U. Sleep in primary enuretic children and controls. *Sleep* 2002;25:579–83
10. Skoog SJ. Editorial: behavior modification in the treatment of enuresis. *J Urol* 1998;160: 861–2
11. Lane W, Robson W, Leung AKC. Secondary nocturnal enuresis. *Clin Pediatr* 2000;39: 379–85
12. Hunsballe J, Rittig S, Pedersen EB, *et al*. Fluid deprivation in enuresis – effect on urine output and plasma arginine vasopressin. *Scand J Urol Nephrol* 1999;33:50–1
13. Skoog SJ. Editorial: primary nocturnal enuresis – an analysis of factors related to its etiology. *J Urol* 1998;159:1338–9
14. Berul C, Murphy JD. Nocturnal enuresis secondary to heart block: report of cure by cardiac pacemaker implantation. *Am Acad Pediatr* 1993;92:284–5
15. Eiberg H. Total genome scan analysis in a single extended family for primary nocturnal enuresis: evidence for a new locus (ENUR3) for primary nocturnal enuresis on chromosome 22q11. *Eur Urol* 1998;33:34–6
16. Hollmann E, Von Gontard A, Eiberg H, *et al*. Molecular genetic, clinical and psychiatric

associations in nocturnal enuresis. *Br J Urol* 1998;81:37–9

17. von Gontard A, Eiberg H, Hollmann E, *et al.* Molecular genetics of nocturnal enuresis: linkage to a locus on chromosome 22. *Scand J Urol Nephrol* 1999;33:76–80

18. Klein NJ. Management of primary nocturnal enuresis. *Urol Nurs* 2001;21:71–5

19. Golbin AZ, Sheldon SH. Parasomnias. In Sheldon SH, Spire JP, Levy HB, eds. *Pediatric Sleep Medicine*. Philadelphia: WB Saunders, 1992:119–35

20. Golbin AZ. *The World of Children's Sleep*. Salt Lake City: Michaelis, 1995

21. Neveus T, Lackgren G, Stenberg A, *et al.* Sleep and night-time behaviour of enuretic and non-enuretics. *Br J Urol* 1998;81:67–71

22. Watanabe H, Kawauchi A. Locus coeruleus function in enuresis. *Scand J Urol Nephrol* 1999;33:14–17

23. Watanabe H. Nocturnal enuresis. *Eur Urol* 1998;33:2–11

24. van Gool JD, Nieuwenhuis E, ten Doeschate IOM, *et al.* Subtypes in monosymptomatic nocturnal enuresis II. *Scand J Urol Nephrol* 1999;33:8–11

25. Kayama Y, Koyama Y. Brainstem neural mechanisms of sleep and wakefulness. *Eur Urol* 1998;33:12–15

26. Kawauchi A, Imada N, Tanaka Y, *et al.* Changes in the structure of sleep spindles and delta waves on electroencephalography in patients with nocturnal enuresis. *Br J Urol* 1998;81:72–5

27. Wolfish N. Sleep arousal function in enuretic males. *Scand J Urol Nephrol* 1999;33:24–6

28. Yeung CK, Chiu HN, Sit FKY. Sleep distrubance and bladder dysfunction in enuretic children with treatment failure: fact or fiction? *Scand J Urol Nephrol* 1999;33:20–3

29. Neveus T. Osmoregulation and desmopressin pharmacokinetics in enuretic children. *Scand J Urol Nephrol* 1999;33:52

30. Neveus T, Stenberg A, Lackgren G, *et al.* Sleep of children with enuresis: a polysomnographic study. *Am Acad Pediatr* 1999;103:1193–7

31. Yeung CK, Sit FKY, To LKC, *et al.* Reduction in nocturnal functional bladder capacity is a common factor in the pathogenesis of refractory nocturnal enuresis. *Br J Urol Int* 2002;90:302–7

32. Cendron M, Klauber G. Combination therapy in the treatment of persistent nocturnal enuresis. *Br J Urol* 1998;81(Suppl 3):26–8

33. Broughton R, Gastaut H. Polygraphic sleep studies of enuresis nocturna. *Electroenceph Clin Neurophysiol* 1964;16:625–6

34. Mikkelsen FJ, Rapaport JL, Nee J, *et al.* Childhood enuresis: sleep patterns and psychopathology. *Arch Gen Psychiatry* 1998;37:1139–44

35. Evans JHC. Nocturnal enuresis. *West J Med* 2001;175:108–13

36. Glazener CMA, Evans JHC. Review: alarm interventions reduce nocturnal enuresis in children. *Evidence-Based Nurs* 2001;4:110

37. Hunsballe J, Rittig S, Pedersen E, *et al.* Single dose imipramine reduces nocturnal urine output in patients with nocturnal enuresis and nocturnal polyuria. *J Urol* 1997;158:830–6

38. Hunsballe J. Sleep studies based on electoencephalogram energy analysis. *Scand J Urol Nephrol* 1999;33:28–30

39. Jensen IN, Kristensen G. Alarm treatment: analyses of response and relapse. *Scand J Urol Nephrol* 1999;33:73–5

40. Monda JM, Husmann DA. Primary nocturnal enuresis: a comparison among observation, imipramine, desmopressin acetate and bed-wetting alarm systems. *J Urol* 1995;154:745–8

41. Gilin JC, Rapaport JL, Mikkelsen FJ, *et al.* EEG sleep patterns in enuretics: a further analysis and comparison with normal controls. *Biol Psychiatry* 1982;17:947–53

13

Nocturnal sleep-related eating (drinking) disorders

Alexander Z. Golbin and Leonid Kayumov

INTRODUCTION

Sleep-related eating problems in infants were known long before they were described in adults. In fact, the International Classification of Sleep Disorders describes this disorder as 'primarily a problem of infancy and early childhood'[1]. In the childhood form of the disorder, the child is usually nursed to sleep (breast or bottle) and then fed repeatedly during the night. The association between nursing (and possibly holding and rocking) and sleep onset is important, but multiple awakenings (typically three to eight) follow throughout the night, at which time the child seems hungry and takes milk or juice eagerly. Large amounts can be consumed at each successive feeding and even more during the night. Wetting may also be excessive (requiring at least one nighttime diaper change) and may be the cause of some of the awakenings.

This disorder is more likely to occur if the caretaker believes that feeding should be continued until no longer 'demanded' by the child or when caretakers have difficulty distinguishing a child's true hunger from habit and continue to feed the child. Sometimes, feeding serves the needs of the caretaker and not those of the child. It may be the only time the caretaker feels important and needed[1].

Parents working long hours may find that the night is the only time available to spend with the child, and the feeding process provides rewards as well as reducing feelings of guilt to the parents.

By 6 months of age or slightly thereafter, full-term, normally growing, healthy infants should acquire the ability to sleep through the night without additional feeding. This development is variable, however. Some children seem to stop waking even though the feedings are never withheld, whereas others continue until the caretakers establish a limit. Children in the latter category may continue waking until they are weaned completely. This is usually achieved when the child is aged 3–4 years. A few polysomnographic studies show normal, but fragmented sleep structures in small children[1].

In 1955 Stunkard and co-workers[2] described a group of adults having strange behaviors called 'nocturnal eating syndrome': a wakening in the middle of the night with the urge to eat or drink, consuming a large amount of food, followed by a sudden awakening or returning to sleep with a varying degree of recollection in the morning. The adult patients in this group were obese with nocturnal hyperphagia, insomnia and diurnal anorexia.

In adults nocturnal sleep-related eating disorders (NSREDs) are distinct from daytime eating disorders. As with all parasomnias, sleep-related behaviors are similar to the daytime ones but have a different clinical picture and physiological nature:

A.C., a 49-year-old physician, requested help for his disturbing habit. In the middle of a bitter divorce, he suddenly found himself awakening in the kitchen in the middle of the night consuming large amounts of food that he took from his refrigerator. On a few occasions in the morning, he had no memory of midnight awakening and coming to the kitchen. The only way he knew about his night trips was by the mess he had made in the kitchen. He had normal dinners and was not hungry before sleep.

Midnight eating episodes happened with increased frequency and became nightly. He was consuming food which he did not like during the day, or food that was not completely cooked. If he woke up while eating, what he was eating would make him feel sick and nauseated. Within the last 6 months he had gained 35 lbs (15.75 kg) and had become depressed.

The polysomnography test discovered fragmented sleep with confusional arousals, multiple outbursts of theta waves on the electroencephalogram (EEG) in the frontal areas, multiple alpha intrusions, rapid eye movement (REM) onsets after awakenings during the night and periodic leg movements. During midnight awakenings, despite a clear alpha rhythm on his EEG, he looked sleepy, his eyes were open, but his blinking reflex was delayed.

Treatment with clonazepam, sertraline and topiramate produced significant improvement. A follow-up after 1 year showed no relapse.

Despite infrequent occurrences, NSREDs are sometimes quite distressing to their victims, challenging for a treating physician and obscure for researchers. Several etiological categories were identified in patients with this condition[3–6] and these are listed below.

NOCTURNAL SLEEP-RELATED EATING DISORDERS

NSREDs are associated with the following:

(1) Familial sleepwalking;

(2) Sleepwalking/periodic limb movement disorder;

(3) Obstructive sleep apnea;

(4) Daytime eating disorders;

(5) REM/sleep arousal disorder;

(6) Restless legs syndrome;

(7) Nocturnal drinking syndrome (hungry wakefulness);

(8) Nocturnal dissociative syndrome;

(9) Medication (triazolam, midazolam, amitriptyline);

(10) Indeterminate.

Understanding NSRED in adults as a sleep problem has an interesting history as described by Schenck and Mahowald[5].

It took 25 years after Stunkard's discovery of the nocturnal eating syndrome for Nadel[6] to suspect that NSRED might be related to parasomnia, as a variant of sleepwalking, but only Oswald and Adam in 1986[7] objectively proved the link between sleep and eating behavior at night. Using polysomnography during the course of six nights (37% males) the latter clearly established that eating occurred during the REM stage of sleep.

Sleepwalking as a basis for nocturnal eating was indicated by Whyte and Kavey[8,9]. In 1994, Italian researchers[10] described ten subjects with adult onset of NSRED in whom obesity was not a predominant feature. Their research confirmed episodes of compulsive food seeking and return to sleep after consumption of large amounts of food. In these cases all subjects were fully awake during episodes and could clearly recall them in the morning. Polygraphic investigation showed low sleep efficiency, high number of awakenings and a strong link between nocturnal eating episodes and non-REM sleep. These were well functioning adults with various psychosomatic problems but medically, neurologically and hormonally intact; occasional co-morbidity with narcolepsy or periodic leg movement was noted.

Schenck and co-workers provided a detailed and intensive review of clinical and polysomnographic correlates in 38 cases[3–5]. Most were females, characterized by frequent nightly sleep-related eating, careless food preparation, complaints of low control and weight gain. Neither daytime binge eating nor obsessive–compulsive disorder was diagnosed in any patient in this group, and the onset of psychiatric disorders was never directly associated with the onset of sleep-related eating. Their major finding was that NSRED is a heterogenic condition characterized by distinct behavior of daytime overeating and involving a sleep physiology. In one of their reports familial cases of NSREDs were described; one of these cases started immediately upon initiation of amitriptyline (200 mg) for migraine headaches. The eating disorder ceased after amitriptyline was discontinued. A few other adult patients woke up sleepwalking combined with periodic leg movements, poor hygiene and obstructive sleep apnea. Only in two cases was NSRED seen in patients with daytime anorexia nervosa and nocturnal eating behavior. Cessation of longstanding alcohol abuse or cigarette smoking was also related to the onset of NSRED. Dissociative disorder was not found in any patient.

Polysomnographic studies showed that NSREDs were associated with arousals from non-REM sleep, but were also seen in REM phases[11–14]. The patients appeared to be not fully awake, and had repetitive chewing, scratching and vocalization. In contrast to patients suffering from injurious sleepwalking who arise from deep delta stages, abrupt arousals with eating occur throughout all stages of non-REM sleep and even during REM sleep. This constitutes an atypical form of sleepwalking.

NSRED is sleep state-dependent. This sleep state-dependent feature justifies the term 'sleep-related eating syndrome'. Other notable features of NSREDs were described as follows[3–5]:

(1) Patients almost never experience hunger despite their compulsive and immediate urge to eat or drink during arousals.

(2) There was no complaint of abdominal pain, nausea, heartburn or hypoglycemic symptoms.

(3) The level of consciousness and degree of subsequent recall varied widely across patients. Typically sleep-related eating is automatic when getting up from bed while asleep or immediately after a partial or full arousal from sleep, going straight to the kitchen with a compulsive 'out of control' urge to eat. Even when there was the simultaneous urge to urinate, patients invariably went first to the kitchen to eat.

(4) Alcohol was not consumed, despite the availability of alcohol in most kitchens or even despite past alcohol abuse in six patients.

(5) There was a strong tendency to drink heavy fluids (whole milk, milk shakes) and to consume carbohydrate-rich foods (peanut butter, ice cream, pies, brownies, candy bars, oatmeal, etc.).

(6) The foods consumed during the night arousals were typically unusual and not of the same type as those eaten during the day.

(7) There was never any purging reported, either during the night or in the morning.

(8) Only a quarter of the patients who smoked cigarettes during the day also smoked during nocturnal arousals.

(9) Sleep-related eating was usually observed during weekdays, vacations and sleeping away from home.

(10) Sleep-related eating might have a lengthy latent period or start suddenly.

The authors conceptualized NSRED as a stress-related disorder. More specifically, NSRED was related to low serotonin levels. They proposed a model of blunted satiety responses linked with low central serotonin activity and of abnormal hedonic responses to food linked with low central dopamine activity. Impressive therapeutic results with dopaminergic (and serotoninergic) agents confirmed this model. Frequent periodic limb movement disorder/restless legs syndrome in patients with NSRED was found to be related to dopaminergic dysfunction.

Many NSRED patients described other parasomnias such as night terrors in their previous or current history. Average age for the onset of sleep-related eating was in their thirties with a mild predominance noted in women. Psychiatric problems were usually within a spectrum of mood disorders such as anxiety and depression; many were seen in otherwise 'normal' people.

Manni and co-workers[13] found about 5.8% of NSREDs among 120 insomniacs characterized by a heterogeneous group of mental and psychiatric disorders. Winkelman[14,15] used self-reports from patients with eating disorders (132 (9%) out-patients and 24 (17%) in-patients) describing eating during nocturnal confusional arousals (predominantly female). Winkelman was not sure if NSREDs were distinct from daytime eating disorders. It is interesting that the level of consciousness was different, ranging from full awake to 'total unconsciousness' in 31.6% of cases. He also found topiramate (γ-aminobutyric acid agonist, glutamatergic antagonist) effective in NSREDs[15].

Video and polysomnographic data demonstrate a common association between NSRED and sleepwalking behavior: looking around as if confused, thrashing about, shouting, sitting up, grabbing at objects, kicking or throwing punches and jumping from the bed – arising abruptly either during uninterrupted stage 3–4 non-REM sleep or from delta non-REM. NSRED may also be characterized by repetitive chewing. Self-awareness of the persons having actually consumed food during polysomnography has ranged from full awakening to not being aware of their actions.

Apart from being a side effect of medications and obstructive sleep apnea syndrome or PLM, NSREDs can be provoked by emotional stress.

The main conclusion of polysomnographic evaluation is that NSRED is a specific sleep disorder[3,14,15,17] which means that it lies in the domain of sleep medicine and should be treated as a 'behavioral, psychiatric complication of a medical condition'. This distinction is important because it allows insurance coverage under a medical code and prevents the patient with NSRED from being stigmatized as suffering from a mental disorder.

TREATMENT

Treatment with behavioral therapy alone is not very helpful. Pharmacological agents, such as dopaminergic agents alone or opioids, in addition to effective stress management techniques, proper sleep hygiene, a balanced diet and sleeping schedule are shown to be useful. Below are the revised suggested treatment protocols for the adult-onset nocturnal eating syndrome[5].

Treatment protocols for the pharmacological control of nocturnal sleep-related eating disorder

Protocol 1

Carbidopa/L-dopa (Sinemet®) 10/100 mg q HS combined with codeine 30 mg q HS. The dose may be doubled if needed. Carbidopa can be substituted by bromocriptine at bedtime. Codeine can be substituted by propoxyphene in case of codeine allergy or intolerance.

Protocol 2

Protocol 1 with the addition of clonazepam 0.25–2.0 mg q HS or alprazolam 0.5–4 mg.

Protocol 3

Anticonvulsants (gabapentin 300–800 mg, tiagabin 4–6 mg or topiramate 25–100 mg/day).

Protocol 4

Fluoxetine (20–60 mg) as a monotherapy or in combination with Protocol 1, 2 or 3.

Protocol 5

Continuous positive airway pressure (CPAP) for patients with obstructive apnea syndrome.

A comprehensive treatment approach would also focus on adjusting psychotropic treatment that may be promoting sleep-related eating, e.g. anticholinergic agents or lithium. Positive responses to CPAP on cessation of nocturnal eating behavior were noted in the patient with obstructive sleep apnea[16]. In addition, proper sleep hygiene, with regular sleep–wake and daytime eating schedules, should be maintained and proper stress management should be suggested.

CONCLUSION

Nocturnal sleep-related eating disorders are another example of episodic parasomnias with a clear and dramatic behavioral picture and obscure pathophysiology. They entail overactivity of the hypothalamic–pituitary–adrenal axis causing exaggerated and shifted-in-time compulsive eating behavior during transitional, mixed sleep–wake states.

More research is needed to understand why transitional stages of consciousness lead to compulsive eating habits and to find methods of restoring normal sleep–wake cycles and good eating habits.

References

1. Lawrence KS. *International Classification of Sleep Disorders: Diagnostic and Coding Manual.* American Sleep Disorders Association. Rochester, MN: Davis Printing, 1997:100–4
2. Stunkard AF, Grace WJ, Wolff HG. The night eating syndrome: a pattern of food intake among certain obese patients. *Am J Med* 1955; 19:78–86
3. Schenck CH, Hurwitz TD, Bandlie SR, Mahowald MW. Sleep related eating disorders: polysomnographic correlates of a heterogeneous syndrome distinct from daytime eating disorders. *Sleep* 1991;14:419–31
4. Schenck CH, Hurwitz TD, O'Connor KA, Mahowald MW. Additional categories of sleep related eating disorders and the current status of treatment. *Sleep* 1993;16:457–66
5. Schenck CH, Mahowald MW. Review of nocturnal sleep related eating disorders. *Int J Eat Dis* 1994;15:343–56
6. Nadel C. Somnambulism, bedtime medications and overeating. *Br J Psychiatry* 1981;139:79
7. Oswald I, Adam K. Rhythms raiding of refrigerator related to rapid eye movement sleep. *Br Med J* 1986;292:589
8. Whyte J, Kavey NB, Gidro-Frank S. Somnambulistic bulimia. *Sleep Res* 1988;17:268 (abstract)
9. Whyte J, Kavey NB. Somnambulistic eating: a report of three cases. *Int J Eat Dis* 1990;9:577–81
10. Spaggiari MC, Granela F, Parrino L, *et al.* Nocturnal eating syndrome in adults. *Sleep* 1994;17:339–44
11. Roper P. Bulimia while sleepwalking; a rebuttal for sane automatism? *Lancet* 1989;2:796
12. Thorpy M. In Thorpy M, ed. *Handbook of Sleep Disorders.* New York: Marcel Dekker, 1990: 551–69
13. Manni R, Ratti MR, Tartata A. Nocturnal eating: prevalence and features in 120 insomniac referrals. *Sleep* 1997;20:734–8

14. Winkelman JW. Clinical and polysomnographic features of sleep-related eating disorders. *J Clin Psychiatry* 1998;59:14–19

15. Winkelman JW. Treatment of nocturnal and sleep related eating with topiramate. *Sleep* 2003;26:A317–18

16. Boone, Allen. Nocturnal eating syndrome. *Sleep Rev* 2001;Winter:24–7

17. Greeno CG, Wing RR, Marcus MD. Nocturnal eating in binge eating disorders and matched-weight controls. *Int J Eat Dis* 1995;18:343–9

14

Static phenomena in sleep

Alexander Z. Golbin

INTRODUCTION

The person sleeps deeply and quietly without moving and without disturbing anyone. Still, his/her sleep may be considered abnormal. Among the peculiarities of sleep, it is important to mention strange body positions, sleep with open eyes, sleep paralysis and sleep-related hallucinations. Static phenomena in sleep are seen in people of all ages and in all cultures.

STRANGE BODY POSITIONS

Ancient medical books emphasize the strange manner in which some people sleep[1]. In recent years, the importance of body positions in sleep has been rediscovered, especially as a risk factor for sudden infant death syndrome (SIDS)[2] and for treatment of obstructive sleep apnea syndrome in adults[3]. Unusual and peculiar positions in sleep are common in children as a part of normal development, but when and what kinds of positions can be considered abnormal?

Body positions in sleep are normally a short-lived feature. If a child sleeps with his head hanging off the bed or his arms twisted in a peculiar way, then it is perceived as being uncomfortable. We know that the child will soon change the position, and if not, we can easily move his head back onto the pillow and his arms back into a more comfortable position. Many unusual positions may be especially favored by the child and look 'cute' to observers. Observations on the dynamics of the body positions in sleep show that there are many and varied sleep positions. They are more or less specific for each person and the dynamics of their changes in the course of the night are individually stable[4].

Sometimes, however, peculiar, unusual and strange positions are maintained for too long. Most importantly, it is difficult to change them. If parents try to put the child's head, for example, back on the pillow, the child immediately slides back down into the same position. If the parents repeat this another time, it will have the same effect. If you forcefully prevent the child from going back to the same position, he/she may wake up, get irritated or exhibit some somatic symptoms. He/she might urinate, start coughing or perspire profusely. Observations made over a period of years convinced us that such positions are mediated by some kind of internal physiological mechanism. This mechanism makes peculiar body positions internally set. What is important is that the children who exhibit strange positions may develop other sleep abnormalities or somatic problems later on[4]. Such specific, strange positions reflect some changes in the integrated activity of the sleeping brain. Some of these, in our experience, may signal or predict the appearance of

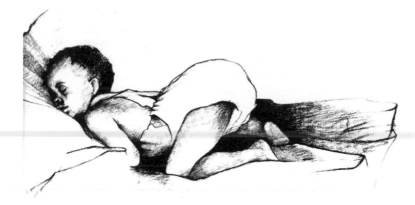

Figure 14.1 'Elbow–knee' position on the stomach with increased muscle tone

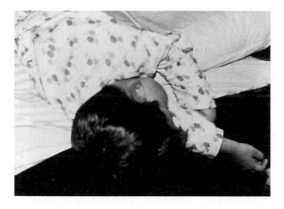

Figure 14.2 'Upside-down' position

later psychosomatic problems. In the case of infants, prolonged and 'fixed' sleeping on the stomach is a high risk for SIDS and other life-threatening events.

Other strange body positions are also important to mention:

(1) 'Elbow–knee' position with increased muscle tone (Figure 14.1). For example, the child looks as if he is bending his arms or legs, and his muscles are very firm. The child pushes or butts his head and arms against the headboard of his bed. This position is usually associated with stage 2 of the first two cycles of non-REM sleep. During the day some of these children display irritability and increased anxiety.

(2) The 'upside-down' position (Figure 14.2). As in other 'fixed' body positions, it is difficult to change this seemingly uncomfortable way of sleeping. In this case, the child remains for a long period of time with his head down and does not change its position. When parents try to put the head back, the child slides down to the same position. Several children with similar sleep patterns were observed in a trauma unit after having experienced concussions from head traumas. We also saw such children develop head banging.

(3) Arched positions (Figure 14.3). These are extreme variants of body positions with muscle hypertone. The whole body is over-extended. Sometimes it looks as if the child is standing on his head and feet. The body seems to be arched in an odd fashion. This position is reminiscent of a symptom called opisthotonus (a symptom of increased intracranial pressure). We observed one of these fixed body positions in a child with severe nocturnal asthma. Lumbar puncture in this case showed no abnormality nor did a thorough neurological examination. This position, just as the 'upside-down' position, was observed in stage 2 of non-REM sleep.

Ornitz and colleagues[5] described a position similar to the arched position in children suffering from vitamin D deficiency.

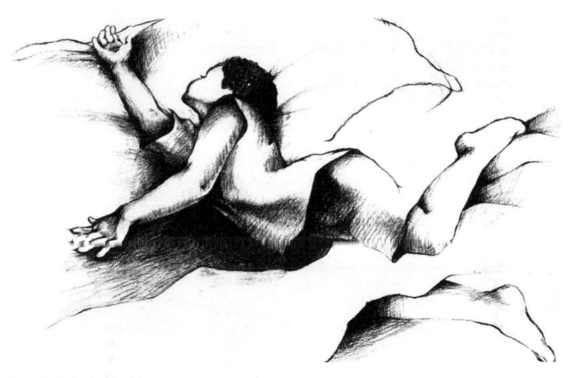

Figure 14.3 'Arched' position

(4) There are body positions that are opposite to the previous ones in terms of muscle tone. All muscles of the body are completely relaxed, and even the chest is not visibly moving. To the observer, it looks as if the child is dead (Figure 14.4). Many mothers, in fact, call them 'dead' positions. Parents often check whether the child is breathing. Sleep recording shows stages 3 and 4 NREM sleep associated with a high amplitude of delta activity. Such positions are seen in bedwetters before they actually urinate and in patients with sleep apnea.

(5) Parents also report sleep with 'stretched arms' (Figure 14.5). The arms are stretched in front of the child when he/she is sleeping on his/her back, and in some cases the child waves them in front of him-/herself. Sleep recording shows stage 3 and 4 NREM sleep. These children are also prone to sleepwalking and/or sleeptalking episodes.

(6) Sleep with open mouth (Figure 14.6) is usually seen in children and adults with nasal obstructions due to adenoids or persons with asthma, COPD or obstructive sleep apnea. Breathing is usually loud. Young children who are chronic mouth breathers typically have large nostrils, bulbous dry lips and bags under the eyes ('adenoidal face'). Bedwetting and other episodic parasomnias are common.

(7) Sleep with open eyes (Figure 14.7) is quite common and normal for newborns and infants but sometimes seen in older children. During the first stages of sleep, the child's eyelids are not completely closed and you can see the eyes between the eyelids. However, in older children and adolescents sometimes the space between the eyelids is large enough to leave an impression that the person is looking at you. Sometimes the eyes are turned up and toward each other, and you can see them clearly. In older children, this has quite a

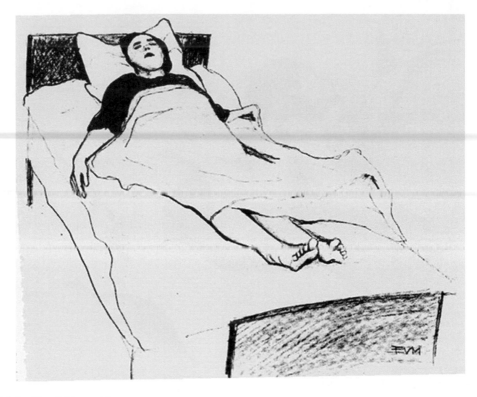

Figure 14.4 'Dead'-like position

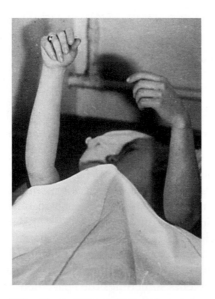

Figure 14.5 Sleep with stretched arms

disturbing appearance characterized as 'rabbit eyes'. It happens during the first two cycles of NREM sleep. This phenomenon is not seen during naps; nor is it observed in REM sleep. The significance of open eyes for the prediction of different disorders is not clear.

(8) Sleep paralysis and pre- and post-sleep hallucinations are typically associated with narcolepsy (see Chapter 9), but may appear in normal conditions under certain circumstances. As temporary phenomena, they are considered benign and need no special treatment other than correction of underlying issues.

Recently, however, sleep paralysis and vivid hallucinations have attracted public attention in connection with cases of 'being taken by aliens' and 'exorcism of possessed persons'[6]. In such cases the persons were in a trance-like state, in which they felt awake, but their bodies were asleep. These states were accompanied by frightening hallucinatory, realistic visions but with an inability to move. The longest

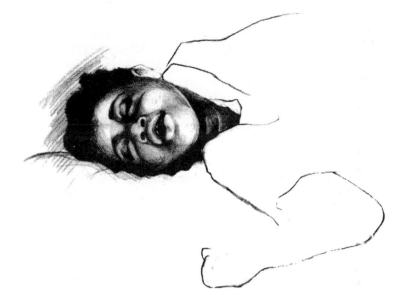

Figure 14.6   Sleep with open mouth

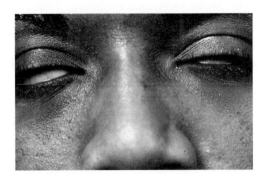

Figure 14.7   Sleep with open eyes

condition reported lasted 6 hours. In the majority of reported cases, the afflicted person had had a traumatic background, was religiously preoccupied and very suggestive.'

There are many other 'fixed' body positions and static phenomena. The cause and meaning of them has yet to be discovered: sleeping with the head covered by a blanket, 'newborn' position in an adult, sleeping sitting on the floor with the head on the bed, sleeping with feet on a cold object, etc. These positions could not be forcefully changed by the family members. The afflicted persons themselves could not explain why they slept so strangely.

ONTOGENETIC DEVELOPMENT OF BODY POSITIONS

Analysis of the dynamics of normal positions developing with age shows that the positions are maturing parallel to the age of the child[4].

The process of 'maturation' is associated with different types of dominant position in sleep. General characteristics of dominant (most common) positions change with age. It is interesting that often the position changes to the opposite type in terms of the muscle tonus as the child gets older. This is called an 'inversion' of positions. For example, newborns have predominantly 'hypertonic' types of position, but after 6 months the child's positions become 'hypotonic' when its muscles are very soft and look as if they are paralyzed. During the second year of life, one position quickly changes into multiple different positions. At the age of 7–8 years, the child appears to find its most favored position. Body position changes in sleep are very sensitive to internal

193

(somatic) and external (psychological) factors. In older children, regression to the position of toddlers may take place, especially if the child becomes sick or depressed.

Strange body positions in sleep seem to be an exaggeration of the 'normal' variants. These strange positions become abnormal when the position becomes fixed and, if forcefully changed, it can result in irritability, somatic symptoms or changes in the quality of awakening, next-day alertness problems, hyperactivity at bedtime and other problems. Is 'upside-down' position a symptom of intracranial pressure or does sleep with the head covered by a blanket reflect a need for hypercapnea? We do not yet know. What we do know is that body positions and other static phenomena have become important clinical signs and are an important parameter of brain function. Major body movements, especially position changes known to occur at the time of the non-REM–REM stage sleep, reflect brain states[7]. The 90-minute pattern of body position reflects normal sleep architecture. Fixed, strange, atypical unchangeable body positions indicate abnormal sleep architecture and might be symptomatic of specific clinical syndromes. Static phenomena in sleep hide many secrets of the sleeping brain

References

1. Avicenna (Abu Ali ibn Sina). *Canon of Medical Science*, 1012 AD, Book 3 (2):180–2. Tauhkent, Uzbek SSR: FAN Publishing, 1981
2. Guntheroth WG. *Crib Death. The Sudden Infant Death Syndrome*, 2nd edn. New York: Futura, 1989:1–323
3. Kryger MH. Management of obstructive sleep apnea/hypopnea syndrome: overview. In Kryger MH, Roth T, Dement WC, eds. *Principles and Practice of Sleep Medicine*, 3rd edn. Philadelphia: WB Saunders, 2000:940–54
4. Golbin AZ. *The World of Children's Sleep*. Salt Lake City: Michaelis Medical Publishing, 1995:1–307
5. Ornitz EM, Ritvo ER, Walter RD. Dreaming sleep in autistic and schizoprenic children. *Am J Psychiatry* 1965;122:419–24
6. Dodzik D. Is sleep paralysis the cause of alien abductions? In *Sleep and Health*. Chicago: Des Plaines Publishing, 2003;4:8
7. Aaronson ST, Rashed S, Biber MP, Hobson JA. Brain state and body position. A time lapse video study of sleep. *Arch Gen Psychiatry* 1982;35:330–5

15

Adaptive theory of parasomnias

Alexander Z. Golbin

A little disorder might be the key to a big order of nature.

Max Planck

Parasomnias are brief disturbances in the body that, by definition, appear in pre-sleep, during sleep and post-sleep periods, as well as during transitional states of vigilance. Phenomena of parasomnias appear as seemingly inadequate behaviors or reflexes. They are often an exaggeration of normal variants of motor or somatic activity ranging from benign and cute habits, such as sucking lip movements and kissing sounds, to bizarre and malignant phenomena, such as violent homicide or sudden death. Parasomnias have recently attracted intensive research; new phenomena have been discovered and more are in the 'pipeline'.

Parasomnias are explained presently as incomplete arousals from non-REM sleep or as exaggerated or disassociated phenomena in non-REM (i.e. periodic limb movements, bruxism) or REM (REM behavior disorder, nightmares) sleep. There is a need for a general integrated theory to explain parasomnias as a separate growing class, and to answer the following key questions:

(1) Why are parasomnias very common and more benign in childhood, but less common and less benign in adults?

(2) Why are parasomnias generally resistant to treatment, but can disappear by themselves?

(3) Why do parasomnias cluster in the same individual or transform from one into another?

(4) Do animals have parasomnias and, if so, could they be used as models for human sleep disorders?

(5) Do parasomnias have any function or are they a by-product of disordered sleep?

It is important to find 'general principles' that explain phenomenologically widely different symptoms and unite them into one class of parasomnias. This chapter presents one such attempt, based on the idea of the adaptive functions of parasomnias.

The first general principle is that parasomnias have a common clinical picture, consisting of the following symptoms:

(1) A clear and usually dramatic main symptom;

(2) Changes of alertness;

(3) Changes in sleep electrographic architecture;

(4) Resistance to direct suppression of the symptoms (treatment);

(5) Spontaneous disappearance of the main symptom (self-cure).

The second principle is a common route, often associated with ontogenetic development, that usually passes through the following phases or periods in the development of parasomnias:

(1) Latent period;

(2) Crystallization period when diffuse symptomatology disappears and the main symptom emerges;

(3) Mono-symptomatic phase, when the main symptoms continue for a long time;

(4) Self-cure (when the main symptoms spontaneously disappear);

(5) Deterioration (when the main symptom becomes more severe or additional symptoms emerge).

The third principle uniting parasomnias is that they are often an exaggeration and deviation of normal variants of motor or somatic activity. They are commonly not a result of the structural organic changes ('hardware'), but are functional deviations ('software').

Thus, parasomnias, despite an exceptionally wide range of main symptoms, have a typical internal structure and common pathways of clinical dynamics. The question is, what is their nature?

Let us start with animals. Phenomena of parasomnias in animals are well known. Animals, like humans, also have rhythmic head and body movements; they scream, run and urinate while sleeping, have narcolepsy and sleep apnea[1–4]. These brief disturbances are described in many animals, especially in those that live with humans, which has led to the idea of the existence of a common biological basis of these 'inadequate behaviors'.

'Biological basis' means that there are some neurophysiological mechanisms that underlie and 'turn on' an unusual and 'stubborn' behavior or a somatic response in immature, deprived or otherwise compromised organisms. In this case, 'stubbornness' (the resistance to treatment) should be analyzed as a physiological phenomenon that the body produces and keeps for some unknown physiological

function. This function might be adaptive, maladaptive or self-destructive.

The fact that brief disturbances in the body could be helpful and even treat some life-threatening diseases has been known for centuries. Let us just mention induced fever spikes, blood-letting, convulsions produced by electric shocks and insulin-induced comas that are recognized and used not only in alternative, but also traditional medicine. Electroconvulsive therapy is now considered the safest treatment for severe depression, even for pregnant women[5], Parkinson's disease and obsessive–compulsive disorders. Botulinum toxin has proved to be effective and safe for many different disorders. Injections into the affected lacrimal glands cure gustatory hyperlacrimation (crocodile tears)[6], and facial muscle paralysis induced by the botulin relieves headaches[7]. How many times have physicians, without knowing the exact mechanism of action, induced a mild disease to prevent a major illness? We could apply the same logic to self-induced (or rather self-produced) behaviors. It is common knowledge that episodic outbursts of anger or tears relieve emotional tension, after which the person calms down for a while.

Parasomnias are not an exception but a good example of self-produced behavior serving adaptive functions. Parasomnias are similar to other brief medical disturbances including spikes of unexplainable night fevers, convulsions, muscle paralysis, bleedings, urination in sleep, etc. At least at the beginning, some of these episodes might serve an adaptive function[8,9].

It is well known to clinicians that many attempts to suppress parasomnias using direct physical manipulations (e.g. forceful awakenings of enuretics) are not very helpful, and frequently have the opposite effect, such as exacerbation of previous phenomena or appearance of other even more undesirable (severe) parasomnias with emotional and behavioral problems during wakefulness. Based on clinical and polysomnographic data (see also Chapters 10–14) we propose a hypothesis that parasomnias, although by themselves symptoms of disorders, serve some important adaptive or compensatory functions[9]. Accepting the usefulness of some externally induced or self-produced disorders such as parasomnias, clinicians and researchers are confronted with paradoxical uncertainty about their nature and neurophysiological mechanisms.

The physiologists of the past century attempted to understand the mechanisms and possible functions of seemingly inadequate behaviors in animals. In 1908 Uchtomsky[10] observed that, in some cases, activity of the nervous system in dogs, together with goal-directed (positive) effects, could result in absolutely senseless (negative) reactions which were resistant to treatment. For example, animals moved away from food when hungry, vomited, scratched themselves without cause, suddenly fell asleep, rocked or urinated, kept turning around for no apparent reason, etc. He called this group 'ultraparadoxical' reactions, inadequate reflexes and explained their existence as 'behind the curtain compensatory dominant'. Kaminsky[11] studied the 'compensatory role of inadequate reflexes' in monkeys, placing them in stressful situations. Vvedensky[12] studied a wide variety of strange, unusual, seemingly absurd body reactions and behaviors, which had some role in survival, and called them 'animal hysterias'. In 1967 Muhametov[13] demonstrated a sigma rhythm on the electroencephalogram (EEG) of animals during rhythmical movements and other reactions, which is usually associated with the sigma state of non-rapid eye movement (non-REM) (light) sleep or altered states of consciousness associated with calmness. This was the first direct evidence that inadequate motor reactions are related to the regulation of stages of vigilance, specifically, helping the brain to calm down. Porshnev[14] collected the most comprehensive material regarding inadequate reflexes and their compensatory role in ontogenetic and evolutional dynamics in animals and humans. Bechtereva and co-workers[15] focused their research on the functional stability of inadequate reflexes and their amazing resistance to treatment.

This group of behavioral patterns, termed 'displacement activities', attracted considerable attention in the zoology community in the West. Tinbergen[16,17] and Kortlandt[18] independently studied 'behavior patterns which appear to be out of context with the behavior that closely precedes or follows them'. Delius[19] studied the displacement activity of black-backed gulls and found it to be a part of their arousal homeostasis, that is a vital mechanism to maintain a narrow comfort zone. Schino and co-workers[20] found primate displacement activities associated with anxiety. Several theories have been put forward to explain a reason for a particular behavioral pattern to appear as a displacement activity[17]. No theory, however, was able to explain the causality of displacement activities and answer the question: why this seemingly disordered behavior is so stable and yet may disappear by itself, while its artificial suppression may be harmful for waking behavior, psychic and somatic health. It is interesting that many naturalists noticed connections between 'inadequate reflexes' or 'displacement activities' and fatigue, sleepiness or other stages of vigilance, but did not focus on this issue. Parasomnias offer multiple examples of displacement activities. The widespread disorder of enuresis (paroxysmal and involuntary bedwetting) is one such example (see Chapter 11). Sleep patterns in enuretics are somewhat different from normal ones: during the first half of the night the REM stage is delayed, while non-REM stages are prolonged and very deep[8]. It is interesting that sleep cycles normalize after enuretic episodes; in some cases enuretic acts reappear several times a night even after forceful awakening and a trip to the toilet[8,9]. After an enuretic episode the cyclicity is normalized but only for that night, so statistically, sleep stages of the enuretic appear to be within the normal range. In this case, the enuretic act itself serves a sleep-stabilizing function.

Rhythmic and paroxysmal disturbances in sleep and transitional stages of vigilance have similar functions and are described in detail in Chapters 10 and 11.

Broughton[21] explained parasomnias as partial arousals related to pathological cardiac and mental activities of subjects. However, despite its clinical relevance, the arousal theory could not explain whether these symptoms have any functional role or just appear as byproducts of incomplete sleep or wakefulness, and did not explain their strong resistance to treatment. For a more integrative theory of parasomnias, capable of explaining their function or absence of function, we need to move one step further. We can do this by applying the concepts of the control system and chaos theories to the analysis of the above-described clinical data. Briefly, there are two types of chaotic behavior:

(1) Destructive, killing, symptomatic of imminent and irreversible structural changes, leading to death of the system as a whole;

(2) Constructive, healing, called 'dynamic deterministic' non-linear chaos that is essential in keeping the system stable as a whole, functional unit.

Research in applying chaos theory to biological and medical problems recently became quite intensive[22–29].

We conclude that parasomnias display chaotic behavior in different physiological systems as an alternative to a serious disease. According to conventional wisdom in medicine (theory of homeostasis), a healthy organism regulates itself to maintain constant rhythm, while erratic behavior of the organism is symptomatic of unfolding disease because it suppresses natural rhythms. However, discoveries over the past decade in mathematics and human physiology prove that chaos in bodily functioning is not necessarily a bad thing. Goldberger and co-workers[22] convincingly demonstrated that a chaotic cardiac pattern is physiologically normal, while a regular, strong periodic pattern would be pathological for the heart. These authors also found scaling (chaotic) behavior in human gait dynamics. As known, dynamic chaos is characterized not only by unpredictability of the response due to strong sensitivity to initial conditions, but also

by structural stability of the nesting system due to the existence of an attractor. The latter property makes dynamic chaos extremely useful for controlling purposes[28,29]. Pecora and Carroll[23] showed how one could effectively synchronize subsystems of a chaotic system by linking them with a common signal. Pecora and Carroll quoted Freeman, who suggested that the brain response should be viewed as a chaotic attractor. Ott and co-workers[24] showed that chaotic motion possesses great inherent flexibility in reacting to different external or internal demands by making small adjustments. They suggested that the presence of chaos in the brain might be not only an advantageous but an absolutely necessary ingredient for controlling purposes. Thus, flexibility of chaotic patterns in the heart and brain allows these organs to perform their regulatory functions. As a result of aging or pathology, an organism may lose these functions. Then, we speculate, such inability of the heart or brain to self-produce chaos may be compensated by dynamic chaos provided by another organ of the organism. Put simply, brief abnormalities in one system (e.g. the urinary system in enuretics) may ensure the stability of the whole organism.

According to this hypothesis, displacement activities of animals, specifically parasomnias, are examples of chaotic behaviors of different parts of their bodies, which set in as an alternative to death or serious disease of the whole organism. In other words, displacement activities, including parasomnias, are an adaptive or maladaptive way of coping with challenge. Parasomnias may be explained as chaotic behaviors of different parts of an organism that re-instate the control function of the brain to produce a normal sleep pattern. Such conclusions are supported by recent observations of Bunde and co-workers[25] that healthy sleep patterns exhibit multifractal correlations. This may explain the resistance of parasomnias to treatment using medications. For example, after the enuretic act, physiological impulses from the bladder stimulate the brain to switch from the non-REM to the REM stage and the sleep architecture returns to normal (see

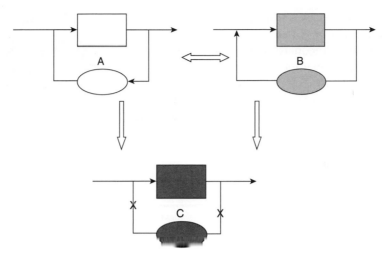

Figure 15.1 Three possible states of an organism considered as an open system with non-linear feedback control between main subsystem □ (MS) and compensatory subsystem ○ (CS). Shades of gray designate the level of chaos in the subsystem. A, healthy organism with normal levels of chaos in MS and CS; B, pathological organism with a strongly chaotic CS that provides chaos to MS; C, pathological organism with conditions of breakdown

Chapter 12). That is, in the case of enuresis the organism turns the bladder into a chaotic state in order to compensate for the dysfunction of the brain. Thus, the adaptive role of bedwetting can be understood as a switch mechanism between different states of sleep and wakefulness. A patient with restless legs syndrome (RLS) starts twitching his/her leg or arm because in this way the body can 'supply' chaos to the spinal brain. Behavioral correlations of rhythmic movements with delta sleep lead to the conclusion that this disorder serves as a 'sleepmaker'. Functional dependence of pathological organisms on displacement activities and inadequate reflexes explains the therapeutic resistance of the latter. Indeed, rejection of treatment by the organism comes as part of its instinct to survive.

When a healthy level of chaos cannot be achieved inside the control organ itself, e.g. the heart, another organ of the organism will be actively turned into a chaotic state to restore the functional level of chaos in the first one. The adaptive nature of the displacement activities (parasomnias) becomes apparent when a biological organism is viewed as the main and compensatory subsystem using ideas of the automatic control system theory (see Figure 15.1).

In summary, parasomnias, at the beginning, may have adaptive and compensatory functions. The benefit of brief disturbances in physiological systems is stability of the organism, structural or functional, as opposed to instability or death. Based on the theory described above, we proposed the principle of compensation and the adaptive role of parasomnias, according to which the loss of controlling function of one immature or defective subsystem may be compensated for by the chaotic behavior of another subsystem, less important for survival of the whole system. Parasomnias are 'helpful' disorders. Application of this principle to biological organisms may bring an explanation of their self-treatment: a mild disorder will be induced in one part of an organism in order to compensate for the loss of control function of another part of the organism. In other words, in order to stabilize the whole organism, one organ may be actively turned into a chaotic state. Such disorder in our case, parasomnias, will be stable and resistant to treatment until the control organ restores its functionality. When the organism matures, parasomnias are not needed any longer and disappear. (Parasomnias may reappear later in life, for example, under stress.)

From this viewpoint, parasomnias at night are similar to habits during the day: the wide range of functional inconsistencies and adaptive disorders (comparable to software problems) in fact may be compensating for structural inconsistencies and diseases (comparable to hardware problems). One can say, for instance, that a limb of an RLS patient or the bladder of an enuretic provides a healthy dose of chaos to the heart or brain[27–29]. Such adaptive disorders stabilize the organism initially, but later on may pose serious health consequences if left untreated.

According to the adaptive theory, treatment of parasomnias should not be directed toward suppressing the symptoms but toward stabilizing the sleep mechanism. Although helpful at the beginning, parasomnias might later 'grow up' to be serious and life-threatening problems[30].

SOME DAYTIME HABITS ARE BORN IN SLEEP

The adaptive theory of parasomnias might be a key to understanding the physiology and pathophysiology of normal and pathological habit formation. Habits are defined as specific, stable, repetitive patterns of behavior, feelings and thoughts. Habits may be simple or elaborate, may appear spontaneously or may be consciously developed. Habits are a normal and necessary part of our functioning, but can be transformed into unnecessary, unhealthy and pathological self-destructive rituals. The deep and intimate relationship between habits and sleep is not easily visible on the surface. Formation of habits has numerous similarities with a natural course of parasomnias, specifically with stereotyped, repetitive rhythmic movements. Habits are 'crystallized' from undifferentiated periods of general instability, have a long 'monosymptomatic' period, are very resistant to change (treatment) and resolve in 'self-cure' or deteriorate to the next level of self-destructive repetitive activity. Motor habits appear and increase during transitional states or heightened hypervigilance.

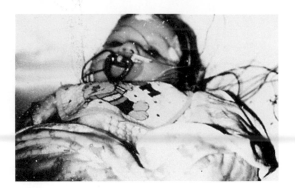

Figure 15.2 Infant during the study of non-nutritive sucking

We analyzed relationships between sleep and habits using the model of non-nutritional sucking in infants (Figure 15.2). Three phases could be differentiated in the appearance of non-nutritional sucking. The child displays diffuse restlessness, irritability and crying (Figure 15.3). At this moment, he/she is noticed to suck intensely on a pacifier. When slow activity develops on the EEG, the sucking movements stop (stabilization phase – Figure 15.4). Sucking movements reappear when the child starts to breathe irregularly with apnea and arousals on the EEG, until rhythmic EEG and regular breathing are restored (resolution phase – Figure 15.5). In children who do not use a pacifier, a substitution is developed in the form of thumb sucking. Finger-sucking movements appear in the same situations as non-nutritional sucking, with the same frequency. When small children have a difficult time falling asleep, finger-sucking before sleep helps them to calm down and to fall asleep. Later, the child begins to suck his/her fingers when he/she is bored or when it is difficult to stay alert and focused. This habit serves as a means of falling asleep or maintaining a certain level of alertness, or dissociating from a frightening reality. While sucking its finger, the child stares unblinkingly into space, does not respond when its name is called, and does not remember what he/she was thinking about when asked later.

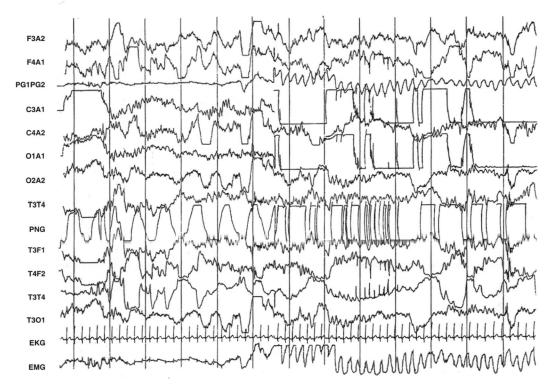

Figure 15.3 Phase 1 (initiation). Sucking movements are intense, i.e. higher frequency (0.2–0.6/s), longer duration (50–60 per cycle) with short intervals (0.5–45 s) negatively correlated with amplitude of electroencephalography reading and positively correlated with large body movements

The fact that some rhythmic movement activity could 'elicit' the brain to work in the same pattern has been known in physiology for a long time. Slow potentials in EEG in the rhythm of finger tremors were first described in 1938 by Jasper and Andrews[31]. In 1961, publications appeared describing the 'chewing' rhythms in EEG from the cortical sensorimotor zones of rabbits[32]. Later, in 1969, Grandstaff[33] discovered, in the EEG of cats, an activity synchronizer with the rhythm of milk licking. In 1974, Voino-Yasenezky[34] performed experiments on newborn rabbits and demonstrated that rhythmic patterns of muscle activity developed ontogenetically before brain activity, and actually induced development of the same patterns in the EEG. Thus, muscle activity during ontogenesis is a 'pacemaker' for the brain.

In 1981, Sologub[35] developed a method of enhancing rhythmic physical and mental performance (i.e. running) using a motor 'pacemaker' to produce the right level of mental meditation (a 'second wind' effect).

Our habits are natural 'switches', 'stabilizers' and 'pacemakers' of the state of alertness. They are born from parasomnias. In this sense, they are 'sleepmakers' and serve as regulators of all stages of vigilance. If natural regulators or pacemakers do not develop or get broken, the next level of unhealthy habits will develop.

DISCUSSION

Parasomnias could be conceptualized as a class of 'helpful' disorders that are produced by the body itself. The adaptive nature of parasomnias could explain predominance of

201

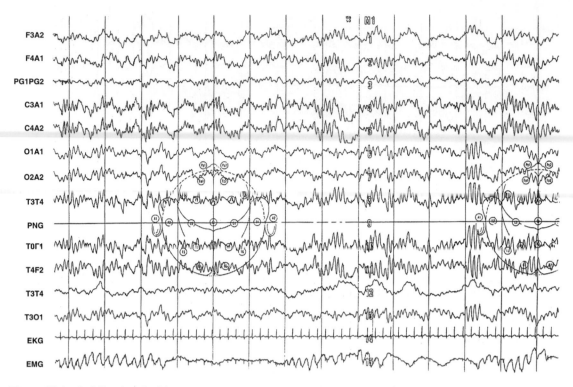

Figure 15.4   Stabilization. Sucking movements (SMs) are formed into a clear pattern: 12 ± 4 movements with 6 ± 2 s intervals. Frequency is 0.7 ± 2 s. On the electroencephalogram hypersynchronized theta (< 4/s) or delta (< 2/s) high amplitude is followed and later synchronized with SMs. SMs are positively correlated with rhythmical movements of fingers

the symptoms in children with immature children and increased frequency and severity in children with brain trauma. When the brain matures the symptom is no longer needed and it disappears by itself. If the situation does not improve, parasomnias get more intense and more severe forms appear.

As in many processes in our body, parasomnias start as an adaptive mechanism or even one advancing survival (like creative writing in our sleep), but later they may move into a maladaptive (e.g. sleepwalking) or even self-destructive phase (e.g. nocturnal wanderings). According to the adaptive theory, parasomnias at night and habits during the day are phenomena of the same nature. In fact, many habits act as 'stimulators' to keep the person alert, active and attentive or 'tranquilizers' to calm down or fall asleep. Some bad habits are clearly started around sleep-time or altered states of consciousness (thumb-sucking, hair

pulling, fire setting, self-mutilating). Persons with such habits usually have night parasomnias also. The adaptive theory of parasomnias postulates the existence of neurophysiological mechanisms that are responsible for 'switching' or 'maintaining' certain stages of sleep as well as stages of wakefulness. (It means, by the way, that stages of wakefulness should be physiologically different as stages of sleep, e.g. quiet wakefulness, attentive alertness, 'super-focused attention', altered states of consciousness, etc.) We already know that the processes of switching from wakefulness to sleep, from delta sleep to the REM stage and from sleep to alertness are active and complex groups of processes. When automatic transmitters do not work, for whatever reason, second mechanisms are turned on to 'switch' or to be a 'pacemaker'. A precise neurophysiological mechanism might be specific for each parasomnia but it involves motor and vestibular pathways[9].

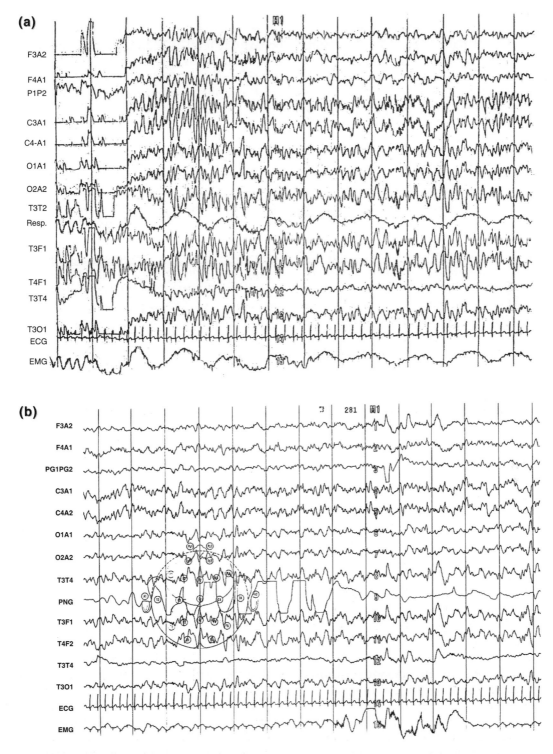

Figure 15.5 Resolution. (a) Termination of sucking movements (SMs). The electroencephalogram reading shows predominantly diffuse slow activity. Behavioral and electrographical sleep. (b) Short episodes of arousal are associated with bursts of SMs followed by the next cycle of slow brain waves

The psychological mechanism of adaptation by parasomnias is also very important. The number of parasomnias, e.g. the number of enuretic episodes, increases after emotional stress and negative experience during the day. If a child is punished by parents for his/her bedwetting and feels guilty, a vicious circle may result whereby every previous episode of bedwetting causes the subsequent episode by increasing the emotional tension.

It looks as if emotional tension, before being realized in parasomnias, causes a sleep structure disorder; a normal sleep structure is only restored after one or a few consequent episodes of parasomnias appear, as if these episodes 'discharge' the emotional tension. However, parasomnias as a very particular pattern of non-verbal (and often stereotyped) behavior determine only a terminal discharge of emotional tension, and later this tension increases once again, thus requiring a new episode of parasomnias for its discharge.

According to this hypothesis, parasomnias remain conversive symptoms that only temporarily help emotional stability. The underlying reason of emotional tension (for instance, an inner emotional conflict or the subconscious feeling of helplessness caused by a subject's inability to solve a problem) cannot be abolished either by conversion or by the parasomnias. Both of them only cover up this emotional tension for a while and actually conserve it. This happens until the subject moves to a higher level of psychological adaptation.

Parasomnias display a palliative way of psychological and behavioral adaptation in conditions when the effective and relevant mechanisms of adaptation demonstrate immaturity and functional insufficiency. Only the maturity of these mechanisms allows a change in the person's attitude toward the traumatic situation, to overcome a tendency to capitulate when confronted with this situation, and as a result to solve the problem that causes the emotional tension. Until this problem is solved, the emotional tension regularly returns and causes the reverberation of parasomnias. One of the major mature mechanisms that helps to solve problems on a psychological and behavioral level is search activity, discussed in detail in this book in Chapter 3. Functionally sufficient REM sleep (with active and vivid dreams), according to this concept, restores search activity in subsequent wakefulness if it is decreased for some reason(s) during wakefulness before sleep, and if the subject 'gave up'[36]. At the same time, a common denominator for all types of parasomnias is functional insufficiency of non-REM and/or REM sleep. After final maturation of the brain mechanisms of search activity and REM sleep, the need for palliative mechanisms that decrease the emotional tension disappears together with the parasomnias.

Another approach to the same problem is available in the opposing concepts of dynamic (constructive) chaos that characterizes normal activity of the mature brain and destructive chaos typical for parasomnias. Destructive chaos, in contrast to constructive chaos, has no positive direction and does not help the subject to adapt to the complicated and polydimensional world, and helps only to limit (for a short period) the reaction to real problems. The level of coping with problems does not change; the clinical symptoms also do not change. If such static and destructive chaos could really substitute for the dynamic chaos of the mature brain, parasomnias would be maintained.

CONCLUSION

Parasomnias are disorders of sleep. Despite an endless variation of symptoms, the internal structure, ontogenetic development and course of parasomnias have common phases and pathways uniting them in a separate clinical entity.

In their early stages, parasomnia phenomena might be protective, compensatory and otherwise adaptive for the developing organism. These 'little' disorders of 'software', like immunizations, may prevent 'big' disorders in the body's 'hardware'. If the underlying problems are not corrected, mild, adequate, protective forms of parasomnias will transform into maladaptive, inadequate and destructive syndromes. What was helpful initially might hurt later on.

The adaptive theory of parasomnia is based on the 'partial arousal' theory by Broughton, and current concepts of control system determinate chaos theory formed around the hypothesis that some of our daytime habits are 'born' from night parasomnias, and as parasomnias serve the function of increasing, decreasing or maintaining alertness and emotional arousal.

As with any theory, especially in the early stage of its creation, the adaptive theory of parasomnias is yet another hypothesis that has its limitations. First, it is applied mostly to pediatric parasomnias. How it is applicable to adults needs to be a focus for future research. Second, adaptive, compensatory functions of parasomnias could be applied to phenomena which are not caused by underlying organic disorders. Third, large multidisciplinary studies are needed to prove or disprove the basic claim of parasomnias as a self-stabilizing function of the sleeping and waking brain.

References

1. Hendricks JC, Morrison AR. Normal and abnormal sleep in mammals. *Am J Vet Res* 1981;178:121–6
2. Hendricks JC, Morrison AR, Fornbach GL, *et al*. A disorder of rapid eye movement sleep in a cat. *J Am Vet Med Assoc* 1980;178:55–7
3. Hendricks JC, Kline LR, Kovalski RJ, *et al*. The English bulldog: a national model of sleep disordered breathing. *J Am Vet Med Assoc* 1983;183
4. Mitler MM, Spave O, Dement WC. Narcolepsy in seven dogs. *J Am Vet Med Assoc* 1976;168:1036–8
5. Fink M. Electroconvulsive therapy in neurological disorders. *Psychiatric Times*. August 2002
6. Montoya FJ, Riddell CE, Caesar R, Hague S. Treatment of gustatory hyperlacrimation (crocodile tears) with injection of botulinum toxin into the lacrimal gland. *Eye* 2002;16:705–9
7. Blumenfeld A. Botulinum toxin found to be effective and cost-effective headache treatment. Annual Meeting of the American Headache Society, Seattle, 2002. *CNS News*. September 2002
8. Golbin AZ. *The World of Children's Sleep*. Salt Lake City, UT: Michaelis Publishing Company, 1995:32
9. Golbin AZ. *Pathological Sleep in Children*. Moscow: Medicina, 1979:244 (in Russian)
10. Uchtomsky AA. Collection of papers. Moscow: Nauka, 1967;16:121–32
11. Kaminsky CD. *Dynamic Pathology of Cortical Brain Activity*. Moscow: Nauka, 1948:39–40 (in Russian)
12. Vvedensky NE. In Porshnev BF. *About the Beginning of Human History (Problems of Paleopsychology)*. Moscow: MISL, 1974:220–78 (in Russian)
13. Muhametov LM. *Investigation of a Sigma Rhythm in the EEG of Mammals*. Moscow: Nauka, 1967 (in Russian)
14. Porshnev BF. *About the Beginning of Human History (Problems of Paleopsychology)*. Moscow: Nauka, 1974:140–312 (in Russian)
15. Bechtereva NP, Kambarova DK, Posteev VK. *Stability of Pathological Condition in Brain Disorders*. Moscow: Medicina, 1978:90–248 (in Russian)
16. Tinbergen NZ. Cited in Porshnev BF. *About the Beginning of Human History. (Problems in Paleo Psychology)*. Moscow: MISL, 1974:384 (in Russian)
17. Tinbergen N. *The Study of Instinct*. Oxford: Oxford University Press, 1951:3–92
18. Kortlandt A. Cited in Porshnev BF. *About the Beginning of Human History. (Problems in Paleo Psychology)*. Moscow: MISL, 1974:271–4 (in Russian)
19. Delius JD. Displacement activities and arousal. *Nature* 1967:214:12–59
20. Schino G, Perretta G, Taglioni AM, *et al*. Primate displacement activities as an ethopharmacological model of anxiety. *Anxiety* 1996;2: 186–91
21. Broughton J. Sleep disorders and disorders of arousal? *Science* 1968;159:1070–8
22. Goldberger AL, Amaral LA, Hausdorff JM, *et al*. Fractal dynamics in physiology: alterations with disease and aging. *Proc Natl Acad Sci USA* 2002;99(Suppl 1):2466–72
23. Pecora LM, Carroll TL. Synchronization in chaotic systems. *Phys Rev Lett* 1990;64:821

24. Ott E, Grebogi C, Yorke JA. Controlling chaos. *Phys Rev Lett* 1990;64:1196
25. Bunde A, *et al*. Correlated and uncorrelated regions in heart-rate fluctuations during sleep. *Phys Rev Lett* 2000;85:3736
26. Kapitsa PL. Pendulum with a vibrating pivot? 'Uspechi Nauki'. Moscow: MISL, 1951;XLIV:7–10 (in Russian)
27. Cabrera JL, Milton JG. On–off intermittency in a human balancing task. *Phys Rev Lett* 2002;89:158702
28. Goodwin JS. Chaos, and the limits of modern medicine. *J Am Med Assoc* 1997;17:1399
29. Milton J, Black D. Dynamic diseases in neurology and psychiatry. *Chaos* 1995;5:8–13
30. Golbin A, Umantzev A. A little disorder may be a key to a big disease. *J Am Med Assoc* 2004, in press
31. Jasper HH, Andrews HL. Brain potentials and voluntary muscle activity in man. *J Neurophysiol* 1938;1:87–8
32. Sadonski B, Longo VG. Electrical activity of the rabbit's brain during conditional elementary reflexes and its modification by drugs. *Excerpta Med* 1961;37:107–10
33. Grandstaff NW. Frequency analysis of EEG during milk drinking. *Clin Neurophysiol* 1969;27:57–63
34. Voino-Yasenezky AV. *Primary Rhythms of Activity in Ontogenesis*. Leningrad: Nauka, 1974:1–147
35. Soedlogub EB. *Cortical Regulation of Movements in Man*. Leningrad: Medicina, 1981.1–101 (in Russian)
36. Rotenberg VS, Arshavsky VV. REM sleep, stress and search activity. Cited in *Waking Sleeping* 1979;3:235–11

Section 4:

Neuropsychiatric disorders and sleep aberrations

16

General concepts of sleep in relation to psychiatry

Eric Vermetten, Elbert Geuze and Joost Mertens

INTRODUCTION

Sleep is a core function of human physiology, controlled by the brain. Two of the major neurotransmitter systems implicated in sleep, the noradrenergic and serotonergic systems, are also implicated in many psychiatric disorders. It therefore seems logical that many psychiatric disorders are associated with reports of sleep complaints and sleep disturbances[1-3]. Whereas insomnia is frequent in the general population, sleep complaints are more commonly reported in psychiatric patients than in the general population[1]. Sleep disorders in psychiatry are primarily considered symptoms of an underlying disorder, but new evidence indicates that sleep disturbances may be one of the critical underlying factors in the pathogenesis of psychiatric disorders themselves[4,5]. Unfortunately, little is known about how the chronicity of insomnia affects this relation and how often patients with chronic insomnia have antecedents of psychiatric disorders. In one large European cohort study, involving telephone interviews with a total of 14 915 individuals aged from 15 to 100 years, the prevalence of insomnia accompanied by impaired daytime functioning was 19.1%. Moreover, the prevalence rate increased significantly with age[6]. More than 90% of these patients had chronic insomnia, 28% of those with insomnia had a current diagnosis of mental disorders and 25.6% had a positive psychiatric history. The presence of severe insomnia, a diagnosis of primary insomnia or insomnia related to a medical condition, and insomnia of more than 1 year's duration were predictors of a psychiatric history. In most cases of mood disorders, the insomnia appeared before (> 40%) or at the same time (> 22%) as mood disorder symptoms. When anxiety disorders were involved, insomnia appeared mostly at the same time as (> 38%) or after (> 34%) the anxiety disorder. This indicates that chronic insomnia can be a residual symptom of a previous mental disorder and places patients at a higher risk of relapse. The Epidemiologic Catchment Area study by the National Institute of Mental Health showed that 32% of the respondents with sleep disturbances suffered from mood disorders, whereas only 5% suffered from anxiety. However, this research did not include a measurement for generalized anxiety disorder[5]. Another cohort study reported a lifetime prevalence of 16.6%[7]. A re-interview 3 years later showed a relationship of prior sleep problems with the later developed mood disorders.

Although sleep-related complaints and electroencephalographic (EEG) changes are

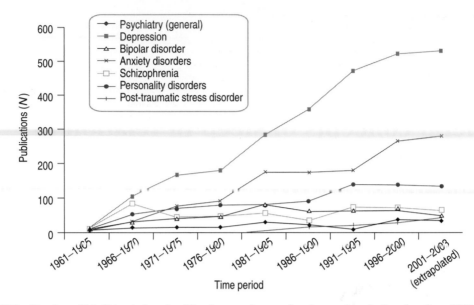

Figure 16.1 Number of MedLine indexed publications on sleep and major psychiatric disorders from 1960 until the present

seen widely across the spectrum of psychiatric disorders, sleep complaints such as insomnia, hypersomnia, nightmares and sleep panic attacks are more common in suicidal patients[8]. Sleep studies report various polysomnographic findings including increased rapid eye movement (REM) time and REM activity in suicidal patients with depression, schizoaffective disorder and schizophrenia. One mechanism responsible for this possible association between suicide and sleep could be the role of serotonin. Serotonergic function is found to be low in patients who have either attempted or completed suicide, particularly in those who used violent methods. Additionally, agents that enhance serotonergic transmission also decrease suicidal behavior. Serotonin plays an important role in the onset and maintenance of slow-wave sleep (SWS) and in REM sleep. Cerebrospinal fluid 5-hydroxytryptamine $(5HT)_{1A}$ levels correlate with SWS in patients with depression as well as schizophrenia. Moreover, $5HT_2$ receptor antagonists improve SWS.

A search of the available literature on sleep and psychiatry reveals scant original contemporary research on the relation of sleep disturbances and psychiatric disorders. With the

discovery of REM sleep and its relationship to sleep and dreaming, psychiatric sleep researchers have been interested in uncovering the complex relationship between disturbed sleep and various psychiatric disorders. Much of our present knowledge is based on research conducted in the 1970s and 1980s, that focused on REM sleep alterations and EEG abnormalities in psychiatric disorders. With the advent of new techniques such as neuroimaging, one might expect more research on this topic. Figure 16.1 shows the number of MedLine indexed publications for physiological concepts of various psychiatric disorders and psychiatry, with only a slight increase in most of the research areas. This increase is probably attributable to the general increase in publications in just about every area of research in the last half-century. Research on physiological concepts of sleep in relation to depression and anxiety increased considerably after the 1960s, but it appears that this increase is now stabilizing. Still, research on sleep in psychiatry should receive our attention. In many instances, a proper psychiatric diagnosis of disordered sleep reveals an underlying psychiatric disorder, which maintains the presenting sleep complaints. If

Table 16.1 Description and characteristics of sleep stages

Stage and description based on EEG	Characteristics
Stage 1 Alpha waves gradually replaced with theta waves	Descending sleep or dozing; 5–10% of sleep time Floating or drifting sensation during transition from drowsiness to sleep onset; insomniacs have longer stage 1 than normal Slow-rolling eye-movements; eyes closed
Stage 2 Theta waves, sleep spindles and K complexes	Unequivocal sleep; 50% of sleep time Slight rolling eye movements Easily awakened, especially sensitive to noise (which evokes K complexes) More frequent in elderly
Stage 3 + 4 Delta waves predominate, theta activity, K complexes	Deep sleep, slow-wave sleep (SWS) or delta sleep; 5–20% of sleep time Subjects hard to arouse Sleepwalking, sleeptalking, night terrors and bedwetting occur during this time
REM Low voltage-random, fast with sawtooth waves	Active sleep, paradoxical sleep, dream-sleep; 20–25% of sleep time Eyeball movement rapid; voluntary muscles relaxed Brain waves quicken; high level of activation of most cerebral systems May be important for psychological health, learning and memory

the disorder is treated properly, the sleep–wake function will improve accordingly. For this reason, psychiatrists view sleep physiology as a window on biological psychiatry, because sleep is one of the few easily quantifiable functions of interest to psychiatrists[9]. Continued developments in sleep research may assist in further understanding of the neuropathophysiology of affective and other psychiatric illnesses. Several psychiatric disorders are related to alterations in sleep–wake cycle, e.g. in circadian rhythms and REM sleep. Physiological alterations between non-rapid eye movement (NREM) and rapid eye movement (REM) sleep (see Table 16.1) as well as alterations in sleep histogram (Figure 16.2) may serve as indicators of physiological functions that are important in evaluating sleep (see Table 16.2). Psychopharmacological treatments, light therapy, electroconvulsive therapy (ECT), sleep deprivation and modern treatments such as transcranial magnetic stimulation (TMS) may well be used to evaluate these parameters in relation to assessing sleep.

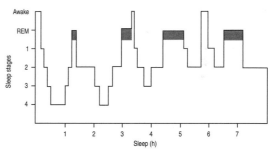

Figure 16.2 Histogram of a typical night's sleep of a normal young adult

PHYSIOLOGICAL CONCEPTS OF SLEEP AND DEPRESSION

Electroencephalographic sleep changes are described in a great number of patients suffering from major depression. The most reliable changes include sleep continuity disturbances such as prolonged sleep latency, and a decrease in delta sleep or SWS, with an abbreviated first REM period relative to sleep onset, and an altered distribution of REM sleep during the night, with a more rapid accumulation of REM sleep in the first third of the night as evidenced by a prolonged first REM period[10]. Although the specificity of such sleep changes in major depression is still a matter of debate, at least some of these changes might have a 'relative' rather than absolute specificity, particularly those related to the first REM period. Reynolds and co-workers[10] investigated the EEG sleep of borderline and primary depressives; both groups had increased sleep latencies and increased REM density, as well as activity, especially during the first REM period.

Major depressive episodes are associated with a dysregulation of various physiological systems. Antidepressant medications administered to depressive patients additionally alter regulation of the hormonal and sleep systems, thus indicating similar physiological mechanisms to those implicated in the sleep–wake cycle[11]. These physiological systems are regulated by three major neurotransmitters, norepinephrine, serotonin and dopamine, all also implicated in the etiology of mood disorders. Manipulations of the sleep system through sleep deprivation can ameliorate depression[12]; see reference 13 for a review. Sleep deprivation has been described in more than three dozen studies published in the past three decades and produces marked, acute antidepressant effects in the majority of depressed individuals[13]. Stress is among the most common causes of transient insomnia, and depression is one of the most common causes of chronic insomnia[4]. As with any disorder, treatment should ideally focus on the cause, not on the symptoms.

Mood disorders produce specific alterations in EEG sleep, including disinhibited REM sleep and suppressed SWS[14]. Sleep underlies homeostatic and circadian mechanisms that interact in complex ways. These relationships have been formalized in electrophysiological, neurochemical and neuroendocrinological models that extend to the pathophysiology of affective illness. Sleep research as a pathophysiological window to the brain contributes extensively to our understanding of the neurobiology of depression and is a substantial guide for the advancement of model-driven clinical and preclinical research. Pharmacological probes of normal and depressed sleep also play an important role. Another strong link between mood disorders and sleep is that depressive symptoms are alleviated by one night of sleep deprivation and recur after sleeping.

Melatonin, an important sleep-inducing hormone, has powerful effects on circadian rhythms and sleep behavior. In addition, melatonin has well-established phase-shifting and sleep-promoting effects, which has implications for neuropsychiatrists[9]. In the research by Kayumov and co-workers[9] the majority of patients with phase delay syndrome were misdiagnosed as having depression. The reason for this error is elucidated in this chapter, and the information concerning the condition may be helpful to many who are relatively unfamiliar with this particular sleep disorder.

It is anticipated that the combination of novel topographic EEG and neuroimaging techniques with traditional experimental methods will provide us with a further insight into the neurobiology of sleep and depression. Nofzinger and co-workers[15] examined REM sleep in unipolar depression. They compared six unipolar depressed subjects to eight healthy subjects with separate 18F-fluorodeoxyglucose (FDG) positron emission tomography scans during waking and during their first REM period of sleep. Clinical and EEG sleep comparisons from an undisturbed night of sleep were also performed. In contrast to healthy control subjects, depressed patients failed to show increases in the regional cerebral metabolic rate of glucose (rCMRglu) in anterior paralimbic structures in REM sleep when compared to waking. Moreover, depressed subjects showed greater increases from waking to REM sleep in rCMRglu in the tectal area and a series of left hemispheric areas including sensorimotor cortex, inferior temporal cortex, uncal gyrus-amygdala and subicular complex than did the control subjects. These observations indicate that changes in limbic and paralimbic function from waking to REM sleep differ significantly from normal in depressed patients.

PHYSIOLOGICAL CONCEPTS OF SLEEP AND BIPOLAR DISORDER

Although physiological alterations in unipolar depression are generally well understood, information concerning sleep and sleep–wake manipulations in bipolar disorder is not as extensive. Studies investigating sleep in bipolar depression suggest that during the depressed phase sleep shows the same stigmata as seen in patients with unipolar depression[16]. In contrast, during the hypomanic or manic phases, REM sleep disinhibition is present and total sleep time is even more reduced, though subjectively this change is not considered disturbing by patients.

An important issue is the question of whether sleep–wake manipulations can also be applied to patients with bipolar depression. It has been suggested that disrupted sleep secondary to psychosocial stressors is a common precipitant of manic episodes in bipolar disorder[17]. However, work by other researchers[16,18] indicates that sleep deprivation and a phase advance of the sleep period is useful in the treatment of bipolar patients during the depressed phase. The risk of a switch into hypomania or mania does not appear more pronounced than the risk with typical pharmacological antidepressant treatment. For patients with mania, on the other hand, sleep deprivation is not an adequate treatment. Rather, treatment strategies aiming at stabilizing a regular sleep–wake schedule are indicated. The sleep–wake cycle of bipolar patients requires monitoring; stabilizing the sleep–wake cycle of bipolar patients may have a beneficial effect on the course of the disease[19].

PHYSIOLOGICAL CONCEPTS OF SLEEP AND ANXIETY DISORDER

As mentioned previously, sleep disorders are common in psychiatric disorders, mostly those characterized by depression. Some studies, however, report an even higher relation of sleep disorder with neurotic, stress-related, somatoform and anxiety disorders (41%), closely followed by affective disorders (31%)[20].

The relation between sleep and anxiety disorders is an intricate, two-way path. In general, anxiety disorders can cause sleep problems, but sleep disturbances by themselves may produce anxiety symptoms. Research on sleep disturbances and anxiety disorders is hampered by methodological difficulties, such as boundary problems with other psychiatric disorders, the large inter-individual variability of the common anxiety disorders, the large co-existence of co-morbidities such as alcohol and drug abuse and, not the least, because sleep disturbances are among the prominent diagnostic features of anxiety disorders, creating a 'chicken and egg' problem. Finally, as anxiety is required to prepare one for fight or flight under 'normal circumstances', it is predictable that sleep function will be suppressed in an anxious situation.

Among the anxiety disorders, generalized anxiety disorder (GAD) is associated with insomnia in 56–70% of the patients[21]. Insomnia associated with an anxiety disorder, mainly GAD, differs from depressive disorder because it is considered a sleep-maintenance insomnia and to a lesser extent a sleep-onset insomnia[22]. Another interesting difference regarding insomnia in depressive versus anxiety disorders is the fact that sleep deprivation has positive therapeutic effects in the former, but not in the latter[23].

Despite these interesting clinical differences, sleep laboratory research in anxiety patients is scant. Almost all polysomnographic studies demonstrate an increased sleep latency in patients with anxiety, compared with normal controls. Also, many report a significant increase in wake time during the total sleep period, more early morning awakening, and a decrease in total sleep and sleep efficiency. Some also show difficulties initiating and maintaining sleep. Others indicate differences in (subjective) sleep efficiency between the home and the laboratory, with patients reporting sleeping better in the latter[24–26]. All anxiety disorders are not the same, and differences are reported between panic disorder with and without agoraphobia, on the one hand, and GAD, social phobia, specific phobia, obsessive–compulsive disorder (OCD) and post-traumatic stress disorder (PTSD) on the other. These diverse observations point toward a more or less identical insomnia in panic disorder and GAD, which differs from the insomniac features in the other disorders. For example, polysomnographic research with patients with panic disorder also shows an increased sleep latency, decreased sleep time and efficacy, as is seen in patients with GAD[27].

The physiology of alterations of sleep function in anxiety disorders is still a relatively young field of research. Some results indicate increased sleep latency, more awakenings and decreased sleep efficiency as the most common observations. As a result, more alertness should affect the patient by generating more problems in resting and falling asleep. Research points toward an increased central nervous system arousal as a pathogenic factor of insomnia in general anxiety disorder.

PHYSIOLOGICAL CONCEPTS OF SLEEP AND POST-TRAUMATIC STRESS DISORDER

In the third edition of the *Diagnostic and Statistical Manual of Mental Disorders* (DSM-III) (APA, 1980), the diagnosis of PTSD was included in the category of anxiety disorders for the first time. Subjective accounts of disturbed sleep in PTSD are numerous, and patients report problems with sleep onset, sleep maintenance and duration of sleep, as well as a higher frequency of nightmares and anxiety dreams[28–30]. However, although various physiological alterations in the sleep of PTSD patients are reported, the objective research findings remain ambiguous and the exact nature of the physiological changes underlying this disorder remain to be clarified[31] (see Chapter 10).

PHYSIOLOGICAL CONCEPTS OF SLEEP AND SCHIZOPHRENIA

In schizophrenia, another of the major psychiatric disorders, physiological alterations of the sleep–wake cycle present commonly. These include impaired sleep continuity and reduced total sleep, reduced amounts of SWS, reduced REM sleep latency and defective REM rebound following REM deprivation[32]. Keshavan and co-workers suggest that reduced SWS may be related to a neurodevelopmental disorder related to the defect state in schizophrenia, but that the pathophysiological significance of the defective REM rebound and the REM sleep abnormalities in schizophrenia remain uncertain. Delta sleep, mediated by thalamocortical circuits, is postulated to be abnormal in schizophrenia[33]. A comparison of 30 unmedicated schizophrenic patients and 30 age- and sex-matched controls for sleep data evaluated by visual scoring as well as automated period amplitude analyses and power spectral analyses showed that schizophrenic patients had reduced visually scored delta sleep[33]. Period amplitude analyses showed significant reductions in delta wave counts but not REM counts; power spectral analyses showed reductions in delta as well as theta power. Delta spectral power was also reduced in the subset of 19 neuroleptic-naive, first-episode schizophrenic patients compared with matched controls. Keshavan and co-workers[33] concluded that the delta sleep deficits that occur in schizophrenia may be related to the primary pathophysiological characteristics of the illness and may not be secondary to previous neuroleptic use.

One interesting paper describes a hypothesis related to the neurochemical background of sleep–waking mental activity[34]. Although sleep–waking mental activity is associated with subcortical structures, it is principally generated in the cerebral cortex. During REM sleep, the monoaminergic neurons, normally active during waking, become silent, with the exception of the dopaminergic neurons. This results in a large disinhibition, while the

Table 16.2   Physiological variability between non-rapid eye movement (NREM) and rapid eye movement (REM) sleep

Variable	NREM	REM
Blood pressure	Lowest during stages 3 and 4; reduced variability	Short increases possible (40 mmHg); magnitude of change greater in hypertensive patients
Heart rate	Decreased	Increased variability; bursts of eye movements accompanied by brief tachycardias, followed by bradycardia
Cardiac activity	Reduced cardiac output; vasodilatation	Transient vasoconstrictions in skeletal muscle circulation; cardiac arrest (during sleep) more frequent during this stage
Cerebral blood flow	Twenty-five per cent reduction of flow to brain stem; reduction to cerebral cortex	Significantly increased blood flow, especially to cochlear nuclei
Temperature	Decreased brain and body temperature	Increased brain temperature; absence of thermoregulation
Respiration	Respiratory rate decreased; upper-airway muscles may be hypotonic, obstructing oxygen flow in patients with sleep apnea	Breathing rapid and may be irregular
Endocrine functions	Growth hormone secretion increased; thyroid stimulating hormone (TSH) and ACTH–cortisol rhythm inhibited	—
Renal function	Decreased urine volume, excretion of sodium, potassium, chloride and calcium	—
Pain	Decreased receptor activity to noxious tactile stimuli	Decreased pain at level of tooth pulp
Sexuality	n/a	Nocturnal penile tumescence: 191 min at age 20 decreasing to 96 min at age 70; lack may be sign of physiological impotence

n/a, not available. Reproduced from Institute for Natural Resources, August 1997, with permission

maintained dopamine influence may be involved in the familiar psychotic-like mental activity of dreaming. The increase of dopamine influence at the prefrontal cortex level could explain the almost total absence of negative symptoms of schizophrenia during dreaming, while an increase in the nucleus accumbens is possibly responsible for hallucinations and delusions, which are regular features of mentation during this sleep stage[34].

Classical analysis of spontaneous sleep EEG in schizophrenia commonly reveals alterations of sleep continuity, number of awakenings, SWS and REM sleep compared to healthy controls; however, this type of conventional analysis cannot help understand dynamic differences of the sleep EEG during different sleep stages[35,36]. Roschke and co-workers measured late components of auditory evoked potentials (AEPs) and visual evoked potentials (VEPs) during different sleep stages of 11 schizophrenic in-patients and in a sex- and age-matched control group[36]. According to linear system theory, they computed the amplitude-frequency characteristic from averaged AEPs and VEPs in different sleep stages. These amplitude-frequency characteristics describe the relation between input and output of the system under study, enabling a characterization of the transfer properties of the schizophrenic brain during sleep. Significant differences were found for the transfer properties during stage 2 and SWS between schizophrenics and controls. During REM a marked enhancement of theta resonance was seen in schizophrenics. Perhaps this observation will allow us to distinguish schizophrenia and depression in EEG studies in the near future.

Carefully designed studies are needed to further characterize the sleep disturbance in schizophrenia and to study it in relation to other, known pathophysiological changes in this disorder.

PHYSIOLOGICAL CONCEPTS OF SLEEP AND PERSONALITY

A considerable body of evidence has appeared over the past decades concerning the physiological alterations of sleep in patients with personality disorders. The bulk of this research has studied individuals with borderline personality disorders, who reveal sleep profiles similar to those of patients with major depression[10]. The co-morbidity of major depression with borderline personality disorder is high[37], so this finding is not surprising. However, Bell and co-workers[38] have demonstrated that borderline patients with and without major depression also have similar sleep profiles. In addition, an Egyptian study, comparing 20 patients with ICD-10 diagnosed borderline disorder without major depression to 20 patients with major depression and 20 healthy controls, revealed that the presumed personality disturbance in the Egyptian culture manifests neurophysiologically as it does

in the Western world[39]. The two patient groups differed significantly from controls in their sleep profiles, especially regarding sleep continuity measures, decreased SWS and REM sleep abnormalities. A high degree of similarity was found in the EEG sleep profiles of the two patient groups, though the changes were more robust in the patients with major depression. However, the similarity between borderline personality disorder patients and patients with major depression does suggest a common biological origin for both conditions.

In borderline personality, positive spikes in the EEG have been associated with impulsivity, and 6/s spike and wave complexes with interpersonal problems[40]. In one study investigating the effects of carbamazepine (CBZ) versus placebo on the dexamethasone suppression test (DST) and sleep EEG in a sample of 20 patients with borderline personality disorder (BPD) without concomitant major depression (MD)[41], CBZ, administered at doses that are therapeutic for epilepsy and affective disorders, had an effect on the DST and sleep EEG in BPD. CBZ significantly increased the post-dexamethasone plasma cortisol values. This did not parallel MD or an increase in the Hamilton depression rating scores. CBZ also increased SWS. The mechanisms by which CBZ increased post-dexamethasone plasma cortisol levels and SWS in BPD are discussed by Hughes[40].

There is some interest in the identification of polysomnographic markers of liability to the mood disorders that may predate the onset of illness in high-risk patients, and/or remain altered after remission[42]. One such putative marker is REM density during the first REM period. In the study by Battaglia and co-workers[42] comparing never-depressed subjects with BPD to age- and gender-matched controls using continuous 48-h ambulatory EEG monitoring, patients with BPD had significantly higher REM density during the first REM period. One man with BPD who later committed suicide had REM density values exceeding the mean value of his group by two standard deviations.

To clarify the effects of anxiety-related personality traits on sleep patterns, polysomnographic examinations were performed over four consecutive nights in normal individuals who tested within the low- or high-anxiety ranges[43]. Six male university students who scored fewer than 45 points (low-anxiety group) were compared to six male university students who scored more than 55 points (high-anxiety group) on the Spielberger's State Trait Anxiety Inventory. The low-anxiety group exhibited a greater change in REM sleep and stage 2 sleep compared to the high-anxiety group. The REM sleep in the low-anxiety group was shorter on the first and second nights compared to the third and fourth nights, and the stage 2 sleep was longer on the first night than on the remaining three nights. Thus, the low-anxiety group showed a first-night effect followed by partial recovery on the second night, whereas the high-anxiety group did not. These results suggest that there is a difference in sleep patterns assessed by consecutive polysomnographics between those with low- and high-anxiety traits, and that anxiety-related personality traits attenuate the occurrence of the first-night effect, reflecting a lower adaptability to a novel environment.

CONCLUSION

From this brief overview of a number of physiological changes seen in psychiatric disorders, it is clear that disturbed sleep is an important feature of many psychiatric disorders. A number of epidemiological studies have described the prevalence of sleep-related psychiatric symptoms in the general population. Therefore, while most psychiatric groups showed significantly reduced sleep efficiency and total sleep time, accounted for by decrements in NREM sleep, no single sleep variable appears to have absolute specificity for any particular psychiatric disorder.

References

1. Benca RM. Sleep in psychiatric disorders. *Neurol Clin* 1996;14:739–64
2. Benca RM, Obermeyer WH, Thisted RA, Gillin JC. Sleep and psychiatric disorders. A meta-analysis. *Arch Gen Psychiatry* 1992;49:651–68; discussion 669–70
3. McCall WV. A psychiatric perspective on insomnia. *J Clin Psychiatry* 2001;62(Suppl 10): 27–32
4. Billiard M, Partinen M, Roth T, Shapiro C. Sleep and psychiatric disorders. *J Psychosom Res* 1994;38(Suppl 1):1–2
5. Ford DE, Kamerow DB. Epidemiologic study of sleep disturbances and psychiatric disorders. An opportunity for prevention? *J Am Med Assoc* 1989;262:1479–84
6. Ohayon MM, Roth T. Place of chronic insomnia in the course of depressive and anxiety disorders. *J Psychiatr Res* 2003;37:9–15
7. Breslau N, Roth T, Rosenthal L, Andreski P. Sleep disturbance and psychiatric disorders: a longitudinal epidemiological study of young adults. *Biol Psychiatry* 1996;39:411–18
8. Singareddy RK, Balon R. Sleep and suicide in psychiatric patients. *Ann Clin Psychiatry* 2001;13:93–101
9. Kayumov L, Zhdanova IV, Shapiro CM. Melatonin, sleep, and circadian rhythm disorders. *Semin Clin Neuropsychiatry* 2000;5:44–55
10. Reynolds CF 3rd, Soloff PH, Kupfer DJ, *et al.* Depression in borderline patients: a prospective EEG sleep study. *Psychiatry Res* 1985;14:1–15
11. Szuba MP, O'Reardon JP, Evans DL. Physiological effects of electroconvulsive therapy and transcranial magnetic stimulation in major depression. *Depress Anxiety* 2000;12:170–7
12. Szuba MP, Baxter LR Jr, Altshuler LL, *et al.* Lithium sustains the acute antidepressant effects of sleep deprivation: preliminary findings from a controlled study. *Psychiatry Res* 1994;51:283–95
13. Wirz-Justice A, Van den Hoofdakker RH. Sleep deprivation in depression: what do we know, where do we go? *Biol Psychiatry* 1999;46:445–53
14. Seifritz E. Contribution of sleep physiology to depressive pathophysiology. *Neuropsychopharmacology* 2001;25(Suppl 5):S85–8
15. Nofzinger EA, Nichols TE, Meltzer CC, *et al.* Changes in forebrain function from waking to REM sleep in depression: preliminary analyses. *Psychiatry Res* 1999;91:59–78

16. Riemann D, Voderholzer U, Berger M. Sleep and sleep–wake manipulations in bipolar depression. *Neuropsychobiology* 2002;45(Suppl 1): 7–12

17. Malkoff-Schwartz S, Frank E, Anderson B, *et al.* Stressful life events and social rhythm disruption in the onset of manic and depressive bipolar episodes: a preliminary investigation. *Arch Gen Psychiatry* 1998;55:702–7

18. Barbini B, Colombo C, Benedetti F, *et al.* The unipolar–bipolar dichotomy and the response to sleep deprivation. *Psychiatry Res* 1998;79: 43–50

19. Leibenluft E, Suppes T. Treating bipolar illness: focus on treatment algorithms and management of the sleep–wake cycle. *Am J Psychiatry* 1999;156:1976–81

20. Saletu B. Sleep disorders, disease entities, symptoms or playing field of specialists? *Wien Klin Wochenschr* 1997;109:377–8

21. Anderson DJ, Noyes R Jr, Crowe RR. A comparison of panic disorder and generalized anxiety disorder. *Am J Psychiatry* 1984;141:572–5

22. Monti JM, Monti D. Sleep disturbance in generalized anxiety disorder and its treatment. *Sleep Med Rev* 2000;4:263–76

23. Labbate LA, Johnson MR, Lydiard RB, *et al.* Sleep deprivation in social phobia and generalized anxiety disorder. *Biol Psychiatry* 1998; 43:840–2

24. Reynolds CF 3rd, Shaw DH, Newton TF, *et al.* EEG sleep in outpatients with generalized anxiety: a preliminary comparison with depressed outpatients. *Psychiatry Res* 1983;8:81–9

25. Akiskal HS, Lemmi H, Dickson H, *et al.* Chronic depressions. Part 2. Sleep EEG differentiation of primary dysthymic disorders from anxious depressions. *J Affect Disord* 1984;6:287–95

26. Papadimitriou GN, Kerkhofs M, Kempenaers C, Mendlewicz J. EEG sleep studies in patients with generalized anxiety disorder. *Psychiatry Res* 1988;26:183–90

27. Mellman TA, Uhde TW. Electroencephalographic sleep in panic disorder. A focus on sleep-related panic attacks. *Arch Gen Psychiatry* 1989;46:178–84

28. Ross RJ, Ball WA, Sullivan KA, Caroff SN. Sleep disturbance as the hallmark of posttraumatic stress disorder. *Am J Psychiatry* 1989; 146:697–707

29. Mellman TA, Kulick-Bell R, Ashlock LE, Nolan B. Sleep events among veterans with combat-related posttraumatic stress disorder. *Am J Psychiatry* 1995;152:110–15

30. Neylan TC, Marmar CR, Metzler TJ, *et al.* Sleep disturbances in the Vietnam generation: findings from a nationally representative sample of male Vietnam veterans. *Am J Psychiatry* 1998;155:929–33

31. Lavie P. Sleep disturbances in the wake of traumatic events. *N Engl J Med* 2001;345:1825–32

32. Keshavan MS, Reynolds CF, Kupfer DJ. Electroencephalographic sleep in schizophrenia: a critical review. *Compr Psychiatry* 1990;31:34–47

33. Keshavan MS, Reynolds CF 3rd, Miewald MJ, *et al.* Delta sleep deficits in schizophrenia: evidence from automated analyses of sleep data. *Arch Gen Psychiatry* 1998;55:113–8

34. Gottesmann C. The neurochemistry of waking and sleeping mental activity: the disinhibition-dopamine hypothesis. *Psychiatry Clin Neurosci* 2002;55:345–51

35. Roschke J, Mann K, Fell J. Non-linear EEG dynamics during sleep in depression and schizophrenia. *Int J Neurosci* 1994;75:271–84

36. Roschke J, Wagner P, Mann K, Prentice-Cuntz T, Frank C. An analysis of the brain's transfer properties in schizophrenia: amplitude frequency characteristics and evoked potentials during sleep. *Biol Psychiatry* 1998;43:503–10

37. Koenigsberg HW, Anwunah I, New AS, *et al.* Relationship between depression and borderline personality disorder. *Depress Anxiety* 1999; 10:158–67

38. Bell J, Lycaki H, Jones D, *et al.* Effect of preexisting borderline personality disorder on clinical and EEG sleep correlates of depression. *Psychiatry Res* 1983;9:115–23

39. Asaad T, Okasha T, Okasha A. Sleep EEG findings in ICD-10 borderline personality disorder in Egypt. *J Affect Disord* 2002;71:11–18

40. Hughes JR. A review of the usefulness of the standard EEG in psychiatry. *Clin Electroencephalogr* 1996;27:35–9

41. De la Fuente JM, Bobes J, Vizuete C, Mendlewicz J. Effects of carbamazepine on dexamethasone suppression and sleep electroencephalography in borderline personality disorder. *Neuropsychobiology* 2002;45:113–19

42. Battaglia M, Ferini Strambi L, Bertella S, *et al.* First-cycle REM density in never-depressed subjects with borderline personality disorder. *Biol Psychiatry* 1999;45:1056–8

43. Kajimura N, Kato M, Sekimoto M, *et al.* A polysomnographic study of sleep patterns in normal humans with low- or high-anxiety personality traits. *Psychiatry Clin Neurosci* 1998; 52:317–20

17

Attention deficit hyperactivity disorder and sleep disorders in children

Peter Dodzik

INTRODUCTION

Attention deficit hyperactivity disorder (ADHD) is a neurobiological disorder that affects 3–6% of school-age children and is one of the most – if not the most – common pediatric disorders to present at out-patient mental health centers[1]. ADHD is generally characterized by one or more of the following developmentally inappropriate symptoms – inattentiveness, hyperactivity and impulsivity.

The disorder itself has a long history and this cluster of symptoms has undergone several name changes since first being identified by G. F. Still in 1902[1]. More recent classifications included minimal brain dysfunction, hyperkinetic reaction of childhood and attention-deficit disorder with or without hyperactivity[1]. With the emergence of the *Diagnostic and Statistical Manual,* 4th Edition[2], the disorder has been renamed attention-deficit/hyperactivity disorder. The current nomenclature was chosen to reflect the importance of the similarity in the etiology of this symptom cluster.

Recent evidence from molecular genetics and epidemiology have begun to suggest an underlying consistency in the transmission of the disorder closely resembling autosomal dominance with heritability rates as high as 0.57[1] when one parent has the disorder and 0.85 when both parents have the disorder[3], with a range of 0.50–0.91. These rates rival those for other strongly genetically determined characteristics such as height and intelligence[3]. Twin studies have been reviewed and have shown 0–29% concordance rates for dizygotic twins and 67–91% for monozygotic twins[1]. Thus, current trends in research on the disorder have centered on identification of the particular genes involved with the disorder and whether sub-classifications based on the predominance of symptoms reflect different genetic presentations[3].

These recent genetic findings have fueled the ongoing controversy over the correct categorization of the disorder. Although initially ADHD was thought of as a childhood disorder, current trends show that perhaps as many as 66% of children reach adulthood with the disorder still present[4]. Barkley[1] and other researchers now believe this rate may be much higher. They cite limitations in the methodology of the DSM-IV classification system as the cause of some of the controversy over adult prevalence. In their view, patients with the disorder continue to lag behind their same-aged peers, displaying such qualities as inattention, impulsivity, distractibility and hyperactivity well into adulthood[3]. In addition, adaptive

Table 17.1 Prevalence of co-morbid psychiatric disorders with attention deficit hyperactivity disorder

Condition	Prevalence (%)	Study
Mood disorders		
Major affective disorders	20–36	Barkley 1998[1]
Anxiety disorders	27–30	Biederman *et al.*, 1991[7]
Anxiety or mood disorders	13–30	Anderson *et al.*, 1987[8]
Major depressive disorder	9–32	Biederman *et al.*, 1991[7]
Bipolar disorder	11	Biederman 1997[9]
Behavior disorders		
Oppositional defiant disorders	54–67	Biederman 1997[9]
Conduct disorder	20–50	Szatmari *et al.*, 1989[10]

functioning in adults who were diagnosed with ADHD is also impaired compared to controls without a history of the disorder in childhood. However, the relative level of disability may vary as the frontal lobes of the brain continue to develop into the twenties[5].

ADHD has also been linked to a number of co-morbid disorders that complicate the diagnostic procedure and resulting treatment plan. When taken together, evidence suggests that at least 44% of children with ADHD will meet criteria for at least one other mental health disorder[6]. The presence of other mental health issues has led to further debate about differences between children with predominantly inattentive symptoms and those with combined or predominantly impulsive/hyperactive symptoms. Children diagnosed with the inattentive type of this disorder tend to show co-morbid mood disorders[3], while children with the impulsive/hyperactive type tend to present with co-morbid behavioral disorders[3]. Table 17.1 provides an overview of co-morbid diagnoses based on a review of recent literature[1,7–10].

These findings highlight the importance of co-morbid conditions with ADHD. However, the causal relationship is less clear. The effects of mood disorders on childhood behavior are well known and their relative impact on sleep may also be an area of concern for the child who presents with ADHD and sleep disturbances.

Results from the MTA Cooperative Group[11] found that 70% of children diagnosed with ADHD had co-morbid conditions when learning and social disabilities were included with other psychiatric disorders. Thus, clinicians should be aware that co-morbidity is likely to be the norm rather than the exception in this population.

Sleep disorders have generally been left out of many of the major texts on ADHD and are often not included among the traditional data on prevalence and co-morbidity. However, with advances in pediatric sleep medicine, more evidence is available to suggest a link between ADHD and sleep disorders. The goal of this chapter is to provide the reader with a relevant review of sleep disorders in children with ADHD and to suggest avenues for intervention. In addition, the co-morbid versus causal relationship of these disorders will be explored, as will diagnostic methods to aid in the differentiation of symptoms of inattentiveness, impulsivity and hyperactivity associated with a primary sleep disorder from those associated with ADHD.

SLEEP DISORDERS ASSOCIATED WITH ADHD

Corkum and colleagues[12] reviewed the literature on ADHD and sleep disorders in 1998. The study found that the method of determination of a sleep disorder varied from study to study, with some relying on questionnaires rather than more objective measurements (e.g. polysomnography, multiple sleep latency tests). In those studies using subjective questionnaires, the prevalence of sleep disorders with ADHD was 25–50% compared to 7% in normal controls. However, the authors point out that few studies have examined the relative rates of sleep disorders in children with other clinical disorders or co-morbid conditions. Thus, it is difficult to determine the relative contribution of other axis-I conditions to the rates of sleep disorders based on these studies alone. In fact, Marcotte and associates found that children with either ADHD, ADHD + a specific learning disability, or learning disability alone differed significantly from children in the community sample with regard to sleep disorders but not from each other[13]. Corkum points out that studies such as this indicate the limitations of using the presence of sleep disorders alone as a marker of ADHD or even as a distinguishing factor from other disorders[14].

In the review of studies that used objective measures of sleep difficulties in children with and without ADHD, Corkum[14] found that several studies (nine out of the ten reviewed) indicated that the total sleep time of children with ADHD did not differ from normal controls. Several studies indicated that children with ADHD tended to display more restless sleep (four out of six studies reviewed). In addition, stimulant medication used to treat the disorder was found to result in prolonged sleep latency and increased length of time to the first rapid eye movement (REM) cycle. However, these changes were thought to be non-pathological. Gruber and colleagues found that the instability of sleep patterns from night to night is the most characteristic feature of sleep in children with ADHD[15].

Studies on ADHD and specific problems in sleep have become more prolific in the past few years, particularly when consideration of individuals' sleep problems, such as apnea and periodic limb movement (PLM) disorders, are considered. The next section looks at prevalence rates for specific sleep-related disorders and ADHD.

Sleep disordered breathing and ADHD

Recent prospective studies have shown associations between sleep disordered breathing (SDB) and daytime symptoms of hyperactivity in children referred to sleep centers. Chervin and Archibold found that children referred to an out-patient sleep clinic had higher scores on measures of hyperactivity when compared to the normative sample for their age group[16]. Conner's ADHD rating scales completed by the parents showed hyperactive symptoms of almost one standard deviation above the normal range. However, of the children referred to the out-patient sleep clinic, children who were found to have SDB did not have significantly higher scores (mean Hyperactivity Index T score 59.5) than those without (mean Hyperactivity Index T score 59.0). Approximately half ($n = 59$) were found to have symptoms of SDB based on polysomnography.

Results from this study indicated that Hyperactivity Index scores showed no significant associations with the rate of apneas and hypopneas, minimum oxygen saturation or most negative esophageal pressure, but they did indicate that scores were positively associated with five or more PLMs per hour ($p = 0.02$). Thus, children referred for SDB did tend to have higher Hyperactivity Index scores, but the presence of the disorder alone could not explain the symptoms. However, PLMs may have been more directly related to the severity of the hyperactive symptoms[16].

Parent questionnaires completed at out-patient child psychiatric clinics and general pediatric clinics have found rates of habitual snoring to be as high as 33% among children diagnosed with ADHD compared to 9–11% for children with other referrals[17]. In addition, higher scores on parent-completed measures of snoring and selected SDB symptoms were associated with higher scores on measures for hyperactivity and inattentiveness. The authors suggest that 81% of habitually snoring children who have ADHD (25% of all children with ADHD) could have their ADHD symptoms eliminated if their habitual snoring and any associated sleep-related breathing disorder were effectively treated. While provocative, this latter statement may reflect the necessity of treating SDB in children prior to treatment of symptoms associated with ADHD.

In one of the most comprehensive studies to date, O'Brien and colleagues[18] used sleep questionnaires with parents referred to an out-patient sleep center. The target group for this study was 5–7-year-old children, and, in addition to standard sleep questions, the parents were also asked whether they believed their child to have symptoms of ADHD. These children were divided into groups, based on their parents' responses, of 'significant' and 'mild' problems. Overnight polysomnography was conducted on the two groups, with 'no symptom' controls.

Results from the study indicated that, while the parents reported snoring as the most significant sleep problem among children diagnosed with ADHD, there was no difference in the presence of obstructive sleep apnea (OSA) as measured by polysomnography between children with 'significant' ADHD (5%) and those with no symptoms of the disorder (5%)[18]. However, the authors noted that for children with 'mild' symptoms of ADHD, OSA was present at much higher rates (26%). Thus, SDB appeared to produce symptoms of mild ADHD as measured by Conner's Parent Rating Scales and could potentially complicate diagnosis and delay proper treatment[18]. The relatively low numbers of children with 'significant' ADHD and SDB would argue against a causal link, but the presence of higher rates of SDB in the 'mild' ADHD cases suggests that ADHD-like symptoms could be produced by SDB in some children.

A relationship between ADHD and SDB is also suggested by studies conducted on the treatment of SDB in an adult sample. Naseem and associates conducted a limited ($n = 3$) case study analysis of three adult patients diagnosed with ADHD and OSA. All three patients in this study were considered overweight and had Respiratory Distress Index (RDI) scores ranging from 7 to 45.6[19]. In addition, all had had longstanding treatment with stimulant medication. Results indicated that all three patients demonstrated improvement in their ADHD symptoms following treatment for their OSA, with two discontinuing their stimulant medication for over 1 year.

Comparable results in a large, well-controlled study in children are lacking. However, Ali and colleagues[20] examined a large group of children aged 6 and older who were awaiting adenotonsillectomy. Twelve were identified as having moderate SDB, and were matched with a second group of children from the waiting list with no evidence of SDB (snoring only) and with a control group awaiting an unrelated surgical procedure. After surgery the SDB group showed reduced aggression, inattention and hyperactivity on Conner's Parent Rating Scales and improved vigilance on the Conner's Continuous Performance Test (CPT). Results further indicated that the snoring group also improved on measures of hyperactivity and vigilance. No changes were observed in the control group[20]. These results suggest that SDB and snoring contribute to the behavioral manifestations of ADHD and would certainly be expected to exacerbate the symptoms in the disorder. However, it should be noted that the subjects in this study were not specifically identified as having ADHD.

Current trends in research suggest that SDB may contribute to the symptoms of ADHD and that the use of rating scales or CPTs may be problematic in children with a family history of ADHD and sleep complaints. Although a causal relationship between ADHD and SDB has yet to be demonstrated, a careful evaluation of the markers of SDB is warranted to rule this out as a co-morbid condition. Treatment of OSA in adults with ADHD with continuous positive airway pressure (CPAP) has been found to reduce the symptoms of ADHD often to subclinical levels[19]. In addition, treatment of SDB and chronic snoring in children with adenotonsillectomy has also been found to reduce symptoms and improve cognitive performance.

Periodic limb movement and restless legs syndrome with ADHD

More research has been published on PLM, restless legs syndrome (RLS) and ADHD than on ADHD and SDB. However, many recent studies using polysomnography with hyperactive patients have failed to demonstrate a relationship with any sleep disorder[21]. Some authors, though, have concluded that this is because of a failure to consider disorders not commonly found in children[21]. Included in this category are PLMs and RLS. Often considered disorders of middle age[41], these syndromes have not been closely studied in children, but have been found to occur in higher rates among children with ADHD when compared to normal controls[21–23]. In addition, children with ADHD have shown improvement in symptoms following dopaminergic treatment for RLS[21].

Several studies have used rating scales for both PLMs and symptoms associated with ADHD to determine the co-morbidity of the disorders. Chervin and co-workers[21] asked parents to complete a Pediatric Sleep Questionnaire (PSQ) for the assessment of PLMs (a six-item subscale), restless legs, growing pains, and several potential confounds between behavior and PLMs or RLS and two common behavioral measures, a DSM-IV-derived inattention/hyperactivity scale (IHS) and the Hyperactivity Index (HI, expressed as a t score) of Conner's Parent Rating Scales. Results from these questionnaires indicated that restless legs were reported in 17% of the subjects by their parents. In addition, a large portion (13%) of the sample were found to have positive HI T scores (> 60, 1 SD above the mean), and of these, 18% had restless legs compared with 11% without elevated HI scores (χ^2 $p < 0.05$).

In the HI T scores > 60 portion, higher (1 standard deviation) overall PLM and restless legs scores, as well as greater growing pains, were found when adjustments for age and gender were made. Results were similar for high IHS scores (> 1.25 standard deviation). The associations between each behavioral measure and the PLM score remained significant after statistical adjustment was made for sleepiness, snoring, restless sleep in general or stimulant use. This latter finding suggests a robust relationship between the behavioral qualities of ADHD (as measured by IHS scores) and PLMs.

Correlational evidence of increased hyperactivity and inattentiveness in conjunction with PLMs and restless legs was acquired using questionnaires. It should be noted that adequate correlations have been found between the PSQ and laboratory-documented PLMs as well[23]. While this is not a causal relationship, the careful consideration of other explanations in this study suggests that some competing possibilities did not show the same relation as PLMs to behavioral symptoms of ADHD.

Retrospective analysis of polysomnography of children with PLMs has also been evaluated by Picchietti and Walters[22]. Of the 129 subjects reviewed, 117 (90.6%) had symptoms of ADHD. The breakdown of the sample included 65 subjects who had 5–10 PLMs per hour, 48 who had 10–25 PLMs per hour and 16 who had > 25 PLMs per hour. Stimulant medication did not seem to play a role in the PLMs according to the authors[22]. Despite the high rates of co-morbidity in this study, causal relationships have not been addressed. In addition, in this retrospective study, withdrawal from stimulant medication and dose-dependent relationships may have produced a misleading picture.

One theory regarding the high rates of RLS and ADHD is that the disorders share a common mechanism. Both have been associated with lower levels of dopamine in the brain, which is associated with faulty motor control, a common problem in both disorders.

Sleep–wake cycles, sleep architecture and ADHD

Problems with the onset and maintenance of sleep have been recognized to occur more often in ADHD[24]. However, onset and maintenance insomnia in children with ADHD has been reported through clinical observations of co-morbidity rather than through scientific rigor[12].

Corkum and colleagues[12] examined medicated and unmedicated children with ADHD, and compared them to clinical and non-clinical control groups for common sleep-related problems. Their findings indicated that involuntary behavior (talking in one's sleep, teeth grinding, restless sleep and jerky movements during sleep) was commonly found in ADHD groups, but not in the controls. However, children with separation anxiety disorder did show similar problems in these areas, suggesting a correlation as opposed to a causal relationship. Corkum and colleagues further suggested that parent reports of children do not always correlate with actigraphs or other findings[12]. These results could indicate that the findings may be related to co-morbid conditions or medications in some cases.

In a study by Trommer and co-workers, parents of ADHD children reported more sleep problems in their offspring, including difficulties in failing asleep (56% versus 23%) and tiredness upon waking (55% versus 27%), than did parents of 30 normal children[23]. Two questionnaire-based studies by Kaplan and associates showed that parents of hyperactive preschool children reported more difficulties with their child's sleep than parents of normally developing children[24]. These results were confirmed in a third study by Ball and Koloian[25], in which sleep diaries identified approximately 25% of children in their ADHD group who had more night wakenings, and shorter daytime naps, but no difference in total sleep time or sleep onset latency when compared to normal control children. Consideration of these findings does suggest avenues for intervention in families of children with some types of sleep disturbance; however, studies have revealed a disparity between parent rating scales and overnight polysomnography findings. This could mean an inaccurate prevalence rate if parent rating scales are used alone.

Corkum considered the cumulative results of the literature on sleep disturbances utilizing objective measures of sleep. Results were often inconsistent. In eight of the studies that assessed sleep onset latency, 33% were found to be longer, 22% shorter and 45% the same[14]. Sleep efficiency was significantly less for the ADHD group in 43% of the studies reviewed (three out of seven) and the remaining 57% did not differ. Sixty-seven per cent of the studies (four out of six) found that the ADHD group displayed more movements during sleep. The number of studies finding differences between the ADHD group and the normal control group in REM and non rapid eye movement (NREM) sleep was the same as those that did not find differences (REM and NREM: 55% and 50% found differences, respectively)[14]. Overall, these results support the claim of Gruber and colleagues that inconsistency is the hallmark of sleep in children with ADHD[15].

There has been some evidence of an increased sleep pressure in children with ADHD as compared to normal controls. Sheldon and colleagues found decreased sleep onset time in children aged 6 to 12 using Multiple Sleep Latency Tests (MSLTs), with the fifth of five naps significantly shorter and an overall trend toward abbreviated sleep onset when compared to normative data for that age group[26]. While the sample was small ($n = 8$), the results also indicated increased frequency of microsleep episodes in naps where sleep onset was prolonged or did not occur. The authors further state that the use of stimulant medications in this population may be contributing to a reduction in this sleep pressure and could be one mechanism of action in the successful treatment of children with ADHD.

DIAGNOSIS AND TREATMENT

The body of research on ADHD and sleep disorders suggests problems in the etiology of symptoms consistent with the disorder. Findings suggest that SDB and PLMs could be seen as both causes and exacerbating factors.

The high rates of SDB in mild, but not in severe, ADHD suggest that there are some children for whom treatment of the SDB may result in reduced symptoms of ADHD and elimination/reduction of the need for stimulant medications. In addition, the frequent, but until recently ignored, co-morbidity of ADHD and PLMs[27] may offer compelling insights into the similarity of the mechanisms of action between the two.

While the presence of sleep disturbances may cloud the diagnostic certainty for practicing clinicians, some changes to the diagnostic procedure are obvious. First, rating scales of ADHD are insufficient to make the diagnosis. Clinicians should carefully rule out all other psychological and psychosocial explanations.

Second, a complete sleep history, including sleep questionnaires, should be completed by parents. Third, when SDB, PLMs or disruptions in sleep–wake cycles are evident, a sleep study should be considered.

Treatment of the sleep condition has been shown in some adult and pediatric studies to reduce the symptomatology of ADHD[19,20]. This could lead to reduced need for medication or more effective control at lower doses. The frequently occurring, but often inconsistent, presence of changes in sleep duration, onset, maintenance and quality indicate that treatment must focus on extrinsic (healthy sleep hygiene) and intrinsic (breathing, limb movements, stimulant medication) factors.

References

1. Barkley RA. *Attention Deficit Hyperactivity Disorder: A Handbook for Diagnosis and Treatment*, 2nd edn. New York: Guilford Press, 1998
2. American Psychiatric Association. *Diagnostic and Statistic Manual of Mental Disorders*, 4th edn. Washington DC: American Psychiatric Press, 2002
3. Barkley RA. Disruptive behavior disorders; attention deficit disorder. Presentation, Chicago, IL, May 2001
4. Fischer M. Persistence of ADHD into adulthood: It depends on who you ask. *ADHD Report* 1997;5:8–10
5. Spreen O, Risser AH, Edgell D. *Developmental Neuropsychology*. London: Oxford Press, 1995
6. Szatmari P, Offord DR, Boyle MH. Ontario Child Health Study: prevalence of attention deficit disorder with hyperactivity. *J Child Psychol Psychiatry* 1989;30:21–230
7. Biederman J, Wozniak J, Kiely K, *et al.* Comorbidity of attention deficit hyperactivity disorder with conduct, depressive, anxiety, and other disorders. *Am J Psychiatry* 1991;148:564–77
8. Anderson JC, Williams S, McGee R, *et al.* DSM-III disorders in preadolescent children. *Arch Gen Psychiatry* 1987;44:69–76
9. Bierdman J. Returns of comorbidity in girls with ADHD. Presented at the annual meeting of the *American Academy of Child and Adolescent Psychiatry*, Toronto, 1997
10. Szatmari P, Boyle M, Offord DR. ADHD and conduct disorder: degree of diagnostic overlap and differences among correlates. *J Am Acad Child Adolesc Psychiatry* 1989;28:865–72
11. MTA Cooperative Group. A 14-month randomized clinical trial of treatment strategies for attention deficit hyperactivity disorder (ADHD). *Arch Gen Psychiatry* 1999;56:1073–86
12. Corkum P, Tannock R, Moldofsky H. Sleep disturbances in children with attention deficit/hyperactivity disorder. *J Am Acad Child Adolesc Psychiatry* 1998;37:637–46
13. Marcotte AC, Thacher PV, Butters M, *et al.* Parental report of sleep problems in children with attentional and learning disorders. *Dev Behav Pediatr* 1998;19:178–86
14. Corkum P. Sleep problems in attention deficit hyperactivity disorder. In Stores G, Wiggs L, eds. *Sleep Disturbance in Children and Adolescents with Disorders of Development: its Significance and Management*. London: Cambridge University Press, 2001:174–80
15. Gruber R, Sadeh A, Raviv A. Instability of sleep patterns in children with attention deficit/hyperactivity disorder. *J Am Acad Child Adolesc Psychiatry* 2000;39:495–501
16. Chervin RD, Archibold KH. Hyperactivity and polysomnographic findings in children evaluated for sleep-disordered breathing. *Sleep* 2001;24:313–20
17. Chervin RD, Dillon JE, Bassetti C, *et al.* Symptoms of sleep disorders, inattention and hyperactivity in children. *Sleep* 1997;20:1185–92

18. O'Brien LM, Holbrook CR, Mervis CB, *et al*. Sleep and neurobehavioral characteristics of 5- to 7-year-old children with parentally reported symptoms of attention-deficit/ hyperactivity disorder. *Pediatrics* 2003;111: 554–63

19. Naseem S, Chaudhary B, Collop N. Attention deficit hyperactivity disorder in adults and obstructive sleep apnea. *Chest* 2001;119:294–6

20. Ali NJ, Pitson D, Stradling JR. Sleep disordered breathing: effects of adenotonsillectomy on behaviour and psychological functioning. *Eur J Pediatr* 1996;155:56–62

21. Chervin RD, Archibold KH, Dillon JE, *et al*. Associations between symptoms of inattention, hyperactivity, restless legs, and periodic leg movements. *Sleep* 2002;25:213–18

22. Picchietti DL, Walters AS. Moderate to severe periodic limb movement disorder in childhood and adolescence. *Sleep* 1999;22:297–300

23. Trommer BL, Hoeppner JB, Rosenberg RS, *et al*. Sleep distrurbance in children with attention deficit disorder. *Ann Neurol* 1988; 24:325

24. Kaplan BJ, McNicol J, Conte RA, *et al*. Sleep disturbance in preschool-aged hyperactive and nonhyperactive children. *Pediatrics* 1987;80: 839–44

25. Ball JD, Koloian B. Sleep patterns among ADHD children. *Clin Psychol Rev* 1995;15: 681–91

26. Sheldon S, Irby J, Applebaum A, *et al*. Sleep pressure in children with attentional deficits. *Sleep Res* 1991;20A:448

27. Golan N, Shauer E, Ravid S, Pillar G. Sleep disorders in children with attention-deficit/ hyperactive disorders. *Sleep* 2004;27:261–6

18

Pervasive developmental disorders and sleep

Victor Kagan, Peter Dodzik and Alexander Z. Golbin

INTRODUCTION

In 1943, Leo Kanner published the first description of autism in 11 children seen at Johns Hopkins Hospital in Baltimore, MD[1]. One year later, a fellow Austrian pediatrician, Hans Asperger, described a group of children who were qualitatively similar but had higher intellectual functioning in a paper entitled 'Autistic Psychopathy in Children'. The difference between Kanner's and Asperger's syndromes has been the source of long and considerable debate[2]. Kanner's autism and Asperger's syndrome, as well as other non-specific, severe and perverse impairments of development, are called 'pervasive developmental disorders', classified under 'communication disorder not otherwise specified'[3].

Pervasive developmental disorders (PDDs) include a wide spectrum of conditions with overlapping symptomatology, multifactorial etiology and complicated pathophysiology. Autism, Asperger's syndrome, Rett's disorder and other autism-like syndromes are neurological disorders with profound effects on language, social development and sensory and emotional regulation that cause impairment in communication, learning, social interaction, empathy, mood and play. In addition to such deficits, the autistic syndromes involve pathologically high levels of repetitive, stereotypic, ritualistic, compulsive or obsessive behaviors together with extreme resistance to cange. Various internal biological factors, as well as deviated sensitivity to socioenvironmental influences, cause a wide range of sleep and circadian rhythm disorders[4–8].

CLASSIFICATION

PDDs are a heterogeneous group. Recently, an etiology-based classification system of PDDs, comparable to that applied to epilepsy, was suggested. Using this classification system, it was possible to reveal a difference in gender preponderance in PDDs as well as diagnostic features[9]. Gabis assigned children with PDDs into three groups – symptomatic, cryptogenic and idiopathic. Children in the symptomatic group were defined as having a clear etiology of the syndrome, along with a chromosomal abnormality or brain damage in which the deficits in language, social interaction and repetitive behavior occurred secondarily to the neurological damage. Those in the cryptogenic group had a suspected underlying neurological etiology, such as abnormal perinatal development, dysmorphic features or other associated findings. The idiopathic group consisted of children who met the criteria for autism and for whom no other neurological disorder was suspected except co-morbid

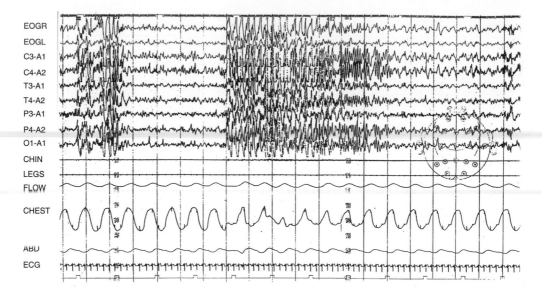

Figure 18.1 Polysomnogram of 13-year-old autistic boy with midnight agitations and abnormal electroencephalogram in non-rapid eye movement sleep

phenomena (e.g. attention deficit hyperactivity disorder or Tourette's syndrome). Figure 18.1 represents a case of idiopathic autism for which EEG revealed nocturnal seizure activity in the absence of any clear neurological insult.

When compared to the idiopathic group, the symptomatic group differed in terms of female predominance and symptomatology, including delay in language and motor milestones, but regression of development was absent. Less frequently, siblings had PDD and autistic features were less severe. Using this classification, Gabis[9] was able to establish that in the symptomatic group, 67% of cases were the result of high-risk pregnancies, while only 26% of children in the idiopathic group were from pregnancies deemed as high risk.

She also found that children who have an underlying neurological syndrome present with less severe PDD. In the symptomatic group 89% of cases were diagnosed with PDD not otherwise specified and none were diagnosed with Asperger's syndrome, while in the idiopathic group autism and Asperger's syndrome were equally represented. Unless etiological findings become more specific, nosological analysis seems to be more acceptable for the majority of researchers because

of the belief that PDDs consist of separate clinical and probably neuroanatomical and pathophysiological entities[8]. Many factors were identified that might cause autism and related disorders, including perinatal problems, vaccination, (see Figure 18.2) malnutrition, genetic, physical and emotional factors, trauma, etc. Figure 18.2 shows a case of suspected vaccination-induced encephalopathy resulting in autistic symptoms.

The prevalence and significance of sleep disorders in children with developmental disabilities such as mental retardation, autism and Asperger's syndrome have also become a focus for researchers and clinicians. General rates of significant sleep disturbances have been estimated at 44.4–89% for people with developmental disabilities[11,12]. Unfortunately, the majority of previous research has focused on undifferentiated participant groups and was conducted without polysomnographic studies that could specify various types of sleep abnormalities.

Dyssomnia seems to be the most frequent among reported problems. Nocturnal arousals, with or without tantrums, were the most commonly cited sleep difficulty within these undifferentiated groups[4–8].

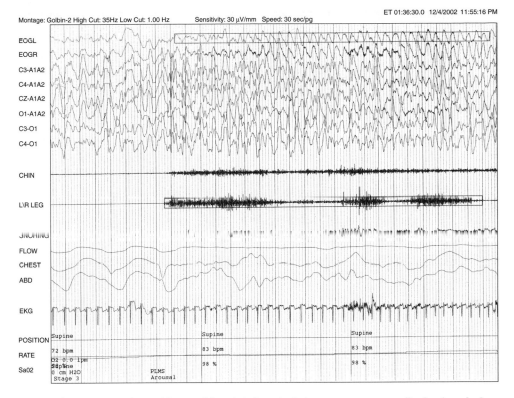

Figure 18.2   Polysomnogram in an 11-year-old autistic boy. Autistic symptoms reportedly developed after measles vaccination. Delta wave hypersynchronization in non-rapid eye movement sleep

Attempts to differentiate and specify connections between types of developmental disability and sleep disorders started with Down's syndrome and, later, with autism.

AUTISM AND RELATED DISORDERS

The most frequently reported sleep disorders within the Down's syndrome population include sleep apnea, night awakenings, increased total sleep time and abnormal sleep architecture[12–14].

Kagan[10] compared clinical observations in children (60 boys and 18 girls diagnosed with childhood schizophrenia; 45 boys and 12 girls with Kanner's syndrome; and 27 boys and nine girls with so-called 'organic' or secondary autism). It is interesting to note that complications in pregnancy and delivery were reported in 91.9% of children with Kanner's syndrome. This was higher than in the group with schizophrenia

(52.7%), and in the group of children where autistic features appeared after an exogenous disease (63.9%) (i.e. organic or secondary autism). Children with Kanner's syndrome were overwhelmingly from the mother's first pregnancy (94.6%); in contrast, only 37.7% of children with childhood schizophrenia were from the first pregnancy. Kagan's hypothesis was that during the first pregnancy some mother–fetus incompatibility may have led to neurodevelopmental complications. This goes along with other signs of neuroanatomical and neurophysiological abnormalities, such as low muscle tone, facial asymmetries, strabismus, dysphasia, motor clumsiness, confused time–space orientation and intolerance of eye contact in the majority of cases. These described symptoms may be related to interhemispheric pathology. There are also data that under-activation of the right hemisphere leads to poor recognition of emotional meanings and speeds up gnosis–praxis'[16,17]. On the other hand, there is a

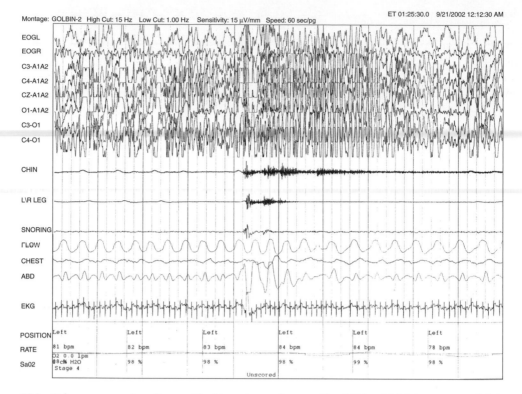

Figure 18.3 Polysomnogram in a 6-year-old with autism and savant-like abilities. Multiple paroxysmal dalta waves observed during trance-like activity

subgroup of high-functioning and creative individuals (savants) among autistic children and adolescents (Figure 18.3).

Unusual neurophysiological circuits might explain paradoxical arousals of children when they are tired (hyperactivity type), agitation when given tranquilizers and paradoxical improvement upon discontinuation of some medications. Electroencephalogram (EEG) evaluation[17] shows that autistic patients have a precocious alpha rhythm, especially in the right hemisphere. Its high amplitude and low reaction was demonstrated on functional tests (i.e. hyperventilation and photo-stimulation).

The daily behavior of autistic children may be close to trance-like states of mind. Taking into account the just partially transparent wall between a child and its environment, as well as the trance-inducing effect of stereotypical activities, this hypothesis seems quite feasible. Kagan's work[10] with high-functioning autistic teenagers indicates that they can be very responsive to trance induction and the use of strategies to employ covert suggestion. Low-functioning, younger children can imitate adults to produce trance-like behavior.

Schreck and Mulick[11] evaluated sleep–wake patterns in four groups of children with autism, mental retardation, those attending special education classes (with no diagnosis of mental retardation) and a normal control group of children of a similar age using parental reports, classroom observation and rating scales. Many authors did not confirm the hypothesis that children with mental retardation sleep more hours per day and per night than other children[18–24]. In contrast, this research demonstrated that total sleep duration in a general population of mentally retarded children is no different from other groups. The authors explained the discrepancy by the restricted age range in their study. Although no difference was found in the quantity of sleep, distinct differences between groups appeared in the quality of sleep and sleep behaviors. Age was also found to have no significant influence in the 5–13-year-old age range.

Parents of children with autism reported sleeping problems in their children significantly more often than parents of any other group[15]. Rating scales and reports did not reveal any specific differences among groups regarding sleep behavior. Although more dyssomnias and severe parasomnias were associated with autism, they included agitated awakenings, disturbing parents and siblings, nightmares and night terrors with screaming, sleepwalking and acting out of dreams. Parents of autistic children, and those with other PDDS, reported more frequent episodes of bruxism and of breathing cessation episodes than those in the special education and control groups[15].

Taira and co-workers[19] found significant sleep disorders, such as parasomnias, in 56 out of 88 Japanese children with autism. Interestingly, 44 of them started to have sleep problems before the age of 3 years. The most common problems were bedwetting, awakenings and motor behaviors. Frequent and intense motor behaviors disrupted parental sleep more frequently and for a longer time (to calm the child down) in a group of autistic children than in mentally retarded or control groups. They also included children sleeping outside their own bedroom, intense fear of noises and bedwetting. Their findings are consistent with autistic children's tendencies to become agitated with seemingly benign changes in their environment[15,24]. Sometimes parents are awakened by the screaming child and try to console the child, assuming that it is awake, even when the child is actually asleep, thus awakening the child. Another interesting difference between children with autism and those with unspecified mental retardation is a type of arousal from sleep. Parents of children with autism reported more disoriented nocturnal awakenings, sluggishness and confusion, than did parents of children with mental retardation[10]. Parents of children with autism reported more difficulties during pre-sleep time and more frequent need for medications to facilitate sleep.

ASPERGER'S DISORDER

Asperger's syndrome is a PDD whose links with high-functioning autism are still in debate. The Diagnostic and Statistical Manual of Mental Disorders (DSM)-IV diagnostic criteria of Asperger's syndrome include altered social interactions, restricted interests, repetitive and stereotyped behaviors as in autism but, contrary to autism, the patient with Asperger's syndrome does not show any significant language abnormalities and, more specifically, any delay in the development of language, psychomotor or cognitive skills[3].

There are very few reports on the neuro anatomical or neurochemical basis of Asperger's syndrome. Thus, researchers and clinicians have to rely on anatomical and brain imaging studies in autism to provide several structural markers for the syndrome, including temporal–occipital systems, frontal lobes, hippocampus and cerebellum. Godbout and co-workers[20] reviewed neurochemical and pharmacological data. The study revealed higher plasma 5-hydroxytryptamine (5-HT) levels (hyperserotoninemia) in more than 50% of children with autism. But this is true only for the high-functioning autistic children (IQ $\geq$ 85). The presence of antibodies directed against 5-HT receptors was also identified in the plasma of high-functioning autistics (possible Asperger's syndrome). These results show that 5-HT neurotransmission is affected in high-functioning autism, a finding that is also true for individuals with Asperger's syndrome. However, Asperger's syndrome and autism are independent clinical entities, so their physiological behavior and cognitive changes should be differentiated[20].

Kanner did not originally believe that autism and schizophrenia were related, but subsequent investigators viewed infantile autism as the earliest manifestation of schizophrenia. Most researchers currently agree with Kanner that autism and schizophrenia are separate entities[21].

A polysomnographic study of sleep in Asperger's syndrome was performed by Godbout and co-workers[20]. Eight patients

(7–53-year-olds) fitting diagnostic criteria for Asperger's syndrome and eight matched control subjects participated in two consecutive polysomnographic studies. Results showed that, as a group, patients with Asperger's syndrome had less sleep in the first two-thirds of the night than the controls and made more entries into rapid eye movement (REM) from a waking state, while the control group had more entries into REM from stage 2 non-rapid eye movement (NREM) sleep. Asperger's syndrome patients had a lower density of spindles in the first and the last third of the night. K complexes in stage 2 sleep were also increased in Asperger's syndrome. Another interesting and important finding was significant increases in the periodic limb movement (PLM) index (12.3 ± 7.1), while the control group did not have such increases. Sleep apnea syndrome was absent in all participants. It is interesting that in one study REM behavior disorder (RBD) was found in about 50% of autistic children. Thus, patients with Asperger's syndrome had difficulties initiating and maintaining sleep, a low incidence of spindles, a high periodic limb movement (PLM) index in non-REM sleep and abnormalities of REM sleep (REM intrusions and dissociations of REM).

Sleep spindles are thought to represent a sleep protective mechanism by deactivation of the thalamocortical loops[23]. Recent studies have suggested that EEG spindle density significantly correlates with selective attention in young healthy persons (see Chapter 2). Thus, decreased spindle density reflects abnormality in the capacity of the thalamocortical loop to contribute to the filtering of inputs, including the perceptual type.

The REM sleep abnormalities may also be related to daytime cognitive difficulties in Asperger's syndrome. In terms of motor activity in REM sleep, data are still very inconsistent: in one study it was normal[20], in another increased[8] and in a third decreased[25]. Increased PLM activity might reflect abnormalities in dopaminergic systems. Elia and associates[8] performed sleep evaluations using polysomnography in 17 male children and adolescents with autistic disorder, in seven patients with mental retardation and fragile X syndrome, and in five age- and gender-matched normal male subjects. They found that the density of REMs was not significantly different in these three groups of subjects. However, some sleep parameters such as time in bed, sleep period time and total sleep time were significantly lower in those with autistic disorder than in normal controls. In contrast, only minor differences were observed between patients with autistic disorder and those with fragile X syndrome with mental retardation. Interestingly, in their study, some neuropsychological measures, such as perception and eye–hand co-ordination, showed a significant correlation with some sleep parameters such as time in bed, sleep latency, stage shifts, first REM latency and wakefulness after sleep onset. Childhood Autism Rating Scale (CARS) scores, such as unusual responses and non-verbal communication, positively correlated with tonic sleep parameters such as sleep period time, wakefulness after sleep onset and total sleep time. Items measuring relations with people and activity level were found to be significantly correlated with REM density. These results showed that sleep changes in autistic children are different from those in subjects with mental retardation and in normal controls.

Sleep studies of mentally retarded subjects[12–15,27–37] found a reduction in the percentage of REM stage and a prolonged latency of the first REM period. Based on the fact that in animals, percentage of REM sleep increases after intensive learning sessions[31], it was hypothesized that the REM stage is involved in the cognitive process and REM sleep itself could be an index of brain plasticity, i.e. the ability of the brain to retain information. This sleep–cognition hypothesis[32] postulates that cognitive defects might be associated with alterations in sleep mechanisms and structure. Mentally retarded patients show a significant reduction in REMs occurring in shorter intervals (< 1 s), as opposed to those separated by longer time intervals (> 23 s).

In normal subjects, high-frequency REMs show marked increases with age and after training[33] and thus are considered an index of the brain's organizational abilities, i.e. the ability to organize information from a random pool of elements into a long-term memory. Pharmacological agents that modify sleep might ameliorate sleep-related psychobiological function[34].

There is no agreement about EEG pathology. Careful EEG studies by a Japanese group from Nakuto University found epileptic discharges in 43% of autistic children in sleep. One-third of these cases had localized spikes, predominantly in mid-frontal areas[35].

DIAGNOSTIC CONSIDERATIONS

EEG and polysomnography evaluations of children with autistic spectrum disorders are very challenging and often require sedation for the child to undergo the study. The Children's National Medical Center in Washington, DC monitored 894 cases over 3.5 years. Three hundred and thirty-eight (37%) were identified as having autistic spectrum disorder and EEG studies were ordered to rule out Landau–Kleffner syndrome, a seizure disorder associated with language problems. Twenty-five per cent of autistic children with acquired aphasia had abnormal EEGs, with 19% (63) exhibiting some form of epileptic activity. Overnight EEG studies confirmed the seizure activity in 56 of these 63 patients, but none of these tracings revealed electrographic status epilepticus during slow-wave sleep, regarded as a diagnostic criterion for Landau–Kleffner syndrome[36]. In a study of polysomnographic phenotypes in different developmental disabilities Harvey and Kennedy[37] tried to identify differences in sleep structure among people with autism, Down's syndrome and fragile X syndrome. According to them, there was an inverse relationship between the severity of mental retardation and the amount of REM time. The presence of autism or Down's syndrome was associated with fewer and briefer bouts of REM sleep and total sleep time. Autism was also associated, in their study, with greater levels of undifferentiated sleep. These findings for autism contrasted with fragile X syndrome, whose sleep architecture

appears to be a function of the degree of mental retardation[38].

In an excellent review, Abril Villalba and co-workers[7] classified disorders of sleep in infantile autism into three types:

(1) Immaturity of sleep, showing destructured polysomnography tracings and a negative correlation with the level of development;

(2) Functional alteration of sleep with early waking and difficulty in going to bed;

(3) Paroxysmal and epileptic form of discharges without motor seizures (not related to Landau–Kleffner syndrome).

Studies of REM sleep in normal and autistic children by Tonguay and co-workers[25] favored the immaturity hypothesis in autism. Discrete REM outbursts in autistic children were similar to those in normal children of much younger age.

In another study by the same group of authors as above[39], 21 autistic subjects between the ages of 4 and 12 without epileptic seizures were assessed; they still found epileptic paroxysmal activity in 66% of cases, all of which appeared in the anterior half of the brain.

Sleep disturbances in children with autism in Kagan's study[10] were represented by disturbances of (1) falling asleep and awakening (67.5%); (2) depth of sleep (35.1%); and (3) deviation of a sleep structure (32.4%)[10]. Very often, parents were concerned with mild night awakening; however, children usually wake up soon after midnight and stay up for a few hours or wake up at about 4–5 a.m. active or even agitated. He observed an interesting phenomenon: medication could normalize a night's sleep, but in this case, behavior during the day became more difficult; and discontinuing of medication improved daytime behavior. Therefore, it is conceivable that spontaneous awakenings compensate for sleep deprivation in the treatment of depression. In other words, some deviations from physiological and statistical norms can be directed to optimize body

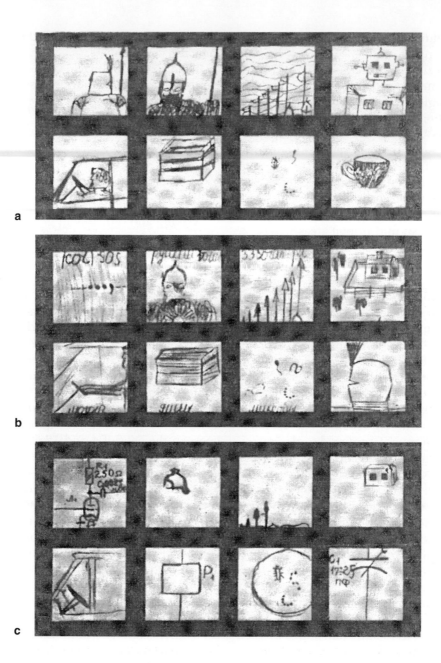

Figure 18.4 Wartegg's test of a 9-year-old autistic boy

function and prevent more severe disturbances. Therefore, sleep disturbances as target symptoms need to be chosen very carefully. A preferable approach is associated with normalizing the sleep–wake pattern as a whole.

Neurological and polysomnographic evaluations of children with PDD might be useful. We also found that children with paroxysmal activity on EEG evaluation are prone to have seizure-like movements in their sleep and during the daytime as well when they are fatigued.

It is also important to mention that periodic limb movement disorders and Giles de la Tourette's syndrome are frequent co-morbidities to autism but not schizophrenia[20]. According to Elia and co-workers[8], polysomnography studies in PDDs might be extremely useful in the differentiation of underlying conditions. They found that sleep structure in autistic children is different from the structure in those with mental retardation.

Actigraphic studies of sleep in autistic children provided a similar level of information to questionnaires alone, and confirmed multiple midnight awakenings and early arousal in the morning[40].

Endocrinological studies, including circadian melatonin, thyroid-stimulating hormone (TSH), prolactin and cortisol, confirmed abnormal circadian patterns in young adults with autism, and correlated with EEG abnormalities[41]. A parallel was evidenced between polysomnography[42] circadian function and impairment in verbal communication. Thus, there appear to be disturbances in various types of neuroendocrinological and circadian abnormalities in autistics. Melatonin, as well as possibly TSH and perhaps prolactin and cortisol, could serve as biochemical markers of the pathophysiology of autistic spectrum disorders[41,42].

TREATMENT OF SLEEP PROBLEMS IN PERVASIVE DEVELOPMENTAL DISORDERS

The successful treatment of sleep problems in autistic children is challenging but possible. Weislap and co-workers[43] reported such success in treating a 5-year-old autistic boy with problems in night settling, nocturnal awakenings and co-sleeping using behavioral principles during three weekly parent training sessions. The parents learned how to use a bedtime routine, reinforcement, effective instructions, partner support strategies and extinction techniques. Once the techniques were implemented, the child learned how to settle himself to bed and how to sleep alone for the entire night. Reportedly, this improvement was maintained at 3- and 12-month follow-ups. Recently, Facilitated Communication Technique has shown promising results. Unfortunately, few cases have such happy endings. Many issues in the treatment and prevention of sleep disorders are still controversial.

Up to now, there is no specific etiological treatment available to cure autism or other PDDs. Pharmacotherapy targets symptom relief. Though psychotropics play a major role in the management of some symptoms, their use needs close monitoring. About half of the subjects with high-functioning autism are currently reported to be on psychotropics (antidepressants, stimulants and anxiolytics), with many of them being on concurrent antipsychotic medication[44]. Despite this high level of psychotropic use, few studies exist investigating specifics of pharmacodynamics or side-effect profiles in this population. Physician–parent communication is essential in managing PDDs. Pharmacotherapy should be used in conjunction with behavioral management techniques. Some symptoms of autism and other PDDs may be responsive to medication (hyperactivity, obsessions, rituals, tics, self-destructive behavior, rocking, etc.), while others may be responsive to behavioral modification but benefit from adjunctive use of medications (anxiety, depression, impulsivity, aggression, some sleep difficulties). Specific skill deficits are usually non-responsive to medication (deficit in academic, sport or social fields). Among medications, the new atypical antipsychotics and selective serotonin reuptake inhibitors are increasingly used in autism with very encouraging results, but a risk–benefit ratio in terms of side-effects is important to consider in each case[45]. Clomipramine, a tricyclic antidepressant with potent serotonin reuptake blocking action, has been shown to be more effective than both placebo and desipramine, a primarily noradrenergic agent, in treating obsessions and compulsions, repetitive and ritualistically stereotyped behaviors in autistic children such as repeated touching and sniffing of objects, ritualistic ordering, checking and collecting, insisting on meaningless routines as well as head banging, hair pulling and nail biting. Amitriptyline was reported to significantly improve emotional contact and communication in young children with PDD[10]. Mildly to moderately positive and relatively equal results were obtained with risperidone, fluoxetine, paroxetine, amitriptyline, duloxetine[45], quetiapine[46] and naltrexone. The use of anticonvuls medication for treatment of behavior problems is very common practice. It is important to mention that any psychopharmacological agent should be used only as a relatively short-course option with drug-free periods; however, if long-term use is necessary it should be carefully monitored. It is also important to recognize that psychotropics can sometimes worsen behavior and can produce iatrogenic symptoms. Certain anti-epileptic medications and psychotropic drugs are metabolized by the same cytochrome P450 iso-enzymes in the liver. In such circumstances, the addition of a psychotropic agent may drastically alter the levels of the anti-epileptic medication and vice versa.

CONCLUSION

Pervasive developmental disorders (PDD) are disorders of the brain's anatomical and functional development. Sleep disorders in people affected by PDD are a reflection of the disorganization of the main biological rhythm of sleep and alertness, and, as such, are an intrinsic part of the pathophysiology of autistic syndromes. Disorganized behavior, cognition and affect are associated with disorganized sleep.

The severity of neurophysiological disorganization of circadian rhythms generally is associated with the severity of developmental retardation. The relationships between different forms of PDD and specific sleep disorders are not simple, but it appears that clinical and polysomnographic studies may help further to define the similarities in these relationships.

The extreme frequency of sleep disturbances in family members makes the topic of sleep disorders in developmental disability a major public health issue.

References

1. Kanner L. Autistic disturbances of affective contact. *Nervous Child* 1943;2:217–50
2. Fritz U, ed. *Autism and Asperger Syndrome*. New York: Cambridge University Press, 1991:247
3. *Diagnostic and Statistical Manual of Mental Disorders*, 4th edn. text revision Washington, DC: American Psychiatric Association, test revision 2000: 69–84
4. Ratzold LM, Richdale AL, Tonge BJ. An investigation into sleep characteristics of children with autism and Asperger's disorder. *J Paediatr Child Health* 1998;34:528–33
5. Ornitz EM. Development of sleep patterns in autistic children. In Clemente CD, Purpura DP, Mayer FE, eds. *Sleep and the Maturing Nervous System*. New York: Academic Press, 1972:364–83
6. Richdale AL, Prior MR. The sleep/wake rhythm in children with autism. *Eur Child Adolesc Psychiatry* 1995;4:175–86
7. Abril Villalba B, Mendez Garcia M, Sans Capdevila O, Valdizan Uson JR. Sleep in infantile autism. *Rev Neurol* 2001;32:641–4
8. Elia M, Ferri R, Musumeci SA, *et al*. Sleep in subjects with autistic disorder: a neurophysiological and psychological study. *Brain Dev* 2000;22:88–92

9. Gabis L. A causative classification of pervasive developmental disorders. *Neuropsychiatry Rev* 2002;12:15–16
10. Kagan V. *Autism in Children*. Leningrad: Medicina, 1981:144 (Russian)
11. Schreck VA, Mulick JA. Parental report of sleep problems in children with autism. *J Autism Dev Disord* 2000;30:127–35
12. Clausen J, Sersen EA, Lidsky A. Sleep patterns in mental retardation: Down's syndrome. *Electroenceph Clin Neurophysiol* 1977;43:183–91
13. Fukuma E, Umezawa Y, Kobayashi K, Motoike M. Polygraphic study on the nocturnal sleep of children with Down's syndrome and endogenous mental retardation. *Folia Psychiatrica Neurologica Japanica* 1974;28:333–45
14. Hamaguchi H, Hashimoto T, Mori K, Tayma M. Sleep in Down's syndrome. *Brain Dev* 1989;11:399–406
15. Petre-Quadens O, Jouvet M. Sleep in the mentally retarded. *J Neurol Sci* 1967;4:354–7
16. Nikolaenko N. Brain pictures: a study on the contribution of the cerebral hemispheres to creativity. Osaka: Katisai University Press, 1998:44–57

17. Kagan V. Functional hemispheric specialization and childhood autism: clinical–physiological aspects. In Mavlov L, ed. *Neuropsychology*. Sophia: Medicina, 1977:155–8

18. Ornitz EM, Ritvo ER, Walter RD. Dreaming sleep in autistic and schizophrenic children. *Am J Psychiatry* 1965;22:419–24

19. Taira M, Takase M, Sasaki H. Sleep disorders in autistic children. *Psychiatry Clin Neurosci* 1998;52:182–3

20. Godbout R, Bergeron C, Limoges E, Stip E, Mottron L. A laboratory study of sleep in Asperger's syndrome. *Neuroreport* 2000;11(1): 127–30

21. Volkmar FR, Cohen DJ. Comorbid association of autism and schizophrenia. *Am J Psychiatry* 1991;148:1705–7

22. Thirumalal SS, Shubin RA, Robinson R. Rapid eye movement disorder in children with autism. *J Child Neurol* 2002;17:173–8

23. Sterade M. Brain electrical activity and sensory processing during waking and sleep states. In Kryger MH, Roth T, Dement WC, eds. *Principles and Practice of Sleep Medicine*, 3rd edn. Philadelphia: WB Saunders, 2000:93–111

24. Musumeci SA, Ferri R, Elia M, *et al*. Sleep neurophysiology in Fragile X patients. *Dev Brain Dysfunct* 1995;8:218–22

25. Tanguay PE, Ornitz EM, Forsythe AB, Ritvo ER. Rapid eye movement (REM) activity in normal and autistic children during REM sleep. *J Autism Child Schizophr* 1976;6:278–88

26. Sun Y, Ming SY, Walters AS. Polysomnographic analysis of sleep disrupted autism patients. *Sleep* 2003;26:A112(abstract)

27. Petre-Quadens O, Jouvet M. Paradoxical sleep in mental retardation. *J Neurol Sci* 1966;3: 608–12

28. Castaldo V, Krynicki V. Sleep patterns and intelligence in functional mental retardation. *J Ment Defic Res* 1973;17:131–5

29. Castaldo V, Krynicki V. Sleep and eye movement patterns in two groups of retardates. *Biol Psychiatry* 1974;9:231–44

30. Grubar JC. Sleep and mental deficiency. *Rev Electroenceph Neurophysiol Clin* 1983;13: 107–14

31. McGrath MJ, Cohen DB. REM sleep facilitation of adaptive waking behavior: a review of the literature. *Psychol Bull* 1978;85:24–57

32. Johnson CR. Sleep problems in children with mental retardation and autism. *Child Adolesc Psychiatr Clin North Am* 1966;5:673–83

33. Petre-Quadens O. Physiologic de sommeil et environment. *Totus Homo* 1980;12:14–22

34. Gigli GL, Grubar JC, Bergonzi P, Maschin MC. Long-term administration of butoctamide succinate on nocturnal sleep of mentally retarded subjects: a polygraphic study versus placebo. *Psychopharmacology* 1995;117:438–42

35. Hashimoto T, Sasaki M, Sugai K, Hanaoka S, Fukumizu M, Kato T. Paroxysmal discharges on EEG in young autistic patients are frequent in frontal regions. *J Med Invest* 2001;48:175–80

36. Pearl P. Routine overnight EEG monitoring not warranted in autistic children. *Am Acad Neurol NewsWise* 2002;4(17):02

37. Harvey M, Kennedy C. Polysomnographic phenotypes in developmental disabilities. *Int J Dev Neurosci* 2002;3–5:443

38. Feinberg I, Braun M, Shulman E. EEG patterns in mental retardation. *Electroenceph Clin Neurophysiol* 1969;27:128–44

39. Valdizan Uson JR, Abril Villalba B, Mendez Garcia M, Sans Capdevila O. Nocturnal polysomnogram in childhood autism without epilepsy. *Rev Neurol* 2002;34:1002 (Spanish).

40. Hering E, Epstein R, Elroy S, Iancu DR, Zelnik M. Sleep pattern in autistic children. *J Autism Dev Disord* 1999;29:143–7

41. Nir I, Meir D, Zilber N, Knobler H, Hadjez J, Lerner Y. Brief report: melatonin, thyroid-stimulating hormone prolactin, and cortisol levels in serum of young adults with autism. *J Autism Dev Disord* 1995;25:641–54

42. Chevvette T, Rolland M, Masse A, *et al*. Sleep wake cycle disorders in autism with mental retardation: effect of melatonin. *Sleep* 2003;26 (abstract 0275E)

43. Weiskop S, Matthewss J, Richdale A. Treatment of sleep problems in a 5 year-old boy with autism using behavioral principles.

44. Santosh PJ, Baird G. Pharmacotherapy of target symptoms in autistic spectrum disorders. *Indian J Pediatr* 2001;68:427–31

45. Wagner KD. Autistic disorder and atypical antipsychotics. *Psychiatric Times* 2002;10:52–4

46. Hardan AY. Quetiapine (Seroquel) in children and adolescents with developmental disorders. *Clin Psychiatr News* 2003;7:31

19

Sleep in seasonal affective disorder

Jianhua Shen, Leonid Kayumov and Colin M. Shapiro

INTRODUCTION

It is of particular interest to consider sleep in seasonal affective disorder (SAD) for several reasons. First, the high sensitivity and specificity of sleep architecture changes in depression make it one of the most important – if not the most important – biological markers in psychiatry. Second, if there is an exceptional pattern in one form of depression then an understanding of this condition will not only have merit in itself but also potentially add to the understanding in this field in general. Third, there is the opportunity to study the subjective and objective sleep congruence in this population.

Epidemiological and clinical population studies suggest that there are primarily two patterns of SAD: winter SAD and summer SAD[1]. Apart from the fact that summer SAD is more likely to have endogenous symptoms with insomnia, few studies regarding summer SAD sleep have been done. Therefore, this review is principally based on sleep in winter-depressive patients.

IS HYPERSOMNIA THE CENTRAL FEATURE OF SAD?

SAD patients whose depressed mood recurs regularly in the winter season often report hypersomnia[2,3], the number being over 80% in some studies[4,5].

We investigated 115 SAD patients with the Seasonal Patterns Assessment Questionnaire (SPAQ). Data were employed to estimate each participant's total sleep hours over a 24-h period across the four seasons. Individuals with SAD reported the most hours of sleep during winter (9.9 ± 2.28) and the fewest hours in summer (7.4 ± 1.22) with intermediate sleep duration in the fall (8.6 ± 1.76) and spring (8.4 ± 1.27)[6].

Complaints of hypersomnia in SAD appear to reflect a combination of earlier sleep onset, difficulty wakening, a low capacity to be awake at unusual times and a lower quality of night-time sleep[7].

However, although SAD patients reported increased sleep during the winter season, hypersomnolence may not be a specific feature of SAD. Studies[8] do document increased amounts of nocturnal sleep during fall and winter in SAD patients, but similar changes are also reported within the general population. The extent of winter/fall oversleeping recorded by SAD patients did not differ dramatically from that reported by the general population. In a 1994 study by Anderson and co-workers[5] covering 1571 individuals from the general population, winter sleep increases of 2 h a day relative to summer were reported by nearly half. Wirz-Justice and co-workers[9] have also reported seasonal variations in sleep length among healthy individuals. These subjects sleep less in May and June but longer in October and November.

In our study sleep time differed significantly as indicated by a one-factor (season) analysis of variance: when entered simultaneously into a multiple regression equation, the entire set of items of the SPAQ accounted for a significant proportion of variance in depressive symptoms. However, examination of the individual β weights for each of the SPAQ items indicated that only social activity levels were significantly related to depressive symptoms. Even when changes in sleep duration were included in the multiple regression analysis, neither this variable nor the other five SPAQ items were significantly related to the severity of depressive symptoms. Although the item concerning hypersomnia in the Hamilton Depression Rating Scale (HDRS) indicated a significant reduction from pre- (1.3 ± 1.23) to post-treatment (0.7 ± 0.93), this was not corroborated by sleep diary data collected just prior to and just after treatment. Total hours of daily sleep did not change significantly (pretreatment 7.5 ± 0.86 versus post-treatment 7.4 ± 0.68). Comparison of mean pretreatment daily hours of sleep did not differ significantly across individuals whose SPAQ responses ranged from 'none' to 'extremely marked' seasonal variation in sleep duration. Similar results were obtained when we examined post-treatment sleep diary information. Total diary sleep hours, as assessed by the sleep diary, were significantly shorter than self-report of sleep duration in the same season on the SPAQ. When SAD patients are asked to provide global retrospective descriptions summarizing sleep over an extended duration there is a pattern of response that concurs with the widely publicized description of SAD. However, the more detailed prospective sleep diary information failed to corroborate this pattern. Interrelations among the seven individual items constituting the SPAQ also failed to support the hypothesized centrality of sleep change in SAD. When all of the seven items were regressed on the HDRS, only the

item corresponding to social activity related significantly to the severity of depressive symptoms. This finding is consistent with extensive literature regarding the behavioral component of SAD. The failure to detect a relation of similar magnitude between depressive symptom severity and sleep behavior as reported on the SPAQ also challenges the assertion that hypersomnia is the central feature of SAD[6].

A number of studies have investigated sleep structure in depressed SAD patients[5,10-14]. In a winter SAD study[5] the polysomnographic (PSG) data were compared with those from the same individuals in summer and those after light therapy, and with age- and gender-matched healthy controls. In this study the sleep changes of SAD patients were decreased delta sleep and decreased sleep efficiency. The total sleep time of SAD patients was significantly longer in winter than in summer. In summer the sleep length of the SAD patients was shorter than that of the controls. As noted above, analysis revealed that the SAD patients demonstrated a significantly lower percentage of delta sleep in winter than in summer; however, among healthy controls there was no difference between winter and summer. Another study[14], though, revealed that SAD patients enjoyed better sleep than the controls, showing higher sleep efficiency, longer total sleep time, and more stage 2 sleep during the entire sleep episode. SAD patients also accumulated less wakefulness during the first 4 h of sleep, whereas rapid eye movement (REM) sleep and slow-wave sleep (SWS) parameters did not differ between the SAD patients and healthy controls. The PSG data collected by Brunner and co-workers[14] did not support the assumption of an involvement of sleep mechanisms in the pathogenesis of winter depression either. When measured on a daily basis, sleep duration of SAD patients in Switzerland does not differ significantly between summer and winter[15,16]. Thus, most PSG sleep data, as well as some data on prospective daily ratings of sleep duration, question the validity of hypersomnia as an intrinsic feature of SAD[14]. The multiple sleep latency test (MSLT) in patients with SAD has also failed to show evidence for increased sleep propensity during the day[17].

Taken together, there is no strong evidence that PSG measures of SAD patients differ from those of healthy controls. None of the sleep electroencephalogram (EEG) studies in SAD[10–13] has found the pattern of sleep EEG changes that characterizes endogenous melancholic depression.

TREATMENTS AND TOTAL SLEEP DEPRIVATION EFFECT ON SLEEP OF SAD PATIENTS

Increased sleep efficiency is the most frequently reported finding in SAD patients after light treatment (LT). Anderson and co-workers[5] found that sleep efficiency was significantly enhanced following a week of bright light treatment compared with the efficiency following room-light exposures. One LT study[18] reported on healthy subjects administered bright light in the afternoon when no phase shifts of circadian rhythms are expected, and concluded that LT could not further improve the good sleep of young subjects. These findings were interpreted as a normalization of decreased sleep efficiency in depressed SAD patients[14].

A curtailment of sleep, possibly related to activation and rebound activities, was documented by the sleep diaries in a group of SAD patients. They reported a reduction of their daily sleep duration by an average of 73 min during LT. In contrast, the controls reported an insignificant increase in their average daily sleep duration[14]. However, these findings differ from ours. Based on a sleep diary report, the sleep duration of our 115 SAD patients following LT was similar to what it had been pre-treatment[6]. The sleep diary recorded by the depressed SAD patients in Switzerland also indicated that their average winter sleep duration (6.9–7.4 h/day) was not significantly different from that following successful LT or found in the summer[9].

Increased SWS was found by Anderson and co-workers[5] using combined morning and evening LT, but not by Brunner and co-workers[14] using midday light. Using morning LT alone, an increase of SWS in the first 3 h of the night has been reported in one study[11], whereas in another no modifications of sleep stage parameters were found[12].

Regarding the effects of LT on power spectra, Brunner and co-workers[14] found that the absolute values of power density did not differ between SAD patients and controls in any frequency bin. The spectral changes were similar for both patient and control groups. In all cases, the recovery nights had increased EEG activity in the low delta band. A slight attenuation of EEG activity was present in the spindle frequencies. The decrease reached significance in the 12.25–14.0 Hz range for the SAD patients. As evaluated by paired comparisons, SAD patients had significantly increased EEG activity in the 0.75–6.0 Hz range for the baseline night whereas the changes in the recovery night did not reach significance in any frequency bin. SAD patients and controls differed significantly in their response to LT in the 1.75–4.0 Hz and 4.75–6.0 Hz bands.

It is clear that there are some variations among the reports regarding the effect of LT. This may be due to differences in the light exposure regimen, such as the duration and the total number of days.

There have been few studies focusing on the efficacy of antidepressant medications on PSG changes in SAD patients despite the fact that antidepressants are a standard treatment for major depression. Shen and co-workers[19] treated nine female winter-depressed patients with nefazodone. The average values of the patients on SPAQ, HRSD-SAD (a 29-item Hamilton Rating Scale for Depression of Seasonal Affective Disorder), Center for Epidemiologic Studies Depression Scale (a 20-item self-report questionnaire for the assessment of depression) and BDI (Beck Depression Inventory, a 21-item self-report questionnaire for depression) were 12.6, 31.1, 25.4 and 19.4, respectively. The total nefazodone treatment period was 8 weeks, and the daily dosages were 100 mg in week 1, 200 mg in week 2, 300 mg in week 3 and 400 mg in weeks 4–8. After taking the medication, the sleep latency of these patients decreased from 39.9 ± 32.7 min at baseline to 16.6 ± 15.3 min at week 8 ($t = 2.739$; $p = 0.025$). Sleep efficiency increased from $78.8 \pm 14.6\%$ at baseline to $91.5 \pm 5.5\%$ at week 8 ($t = -2.569$; $p = 0.033$). Stage 1 sleep decreased from $4.9 \pm 1.9\%$ at baseline to $3.4 \pm 2.6\%$ at week 8 ($t = 3.9$; $p = 0.005$). Arousal index increased from 8.2 ± 3.6 at baseline to 12.2 ± 7.1 at week 8 ($t = -2.311$, $p = 0.05$). The results indicate that nefazodone has predominately positive effects on PSG sleep in this population.

Some researchers have found no difference between SAD patients and other subgroups of major depression in their response to total sleep deprivation (TSD)[20]. TSD increases total sleep time, sleep efficiency, SWS and total minutes of REM sleep; it also reduces sleep latency, the amount of wakefulness and stage 1 sleep[14]. However, in a study evaluating sleep deprivation in SAD patients and normal controls, several other changes were found in both groups, including that REM latency of the SAD patients was markedly reduced. In other studies this phenomenon was also found after sleep deprivation in elderly men and women[21], but not in healthy young men[22,23]. Since a delayed onset of REM sleep is often seen in disrupted sleep, TSD may reduce REM sleep latency by consolidating sleep in the middle-aged and elderly. In female SAD patients, power spectra of non-REM sleep were changed by TSD. The power spectra changes were nearly identical to those found in healthy young men[22–24]. Increased EEG activity in all frequencies below 11 Hz was accompanied by slightly attenuated values in the spindle frequencies (12.25–14.0 Hz). The increase of power density in the low delta frequencies is comparable to, or even larger than, that reported after TSD in healthy young men[22,23].

POSSIBLE PATHOPHYSIOLOGICAL MECHANISMS RELATIVE TO SAD SLEEP

Hypotheses about the pathophysiology of SAD have focused on abnormalities in circadian pacemaker function, such as a phase delay[25,26], diminished amplitude of circadian rhythms during winter[27,28] and/or abnormal photoperiodic response[2]. Accordingly, the therapeutic effects of bright light have been attributed to its ability to normalize aberrant circadian rhythms.

Lewy and co-workers[25] hypothesized that most SAD patients have a phase-delay in their endogenous circadian rhythm relative to sleep, and that the antidepressant effect of light may be mediated by the phase-advancing effect of morning light. They found the circadian rhythm of melatonin to be phase-delayed relative to sleep in winter depressives compared to non-depressed controls. Terman and co-workers[29] have also found phase-delayed melatonin rhythms in SAD. Although some researchers[30,31] did not find that extraocular light induces a phase shift of the circadian pacemaker, it is generally thought that properly timed bright light causes a significant phase-advance[26,32]. Morning light produced phase advances of the melatonin rhythm, while evening light produced delays, the magnitude depending on the interval between melatonin onset and light exposure, or circadian time. Early-morning administration in circadian time increases the antidepressant effect of light. The optimal time is about 8.5 h after melatonin onset or 2.5 h after the sleep midpoint[33]. Timed bright light can also increase the amplitude of the temperature rhythm. Thus, Czeisler and co-workers[27] have proposed a hypothesis that the endogenous circadian amplitude is low in SAD and that bright light therapy increases the amplitude to normal levels.

Avery and co-workers[34] assessed circadian temperature, cortisol and thyroid-stimulating hormone (TSH) rhythms during constant-routine research in female hypersomnic SAD patients and controls before and after morning bright light treatment. After sleep was standardized for 6 days, the subjects were sleep-deprived and at bed rest for 27 h while rectal temperature, cortisol and TSH levels were assessed. The minimum of the fitted rectal temperature rhythm was phase-delayed in the SAD group compared to the controls (5.42 a.m. versus 3.16 a.m.). With bright light treatment, the minimum advanced from 5.42 a.m. to 3.36 a.m. The minimum of the cortisol rhythm was phase-delayed in the SAD group compared to the control group (00.11 a.m. versus 11.03 p.m.). With bright light treatment, the minimum advanced from 00.11 a.m. to 11.38 p.m. The peak-phase of the TSH rhythm was not significantly phase-delayed in SAD subjects compared to controls, though the trend appeared to be toward a phase-delay. After bright light therapy, the TSH peak-phase was not significantly different in the SAD subjects, the trend was a phase-advance. These results suggest that circadian rhythms are phase-delayed relative to sleep in SAD patients and that morning bright light phase-advances those rhythms.

In a study of ambulatory monitoring of rectal temperature, Rosenthal and co-workers[35] found that the temperature amplitude of SAD subjects was similar to that of controls. Although there was no systematic shift in phase with the photo-period extension, temperature minimum was advanced in six of ten SAD patients and delayed in four of ten. Those SAD patients who advanced their rhythms with LT tended to experience more hypersomnia at baseline, a greater increase in temperature amplitude with light treatment and a better antidepressant response. Those whose temperature rhythms were phase-delayed with bright light tended to have early morning awakening, reducing amplitude increase and inferior antidepressant response. In SAD patients LT lowers core temperature during sleep in proportion to its antidepressant efficacy[36]. When the SAD patients and controls were restudied in the summer, the amplitudes were not different, but the overall mean temperature across the 24-h period was lower for both groups[37]. In contrast to endogenous-melancholic depressed in-patients who usually have high nocturnal temperatures and low temperature amplitude[34], SAD patients do not frequently show these abnormalities either in an ambulatory study[35] or in constant-routine study.

The circadian rhythms of cortisol obtained without a constant routine were found to be similar in SAD patients compared to controls in both phase and amplitude; the rhythms did not change with successful bright light[38]. Since sleep has a suppressing effect on cortisol[39], those cortisol data do not reflect the unmasked endogenous circadian rhythm of cortisol. SAD patients had normal cortisol and adrenocorticotropic hormone (ACTH) levels, but their responses to corticotropin-releasing hormone (CRH) were delayed and significantly reduced[38,40]. With bright light therapy, the responses of cortisol and ACTH to CRH significantly increased.

Raitiere[41] found that 35% (17) of 49 SAD patients had elevated TSH compatible with mild primary hypothyroidism, and that this proportion was significantly greater than that seen in non-seasonal depressed patients. Circadian profiles without a constant routine have shown no differences between SAD patients and controls, but with bright light treatment the nocturnal TSH values decreased significantly. It has been shown that responsiveness of TSH to thyrotropin-releasing hormone (TRH) stimulation is reduced in SAD patients[42].

Overall, the data generally support the hypothesis that the circadian rhythms obtained under constant-routine conditions are phase-delayed in SAD subjects compared to controls, and that morning bright light treatments phase-advance those circadian rhythms. However, there are some discrepancies among the reports. The cortisol data offer some support for the low circadian amplitude hypothesis. These data suggest that the phase-delay hypothesis and the low circadian amplitude hypothesis are not mutually exclusive.

CONCLUSION

This review suggests that an impairment of circadian rhythm is part of the pathogenesis of SAD and that there is a pattern of delayed sleep phase in such patients. The relationship between circadian rhythm and modifier in the treatment of SAD patients requires further study.

References

1. Wehr TA, Giesen HA, Schulz PM, *et al*. Contrasts between symptoms of summer depression and winter depression. *J Affect Disord* 1991;23:173–83
2. Rosenthal NE, Sack DA, Gillin JC, *et al*. Seasonal affective disorder: a description of the syndrome and preliminary findings with light therapy. *Arch Gen Psychiatry* 1984;41:72–80
3. Thompson C, Stinson D, Fernandez M, *et al*. A comparison of normal, bipolar and seasonal affective disorder subjects using the Seasonal Pattern Assessment Questionnaire. *J Affect Disord* 1988;14:257–64
4. Rosenthal NE, Wehr TA. Seasonal affective disorder. *Psychiatr Ann* 1987;17:670–4
5. Anderson JL, Rosen LN, Mendelson WB, *et al*. Sleep in full/winter seasonal affective disorder: effects of light and changing seasons. *J Psychosom Res* 1994;38:323–37
6. Shapiro CM, Devins GM, Feldman B, Levitt AJ. Is hypersomnolence a feature of seasonal affective disorder? *J Psychosom Res* 1994;38 (Suppl 1):49–54
7. Putilov AA, Booker JM, Danilenko KV, Zolotarev DY. The relation of sleep–wake patterns to seasonal depressive behavior. *Arctic Med Res* 1994;53:130–6
8. Rosen LN, Targum SD, Terman M, *et al*. Prevalence of seasonal affective disorder at four latitudes. *Psychiatry Res* 1990;31:131–44
9. Wirz-Justice A, Wever RA, Aschoff J. Seasonality in freerunning circadian rhythms in man. *Naturwissenschaften* 1984;71:316–19
10. Rosenthal NE, Skwerer RG, Levendosky BA, *et al*. Sleep architecture in seasonal affective disorder: the effects of light therapy and changing seasons. *Sleep Res* 1989;18:440
11. Endo T. Morning bright light effects on circadian rhythms and sleep structure of SAD. *Jikeikai Med J* 1993;40:295–307
12. Partonen T, Appelberg B, Partinen M. Effects of light treatment on sleep structure in seasonal affective disorder. *Eur Arch Psychiatry Clin Neurosci* 1993;242:310–13
13. Kohsaka M, Honma H, Fukuda N, *et al*. Does bright light change sleep structures in seasonal affective disorder? *Soc Light Ther Biol Rhythms* 1994;6:32
14. Brunner DP, Kräuchi K, Dijk D-J, *et al*. Sleep electroencephalogram in seasonal affective disorder and in control women: effects of midday light treatment and sleep deprivation. *Biol Psychiatry* 1996;40:485–96
15. Brunner DP, Kräuchi K, Leonhardt G, *et al*. Sleep parameters in SAD: effects on midday light, season, and sleep deprivation. *Sleep Res* 1993;22:396
16. Kräuchi K, Wirz-Justice A, Graw P. High intake of sweets late in the day predicts a rapid and persistent response to light therapy in winter depression. *Psychiatry Res* 1993;46:107–17
17. Putilov AA, Danilenko KV, Palchikov VE, Schergin SM. The multiple sleep latency test in seasonal affective disorder: no evidence for increased sleep propensity. *Soc Light Treat Biol Rhythms* 1995;7:30
18. Carrier J, Dumont M. Sleep propensity and sleep architecture after bright light exposure at three different times of day. *J Sleep Res* 1995;4:202–11
19. Shen J, Chang J, Levitan R, *et al*. Nefazodone effects on women with seasonal affective disorder: clinical and polysomnographic analysis. *J Psychiatry Neurosci* 2003;in press
20. Graw P, Haug HJ, Leonhardt G, Wirz-Justice A. Sleep deprivation response in seasonal affective disorder during a 40-h constant routine. *J Affect Disord* 1998;48:69–74
21. Reynolds CF, Kupfer DJ, Hoch CC, *et al*. Sleep deprivation in healthy elderly men and women: effects on mood and on sleep during recovery. *Sleep* 1986;9:492–501
22. Borbély AA, Baumann F, Brandeis D, *et al*. Sleep deprivation: effect on sleep stages and EEG power density in man. *Electroenceph Clin Neurophysiol* 1981;51:483–93
23. Dijk DJ, Hayes B, Czeisler CA. Dynamics of electroencephalographic sleep spindles and wave activity in men: effect of sleep deprivation. *Brain Res* 1993;626:190–9
24. Dijk DJ, Brunner DP, Beersma DG, Borbely AA. Electroencephalogram power density and slow wave sleep a function of prior waking and circadian phase. *Sleep* 1990;13:430–40
25. Lewy AJ, Sack RL, Singer CM. Treating phase-typed chronobiologic sleep and mood disorders using appropriately timed bright artificial light. *Psychopharmacol Bull* 1985;21: 368–72
26. Lewy AJ, Sack RL, Miller LS, Hoban TM. Antidepressant and circadian phase-shifting effects of light. *Science* 1987;235:352–4
27. Czeisler CA, Kronauer RE, Mooney JJ, *et al*. Biologic rhythm disorders, depression, and phototherapy: a new hypothesis. *Psy Clin North Am* 1987;10:687–709
28. Czeisler CA, Kronauer RE, Allan JS, *et al*. Bright light induction of strong (type 0) resetting of the human circadian pacemaker. *Science* 1989;244:1328–33
29. Terman M, Terman JS, Quitkin FM, *et al*. Response of the melatonin cycle to phototherapy for seasonal affective disorder. *J Neural Transm* 1988;72:147–65

30. Cajochen C, Brunner DP, Krauchi K, *et al*. EEG and subjective sleepiness during extended wakefulness in seasonal affective disorder: circadian and homeostatic influences. *Biol Psychiatry* 2000;47:610–17

31. Koorengevel KM, Gordijn MC, Beersma DG, *et al*. Extraocular light therapy in winter depression: a double-blind placebo-controled study. *Biol Psychiatry* 2001;50:691–8

32. Sack RL, Lewy AJ, White DM, *et al*. Morning versus evening light treatment for winter depression: evidence that the therapeutic effects of light are mediated by circadian phase shifting. *Arch Gen Psychiatry* 1990;47:343–51

33. Terman JS, Terman M, Lo ES, Cooper TB. Circadian time of morning light administration and therapeutic response in winter depression. *Arch Gen Psychiatry* 2001;58:60–75

34. Avery DH, Dahl K, Savage MV, *et al*. Circadian temperature and cortisol rhythms during a constant routine are phase-delayed in hypersomnic winter depression. *Biol Psychiatry* 1997; 41:1109–23

35. Rosenthal NE, Levendosky AA, Skwerer RG, *et al*. Effects of light treatment on core body temperature in seasonal affective disorder. *Biol Psychiatry* 1990;27:39–50

36. Schwartz PJ, Rosenthal NE, Wehr TA. Serotonin 1A receptors, melatonin, and the proportional control thermostat in patients with winter depression. *Arch Gen Psychiatry* 1998;55:897–903

37. Levendosky AA, Joseph-Vanderpool JR, Hardin T, *et al*. Core body temperature in patients with seasonal affective disorder and normal controls in summer and winter. *Biol Psychiatry* 1991;29:524–34

38. Joseph-Vanderpool JR, Rosenthal NE, Chrousos GP, *et al*. Abnormal pituitary–adrenal responses to corticotropin-releasing hormone in patients with seasonal affective disorder: clinical and pathophysiological implications. *J Clin Endocrinol Metab* 1991;72:1382–7

39. Weitzman E, Zimmerman JC, Czcislcr CA, Ronda J. Cortisol secretion is inhibited during sleep in normal man. *J Clin Endocrinol Metab* 1983;66:1352–8

40. Partonen T. A mechanism of action underlying the antidepressant effect of light. *Med Hypotheses* 1995;45:33–4

41. Raitiere MN. Clinical evidence for thyroid dysfunction in patients with seasonal affective disorder. *Psychoneuroendocrinology* 1992;17:231–41

42. Coiro V, Colp R, Marchesi C, *et al*. Lack of seasonal variation in abnormal TSH secretion in patients with seasonal affective disorder. *Biol Psychiatry* 1994;35:36–41

20

Disordered sleep in post-traumatic stress disorder: clinical presentation, research findings and implications for treatment

Elbert Geuze and Eric Vermetten

and a dream full of horror has not ceased to visit me, at sometimes frequent, sometimes longer, intervals. It is a dream within a dream, varied in detail, one in substance. I am sitting at a table with my family... apparently without tension or affliction; yet I feel a deep and subtle anguish, the definite sensation of an impending threat, ...everything collapses and disintegrates around me... Now everything has turned to chaos; I am alone in the centre of a grey and turbid nothing, and now, I know what this thing means, and I also know that I have always known it; I am in the Lager once more, and nothing is true outside the Lager... Now this inner dream, this dream of peace, is over, and in the outer dream, which continues, gelid, a well-known voice resounds: a single word, not imperious, but brief and subdued. It is the dawn command of Auschwitz, a foreign word, feared and expected: get up,'Wstawàch.

Primo Levi, *The Truce*

INTRODUCTION

Sleep complaints are among the most frequently reported symptoms associated with many psychiatric disorders[1,2]. Post-traumatic stress disorder (PTSD) is no exception to this. In fact, in PTSD, sleep disturbances are manifested symptoms of the disease. Moreover, on the basis of sleep complaints as early as 1 month after the trauma, it is possible to predict those individuals who will later develop chronic PTSD[3]. Sleep disturbances affect about 70% of all PTSD patients, with reports of violent or injurious behavior during sleep, as well as sleep paralysis, sleeptalking, hypnagogic and hypnopompic hallucinations being among those disturbances most frequently cited[4]. The following discussion commences by describing the symptom clusters of PTSD, followed by an account of the subjective and objective research findings of disordered sleep in PTSD. The chapter closes with a discussion of treatment options for the sleep disturbances caused by PTSD and contains a number of conclusions.

SYMPTOM CLUSTERS OF POST-TRAUMATIC STRESS DISORDER

Society is increasingly affected by global, as well as personal, types of human violence including wars, terrorism, natural disasters, bombings, murders, suicides, rapes, shootings, robberies, assaults and accidents. These events can and do leave individuals (and societies) with feelings of intense terror, fear and paralyzing helplessness. Approximately 60% of men and 50% of women experience significant psychological trauma (defined as threat to life of self or significant other) at some time in their lives[5]. The predictive value of PTSD is dependent on the type of trauma, e.g. witnessing assault is less likely to result in PTSD than witnessing rape or exposure to a theater of war. Estimates of the lifetime prevalence of PTSD range from 7.8% to 9.2%[6]. PTSD is twice as common in women than in men[5]. This figure is more than twice the prevalence of bipolar disorder or schizophrenia. Among traumatized individuals the lifetime prevalence is even higher: 8% in men and 20% in women. More than one-third of individuals with an index episode of PTSD fail to recover even after many years[5]. PTSD has long been recognized as being related to wartime experiences and more recently as being associated with other types of trauma[6–9]. It is also increasingly acknowledged that PTSD is present in diverse cultures[10].

The diagnosis of PTSD was first included in the third edition of the Diagnostic and Statistical Manual of Mental Disorders (DSM-III) in 1980[11], where it was categorized as an anxiety disorder. Its first appearance in the International Classification of Diseases (ICD) is more recent[12]. PTSD is the only psychiatric condition whose definition demands that a particular stressor precede its appearance[13]. It is characterized by specific symptoms, which develop following exposure to psychological trauma and where the person's response involved (at the time of exposure) intense fear, helplessness or horror. The symptoms of PTSD are divided into three categories:

(1) Re-experiencing of the event;

(2) Avoidance of stimuli;

(3) Persistent symptoms of increased arousal (for an overview of the diagnostic criteria of PTSD according to DSM-IV[13], see the Appendix).

Chronic combat-related PTSD is frequently associated with other psychiatric disorders. However, the onset of PTSD in relation to co-morbidity often shows that, unlike generalized anxiety disorder and past substance abuse, the mean onset of co-morbid disorders occurs later than PTSD[14]. PTSD almost always emerges soon after exposure to the trauma. Lifetime PTSD appears to be associated with increased risk of lifetime panic disorder, major depression, alcohol abuse or alcohol dependence, and social phobia. Current PTSD is associated with an increased risk of current panic disorder, dysthymia, social phobia, major depression and generalized anxiety disorder. Relative to PTSD, the onset of the co-morbid disorders during the course of illness in a prisoner of war sample is: major depression, alcohol abuse or alcohol dependence, agoraphobia, social phobia and panic disorder[15].

The rapid pace at which knowledge of stress processing expanded in the past decade led to an increase in our understanding of the psychopathology of PTSD. In addition to results from preclinical studies that used a variety of animal models of traumatic stress, other factors have guided recent advances in the neurobiology of PTSD. These include: utilization of functional brain imaging; the incorporation of cross-system research (including neuroendocrine, neurochemical and neuro-immunological systems); and digression from exclusively studying combat veterans to include PTSD in patients suffering from non-combat-related traumas[16].

The basic and underlying pathophysiology of PTSD reflects long-lasting changes in the biological stress response systems that underlie many of the symptoms of PTSD and other trauma-related disorders[17–21]. Critical underlying psychobiological processes that have been defined include stress sensitization, fear conditioning and failure of extinction[22]. Specific brain areas including the hippocampus, amygdala, hypothalamus, medial prefrontal cortex and the cingulate gyrus[21,23,24] play an important role in mediating the biological stress response. In addition, they are also involved in processes of learning and memory, and are preferentially affected by stress.

CLINICAL PRESENTATION OF SLEEP DISTURBANCES IN POST-TRAUMATIC STRESS DISORDER

Disordered sleep in general

As early as 1666, Samuel Pepys reported that he suffered from seriously disturbed sleep and nightmares in the wake of the Great Fire of London[25]. Similar sleep disturbances have been reported in traumatized adults[26,27], and children[28], after World War II. In general, subjective accounts of the immediate and long-term sleep effects of traumatic occurrences are quite consistent. Individuals from a variety of populations and circumstances report frequent awakenings; difficulty falling asleep; decreased total sleep time; higher frequency of nightmares and anxiety dreams; and restless sleep[29–34]. Two of these studies[32,33] evaluated sleep disturbances in victims of Hurricane Andrew. Hurricane Andrew was a small and ferocious Cape Verde hurricane that brought unprecedented economic devastation along a path through the north-western Bahamas, the southern Florida peninsula and south-central Louisiana in 1992. Hurricane Andrew resulted in 35 deaths and left up to 250 000 people temporarily homeless. The study by Mellman and co-workers[32] provides us with an account of sleep disturbances shortly after Hurricane Andrew. These type of data are usually obtained years after the original traumatic event and, like other data collected retrospectively, are not as trustworthy. Subjects with active psychiatric morbidity (in Mellman's sample mostly PTSD and some depression) reported a range of sleep-related complaints such as:

(1) Significantly fewer hours of sleep;

(2) More problems with insomnia and non-restorative sleep;

(3) More problems with sleep maintenance (or middle insomnia);

(4) More parasomnia-like events, such as nightmares, thrashing movements and panic-like awakenings[32].

Six months prior to Hurricane Andrew, none of these patients had psychiatric illnesses. It is interesting to note that the patients with an active psychiatric morbidity reported greater frequencies of sleep disturbances and nightmares before the traumatic event than traumatic controls did.

Sleep disturbances have also been reported by children in the wake of traumatic events. In a comprehensive review of the psychological adjustment of 57 children (age range, 3 to 12 years) who sustained mutilating traumatic injuries to the face or upper or lower extremities, 21% matched the criteria of PTSD after a 12-month follow-up visit[35]. Typical symptoms reported by these children included flashbacks, mood disorders, anxiety, nightmares and sleep disturbances. A similar assessment of post-traumatic stress symptoms after road traffic accidents in children reported sleep difficulties and nightmares in 17% of children who had endured a road traffic accident in the previous 7 months[36]. Younger children, those who had not fully recovered from their accident injuries and children who also had a parent involved in the same accident were most at risk. In a review of 82 children and adolescents, aged between 30 months and 20 years, with burn injuries, Kravitz and co-workers[37] reported profound sleep disorders. One year or more after burn injury, 37% experienced nightmares, 24% bedwetting, and 18% suffered from sleepwalking. Dream content was related to burn injury in 7% of the children, and to burn treatment in 6%. Fifty-five per cent experienced dreams related to normal childhood topics. Daytime naps were reported in 63% of the children, although 92% were well beyond the normal age associated with napping. It is also important to note that no relationship was found between age at time of the burn injury, length of time after the burn injury, cause of the burn injury, family history of nightmares, or patient history of bedwetting and the incidence of nightmares.

Nightmares in post-traumatic stress disorder

One of the most frequently reported symptoms in PTSD is the presence of recurring nightmares. Indeed, 'recurrent distressing dreams of the event' is also one of the re-experiencing criteria of PTSD. The nightmare described by Primo Levi at the end of his book *The Truce*, related at the beginning of this chapter, is an enthralling subjective account of this re-experiencing phenomenon. Nightmares have been described by many different populations suffering from PTSD, including survivors of concentration camps[38], perpetrators of crimes[39], children[36], the aged[40], combat-related PTSD[30], child abuse-related PTSD[41], shortly after the trauma[42] and years after the trauma[34,43]. The variety of populations suffering from nightmares and the frequency with which this is reported makes it clear that nightmares truly represent a hallmark of PTSD.

It has been hypothesized, especially in patients with a history of major psychological trauma, that nightmares and sleepwalking are symptomatic of a protective dissociative mechanism. During sleep, intolerable impulses, feelings and memories can escape. Control of mental defense mechanisms can diminish, and these feelings, memories and impulses can erupt in a limited motor or affective form, with restricted awareness and subsequent amnesia for the event. Mellman and co-workers[44] have also suggested that rapid eye movement (REM) sleep may be a mechanism by which details of trauma memories are incorporated into less threatening scenarios; therefore, the dream content of someone with PTSD is more likely to be unmodified compared to a traumatized person without PTSD. A history of psychological trauma exists only in a minority of adult patients presenting with sleepwalking or night terror syndrome, although the trauma appears to dictate the subsequent content of the attacks in this subgroup[45].

One of the first questions to intrigue health-care workers who deal with patients exhibiting PTSD is the content of these nightmares. Do these recurring nightmares resemble the trauma, or are they unrelated? Are we really looking at re-experiencing phenomena? In an attempt to determine an answer to questions like these, Esposito and co-workers[46] developed a dream rating scale for combat-related PTSD. This dream rating scale included parameters previously incorporated in an earlier dream content analysis by Hall and van de Castle[47], such as setting, characters and objects in the dream; degree of overt threat to the dreamer; contemporaneity; and degree of distortion from actual or plausible events. Inter-rater reliability and internal consistency were established; four investigators reviewed the dreams of 19 Vietnam combat veterans. Settings, characters or objects characteristic of combat were reported in 47% of subjects, 53% of the dreams were set at least partially in the present, and only three of the dreams were rated as low in threat setting. As much as 79% of the dreams contained distorted elements; 21% of the dreams exactly replicated a prior event.

In the 1980s, Kramer and co-workers[48,49] also reported that military content was found in the dreams of approximately half of Vietnam war veterans. These authors concluded that target dreams of combat veterans with PTSD vary with regard to replication of trauma and elements normally associated with dreaming, but typically are threatening[49]. Although the evaluation of dream content in children with burn injuries by Kravitz and associates[37] was not as thoroughly evaluated as in Esposito's study[46], they found that 55% of dream content was related to normal childhood topics[37].

In another attempt to evaluate dream content, Schreuder and co-workers[43] developed a Nocturnal Intrusions after Traumatic Events (NITE) self-report questionnaire. Armed with the NITE, they investigated dream content in civilian war victims and veterans with PTSD after the occurrence of a post-traumatic nightmare. In their study, a post-traumatic nightmare was defined as any anxiety dream from which the sleeper wakes, and where the content relates to traumatic war experiences. Although nightmares occurred with almost equal frequency in both groups, this study was able to differentiate between veterans and civilian war victims. In veterans with PTSD, the content of the post-traumatic nightmares corresponded significantly more often with the original traumatic event than among civilian war victims with PTSD. However, in both groups, recalled dream content was strongly associated with war experiences, and the original traumatic event was often experienced in an exact replay of that event. These findings were not only limited to PTSD, but were also found in trauma victims in general. Even more than 40 years after war trauma, as many as 56% of war victims and veterans report post-traumatic nightmares[34,50]. PTSD in holocaust victims may also be a risk factor for the onset of PTSD in their offspring[51].

Re-experiencing, traumatic recall, flashbacks and flashbulb memories in post-traumatic stress disorder

Some of the most intriguing aspects of trauma disorders are the re-experiencing phenomena. Numerous labels and descriptions are applied to such phenomena[52], including flashbacks, traumatic recall or flashbulb memories. Traumatic recall paradigms form a unique opportunity to study the nightmares that occur in PTSD patients. It is as yet impossible to induce a nightmare in a sleeping person, but it has been shown that flashbacks, another of the re-experiencing phenomena, can be experimentally induced through the presentation of slides and sounds[24], a verbally presented script[23] or odors[53,54] related to the trauma. Traumatic recall can be defined as imaginary (or virtual) re-exposure to a traumatic event in which the person experienced, witnessed or was confronted by death or serious injury to self or others, and responded with intense fear, helplessness or horror, and during which a re-experience of similar emotional responses occur[13]. Previously, traumatic recall was also described as a 'flashback', the

reliving of the traumatic event with strong emotional involvement[55]. Flashbacks often lead to sleeping problems, irritability, feeling worse because of traumatic reminders, and secondary avoidance. They are distinct from common (autobiographical) memories in their emotional involvement. Typically, they recall the helplessness and uncontrollability of the situation at that time, and can narrow the attention so that 'it feels like being back there' (i.e. when and where the traumatic event occurred). There can be a sense of loss of control, or of self-agency ('that's not who I am' or 'it is not me to whom that happened'). Often there is an autonomic response (such as tachycardia, tachypnea and diaphoresis) that can lead to a feeling of panic ('I'm losing it again'). The recall may be triggered by a variety of markers related to the trauma, thoughts about the trauma, information about the trauma, trauma-related images or sounds, and smells, of which the person does not have to be consciously aware. Veterans reveal this effect potently when exposed to darkness and demonstrate augmented startle reflexes[56]. For a long time flashbacks were assumed to lack a recognizable neurophysiological correlate – therefore they were thought to be at least as likely to be figments of the imagination as of memory[55]. In a recent study of 62 PTSD patients comparing flashbacks with ordinary autobiographical memory performance on cognitive tasks, flashback periods were associated with a specific decrement in visuospatial processing, and not with specific decrements on a verbal processing task. Flashback periods were also found to be associated with increases in a wide range of autonomic and motor behaviors[57].

Flashbacks share a phenomenology with what was described as 'flashbulb memory', to refer to the vivid recollections that humans may have of events considered to be of particular significance to the individual. These memories were described as having a photographic quality and as being accompanied by a strong apparel of contextual information (weather, background music, clothes worn, etc.) pertaining to the time and place where

Table 20.1   Objective research findings on sleep disturbances in post-traumatic stress disorder (PTSD)

Study	Findings	Type of finding
Kramer et al., 1984[48],	↑ REM latency	
Glaubman et al., 1990[65],	↑ REM latency	
Kaminer and Lavie, 1991[66]	↑ Sleep latency	
Ross et al., 1994[67,68]	↑ Eye movements during REM, ↑ REM sleep	
Reist et al., 1995[69]	↓/↑ REM latency	
Mellman et al., 1997[70]	↓ REM sleep time, ↑ eye movements during REM	REM sleep
Mellman et al. 2002[44]	Development of PTSD symptoms associated with ↓ REM sleep	
Woodward et al., 2000[71]	Inverse correlation between REM–NREM sleep HR difference and REM per cent of sleep in PTSD patients	
Mellman et al., 1995[72]	↑ Nocturnal excretion of MHPG in PTSD patients	
Dagan et al., 1991[73]	↑ Awakening thresholds, ↑ latencies to the arousal response	
Pittman et al., 1999[74]	Deepening of sleep compared to controls	Hormonal findings
Hurwitz et al., 1998[75]	No significant differences on sleep measures – laboratory values	Polysomnograph measures
Klein et al., 2002[76]	No significant differences on any of the polysomnograph measures	
Peters et al., 1990[77]	Global sulcal widening correlated significantly with number of awakenings and time spent asleep	
Phan et al., 2002[78]	Implicates mPFC, amygdala, OC, subcallosal gyrus and ACC in traumatic recall	Neuroimaging

mPFC, medial prefrontal cortex; OC, occipital cortex; ACC, anterior cingulate cortex

the event first occurred. From a memory point of view, we now know that such memories are not perfectly accurate and are subject to decay, but what does not decay is their capacity to evoke emotions similar to the ones felt when first exposed to these contextual qualities[58]. It was suggested that flashbulb memories are formed by the activity of an ancient brain mechanism evolved to capture emotional and cognitive information relevant to the survival of the individual. Some of the original assumptions have since been challenged, but the phenomenon in question remains an important area of research[59,60]. The experiences share clinical features such as involuntary paroxysmal repetition, sensory vividness, and a capacity to trigger emotions such as anxiety, shame or anger.

SLEEP-RELATED BIOLOGICAL MARKERS

The current interest in the biological basis of psychiatric disorders led to a large increase in studies looking at the biological correlates of PTSD[22,61–64]. Research on the biological basis of disordered sleep in PTSD is also benefiting from this surge of interest (see Table 20.1). Like other DSM-IV[13] disorders, the DSM-IV criteria of PTSD have not been validated with objective sleep assessment technology. Neither have they incorporated nosological constructs from the field of sleep medicine, nor adequately addressed the potential for PTSD sleep problems to manifest as primary physical disorders, requiring independent medical assessment and therapy. The understanding of sleep problems in PTSD may be limited by use of such terms as 'insomnia related to another mental disorder' or 'psychiatric insomnia'[79].

A number of groups have studied disordered sleep in PTSD patients and looked at the biological alterations in sleep-related biological markers, including alterations in electroencephalographic recordings during sleep, and alterations in the neuroendocrine system.

Sleep laboratory findings

Sleep research clearly benefits a great deal from the electroencephalogram (EEG), which was first demonstrated by the German psychiatrist Hans Berger[80]. EEGs distinguish between different states of consciousness, and delineate sleep into four non-rapid eye movement (NREM) sleep stages and rapid eye movement (REM) sleep, each with more or less distinctive patterns of physiological variables and brain activity[81]. In healthy adults, progression through these stages is cyclic, with each cycle lasting approximately 90 min[82]. Electromyograms (EMGs) and electro-oculograms (EOGs) aid in describing healthy sleep and distinguishing it from disordered sleep.

Although the subjective accounts of sleep disturbances in PTSD are numerous and well documented, and provide a consistent body of evidence, identifying sleep disturbances in a sleep laboratory is not easy[42], because available evidence is not in agreement. Some studies identify severely disturbed sleep patterns, such as increased sleep latency, recurrent awakenings from REM sleep accompanied by anxiety dreams, and decreased total sleep time[31,73,83]. Patients with combat-related PTSD had a greater number of arousals and entries into stage 1 sleep than controls did[31]. Other reports show lower arousal rates in patients with PTSD[67,75], or fail to find significant differences in sleep-laboratory values of patients with PTSD compared to controls[67,70,75].

Polysomnography remains a popular method to assess disordered sleep. Studies using this method find that REM sleep is related to the pathophysiology of sleep[67,70,84]. Similarly, REM density correlates positively with both the PTSD symptom of re-experiencing trauma and with global distress[31,32]. However, data from studies of REM sleep differ considerably. Whereas a number of studies described increased REM latency[48,65,66], other studies showed the opposite, namely reduced or normal REM latency[69]. Some studies report an increase in total time spent in REM sleep[67]; others find a decrease in total REM sleep time[70]. Polysomnographic studies reveal that PTSD patients have increased awakenings, reduced sleep time and increased motor activity, or in some cases, paradoxical deepening of sleep compared to controls[74].

Some studies find an increased frequency of rapid eye movements during REM sleep in patients with PTSD[31,67,68,74]. The rapid eye movements appear to be related to leg muscle twitches in these patients[68], which is surprising, since normally REM sleep is associated with near paralysis of body musculature. Patients with other psychiatric disorders also display an increased frequency of eye movements during REM sleep, possibly as a result of coexisting psychiatric illness in PTSD[42,85]. Despite these findings, none of these pathophysiological alterations can be used for diagnostic screening; the studies do not account for co-morbid conditions; the findings are not unique. Moreover, the sensitivity, specificity and predictive value of these tests give them only marginal diagnostic value.

In an effort to clarify some of the ambiguities surrounding sleep findings in the acute phase preceding PTSD, Mellman and co-workers obtained polysomnographic recordings during the acute period following a life-threatening experience[44]. They examined 21 injured subjects within a month of injury and assessed PTSD symptoms concurrently and 6 weeks later. Sleep measures were compared among injured subjects with and without significant PTSD symptoms at follow-up, and among ten non-injured comparison subjects. Mellman's research found evidence for increased wake time after the onset of sleep in injured, trauma-exposed patients compared to non-injured comparison subjects. The development of PTSD symptoms was also associated with a shorter average duration of REM sleep before a change in sleep stage. Mellman and co-workers[44] concluded that the development of PTSD symptoms after traumatic injury is associated with a more fragmented pattern of REM sleep. However, another recent study on the development of sleep disturbances in PTSD reported that there were no significant differences between PTSD and non-PTSD patients on any of the polysomnograph measures[76]. Also, in this study, the PTSD and non-PTSD groups did not differ significantly from each other with respect to awakening thresholds during REM sleep. Klein and co-workers[76] suggested that altered sleep perception rather than sleep disturbances *per se* are responsible for the subjective sleep complaints of PTSD patients, and that this may explain the discrepancy between objective and subjective research.

One could imagine that, at least in the case of combat-related PTSD, the awakening threshold is lowered, owing to an overall increase in the arousal function. After all, PTSD is associated with 'persistent symptoms of increased arousal'[71]. Such a lowered awakening threshold would have survival value in combat situations, and is compatible with other research findings linking combat-related PTSD to heightened arousal and reduced sensory gating[86,87]. Although little research has been done on awakening thresholds in PTSD, an early study on awakening thresholds in combat-related PTSD is available[73]. Contrary to what one might expect, patients had significantly higher awakening thresholds and significantly longer latencies to an arousal response than normal controls. These results were interpreted to suggest modifications in the depth of sleep as one of the long-term sequelae of traumatic events. Polysomnographic studies in PTSD patients also provide some support for the occurrence of sleep disruption related to arousal regulation[84].

Woodward and co-workers studied symptoms of arousal under conditions in which effects of anticipatory anxiety could be ruled out[71]. In this study, heart rate and electroencephalogram spectral power were assessed during sleep, a state free of most sources of artifact contaminating indices of tonic arousal. Fifty-six unmedicated non-apneic Vietnam combat-related in-patients with PTSD and 14 controls spent 3 or more nights in the sleep laboratory during which their electrocardiograms and electroencephalograms were continuously recorded. PTSD patients exhibited a trend toward reduced low-frequency electroencephalogram spectral power during NREM sleep. This reduction

was significant during slow-wave sleep in those subjects producing scoreable slow-wave sleep. The relationship of REM beta-band power to NREM beta-band power was different in PTSD patients and controls, with patients exhibiting more beta-band power in REM versus NREM sleep than did controls. In patients, NREM sleep sigma-band electroencephalogram spectral power exhibited a positive correlation with subjective hyperarousal. Finally, a novel and surprisingly strong inverse correlation between REM–NREM sleep heart rate difference and REM per cent of sleep was observed in PTSD patients only, suggesting that more consideration should be directed to mechanisms of central arousal in PTSD.

Krakow and co-workers[79] argued that post-traumatic sleep disturbance frequently manifests with the combination of insomnia and a higher than expected prevalence of sleep-disordered breathing (SDB). In this model of complex sleep disturbance, the underlying sleep pathophysiology interacts with PTSD and related psychiatric distress. This relationship appears to be very important, as demonstrated by improvement in insomnia, nightmares and other post-traumatic stress symptoms, with successful SDB treatment, which was independent of other psychiatric interventions.

The noradrenergic system

The major role of the central noradrenalin axis and the locus ceruleus in sleep was established through the efforts of Hobson and co-workers[88]. With a heightened arousal and a high occurrence of sleep disturbances in PTSD, the implication of the central noradrenergic system in PTSD is not entirely unexpected[61–63,89,90]. As central noradrenergic systems have a role in regulating arousal levels during sleep, and heightened arousal frequently manifests in relation to sleep in PTSD, it would be interesting to evaluate noradrenergic production in relation to sleep and waking activity in PTSD patients. Mellman has examined daytime and nocturnal catecholamine measures in combat-related PTSD patients and normal controls[31,32]. Although 24-h norepinephrine and 3-methoxy-4-hydrophenylglycol (MHPG) (the more centrally derived metabolite) levels did not differ between patients and controls, PTSD patients had elevated nocturnal excretion of MHPG (comparing the average of two daytime values) as opposed to controls who had decreased nocturnal excretion of MHPG. This difference was significant between the two groups, thus supporting a relationship of undiminished central noradrenergic activity at night, and sleep disturbance in chronic, combat-related PTSD. Other important neurotransmitter systems involved in PTSD include the serotonergic system, the hypothalamic–pituitary–adrenal axis and various neuropeptides. However, a discussion of these neurotransmitter systems is beyond the scope of this chapter (for a review see Vermetten and Bremner[62,63]).

Relation to other disorders

Although PTSD overlaps major depression (MD) clinically, and REM density is increased in both patient groups, the amount of REM sleep in PTSD patients is significantly reduced in comparison to MD patients, suggesting that different underlying mechanisms are responsible in these disorders[70]. In a study comparing patients with PTSD and MD to patients with PTSD only, patients with PTSD and MD failed to exhibit shorter REM latencies, greater REM percentages of sleep or greater REM densities than patients with PTSD only, but these patients did exhibit less slow-wave sleep[91]. PTSD patients with co-morbid MD also exhibited less facial electromyographic activity.

One study points out that there may be a link between REM sleep behavior disorder (RBD), a parasomnia in which there is often violent enactment of dream mentation, and PTSD[68,92]. Although RBD is sometimes associated with neurological disorders, psychiatric co-morbidity is not typical. The authors present a unique series of veterans with RBD,

with a high incidence of co-morbidity with PTSD. They suggest the possibility that similar neuropathological processes are responsible for both conditions, at times in the same patient.

Neuroimaging

In the past decade, a number of neuroimaging studies revealed some of the structural and functional brain aberrations present in PTSD[93–97]. For example, volumetric analysis of the brain with magnetic resonance imaging demonstrates reduced hippocampal volume in PTSD[98,99]. Symptom provocation studies found decreased regional cerebral blood flow in the medial prefrontal cortex. For researchers interested in disordered sleep in PTSD, it would also have been interesting to examine the affinity of noradrenergic receptor binding in PTSD patients with heightened arousal and disordered sleep. To our knowledge, such a study has not yet been performed. One imaging study examined the relation of the sleep disturbances found in combat-related PTSD to brain abnormalities[77]. These authors examined former American prisoners of war (POWs) captured by the Japanese in World War II, who later complained of sleep disturbances and PTSD. Sleep EEG and computerized axial tomographic (CT) scans were obtained in all subjects. Six of the ten subjects exhibited no stage 4 sleep and had significantly higher mean ventricular brain ratios (VBRs). Structural brain measures such as VBRs and global sulcal widening (GSW) correlated significantly with the number of awakenings; GSW also correlated significantly with time spent asleep. A major drawback of this study, and probably also the reason why these results have never been replicated, is the absence of a control group. It is possible that these changes are not specific to PTSD, but rather that they are associated with normal aging.

As stated earlier, although it is not yet possible to study nightmares *in vivo*, it is possible to study another of the re-experiencing criteria, traumatic recall, or

Table 20.2 Brain areas involved in traumatic recall

Brain area	Involved in
Medial prefrontal cortex	General role in emotional processing
Amygdala	Specific role in fear processing
Medial prefrontal cortex/subcallosal gyrus (area 25)	Involved in the processing of sadness
Occipital cortex and amygdala	Activation by emotional induction of visual stimuli
Anterior cingulate cortex (area 32) and insula	Induction of emotional recall/imagery and induction of emotional tasks with cognitive demand medial prefrontal cortex

general emotional activation, in considerable depth. In a meta-analysis of positron emission tomography (PET) and functional magnetic resonance imaging (fMRI) studies of general emotional activation, which reviewed 43 PET and 12 fMRI activation studies spanning almost a decade of research, Phan and co-workers[78] describe brain areas that are involved in emotion induction with cognitive demand, typical paradigms of the recall of autobiographical elements or visual imagery. The brain areas described are shown in Table 20.2. Perhaps these brain areas also play a role in the other re-experiencing criteria. According to the activation–synthesis model developed by Hobson and McCarley[100], dreaming is the subjective awareness of brain activation in sleep. One could reasonably postulate that the same brain areas involved in traumatic recall are also activated during nightmares, with the distinction that in nightmares, the external sensory input and motor output are actively blocked by neurophysiological mechanisms.

TREATMENT

Despite inconclusive and inconsistent objective research findings, the subjective experience of PTSD patients is very real indeed and demands treatment. In the treatment of sleep disorders, two methods may be employed:

pharmacological interventions, or behavioral and psychological interventions. We will first discuss pharmacological treatments proven to be effective in treating the sleep disturbances (see Table 20.3): tricyclic antidepressants and benzodiazepines; selective serotonergic reuptake inhibitors; serotonin antagonists; serotonin antagonist reuptake inhibitors; antipsychotic and anticonvulsant augmentation; and the agents prazosin and mirtazapine. Behavioral and psychological interventions will sum up this discussion of the treatment of disordered sleep in PTSD.

Tricyclic antidepressants

Tricyclic antidepressive agents are effective in the treatment of sleep disorders in PTSD patients[101]. In a study illustrating that the timely diagnosis and treatment of trauma-related symptoms significantly stalls the development of PTSD, Robert and co-workers[102] also established that imipramine proves to be helpful in the treatment of hyperarousal and intrusive re-experiencing symptoms. They treated 25 pediatric patients with acute burns. Eighty per cent of the children experienced remission of hyperarousal symptoms (e.g. trouble staying asleep, trouble falling asleep) and intrusive re-experiencing symptoms (e.g. nightmares) after being treated with imipramine. Twelve per cent of the children experienced a decrease in the frequency or intensity of acute stress disorder symptoms. This finding also demonstrated that proper and timely treatment of acute stress disorder symptoms may prevent the development of PTSD.

Benzodiazepines

Historically, many PTSD patients were treated with high dosages of benzodiazepines[103]. The risks attendant on benzodiazepine management of PTSD, coupled with poor clinical outcome, have led clinicians to explore alternative treatment. The administration of temazepam, a benzodiazepine hypnotic, within 1–3 weeks of trauma exposure revealed

Table 20.3 Pharmacological treatment in post-traumatic stress disorder (PTSD)

	Drug	N	Type of trauma	Type of study	Study
Tricyclic antidepressants	Tricyclic antidepressants	3	Torture and war victims	Case study	Brimstedt and Ansehn, 1991[101]
	Imipramine	25	Children with acute burns	Open-label	Robert et al., 1999[102]
SSRIs and serotonin antagonists	Clonidine SSRIs, anticonvulsants	632	Mainly combat-related	Review	Viola et al., 1997[103]
			Combat-related	Open-label	Neylan et al., 2001[105]
	Fluvoxamine	21	Combat-related		
	Fluvoxamine	24	Combat-related	Open-label	De Boer et al., 1992[106]
Benzodiazepine	Temazepam	4	Mainly surgical trauma	Pilot study	Mellman et al., 1998[104]
Serotonin antagonist reuptake inhibitors	Nefazodone	12	Combat-related	Open-label	Gillin et al., 2001[107]
	Trazodone	74	Combat-related	Open-label/ retrospective	Warner et al., 2001[108]
Antipsychotics	Olanzapine augmentation	19	Combat-related	Double-blind, placebo-controlled	Stein et al., 2002[109]
Anticonvulsants	Gabapentin augmentation	30	Various	Retrospective	Hamner et al., 2001[110]
	Topiramate augmentation	35	Civilian PTSD	Open-label	Berlant and van Kammen, 2002[111]
Adrenergic antagonist agents	Prazosin	5	Civilian PTSD	Open-label	Taylor and Raskind 2002[112]
	Prazosin	10	Combat-related	Double-blind crossover, placebo-controlled study	Raskind et al., 2003[113]
	Mirtazepine	300	War trauma in refugees	Retrospective	Lewis, 2002[114]

SSRIs, selective serotonin reuptake inhibitors

improved sleep and reduced PTSD symptoms, further illustrating the beneficial effect of early intervention[104].

Selective serotonin reuptake inhibitors and serotonin antagonists

Selective serotonin reuptake inhibitors (SSRIs) are also effective in treating poor sleep quality in PTSD[105,106]. A study assessing the efficacy of fluvoxamine treatment on different domains of subjective sleep quality in Vietnam combat veterans with chronic PTSD found that fluvoxamine treatment led to improvements in PTSD symptoms in general, and in all domains of subjective sleep quality[105]. The strongest effect was for dreams linked to the traumatic experience in combat. In contrast, generic unpleasant dreams showed only a modest response to treatment. Sleep maintenance insomnia and

'troubled sleep' showed a large treatment response, whereas sleep onset insomnia improved less substantially.

Cyproheptadine, a serotonin 2 ($5HT_2$) antagonist has been an accepted treatment for nightmares in PTSD for some time. The addition of cyproheptadine to antidepressants orally at night controls nightmares[115–117]. Bedtime treatment of 4–12 mg of cyproheptadine provides relief from nightmares, decreasing their intensity and frequency, and providing complete remission in some instances[116–118]. However, a recent double-blind, randomized, placebo-controlled trial of cyproheptadine for treating sleep problems in 69 patients with combat-related PTSD found that drug and placebo groups did not differ significantly on sleep-related symptoms[119]. In contrast, sleep problems were slightly (though not significantly) exacerbated in the treatment group. The authors rightly assert the need for skepticism about open-label and anecdotal findings, and the need for careful scientific trials to replicate uncontrolled studies.

Serotonin and noradrenergic reuptake inhibitors (nefazodone) and serotonin-2 antagonist and serotonin reuptake inhibitor (trazodone)

Serotonin and noradrenergic reuptake inhibitors (SNRIs), such as nefazodone, and serotonin-2 antagonist and serotonin re-uptake inhibitors (SASRIs), such as trazodone, are also effective in the treatment of nightmares and disordered sleep in PTSD. Both agents act by strongly blocking $5HT_{2A}$ receptors, combined with less potent serotonin reuptake inhibitor properties, and weak α_1-adrenergic blocking capacity. Nefazodone has the added advantage of weak noradrenergic reuptake inhibition. Nefazodone's effectiveness in treating nightmares in PTSD is well established[107,120–122], and is associated with significant improvements in intrusive recollections, avoidance, hyperarousal clusters on a global PTSD scale and early improvements in nightmares and general sleep disturbance[123,124]. One study compared effects of nefazodone on polysomnographic sleep measures, subjective reports of sleep quality, nightmares, and other symptoms in patients with chronic combat-related PTSD during a 12 week, open-label clinical trial[125]. Significant improvement of subjective symptoms of nightmares and sleep disturbance, as well as depression and PTSD symptoms were noted. Nevertheless, objective polysomnographic sleep measures did not change. Unfortunately, the use of nefazodone has dropped, owing to its side-effects. In some patients it caused serious liver problems and it has been taken off the market in some European countries.

To date, the literature has reported little on the use of trazodone in the treatment of insomnia and nightmares in PTSD, even though it is commonly used[108]. An early study reported that sleep was the first symptom to improve at 2–3 months[126]. Patients were started on 50 mg per day, and the dosage was titrated up to 400 mg per day until response was maximal. Seventy-two per cent of 60 patients using trazodone found it to be helpful in decreasing nightmares, from an average of 3.3–1.3 nights per week, 92% found it helped with sleep onset and 78% reported improvement with sleep maintenance[108]. The effective dose range of trazodone for 70% of patients was 50–200 mg nightly. There was a higher than expected occurrence of priapism in patients taking trazodone, warranting the need for clinicians to ask directly about this side-effect. However, these findings need to be confirmed by using a larger sample in a double-blind, placebo-controlled study.

Antipsychotic and anticonvulsant augmentation

PTSD symptoms may improve significantly with antidepressant medications; however, some phenomena can remain refractory to the most commonly used treatments, especially sleep disturbances, such as insomnia and nightmares. In combat-related PTSD, standard pharmacological interventions with selective serotonin reuptake inhibitors do not always have the desired effect. Recent evidence suggests that augmentation with atypical antipsychotics may especially benefit the treatment of sleep symptoms[109]. Nineteen patients with PTSD were assessed in a double-blind, placebo-controlled study of olanzapine augmentation with SSRIs. This study showed that olanzapine augmentation was associated with a statistically significant greater reduction than placebo in specific measures of post-traumatic stress, and depressive and sleep disorder symptoms.

Gabapentin, a novel anticonvulsant agent, has been of interest as a potential anxiolytic agent, and may also play a role in augmenting SSRIs in order to relieve sleep-related symptoms of PTSD. In a retrospective study of gabapentin augmentation in 30 patients, 77% showed moderate or great improvement in duration of sleep, and most noted a decrease in the frequency of nightmares at a dose range of 300–3600 mg/day[110]. Sedation and mild dizziness were the most commonly reported side-effects. The rationale for use of anticonvulsants as a treatment for PTSD is based on the hypothesis that exposure to traumatic events may sensitize or kindle limbic nuclei. However, double-blind placebo-controlled studies have not yet been performed.

Another anticonvulsant, topiramate, may also reduce or even eliminate trauma-related intrusive memories and nightmares in previously treatment-refractory patients[127]. An open-label study that investigated topiramate's effectiveness as monotherapy or add-on in 35 patients with PTSD found that topiramate decreased nightmares in 79% (19/24) and flashbacks in 86% (30/35) of patients, with full suppression of nightmares in 50% and of intrusions in 54% of patients with these symptoms[111]. Nightmares or intrusions partially improved in a median of 4 days and were fully absent in a median of 8 days. Ninety-one per cent of the full responders required a dosage of 100 mg/day or less, demonstrating that topiramate is effective both as an add-on and as monotherapy for PTSD, with rapid onset of action, and minimal dose-related side-effects. These early reports of successful reduction in the frequency of nightmares and occurrences of sleep disturbances in PTSD by anticonvulsant medication are impressive, but need to be confirmed with double-blind placebo-controlled studies.

Prazosin and mirtazepine

Of late, the use of the α_1-adrenergic antagonist, prazosin, to treat combat trauma nightmares in veterans with PTSD has attracted attention. As mentioned previously, central nervous system (CNS) adrenergic hyper-responsiveness may be involved in the pathophysiology of PTSD. During treatment of two Vietnam combat veterans with PTSD for symptoms of benign prostatic hypertrophy, with prazosin, these patients unexpectedly reported elimination of combat trauma nightmares. This observation prompted an open-label feasibility trial of prazosin

for combat trauma nightmares in chronic combat-induced PTSD[128]. To date, two open-label studies have provided support for the use of prazosin in such cases. In a retrospective chart review study, Raskind and co-workers analyzed data from 59 consecutive combat veterans with previously treatment-resistant chronic PTSD (*DSM-IV* criteria[13]) and severe intractable trauma content nightmares to whom prazosin had been prescribed[113,129]. Nightmare severity was quantified using the recurrent distressing dreams item of the Clinician Administered PTSD Symptom Scale (CAPSS). Mean recurrent distressing dreams item scores improved significantly in the 36 patients who completed at least 8 weeks of prazosin treatment at their maximum titrated dose. The mean maximum prazosin dose used in these 36 patients was 9.6 ± 0.9 mg per day. Recurrent distressing dreams scores also improved in the total group who filled their prazosin prescriptions ($n = 51$). No significant change in CAPSS recurrent distressing dreams score was noted in a comparison group of eight patients who did not fill their prazosin prescriptions, but continued in outpatient treatment. There were also no serious adverse effects attributable to prazosin. In order to provide authoritative scientific evidence for the efficacy of prazosin in reducing nightmares in PTSD, Raskind and co-workers[113] completed a double-blind crossover, placebo-controlled study. Ten Vietnam combat veterans with chronic PTSD and severe trauma-related nightmares each received prazosin and placebo in a 20 week double-blind crossover protocol. Prazosin (mean dose of 9.5 mg nightly) was superior to placebo for the three primary outcome measures: scores on the recurrent distressing dreams item; the difficulty falling and staying asleep item of the CAPSS; and the change in overall PTSD severity and functional status according to the Clinical Global Impression of change. Total score and symptom cluster scores for re-experiencing, avoidance and numbing, and hyperarousal on the CAPSS were also significantly improved and the drug was well tolerated. Prazosin may also reduce trauma-related nightmares in elderly men with chronic PTSD[130].

Mirtazepine, a noradrenergic and specific serotonergic antidepressant, is an α_2-antagonist that also blocks the $5HT_{2A}$, $5HT_{2C}$ and $5HT_3$ receptors. It is effective in PTSD[114]. Lewis published a preliminary report of mirtazepine administered to more than 300 refugees suffering from nightmares characteristic of PTSD[114]. He estimated that 75% of the patients have reported improvement due to the reduction of the frequency and intensity of nightmares. In a substantial minority of the patients the nightmares were absent altogether. Reports of side-effects were extremely rare. Carefully planned research is necessary to prove that these preliminary findings are indeed correct.

Psychological treatments of disordered sleep in post-traumatic stress disorder

Psychological and behavioral therapies, such as imagery rehearsal therapy, muscle relaxation, paradoxical intention, sleep hygiene, sleep restriction, hypnotic procedures, stimulus control, and also eye movement desensitization and reprocessing (EMDR) are frequently used to treat disordered sleep in PTSD[41,131,132]. In the treatment of PTSD, individual psychotherapy and group techniques focusing on denial, trust, loss, survivor guilt and reparation are well established (see Rabois and co-workers[133] and Allodi[134] for a review). The review article of Rabois and co-workers[133] provides an interesting attempt to initiate dialog among those conducting research on the biological aspects of PTSD and clinicians and researchers concerned with developing effective psychological treatments for PTSD. They discuss the impact and implications of biological findings for psychological treatment and provide important bridging work between these two paradigms.

Rothbaum and Mellman[131] have reviewed the use of dreams and exposure therapy in PTSD. Exposure therapy is a well established treatment for PTSD that requires the patient to focus on and describe the details of a traumatic experience. As we have established earlier, nightmares that refer to or replicate traumatic experiences are prominent and distressing symptoms of PTSD and appear to exacerbate the disorder. Nightmares that replay the trauma and disrupt sleep do not meet requirements for therapeutic exposure, whereas other dreaming may aid in the recovery from trauma. An open-label trial of cognitive behavior therapy also showed that this treatment was successful in reducing insomnia and nightmares in crime victims[135–138].

Imagery rehearsal therapy has also been used for the treatment of chronic nightmares. The efficacy of imagery rehearsal therapy has been established in a sample of adolescent girls with sexual abuse-related PTSD, suffering from nightmares, sleep complaints and other post-traumatic stress symptoms[42,139,140]. Imagery rehearsal therapy consists of three steps, all of which are performed in the waking state:

(1) Select a nightmare;

(2) 'Change the nightmare any way you wish';

(3) Rehearse the images of the new version ('new dream') 5–20 min each day.

After 3 months of therapy, self-reported retrospectively assessed nightmare frequency decreased by 57%, and 71% in the treatment group, compared to no significant changes in the control group. Another large meta-analytical study of behavioral studies demonstrated that these psychological interventions provide reliable and durable changes in the sleep patterns of patients with chronic insomnia[141].

EMDR is another psychological technique that has been used in the treatment of PTSD for some time; its efficacy and use have been reviewed recently[136,137]. The biological basis of this intervention is recognized by a number of researchers and a theory of the biological mechanism of EMDR has been proposed to serve as an explanation of current results[136,142]. However, long-term follow-up studies on the efficacy of this intervention are still lacking.

Other non-pharmacological and non-psychotherapeutic treatment interventions

A separate line of treatment is the continuous positive airway pressure (CPAP) treatment in PTSD. Patients with sleep disordered breathing (SDB) have reduced electroencephalographic arousals and sleep fragmentation, symptoms which are usually attributed to central nervous system or psychophysiological processes. An arousal-based mechanism, perhaps initiated by post-traumatic stress and/or chronic insomnia, is thought to underlie the development of SDB in PTSD and perhaps also in other patients with chronic insomnia[66,143]. White noise has also been mentioned as a simple, safe, cost-effective alternative to hypnotic medication in PTSD. It is thought to be based on the reduction of the signal-to-noise ratio of ambient sound[144]. It has also been proposed that sleep dynamic therapy (SDT), an integrated program of primarily evidence-based, non-pharmacological sleep medicine therapies coupled with standard clinical sleep medicine instructions, is effective in reducing sleep disturbance in PTSD. In an uncontrolled study, Krakow and co-workers reported improvements in sleep disturbance, post-traumatic stress, anxiety and depression 12 weeks after initiating treatment in 66 adults, 10 months after the Cerro Grande Fire that occurred in May 2000, in New Mexico[145].

CONCLUSIONS

PTSD can be and often is a chronic, devastating disorder that may progressively worsen over time, affecting crucial aspects of life, including work, interpersonal relationships, physical health and view of self[146]. Although generally understood as a psychological disorder, PTSD may also be viewed from a biological perspective. Enough evidence has now accumulated to suggest that severe psychological trauma can cause alterations in the human organism's neurobiological response to stress, even years after the original insult[61,63]. Long-standing alterations in the biological response to stress may contribute to a number of complaints commonly expressed by patients with PTSD. For example, increased sensitivity and sensitization of the noradrenergic system may leave the individual in a hyperaroused, vigilant, sleep-deprived and, at times, explosive state that worsens over time. To quiet these symptoms of hyperarousal, PTSD patients often abuse substances, particularly central nervous system depressants that suppress peripheral and central catecholamine function. Alterations in other neurobiological systems may further contribute to multiple symptoms, such as intrusive memories, dissociative phenomena and numbing. Characterization of the biological underpinnings of PTSD relies to a large degree on available neurobiological technology. At present PTSD is thought to be associated with a dysfunction of the prefrontal cortex, which, through failure of inhibition of amygdala function, may mediate failure of the extinction of fear responses. Perhaps similar mechanisms are responsible for the nightmares observed in PTSD, although the triggering mechanism for nightmares remains unclear. Complaints of REM-related sleep symptoms could be an indication of an underlying problem stemming from PTSD-related pathology. It is possible that by processing fear-related memory content, memory consolidation may sensitize or kindle limbic nuclei.

Considerable research has examined sleep disturbances in PTSD. Subjective accounts of disordered sleep in PTSD consistently report frequent awakenings, difficulty falling asleep, decreased total sleep time, higher frequency of nightmares and anxiety dreams, and restless sleep[29–32,34]. The subjective sleep disturbances experienced by children mirror the sleep disturbances seen in adults in the wake of traumatic events. One of the re-experiencing criteria of PTSD, nightmares, are also frequently reported in child and adult populations suffering from PTSD. These nightmares usually mirror the original traumatic event or include elements from schemas related to the original traumatic experience. Nightmares are difficult to study *in vivo*, but the traumatic recall paradigm provides us with an opportunity to study a variation of the re-experiencing criteria.

Whereas the subjective accounts of disordered sleep in PTSD are unambiguous, objective evidence from sleep-laboratory research is far from consistent. Some studies report severely disordered sleep after traumatic events, whereas others find very little objective evidence of sleep disturbances[42]. Similar ambiguous results exist in relation to the amount of REM sleep in patients with PTSD. Various explanations have been put forth for this discrepancy between subjective experience and objective evidence. Some suggest that altered sleep perception, rather than sleep disturbance *per se*, may be the key problem in PTSD[76]. Others turn to discrepancies in methodology. Woodward[147] suggests three sources of error that could interfere with the observation of sleep continuity and depth deficits in PTSD patients when using traditional polysomnographic analyses. Firstly, standard polysomnographic analysis filters out awakenings or movements lasting less than 15 s. Secondly, traditionally scoring short-wave sleep involves spectral estimation based on visual analysis of the EEG waveform, which is very difficult to standardize. Thirdly, the sleep laboratory itself may exert an ameliorative effect on sleep in PTSD. Under such circumstances, absence of sleep disturbances in the laboratory does not mean that these sleep disturbances do not occur. An ideal experiment would observe patients with PTSD for a longer time period (1 week to 1 month), at home, with computer-aided spectral estimation of digitized EEG data, without filtering out movements and awakenings of less than 15 s. Although such an experiment would be ideal, like many ideal experiments, it is much harder to realize.

Neuroimaging techniques challenge the integration of ever more complex neurobiological models across many neurochemical systems and structures into a cohesive understanding of PTSD. With further advances in brain imaging, it will soon be possible to better delineate acute and long-term stress-induced changes in central and peripheral nervous system functioning. *In vivo* neuroimaging of nightmares is not yet possible, but an interesting alternative exists. Traumatic recall paradigms, which induce flashbacks through the presentation of combat-related sounds, slides, or smells, may show which brain areas are involved in the nightmares. A number of reports on the neuroimaging of NREM sleep[148,149] and REM sleep[148] have been published. Perhaps neuroimaging data on nightmares will be available in the near future.

Whether the sleep disturbances experienced by patients with PTSD are real or imagined, the presence of sleep disturbances in their subjective experience demands treatment. Whereas the treatment of choice previously included benzodiazepine medications or tricyclic antidepressants, of late a larger variety of medications is available to treat disordered sleep in PTSD. Selective serotonin reuptake inhibitors, imipramine, temazepam, trazadone, mirtazapine and prazosin have all been shown to be effective in reducing nightmares and sleep disturbances. Other studies report the use of antipsychotics (olanzapine) and anticonvulsants (gabapentin and topiramate) to augment SSRIs in reducing nightmares and night terrors in PTSD. Behavioral therapies such as progressive muscle relaxation, exposure therapy, imagery rehearsal therapy, sleep hygiene, sleep restriction, hypnotic procedures and EMDR are also effective in reducing disordered sleep in PTSD. However, there is a dearth of double-blind placebo-controlled studies with adequate study samples.

Our understanding of PTSD and its symptoms is constantly being updated, and an increasing knowledge base is developing. Theories concerning predisposing and sustaining factors, etiology and treatment all profit from the surge of publications in neurobiology. Currently a discrepancy exists in subjective experience and objective research findings on disordered sleep in PTSD. Nonetheless, considering the relatively high prevalence of PTSD and its important co-morbidity with other sleep and psychiatric disorders, an assessment of sleep disturbances should be part of a clinician's routine inquiry in order to limit chronicity and maladjustment following traumatic events. Both pharmacological and psychological treatments are available and have proved effective in treating the sleep disturbances associated with PTSD. It is unlikely that traumatic events will ever cease in human society, and sleep disturbances will continue to affect a considerable portion of those exposed to them. Fortunately, the ever-increasing treatment possibilities considerably relieve the deleterious effects of trauma for many individuals with PTSD.

APPENDIX: DIAGNOSTIC CRITERIA FOR POST-TRAUMATIC STRESS DISORDER

(1) The person has been exposed to a traumatic event in which both of the following were present:

  (a) The person experienced, witnessed or was confronted with an event or events that involved actual or threatened death or serious injury, or a threat to the physical integrity of self or others;

  (b) The person's response involved intense fear, helplessness or horror.

Note: In children, this may be expressed by disorganized or agitated behavior instead.

(2) The traumatic event is persistently re-experienced in at least one of the following ways:

  (a) Recurrent and intrusive distressing recollections of the event, including images, thoughts or perceptions;

Note: In young children, repetitive play may occur in which themes or aspects of the trauma are expressed.

  (b) Recurrent distressing dreams of the event;

Note: In children there may be frightening dreams without recognizable content.

  (c) Acting or feeling as if the traumatic event were recurring (includes a sense of reliving the experience, illusions, hallucinations and dissociative flashback episodes, including those that occur on awakening or when intoxicated).

Note: In young children, trauma-specific reenactment may occur.

  (d) Intense psychological distress at exposure to internal or external cues that symbolize or resemble an aspect of the traumatic event;

  (e) Physiological reactivity on exposure to internal or external cues that resemble an aspect of the traumatic event.

(3) Persistent avoidance of stimuli associated with the trauma and numbing of general responsiveness (not present before the trauma), as indicated by three (or more) of the following:

  (a) Efforts to avoid thoughts, feelings or conversations associated with the trauma;

  (b) Efforts to avoid activities, places or people that arouse recollections of the trauma;

  (c) Inability to recall an important aspect of the trauma;

  (d) Markedly diminished interest or participation in significant activities;

  (e) Feeling of detachment or estrangement from others;

  (f) Restricted range of affect (e.g. unable to have loving feelings);

  (g) Sense of a foreshortened future (e.g. does not expect to have a career, marriage, children or a normal life span).

(4) Persistent symptoms of increased arousal (not present before the trauma), as indicated by two (or more) of the following:

    (a) Difficulty falling or staying asleep;

    (b) Irritability or outbursts or anger;

    (c) Difficulty concentrating;

    (d) Hypervigilance;

    (e) Exaggerated startle response.

(5) Duration of the disturbance (symptoms in Criteria 2, 3 and 4) is more than 1 month.

(6) The disturbance causes clinically significant distress or impairment in social, occupational or other important areas of functioning;

    (a) Specify if: **Acute**: if duration of symptoms is less than 3 months
    Chronic: if duration of symptoms is 3 months or more

    (b) Specify if: **With delayed onset**: if onset of symptoms is at least 6 months after the stressor.

Reproduced from *DSM-IV Diagnostic and Statistical Manual of Mental Disorders*, 4th edn. Copyright American Psychiatric Association, 1994.

References

1. Benca RM, Obermeyer WH, Thisted RA, *et al.* Sleep and psychiatric disorders. A meta-analysis. *Arch Gen Psychiatry* 1992;49:651–68; discussion 669–70

2. Benca RM. Sleep in psychiatric disorders. *Neurol Clin* 1996;14:739–64

3. Koren D, Arnon I, Lavie P, *et al.* Sleep complaints as early predictors of posttraumatic stress disorder: a 1-year prospective study of injured survivors of motor vehicle accidents. *Am J Psychiatry* 2002;159:855–7

4. Ohayon MM, Shapiro CM. Sleep disturbances and psychiatric disorders associated with posttraumatic stress disorder in the general population. *Compr Psychiatry* 2000;41:469–78

5. Kessler RC, Sonnega A, Bromet E, *et al.* Posttraumatic stress disorder in the National Comorbidity Survey. *Arch Gen Psychiatry* 1995; 52:1048–60

6. Breslau N, Kessler RC, Chilcoat HD, *et al.* Trauma and posttraumatic stress disorder in the community: the 1996 Detroit Area Survey of Trauma. *Arch Gen Psychiatry* 1998;55:626–32

7. Weisaeth L, Eitinger L. Posttraumatic stress phenomena: common themes across wars, disasters, and traumatic events. In Wilson JP, Raphael B, eds. *International Handbook of Traumatic Stress Syndromes.* New York: Plenum, 1993:69–77

8. Wilson JP. The historical evolution of PTSD diagnostic criteria: from Freud to DSM-IV. *J Trauma Stress* 1994;7:681–98

9. Saigh PA, Bremner JD. The history of posttraumatic stress disorder. In Saigh PA, Bremner JD, eds. *Posttraumatic Stress Disorder: A Comprehensive Text.* Needham Heights, MA: Allyn and Bacon, 1999

10. Kleber RJ, Figley CR, Gersons BPR, eds. *Beyond Trauma: Cultural and Societal Dynamics.* New York: Plenum, 1995

11. APA. *Diagnostic and Statistical Manual of Mental Disorders*, 3rd edn. Washington, DC: American Psychiatric Association, 1980

12. WHO. *ICD-10 Classification of Mental and Behavioral Disorders: Clinical Descriptions and Diagnostic Guidelines.* Geneva: World Health Organization, 1992

13. APA. *Diagnostic and Statistical Manual of Mental Disorders*, 4th edn. Washington, DC: American Psychiatric Association, 1994

14. Mellman TA, Randolph CA, Brawman-Mintzer O, *et al.* Phenomenology and course of psychiatric disorders associated with combat-related posttraumatic stress disorder. *Am J Psychiatry* 1992;149:1568–74

15. Engdahl B, Dikel TN, Eberly R, *et al.* Comorbidity and course of psychiatric disorders in a community sample of former prisoners of war. *Am J Psychiatry* 1998;155:1740–5

16. Newport DJ, Nemeroff CB. Neurobiology of posttraumatic stress disorder. *Curr Opin Neurobiol* 2000;10:211–18

17. Friedman MJ, Charney DS, Deutch AY. *Neurobiological and Clinical Consequences of Stress: from Normal Adaptation to PTSD.* New York: Raven Press, 1995

18. Charney DS, Grillon CC, Bremner JD. The neurobiological basis of anxiety and fear: circuits, mechanisms, and neurochemical interactions (Part I). *Neuroscientist* 1998;4:35–44

19. Charney DS, Grillon CC, Bremner JD. The neurobiological basis of anxiety and fear: circuits, mechanisms, and neurochemical

interactions (Part II). *Neuroscientist* 1998;4: 122–32

20. Charney DS, Bremner JD. Psychobiology of posttraumatic stress disorder. In Bunney S, Nestler E, Charney DS, eds. *Neurobiology of Psychiatric Disorders*. New York: Oxford University Press, 1999:494–517

21. McEwen BS. The neurobiology of stress: from serendipity to clinical relevance. *Brain Res* 2000;886:172–89

22. Charney DS, Deutch AY, Krystal JH, *et al.* Psychobiologic mechanisms of posttraumatic stress disorder. *Arch Gen Psychiatry* 1993;50: 295–305

23. Bremner JD, Narayan M, Staib LH, *et al.* Neural correlates of memories of childhood sexual abuse in women with and without posttraumatic stress disorder. *Am J Psychiatry* 1999;156:1787–95

24. Bremner JD, Staib LH, Kaloupek D, *et al.* Neural correlates of exposure to traumatic pictures and sound in Vietnam combat veterans with and without posttraumatic stress disorder: a positron emission tomography study. *Biol Psychiatry* 1999;45:806–16

25. Daly RJ. Samuel Pepys and post-traumatic stress disorder. *Br J Psychiatry* 1983;143:64–8

26. Kardiner A. *The Traumatic Neuroses of War*. New York: Hober, 1941

27. Grinker RG, Spiegel JP. *Men under Stress*. Philadelphia: Blackstone, 1945

28. Bradner T. Psychiatric observations among Finish children during the Russia-Finnish War of 1939–1940. *Nervous Child* 1943;2: 313–19

29. Neylan TC, Marmar CR, Metzler TJ, *et al.* Sleep disturbances in the Vietnam generation: findings from a nationally representative sample of male Vietnam veterans. *Am J Psychiatry* 1998;155:929–33

30. Silva C, McFarlane J, Soeken K, *et al.* Symptoms of post-traumatic stress disorder in abused women in a primary care setting. *J Womens Health* 1997;6:543–52

31. Mellman TA, Kulick-Bell R, Ashlock LE, *et al.* Sleep events among veterans with combat-related posttraumatic stress disorder. *Am J Psychiatry* 1995;152:110–15

32. Mellman TA, David D, Kulick-Bell, R, *et al.* Sleep disturbance and its relationship to psychiatric morbidity after Hurricane Andrew. *Am J Psychiatry* 1995;152:1659–63

33. David D, Mellman TA, Mendoza LM, *et al.* Psychiatric morbidity following Hurricane Andrew. *J Trauma Stress* 1996;9:607–12

34. Schreuder BJ, Kleijn WC, Rooijmans HG. Nocturnal re-experiencing more than forty years after war trauma. *J Trauma Stress* 2000; 13:453–63

35. Rusch MD, Grunert BK, Sanger JR, *et al.* Psychological adjustment in children after traumatic disfiguring injuries: a 12-month follow-up. *Plast Reconstr Surg* 2000;106:1451–8; discussion 1459–60

36. Ellis A, Stores G, Mayou R. Psychological consequences of road traffic accidents in children. *Eur Child Adolesc Psychiatry* 1998;7:61–8

37. Kravitz M, McCoy BJ, Tompkins DM, *et al.* Sleep disorders in children after burn injury. *J Burn Care Rehabil* 1993;14:83–90

38. Kinzie JD, Fredrickson RH, Ben R, *et al.* Posttraumatic stress disorder among survivors of Cambodian concentration camps. *Am J Psychiatry* 1984;141:645–50

39. Rogers P, Gray NS, Williams T, *et al.* Behavioral treatment of PTSD in a perpetrator of manslaughter: a single case study. *J Trauma Stress* 2000;13:511–19

40. Kuch K, Cox BJ. Symptoms of PTSD in 124 survivors of the Holocaust. *Am J Psychiatry* 1992;149:337–40

41. Krakow B, Sandoval D, Schrader R, *et al.* Treatment of chronic nightmares in adjudicated adolescent girls in a residential facility. *J Adolesc Health* 2001;29:94–100

42. Lavie P. Sleep disturbances in the wake of traumatic events. *N Engl J Med* 2001;345:1825–32

43. Schreuder BJ, van Egmond M, Kleijn WC, *et al.* Daily reports of posttraumatic nightmares and anxiety dreams in Dutch war victims. *J Anxiety Disord* 1998;12:511–24

44. Mellman TA, Bustamante V, Fins AI, *et al.* REM sleep and the early development of posttraumatic stress disorder. *Am J Psychiatry* 2002; 159:1696–701

45. Hartman D, Crisp AH, Sedgwick P, *et al.* Is there a dissociative process in sleepwalking and night terrors? *Postgrad Med J* 2001;77:244–9

46. Esposito K, Benitez A, Barza L, *et al.* Evaluation of dream content in combat-related PTSD. *J Trauma Stress* 1999;12:681–7

47. Hall CS, van de Castle RL. *The Content Analysis of Dreams*. New York: Appleton-Century-Crofts, 1966

48. Kramer M, Schoen LS, Kinney L. Psychological and behavioral features of disturbed dreamers. *Psychiatr J Univ Ott* 1984;9: 102–6

49. Kramer M, Schoen LS, Kinney L. *et al.* Nightmares in Vietnam veterans. *J Am Acad Psychoanal* 1987;15:67–81

50. Lee KA, Vaillant GE, Torrey WC, *et al.* A 50-year prospective study of the psychological sequelae of World War II combat. *Am J Psychiatry* 1995;152:516–22

51. Yehuda R, Schmeidler J, Giller EL, *et al.* Relationship between posttraumatic stress disorder characteristics of holocaust survivors and

their adult offspring. *Am J Psychiatry* 1998; 155:841–3

52. Van Oyen Witvliet C. Traumatic intrusive imagery as an emotional memory phenomenon: a review of research and explanatory information processing theories. *Clin Psychol Rev* 1997;17:509–36

53. Kline NA, Rausch JL. (1985). Olfactory precipitants of flashbacks in posttraumatic stress disorder: case reports. *J Clin Psychiatry* 1985; 46:383–4

54. Vermetten E, Schmahl C, Siddiq S, *et al.* Neural correlates of olfactory induced emotions in veterans with and without combat related posttraumatic stress disorder. 2003;in review

55. Frankel FH. The concept of flashbacks in historical perspective. *Int J Clin Exp Hypn* 1994;42:321–36

56. Grillon C, Southwick SM, Charney DS. The psychobiological basis of posttraumatic stress disorder. *Mol Psychiatry* 1996;1:278–97

57. Hellawell SJ, Brewin CR. A comparison of flashbacks and ordinary autobiographical memories of trauma: cognitive resources and behavioural observations. *Behav Res Ther* 2002;40:1143–56

58. Conway MA, Anderson SJ, Larsen SR, *et al.* The formation of flashbulb memories. *Mem Cognit* 1994;22:326–43

59. Davidson PS, Glisky EL. Is flashbulb memory a special instance of source memory? Evidence from older adults. *Memory* 2002;10:99–111

60. Sierra M, Berrios GE. Flashbulb memories and other repetitive images: a psychiatric perspective. *Compr Psychiatry* 1999;40:115–25

61. Southwick SM, Bremner D, Krystal JH, *et al.* Psychobiologic research in post-traumatic stress disorder. *Psychiatr Clin North Am* 1994; 17:251–64

62. Vermetten E, Bremner JD. Circuits and systems in stress. I. Preclinical studies. *Depress Anxiety* 2002;15:126–47

63. Vermetten E, Bremner JD. Circuits and systems in stress. II. Applications to neurobiology and treatment in posttraumatic stress disorder. *Depress Anxiety* 2002;16:14–38

64. Van der Kolk BA, Fisler RE. The biologic basis of posttraumatic stress. *Prim Care* 1993;20: 417–32

65. Glaubman HM, Miculincer M, Porat A, *et al.* Sleep of chronic post-traumatic patients. *J Trauma Stress* 1990;3:255–63

66. Kaminer H, Lavie P. Sleep and dreaming in Holocaust survivors. Dramatic decrease in dream recall in well-adjusted survivors. *J Nerv Ment Dis* 1991;179:664–9

67. Ross RJ, Ball WA, Dinges DF, *et al.* Rapid eye movement sleep disturbance in posttraumatic stress disorder. *Biol Psychiatry* 1994;35:195–202

68. Ross RJ, Ball WA, Dinges DF, *et al.* Motor dysfunction during sleep in posttraumatic stress disorder. *Sleep* 1994;17:723–32

69. Reist C, Kauffmann CD, Chicz-Demet A, *et al.* REM latency, dexamethasone suppression test, and thyroid releasing hormone stimulation test in posttraumatic stress disorder. *Prog Neuropsychopharmacol Biol Psychiatry* 1995;19: 433–43

70. Mellman TA, Nolan B, Hebding J, *et al.* A polysomnographic comparison of veterans with combat-related PTSD, depressed men, and non-ill controls. *Sleep* 1997;20:46–51

71. Woodward SH, Arsenault NJ, Murray C, *et al.* Laboratory sleep correlates of nightmare complaint in PTSD inpatients. *Biol Psychiatry* 2000;48:1081–7

72. Mellman TA, Kumar A, Kulick-Bell R, *et al.* Nocturnal/daytime urine noradrenergic measures and sleep in combat-related PTSD. *Biol Psychiatry* 1995;38:174–9

73. Dagan Y, Lavie P, Bleich A. Elevated awakening thresholds in sleep stage 3–4 in war-related post-traumatic stress disorder. *Biol Psychiatry* 1991;30:618–22

74. Pitman RK, Orr SP, Shalev AY, *et al.* Psychophysiological alterations in post-traumatic stress disorder. *Semin Clin Neuropsychiatry* 1999;4:234–41

75. Hurwitz TD, Mahowald MW, Kuskowski M, *et al.* Polysomnographic sleep is not clinically impaired in Vietnam combat veterans with chronic posttraumatic stress disorder. *Biol Psychiatry* 1998;44:1066–73

76. Klein E, Koren D, Arnon I, *et al.* No evidence of sleep disturbance in post-traumatic stress disorder: a polysomnographic study in injured victims of traffic accidents. *Isr J Psychiatry Relat Sci* 2002;39:3–10

77. Peters J, van Kammen, DP, van Kammen WB, *et al.* Sleep disturbance and computerized axial tomographic scan findings in former prisoners of war. *Compr Psychiatry* 1990;31: 535–9

78. Phan KL, Wager T, Taylor SF, *et al.* Functional neuroanatomy of emotion: a meta-analysis of emotion activation studies in PET and fMRI. *Neuroimage* 2002;16:331–48

79. Krakow B, Melendrez D, Warner TD, *et al.* To breathe, perchance to sleep: sleep-disordered breathing and chronic insomnia among trauma survivors. *Sleep Breath* 2002;6:189–202

80. Hobson JA. *Sleep*. New York: Scientific American Library, 1995

81. Ross RJ, Ball WA, Sullivan KA, *et al.* Sleep disturbance as the hallmark of posttraumatic stress disorder. *Am J Psychiatry* 1989;146:697–707

82. Stickgold R, Hobson JA, Fosse R, *et al.* Sleep, learning, and dreams: off-line memory reprocessing. *Science* 2001;294:1052–7

83. Lavie P, Katz N, Pillar G, *et al*. Elevated awaking thresholds during sleep: characteristics of chronic war-related posttraumatic stress disorder patients. *Biol Psychiatry* 1998;44:1060–5

84. Mellman TA. Psychobiology of sleep disturbances in posttraumatic stress disorder. *Ann NY Acad Sci* 1997;821:142–9

85. Dow BM, Kelsoe JR Jr, Gillin JC. Sleep and dreams in Vietnam PTSD and depression. *Biol Psychiatry* 1996;39:42–50

86. Paige SR, Reid GM, Allen MG, *et al*. Psycho physiological correlates of posttraumatic stress disorder in Vietnam veterans. *Biol Psychiatry* 1990;27:419–30

87. Neylan TC, Fletcher DJ, Lenoci M, *et al*. Sensory gating in chronic posttraumatic stress disorder: reduced auditory P50 suppression in combat veterans. *Biol Psychiatry* 1999;46: 1656–64

88. Steriade M, Datta S, Pare D, *et al*. Neuronal activities in brain-stem cholinergic nuclei related to tonic activation processes in thalamocortical systems. *J Neurosci* 1990;10:2541–59

89. Southwick SM, Bremner JD, Rasmusson A, *et al*. Role of norepinephrine in the pathophysiology and treatment of post-traumatic stress disorder. *Biol Psychiatry* 1999; 46:1192–204

90. Bremner JD, Vermetten E. Stress and development: behavioral and biological consequences. *Dev Psychopathol* 2001;13:473–89

91. Woodward SH, Friedman MJ, Bliwise DL. Sleep and depression in combat-related PTSD inpatients. *Biol Psychiatry* 1996;39:182–92

92. Husain AM, Miller PP, Carwile ST. REM sleep behavior disorder: potential relationship to post-traumatic stress disorder. *J Clin Neurophysiol* 2001;18:148–57

93. Bremner JD. Neuroimaging studies in post-traumatic stress disorder. *Curr Psychiatry Rep* 2002;4:254–63

94. Villarreal G, King CY. Brain imaging in post-traumatic stress disorder. *Semin Clin Neuropsychiatry* 2001;6:131–45

95. Grossman R, Buchsbaum MS, Yehuda R. Neuroimaging studies in post-traumatic stress disorder. *Psychiatr Clin North Am* 2002;25: 317–40, vi

96. Rauch SL, Shin LM. Functional neuroimaging studies in posttraumatic stress disorder. *Ann NY Acad Sci* 1997;821:83–98

97. Hull AM. Neuroimaging findings in post-traumatic stress disorder. Systematic review. *Br J Psychiatry* 2002;181:102–10

98. Bremner JD, Randall P, Scott TM, *et al*. MRI-based measurement of hippocampal volume in patients with combat-related posttraumatic stress disorder. *Am J Psychiatry* 1995;152: 973–81

99. Bremner JD, Randall P, Vermetten E, *et al*. Magnetic resonance imaging-based measurement of hippocampal volume in posttraumatic stress disorder related to childhood physical and sexual abuse – a preliminary report. *Biol Psychiatry* 1997;41:23–32

100. Hobson JA, McCarley RW. The brain as a dream state generator: an activation–synthesis hypothesis of the dream process. *Am J Psychiatry* 1977;134:1335–48

101. Brimstedt L, Ansehn B. Tricyclic antidepressive agents are effective in the treatment of sleep disorders among torture and war victims. *Lakartidningen* 1991;88:521–2, 524

102. Robert R, Meyer WJ 3rd, Villarreal C, *et al*. An approach to the timely treatment of acute stress disorder. *J Burn Care Rehabil* 1999;20: 250–8

103. Viola J, Ditzler T, Batzer W, *et al*. Pharmacological management of post-traumatic stress disorder: clinical summary of a five-year retrospective study, 1990–1995. *Mil Med* 1997;162:616–19

104. Mellman TA, Byers PM, Augenstein JS. Pilot evaluation of hypnotic medication during acute traumatic stress response. *J Trauma Stress* 1998;11:563–9

105. Neylan TC, Metzler TJ, Schoenfeld FB, *et al*. Fluvoxamine and sleep disturbances in post-traumatic stress disorder. *J Trauma Stress* 2001;14:461–7

106. De Boer M, Op den Velde W, Falger PJ, *et al*. Fluvoxamine treatment for chronic PTSD: a pilot study. *Psychother Psychosom* 1992;57: 158–63

107. Gillin JC, Smith-Vaniz A, Schnierow B, *et al*. An open-label, 12-week clinical and sleep EEG study of nefazodone in chronic combat-related posttraumatic stress disorder. *J Clin Psychiatry* 2001;62:789–96

108. Warner MD, Dorn MR, Peabody CA. Survey on the usefulness of trazodone in patients with PTSD with insomnia or nightmares. *Pharmacopsychiatry* 2001;34:128–31

109. Stein MB, Kline NA, Matloff JL. Adjunctive olanzapine for SSRI-resistant combat-related PTSD: a double-blind, placebo-controlled study. *Am J Psychiatry* 2002;159:1777–9

110. Hamner MB, Brodrick PS, Labbate LA. Gabapentin in PTSD: a retrospective, clinical series of adjunctive therapy. *Ann Clin Psychiatry* 2001;13:141–6

111. Berlant J, van Kammen DP. Open-label topiramate as primary or adjunctive therapy in chronic civilian posttraumatic stress disorder: a preliminary report. *J Clin Psychiatry* 2002; 63:15–20

112. Taylor F, Raskind MA. The alpha1-adrenergic antagonist prazosin improves sleep and

nightmares in civilian trauma posttraumatic stress disorder. *J Clin Psychopharmacol* 2002; 22:82–5

113. Raskind MA, Peskind ER, Kanter ED, *et al*. Reduction of nightmares and other PTSD symptoms in combat veterans by prazosin: a placebo-controlled study. *Am J Psychiatry* 2003;160:371–3

114. Lewis JD. Mirtazapine for PTSD nightmares. *Am J Psychiatry* 2002;159:1948–9

115. Brophy MH. Cyproheptadine for combat nightmares in post-traumatic stress disorder and dream anxiety disorder. *Mil Med* 1991; 156:100–1

116. Gupta S, Austin R, Cali LA, *et al*. Nightmares treated with cyproheptadine. *J Am Acad Child Adolesc Psychiatry* 1998;37:570–2

117. Gupta S, Popli A, Bathurst E, *et al*. Efficacy of cyproheptadine for nightmares associated with posttraumatic stress disorder. *Compr Psychiatry* 1998;39:160–4

118. Rijnders RJ, Laman DM, Van Diujn H. Cyproheptadine for posttraumatic nightmares. *Am J Psychiatry* 2000;15:1524–5

119. Jacobs-Rebhun S, Schnurr PP, Friedman MJ, *et al*. Posttraumatic stress disorder and sleep difficulty. *Am J Psychiatry* 2000;157: 1525–6

120. Hertzberg MA, Feldman ME, Beckham JC, *et al*. Open trial of nefazodone for combat-related posttraumatic stress disorder. *J Clin Psychiatry* 1998;59:460–4

121. Mellman TA, David D, Barza L. Nefazodone treatment and dream reports in chronic PTSD. *Depress Anxiety* 1999;9:146–8

122. Davidson JR, Weisler RH, Malik ML, *et al*. Treatment of posttraumatic stress disorder with nefazodone. *Int Clin Psychopharmacol* 1998;13:111–13

123. Davidson *et al*. 1998b

124. Zisook S, Chentsova-Dutton YE, Smith-Vaniz A, *et al*. Nefazodone in patients with treatment-refractory posttraumatic stress disorder. *J Clin Psychiatry* 2000;61:203–8

125. Gillin *et al*. 2001b

126. Hertzberg MA, Feldman ME, Beckham JC, *et al*. Trial of trazodone for posttraumatic stress disorder using a multiple baseline group design. *J Clin Psychopharmacol* 1996;16:294–8

127. Berlant JL. Topiramate in posttraumatic stress disorder: preliminary clinical observations. *J Clin Psychiatry* 2001;62(Suppl 17):60–3

128. Raskind MA, Dobie DJ, Kanter ED, *et al*. The alpha1-adrenergic antagonist prazosin ameliorates combat trauma nightmares in veterans with posttraumatic stress disorder: a report of 4 cases. *J Clin Psychiatry* 2000;61: 129–33

129. Raskind MA, Thompson C, Petrie EC, *et al*. Prazosin reduces nightmares in combat veterans with posttraumatic stress disorder. *J Clin Psychiatry* 2002;63:565–8

130. Peskind ER, Bonner LT, Hoff DJ, Raskind MA. Prazosin reduces trauma-related nightmares in older men with chronic posttraumatic stress disorder. *J Geriatr Psychiatry Neurol* 2003;16:165–71

131. Rothbaum BO, Mellman TA. Dreams and exposure therapy in PTSD. *J Trauma Stress* 2001;14:481–90

132. Evans FJ. Hypnosis and sleep: the control of altered states of awareness. *Ann NY Acad Sci* 1977;296:162–74

133. Rabois D, Batten SV, Keane TM. Implications of biological findings for psychological treatments of post-traumatic stress disorder. *Psychiatr Clin North Am* 2002;25:443–62, viii

134. Allodi FA. Assessment and treatment of torture victims: a critical review. *J Nerv Ment Dis* 1991;179:4–11

135. Krakow B, Johnston L, Melendrez D, *et al*. An open-label trial of evidence-based cognitive behavior therapy for nightmares and insomnia in crime victims with PTSD. *Am J Psychiatry* 2001;158:2043–7

136. Stickgold R. EMDR: a putative neurobiological mechanism of action. *J Clin Psychol* 2002; 58:61–75

137. Shapiro F. EMDR 12 years after its introduction: past and future research. *J Clin Psychol* 2002;58:1–22

138. Rogers S, Silver SM. Is EMDR an exposure therapy? A review of trauma protocols. *J Clin Psychol* 2002;58:43–59

139. Krakow B, Hollifield M, Johnston L, *et al*. Imagery rehearsal therapy for chronic nightmares in sexual assault survivors with posttraumatic stress disorder: a randomized controlled trial. *J Am Med Assoc* 2001;286: 537–45

140. Forbes D, Phelps A, McHugh T. Treatment of combat-related nightmares using imagery rehearsal: a pilot study. *J Trauma Stress* 2001; 14:433–42

141. Morin CM, Culbert JP, Schwartz SM. Nonpharmacological interventions for insomnia: a meta-analysis of treatment efficacy. *Am J Psychiatry* 1994;151:1172–80

142. Hassard A. Reverse learning and the physiological basis of eye movement desensitization. *Med Hypotheses* 1996;47:277–82

143. Krakow B, Melendrez D, Johnson L, *et al*. Sleep-disordered breathing, psychiatric distress, and quality of life impairment in sexual assault survivors. *J Nerv Ment Dis* 2002;190:442–52

144. Lopez HH, Bracha AS, Bracha HS. Evidence based complementary intervention for insomnia. *Hawaii Med J* 2002;61: 192, 213.

145. Krakow BJ, Melendrez DC, Johnston LG, *et al*. Sleep dynamic therapy for Cerro Grande Fire evacuees with posttraumatic stress symptoms: a preliminary report. *J Clin Psychiatry* 2002;63:673–84

146. Bremner JD, Brett E. Trauma-related dissociative states and long-term psychopathology in posttraumatic stress disorder. *J Trauma Stress* 1997;10:37–49

147. Woodward SH. Neurobiological perspectives on sleep in post-traumatic stress disorder. In Friedman MJ, Charney AY, eds. *Neurobiological and Clinical Consequences of Stress: From Normal Adaptation to PTSD.* Philadelphia: Lippincot-Raven Publishers, 1995

148. Kjaer TW, Law I, Wiltschiotz G, *et al*. Regional cerebral blood flow during light sleep – a H(2)(15)O-PET study. *J Sleep Res* 2002;11: 201–7

149. Smith MT, Perlis ML, Chengazi VU, *et al*. Neuroimaging of NREM sleep in primary insomnia: a Tc-99-HMPAO single photon emission computed tomography study. *Sleep* 2002;25:325–35

21

Sleep and general neurology

Steven L. Meyers

Disorders of sleep are ubiquitous in general neurological practice. Realistically speaking, most common neurological disorders are associated with sleep disturbances, either related to pain, immobility, the effects of medications, or related to the pathophysiology of the underlying disease. At times the sleep disturbance may be the most troublesome and debilitating aspect of the illness, from the point of view of either the patient or the family. There may be difficulty determining whether an abnormal behavior during sleep represents a sleep disorder or paroxysmal neurological event such as a seizure or movement disorder. Not only can sleep disorders complicate or coexist with neurological disease, there is growing evidence to indicate that certain sleep disorders may predispose to or be risk factors for the development of neurological disease, specifically cerebrovascular disease. This chapter reviews the common sleep disorders seen in general neurological practice, including movement disorders, epilepsy, cerebrovascular disease and headache.

SLEEP AND MOVEMENT DISORDERS

The relationship between movement disorders and sleep is two-fold. First, many of the classic movement disorders such as Parkinson's disease may be complicated at some point with disruption of normal sleep; and second,

certain movement disorders present as sleep problems. In addition, episodic neurological disorders, epilepsy being a good example, often involve abnormal motor activity during sleep. These movements can result in diagnostic confusion and need to be considered in any differential diagnosis of abnormal movements occurring during sleep. The relationship between epilepsy and sleep is reviewed in the next section.

Sleep disorders in persons with movement disorders

Parkinson's disease

Parkinson's disease is a common neurological disorder primarily affecting the elderly. The condition is characterized by the cardinal signs of resting tremor, bradykinesia or slowness of movement, cogwheel rigidity and loss of postural reflexes. Additional features may include depression and progressive dementia. A variety of sleep difficulties may be seen at any stage of the illness. The cause of Parkinson's disease remains unknown. Pre- and postzygotic genetic aberrations, environmental toxins and degenerative factors may all contribute. The underlying pathophysiology involves loss of dopamine-containing neurons in the substantia nigra, with subsequent loss of the dopamine content in the basal ganglia. Whereas loss of neurons in the substantia nigra seems to relate to the cardinal motor features of the disease, involvement of other brain regions and neurotransmitter systems may underlie the sleep problems *per se*. Reductions in the number of serotonergic neurons in the dorsal raphe, cholinergic neurons in the pedunculopontine nucleus and noradrenergic neurons in the locus ceruleus may relate to these sleep changes[1,2].

The sleep disturbances characteristic of Parkinson's disease can be broadly grouped into three categories. First, the motor disturbance of Parkinson's disease may directly interrupt sleep. The stiffness and immobility may make it difficult for patients to move in bed, resulting in both difficulty falling asleep and frequent awakenings. On occasion, tremor may be severe enough to interrupt sleep. Second, the medications used to treat Parkinson's disease can cause insomnia, vivid dreaming and nocturnal hallucinations. Third, Parkinson's disease can be associated with specific sleep disorders such as rapid eye movement (REM) sleep behavior disorder (RBD) and periodic limb movement disorder, which will be discussed later. Finally, depression and dementia, which frequently complicate Parkinson's disease, exacerbate these problems and are associated with sleep disruption *per se*.

Treatment of the sleep disorders can be quite complicated, as not infrequently treatment may produce its own problems with sleep. Frequently, trial and error may be necessary, as may be the need for re-evaluation. Difficulty falling asleep or frequent arousals that seem to be related to immobility, stiffness or tremor may respond to bedtime dosing with L-dopa or dopamine agonists. Unfortunately, these medications may be accompanied by nocturnal hallucinations, nightmares and agitation. In other patients reduction of nighttime medications may be necessary to eliminate nocturnal agitation or hallucinations. Specific sleep disorders such as REM behavior disorder and periodic limb movement disorder can be treated as in a patient without Parkinson's disease and will be discussed later in this chapter.

Other Parkinsonian syndromes

A variety of other degenerative neurological diseases exist which are much less common than Parkinson's disease. These conditions are frequently referred to as Parkinsonian in nature, as they share the core features of akinesia and rigidity with Parkinson's disease. These disorders share many of the same sleep problems with Parkinson's disease although specific disorders may be associated with unique features. These disorders are discussed only briefly. Progressive supranuclear palsy is frequently associated with insomnia[3]. Polysomnography demonstrates absent sleep spindles and decreased amounts of REM sleep associated with increased amounts of slow waves during REM. The Shy–Drager syndrome and olivopontocerebellar atrophy are associated with RBD. Olivopontocerebellar atrophy has also been associated with absent REM and stage 4 sleep and increased frequency of both central and obstructive sleep apnea[4].

Tourette's syndrome

Tourette's syndrome is a childhood-onset, neurological disorder characterized by multiple motor and vocal tics. By definition the age of onset is prior to age 21. Tourette's syndrome can be associated with obsessive–compulsive disorder and attention-deficit–hyperactivity disorder (ADHD). The etiology is unknown, but a genetic etiology is most likely.

Tourette's syndrome is frequently associated with sleep disorders. Sleepwalking, sleeptalking, night terrors, nightmares and insomnia have all been reported to be more common in Tourette's syndrome patients than in controls[5,6]. Whether these sleep problems are inherent to the syndrome or are related to the frequently co-morbid condition of ADHD is not certain.

The medications used to treat Tourette's syndrome and the co-morbid conditions can also affect sleep. The stimulants used to treat ADHD can result in insomnia. Neuroleptics used to suppress tics tend to be sedating and can produce daytime sleepiness.

Table 21.1[7]   Diagnostic criteria for restless legs syndrome (International Restless Legs Syndrome Study Group, 1995)

Essential features	*Common but not essential*
1. Desire to move the legs usually caused by or accompanied by uncomfortable or unpleasant sensations in the legs 2. The urge to move begins during periods of rest or inactivity 3. The urge to move or unpleasant sensation is at least partially alleviated by movement 4. The symptoms must be worse in the evening or at night	1. Sleep disturbance 2. Periodic limb movements 3. Progressive course 4. Response to dopaminergic drugs 5. Positive family history

Movement disorders presenting as sleep disorders

There are a number of conditions characterized by abnormal, involuntary movements that interfere with sleep. While many of these disorders occur commonly in individuals with other movement disorders as described above, they can all occur in the absence of other neurological diseases. Some of these disorders are very common in the general population and as a group they are under-recognized and under-diagnosed. Some may pose diagnostic dilemmas being confused with epilepsy and, therefore, treated inappropriately.

Restless legs syndrome

Restless legs syndrome (RLS) was first described in the 17th century by the English physician Thomas Willis. The International Restless Legs Syndrome Study Group has published diagnostic criteria which include essential and supportive features (Table 21.1)[7]. The primary symptom is an unpleasant, at times painful, sensation in the legs at rest. The discomfort is described as any combination of cramps, pins and needles, drawing sensations, and occasionally shooting pains. These abnormal sensations worsen or may be present only later in the day or night. Typically a patient will move the legs or walk about to alleviate the discomfort. Most patients complain of difficulty falling asleep because of discomfort, though an occasional individual reports falling asleep easily only to awaken multiple times nightly because of the abnormal sensations. In more severe cases discomfort may occur whenever the person is at rest, making attending the theater or watching movies difficult.

RLS is one of the most common sleep disorders, with recent surveys indicating that 10–15% of the population may suffer some degree of this condition[8]. RLS affects people of all ages, although age of onset is typically between the ages of 20 and 40. Prevalence increases with age.

RLS has been reported in association with other medical conditions. Whether the underlying illness causes the RLS or not is a matter of some debate. RLS is reported to occur more frequently in persons with peripheral neuropathy, although this observation may reflect the high incidence of peripheral neuropathy in the elderly population[9]. No specific type of neuropathy is associated with RLS. Examination of patients with RLS for the presence of neuropathy is called for, but extensive diagnostic testing such as nerve conduction studies are rarely indicated.

Iron deficiency anemia is also more common in RLS patients[10]. Treatment with iron supplements leads to improvement in some patients[11]. Screening for iron deficiency with serum ferritin levels seems reasonable, but empiric treatment with iron supplementation in the absence of documented iron deficiency is not recommended. RLS is

Table 21.2 Drugs used to treat restless legs syndrome

Drug	Typical dose range	Adverse effects
Dopamine agonists		
Pramipexole	0.125–1.5 mg qHS	nausea, orthostasis, hallucinations
Ropinirole	0.25–5 mg qHS	
Pergolide	0.1–1 mg qHS	
Bromocriptine	2.5–10 mg qHS	
Dopamine precursors		
Levodopa with carbidopa	25/100–50/200 qHS	rebound, augmentation, nausea, hallucinations
Benzodiazepines		
Clonazepam	0.5–2.0 mg qHS	daytime drowsiness, tolerance
Temazepam	15–30 mg qHS	
Lorazepam	1–4 mg qHS	
Opiates		
Oxycodone	5–10 mg qHS may need to repeat during night	daytime drowsiness, tolerance, constipation
Propoxyphene	50–200 mg qHS	
Codeine	15–60 mg qHS	
Anticonvulsants		
Carbamazepine	200–400 mg qHS	bone marrow suppression, nausea, dizziness
Gabapentin	100–800 mg qHS	drowsiness, dizziness

associated with uremia and hemodialysis[12] in a significant number of patients[13]. Less well-documented associations include fibromyalgia[14], magnesium deficiency[15], rheumatoid arthritis[16] and childhood ADHD[17]. Medications including lithium carbonate, tricyclic antidepressants and serotonin reuptake inhibitors may induce or exacerbate symptoms. This is particularly important to remember, as many patients are prescribed these antidepressants to treat insomnia, which may be due to RLS.

The diagnosis of RLS can usually be made based on history. When the diagnosis is not clear or when other sleep disorders coexist, polysomnography should be considered. In view of the above associations it is reasonable to obtain iron, ferritin, magnesium and vitamin B_{12} levels. Careful clinical examination to exclude peripheral neuropathy should be performed in all patients, whereas electrodiagnostic testing should not be performed in the absence of clinical findings to suggest neuropathy.

RLS responds to four classes of medication. Dopaminergic agents, benzodiazepines, opioids and anticonvulsant medications have all demonstrated efficacy in this condition (Table 21.2). Initial treatment should be with a dopaminergic agent. Dopaminergic agents include dopamine agonists and L-dopa. Dopamine agonists are the preferred agents, as L-dopa has a tendency to produce early morning restlessness and to exacerbate periodic limb movements. Additionally, many people treated with L-dopa begin to experience RLS symptoms earlier in the day, a phenomenon referred to as augmentation[18]. Dopamine agonists do not appear to cause these problems. The older agonists (bromocriptine and pergolide) can be difficult to tolerate, owing to nausea and orthostatic hypotension. The newer agents pramipexole and ropinirole are better tolerated and have become the initial treatment of choice[19,20].

The benzodiazepines, including clonazepam, lorazepam and temazepam, have demonstrated efficacy in alleviating RLS

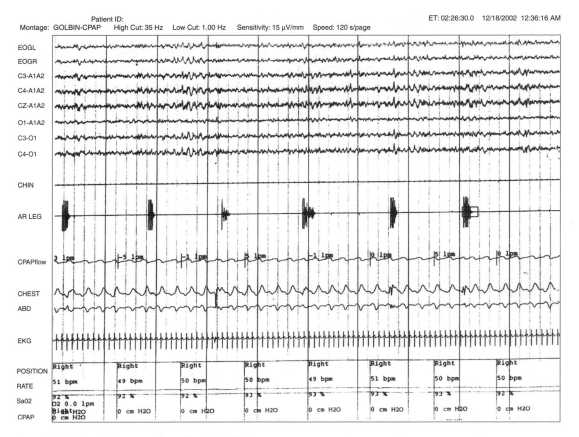

Figure 21.1 Typical presentation of periodic limb movements, stage 2 non-rapid eye movement sleep

symptoms[21]. However, these agents are potentially habit forming and can result in excessive daytime drowsiness, thus making them less attractive. Benzodiazepines have been associated with falls in the elderly and may also exacerbate obstructive sleep apnea. Clonazepam is the next option in persons unable to tolerate dopaminergic agents.

In the original description of RLS by Thomas Willis, symptom amelioration by opioids was noted. A variety of opiates are helpful, albeit with the usual concern over abuse and addiction. In the absence of a history of abuse, however, the risks appear to be very low. Indeed, the addition of a small dose of an opiate at bedtime can be quite helpful[22,23] in those individuals who do not respond adequately to dopaminergic agents or benzodiazepines.

The anticonvulsant gabapentin can be effective, particularly when dysesthetic pain is a prominent feature[24]. The lack of drug interaction makes gabapentin an attractive option in the elderly who may be taking a number of other medications. Carbamazepine has also been found to be effective in some studies[25] but overall it appears less effective than other alternatives. It may be particularly helpful in eliminating lancinating pain when this is present.

Periodic limb movements during sleep

This condition is closely linked to RLS. While most patients with RLS demonstrate periodic limb movements during sleep (PLMS), this can occur in the absence of RLS and thus represents a distinct disorder (Figure 21.1). Like

RLS, the prevalence of PLMS increases with age and may be found in up to 44% of persons above age 65.

PLMS consists of rhythmic movements of the lower extremities of variable intensity. The movements are brief but can occur in succession lasting from minutes to hours. Movements are most common early in sleep, though they may persist throughout the night. Not infrequently these movements are asymptomatic but they can cause nocturnal arousals leading to excessive daytime sleepiness. At times it may be the bed partner who is most bothered by the movements. Treatment is the same as for RLS.

REM sleep behavior disorder

RBD is a fascinating disorder consisting of violent motor behaviors during REM sleep. This abnormal activity can result in injury to either the patient or the bed partner.

Normal REM sleep is associated with muscle atonia affecting all voluntary muscles except the extraocular muscles and diaphragm. This state appears to be mediated by active inhibition originating in the region of the locus ceruleus of the brainstem. RBD appears to represent failure of this inhibitory mechanism resulting in abnormal motor activity during REM sleep.

RBD can occur during ethanol withdrawal[26] and is also reported in patients receiving a variety of antidepressants[27,28]. Most cases, however, are either idiopathic or associated with other neurological disorders, primarily degenerative conditions. RBD may be the initial symptom of several Parkinsonian conditions including idiopathic Parkinson's disease, progressive supranuclear palsy and multisystem atrophy. RBD may antedate the more typical motor symptoms of these disorders by many years. In one series, approximately one-third of men originally diagnosed as having idiopathic RBD ultimately developed Parkinson's disease[29].

RBD is associated with a variety of other conditions[30]. Persons with narcolepsy have RBD at a higher incidence than expected.

RBD has been seen in Tourette's syndrome, Alzheimer's disease, amyotrophic lateral sclerosis and diffuse Lewy body dementia. Additionally, the use of cholinergic medications in Alzheimer's disease has been reported to induce RBD.

Clonazepam is usually dramatically effective at treating RBD. Bedtime doses of 0.5–1.0 mg are effective for the vast majority of patients. Tolerance does not appear to be a problem. Relapses typically occur after missing even a single evening dose. In those patients who do not respond to or cannot tolerate clonazepam, useful alternatives include desipramine, imipramine, clonidine, L-dopa, melatonin and gabapentin[30].

SLEEP AND EPILEPSY

Sleep and seizures are closely related phenomena. It is well established that the occurrence of seizures is increased during sleep and that sleep deprivation can trigger seizures. This is why sleep deprivation is a routinely utilized activating procedure in electroencephalography (EEG) laboratories and why obtaining sleep is so important during routine EEG studies. It is also well established that sleep deprivation can increase the frequency of parasomnias, many of which can be difficult to differentiate from seizures on clinical grounds alone. On the other hand, seizures can disturb normal sleep architecture, leading to complaints of insomnia or excessive daytime sleepiness.

Parasomnias and seizures both produce abnormal behaviors that can closely mimic each other. They both have many features in common. They begin suddenly and are usually associated with some degree of confusion or alteration in awareness. Persons with parasomnias and seizures are typically amnestic for the events. The age of onset while quite variable is most common during childhood and adolescence for both disorders. The types of abnormal behaviors overlap considerably making diagnosis based solely on description of the behaviors difficult.

Epidemiology

The incidence of epilepsy varies based upon the population being studied. There is a higher incidence in developing countries compared to developed countries. Younger populations tend to have a higher incidence. In the United States there are approximately 2.5 million persons diagnosed with epilepsy. The lifetime incidence is between 1.3 and 3.1% of the population[31]. Approximately 40% of seizures are generalized and the remaining 60% are focal or localization-related. The incidence of parasomnias is more difficult to measure. The prevalence of sleepwalking is between 3 and 10% and that of RBD is estimated as 0.5%[32,33].

Sleep disorders confused with epilepsy

Several normal sleep behaviors can be confused with seizure activity. Sleep starts, consisting of sudden jerks of the body, commonly occur during the transition from waking into sleep. Occasionally, sleep starts may consist of visual phenomena, such as flashes of light or even brief visual hallucinations, loud banging sounds, or unusual sensory phenomena such as pain or floating sensations without any motor activity[34,35]. Nightmares are unpleasant, frightening dreams that usually occur during REM sleep. Nightmares are not typically associated with motor activity or vocalizations. Unlike other parasomnias, nightmares usually fully awaken the sleeper and there is memory of the event[36].

In a person not known to be suffering from epilepsy the complaint of hypersomnia would not ordinarily lead to an evaluation for seizures. However, nocturnal seizures may only result in arousals, which if frequent enough, may cause sleep fragmentation to a degree severe enough to produce excessive daytime sleepiness. These seizures may not be associated with prominent motor activity and therefore, may escape detection[37]. Many patients being treated for epilepsy complain of excessive sleepiness. This is very frequently attributed to the anticonvulsant medications the patient is taking, leading to dosage adjustments or medication changes, with the resultant possibility of poor seizure control and/or non-compliance. One study looking at objective measures of sleepiness in children with epilepsy found no correlation between the degree of sleepiness and whether they were taking medication or not[38].

The parasomnias as previously discussed have the most similarity with epilepsy and create the greatest diagnostic challenges. Disorders of arousal are the most common parasomnias and include confusional arousals, sleepwalking and sleep terrors. Similar to many seizure disorders, disorders of arousal are associated with a positive family history, tend to occur early in the night during stage 3 and 4 non-REM sleep, and tend to begin in childhood and lessen with age[39–41]. Disorders of arousal and seizures can mimic each other and can be difficult to differentiate. It is a misconception that the preservation of awareness during a nocturnal spell indicates a sleep disorder or psychogenic condition[42]. Seizures manifesting as episodes of laughing (gelastic epilepsy) or crying (dacrystic epilepsy) can easily be confused with confusional arousals, night terrors, or psychogenic spells[43,44].

RBD and PLMS were discussed above in relation to movement disorders. It is easy to see how these conditions could be confused with a nocturnal seizure or psychogenic spells. Alternatively, particularly in someone with a predisposing movement disorder, a nocturnal seizure could be misdiagnosed as RBD or PLMS[45,46].

Enuresis or bedwetting is a common childhood problem that typically resolves with age. It can be the manifestation of both physical and psychological problems. Enuresis may be the only sign of a nocturnal seizure[47]. Particularly in adults, the sudden appearance of enuresis should prompt an evaluation for nocturnal seizures.

Seizures confused with sleep disorders

The behavioral manifestation of nocturnal seizures can be quite bizarre and can mimic parasomnias or psychogenic conditions. Seizures that arise from the frontal lobes in particular can produce unusual behaviors and may be impossible to detect with routine surface EEG[48]. Frontal lobe seizures have been documented to produce such unusual activities as running, bicycling, vocalizations and swearing. Frontal lobe epilepsy occurring exclusively during sleep is easily misdiagnosed as RBD or a psychogenic spell[49–52].

Episodic nocturnal wanderings is a condition in which patients walk about, vocalize and may display violent behaviors. The clinical description may be confused with sleepwalking or sleep terrors. This condition responds to anticonvulsants. Some patients, though not all, have abnormal waking EEGs and it is likely that this condition represents an epileptic condition[32,53,54].

Nocturnal paroxysmal dystonia consists of nocturnal episodes of tonic limb movements that can recur repetitively throughout the night. On occasion the movements can be associated with vocalizations or laughing. Interictal EEGs are normal. EEGs during the episode are commonly obscured by movement artifact and typically clear epileptiform activity is not seen[55]. Carbamazepine is usually very effective at controlling the episodes. While uncertainty exists the evidence is mounting that nocturnal paroxysmal dystonia is an epileptic disorder[56,57].

Evaluation and management

As has already been stated, the differentiation between nocturnal seizures and sleep disorders based upon clinical phenomenology may be impossible. Both types of disorder must be considered in the differential of recurrent, stereotyped behaviors no matter how bizarre they may appear. The assumption that behaviors that do not fit into standard diagnostic categories represent psychiatric disorders must be avoided. Routine and sleep-deprived EEGs are frequently inadequate for evaluating sleep-related disorders. As stated earlier, many nocturnal epileptic conditions may have normal interictal studies.

All-night polysomnographic evaluation utilizing video recording and complete seizure montages may be necessary for proper diagnosis (Figure 21.2). Specific diagnosis is critical in order to choose appropriate therapy and to avoid unnecessary and potentially toxic drugs and to avoid the improper labeling of a patient with epilepsy with the unfortunate, attendant psychosocial ramifications.

Most parasomnias do respond to therapy if the correct diagnosis is made. Treatment of nocturnal seizures is the same as for other forms of epilepsy and is outside the scope of this chapter. Treatment of the various parasomnias and other sleep disorders is discussed in the appropriate chapters of this text.

SLEEP AND STROKE

It has been demonstrated that the incidence of stroke is greatest in the morning hours and that the first hour after waking is the period of greatest risk[58,59]. Many physiological functions demonstrate circadian fluctuations which affect the vascular system. Endocrine function, thermoregulation, respiratory control, heart rhythm, hematological and immune function, and drug metabolism all undergo diurnal fluctuations which have widespread physiological effects, and in conjunction with other risk factors may precipitate vascular events.

During non-REM sleep there is an increase in parasympathetic tone resulting in decreased heart rate, respiratory rate, peripheral vascular resistance, blood pressure and cardiac output. REM sleep is characterized by variability in sympathetic and parasympathetic activity resulting in fluctuations of these same parameters. In a tenuous vascular system these alterations may be enough to trigger a stroke.

In addition to these hemodynamic changes, hemostatic changes favoring thrombosis also occur in the early morning hours. Fibrinolytic activity is decreased and platelet aggregability is enhanced in the morning[60,61].

Sleep-related breathing disorders are increasingly appearing to be significant risk

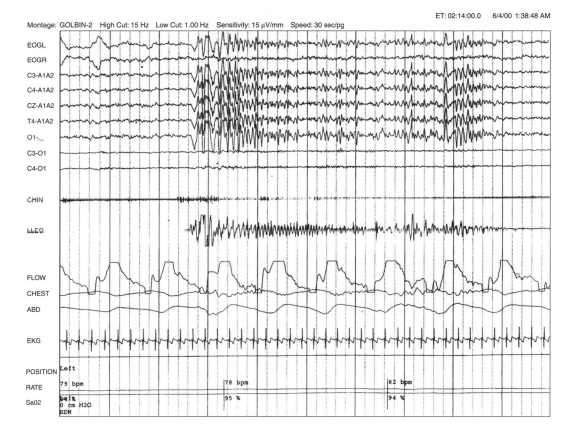

Figure 21.2 Paroxysmal theta and delta activity in rapid eye movement stage

factors for stroke. Snoring, which is frequently associated with sleep-disordered breathing (SDB), has been found to be a risk factor for stroke, hypertension and ischemic heart disease[62,63]. In one study the relative risk for stroke in persons with snoring and sleep apnea was approximately 2. The risk correlated with the severity of the apnea, approaching 10 in the most severely affected persons[63]. Treatment of SDB may improve hypertensive control[64], and in one study tracheostomy appeared to lower the incidence of stroke in a population of patients with sleep apnea[65].

The mechanism by which SDB contributes to stroke risk is a matter of conjecture at this time. Several mechanisms have been postulated, although none have been proved. As has already been mentioned, SDB and obstructive sleep apnea are associated with hypertension[66,67], a well-established risk factor for stroke. Another mechanism by which obstructive sleep apnea may contribute to stroke risk is through its association with myocardial infarction and arrythmia[62]. It has been postulated that sleep apnea may contribute to diabetes mellitus, increased platelet aggregability and decreased fibrinolysis, all of which would increase the risk of thrombosis[68]. Periods of apnea can result in either hypotension or hypertension, cardiac arrhythmias and decreased cardiac output. The hypoxia and hypercarbia that occur during apnea can lead to cerebral vasodilatation and increased intracranial pressure[69]. The combination of hypotension and cerebral vasodilatation results in decreased cerebral perfusion pressure. In the presence of a compromised vascular bed these changes could result in stroke.

It is commonplace today to screen patients for vascular risk factors on a regular basis. Evaluating blood pressure and cardiac rhythm, auscultating for carotid bruits and heart murmurs, and obtaining blood for glucose, lipid and coagulation studies have become routine. Screening for SDB has not. Screening may be as simple as questioning the patient about whether they snore regularly or inquiring from bed partners information regarding apnea at night. The growing evidence would suggest that it is time to add SDB and obstructive sleep apnea to the list of treatable vascular risk factors.

SLEEP AND HEADACHE

Headache is one of the most common complaints in neurological practice and in general medicine. The association between sleep and headache is well established. Sleep affects headache in a variety of ways, both positively and negatively. Certain sleep disorders may cause headache or worsen headache in someone prone to them. Specific headache types may be more common during sleep or may occur exclusively at night. Sleep complaints are very common in the chronic headache population and contribute significantly to poor quality of life[70,71].

The most commonly seen and well-known effect of sleep on headache is the amelioration of migraine by sleep. Even brief naps may be sufficient to completely abort migraine attacks[72].

Sleep deprivation frequently results in non-specific headache[73]. Any alteration in the usual sleep pattern can trigger headaches, particularly migraine. Over-sleeping, under-sleeping and schedule changes can all trigger migraine[74].

Cluster headache is an idiopathic headache disorder characterized by severe, unilateral attacks of pain typically centered in or around one orbit. The attacks are associated with a variety of autonomic symptoms including ptosis, unilateral tearing, conjunctival injection and nasal congestion or rhinorrhea on the side of the pain. Cluster attacks are brief, lasting between 15 and 180 minutes. They can occur from once to several times daily particularly at night. In any given individual they tend to occur at similar times daily and frequently awaken the patient from sleep, typically coinciding with the first REM period[75,76].

Hypnic headache is a recently described, rare headache disorder occurring in older patients. The headache is moderately severe and awakens the patient after sleeping for a few hours. Attacks can recur during the night and can interrupt daytime naps[77,78]. Etiology is unknown. Treatment with nighttime doses of lithium carbonate usually controls the attacks[77]. If not tolerated, caffeine before sleep has been reported to be useful[78].

Headache sufferers have a higher incidence of other conditions which may be linked through common pathophysiological factors. Depression and anxiety are frequently co-morbid with headache, particularly in daily headache sufferers. These individuals commonly report insomnia and early morning wakenings[79,80]. Fibromyalgia is another common syndrome seen in the chronic headache population that is associated with insomnia and poor-quality sleep[80].

Medications are another common cause of sleep disturbance in the headache population. Sleep disturbances can be seen with many of the medications used to prevent migraine. Perhaps more insidious is the over-use of symptomatic medications which is frequently seen in the chronic headache population. The over-use of analgesics, ergots, barbiturates and caffeine-containing compounds frequently leads to rebound headaches[81]. The short duration of action of these medications results in the common scenario of a patient routinely being awakened in the early morning hours with a severe headache and needing to take additional doses of the offending agent in order to fall back to sleep[80].

Headache can also be a symptom of a primary sleep disorder. Morning headaches are seen frequently in obstructive sleep apnea and snoring[82]. These headaches tend to be dull and generalized, usually lasting for 1–2 h after awakening[83]. The mechanism is felt to be related to cerebral hypoxia, hypercapnia and cerebral vasodilatation as well as sleep fragmentation[84]. Periodic limb movement disorder has also been reported to cause headaches[80], presumably owing to sleep fragmentation.

CONCLUSION

Understanding and recognizing the inter-relationship between neurological disease and sleep disorders is critical to the successful management of these common disorders. Failure to recognize the importance of dis-ordered sleep leads to suboptimal treatment and reduced function and quality of life for the patient and frequently for the family as well. Misdiagnosis can lead to inappropriate and potentially harmful treatments, such as treating a parasomnia as epilepsy. Incorrectly attributing complaints of excessive fatigue to the neurological disease or medication effects

can lead to unnecessary adjustments in therapy and less optimal disease management. Inadequate treatment leads to greater dis-ability and in some cases may result in loss of employment or other social roles. Treatment of an underlying sleep disorder can result in improved symptom control, as in patients with chronic headache or Parkinson's disease. Failure to recognize and look for sleep dis-orders can result in a missed opportunity to prevent illness, as in the case of sleep apnea and the possible prevention of hypertension and subsequent vascular disease.

Many neurological diseases are not curable at the present time. Some may be preventable. Frequently the goal of neurological therapy is to maximize functioning, increase independence and to delay future disability whenever possible, and always to improve the quality of life of persons with neurological disease. Any opportunity to do so should not be missed. The importance of proper sleep to neurological functioning cannot be overestimated.

References

1. Jellinger K. Pathology of parkinsonism. In Fahn S, Marsden CD, Jenner P, et al. eds. *Recent Developments in Parkinson's Disease*. New York, NY: Raven Press, 1986:33–66

2. Zweig RM, Jankel WR, Hedreen JC, et al. The pedunculopontine nucleus in Parkinson's disease. *Ann Neurol* 1989;26:41–6

3. Aldrich MS, Foster NL, White RF, et al. Sleep abnormalities in progressive supranuclear palsy. *Ann Neurol* 1989;25:577–81

4. Neil JF, Holzer BC, Spiker DG, et al. EEG sleep alterations in olivopontocerebellar degenera-tion. *Neurology* 1980;30:660–2

5. Barabas G, Matthews WS, Ferrari M. Somnambulism in children with Tourette's syn-drome. *Dev Med Child Neurol* 1984;26:457–60

6. Allen RP, Singer HS, Brown JE, et al. Sleep disorders in Tourette syndrome: a primary or unrelated problem? *Pediatr Neurol* 1992;8: 275–80

7. The International Restless Legs Syndrome Study Group. Towards a better definition of the restless legs syndrome. *Mov Disord* 1995;10: 634–42

8. Lavigne G, Montplaisir J. Restless legs syn-drome and sleep bruxism: prevalence and association among Canadians. *Sleep* 1994;17: 739–43

9. Ondo W, Jankovic J. Restless legs syndrome: clinicoetiologic correlates. *Neurology* 1996;47: 1435–41

10. Matthews WB. Iron deficiency and restless legs syndrome. *Br Med J* 1976;1:898

11. O'Keeffe ST, Gavin K, Lavan JN. Iron status and restless legs syndrome in the elderly. *Age Ageing* 1994;23:200–3

12. Trenkwalder C, Walters AS, Hening W. Periodic limb movements and restless legs syn-drome. *Neurol Clin* 1996;14:629–49

13. Wetter TC, Stiasny K, Kohnen R, et al. polysomnographic sleep measures in patients with uremic and idiopathic restless legs syn-drome. *Mov Disord* 1998;13:820–4

14. Yunus MB, Aldag JC. Restless legs syndrome and leg cramps in fibromyalgia syndrome: a controlled study. *Br Med J* 1996;312:1339

15. Popoviciu L, Asgian B, Popoviciu DP, et al. Clinical, EEG, electromyographic and

polysomnographic studies in restless legs syndrome caused by magnesium deficiency. *Rom J Neurol Psychiatr* 1993;31:55–61

16. Reynolds G, Blake DR, Pall HS, *et al*. Restless legs syndrome and rheumatoid arthritis. *Br Med J* 1986;292:659–60

17. Picchieti DL, Walters AS. Restless legs syndrome and periodic limb movement disorders in children and adolescents. *Child Adolesc Clin North Am* 1996;5:729–40

18. Allen RP, Earley CJ. Augmentation of the restless legs syndrome with carbidopa/levodopa. *Sleep* 1996;19:205–13

19. Montplaisir J, Nicolas A, Denesle R, *et al*. Restless legs syndrome improved by pramipexole: a double-blind randomized trial. *Neurology* 1999;52:938–43

20. Ondo W. Ropinirole for restless legs syndrome. *Mov Disord* 1999;14:138–40

21. Hening W, Allen R, Earley C, *et al*. The treatment of restless legs syndrome and periodic limb movement disorder: an American Academy of Sleep Medicine Review. *Sleep* 1999; 22:970–99

22. Walters AS, Wagner ML, Hening WA, *et al*. Successful treatment of the idiopathic restless legs syndrome in a randomized double-blind trial of oxycodone versus placebo. *Sleep* 1993; 16:327–32

23. Trzepacz PT, Violette EJ, Sateia MJ. Response to opioids in three patients with restless legs syndrome. *Am J Psychiatry* 1984;141:993–5

24. Mellick GA, Mellick LB. Successful treatment of restless legs syndrome with gabapentin. *Sleep* 1995;24:290

25. Telstad W, Sorensen O, Larsen W, *et al*. Treatment of the restless legs syndrome with carbamazepine: a double blind study. *Br Med J* 1984;89:1–7

26. Tachibana M, Tanaka K, Hishikawa Y, *et al*. A sleep study of acute psychotic states due to alcohol and meprobamate addiction. *Adv Sleep Res* 1975;2:177–205

27. Besset A. Effect of antidepressants on human sleep. *Adv Biosci* 1978;21:141–8

28. Schutte S, Doghramji K. REM behavior disorder seen with venlafaxine (Effexor). *Sleep Res* 1996;25:364

29. Schenk CH, Bundlie SR, Mahowald MW. Delayed emergence of a parkinsonian disorder in 38% of 29 older men initially diagnosed with idiopathic rapid eye movement sleep behavior disorder. *Neurology* 1996;46:388–93

30. Mahowald MW, Schenk CH. REM sleep parasomnias. In Kryger MH, Roth T, Dement WC, eds. *Principles and Practice of Sleep Medicine*, 3rd edn. New York: WB Saunders, 2000: 724–41

31. Hauser WA. Overview: epidemiology, pathology, and genetics. In Engel J Jr, Pedley TA, eds. *Epilepsy: A Comprehensive Textbook*, Vol. 1. Philadelphia, PA: Lippincott-Raven, 1997:11–14

32. Ohayon MM, Caulet M, Priest RG. Violent behavior during sleep. *J Clin Psychiatry* 1997; 58:369–76

33. Goldin PR, Rosen RC. Epidemiology of nine parasomnias in young adults. *Sleep Res* 1997; 26:367

34. Lugaresi E, Coccagna G, Cirignotta F. Phenomena occurring during sleep onset in man. In Popoviciu L, Asgian B, Badiu G, eds. *Sleep 1978. Fourth European Congress on Sleep Research, Tirgu-Mures*. Basel, Switzerland: S. Karger, 1980:24–7

35. Shouse MN, Mahowald MW. Epilepsy and sleep disorders. In Kryger MH, Roth T, Dement WC, eds. *Principles and Practice of Sleep Medicine*, 3rd edn. New York: WB Saunders, 2000:712

36. Diagnostic Classification Steering Committee. *International Classification of Sleep Disorders: Diagnostic and Coding Manual*. Rochester: American Sleep Disorders Association, 1990

37. Zucconi M, Oldani A, Ferini-Stambi L, *et al*. Nocturnal paroxysmal arousals with motor behaviors during sleep: frontal lobe epilepsy or parasomnias? *J Clin Neurophysiol* 1997;14: 513–22

38. Palm L, Anderson H, Elmqvist D, *et al*. Daytime sleep tendency before and after discontinuation of antiepileptic drugs in preadolescent children with epilepsy. *Epilepsia* 1992;33:687–91

39. Abe K, Amatomi M, Oda N. Sleepwalking and recurrent sleep talking in children of childhood sleepwalkers. *Am J Psychiatry* 1984;141: 800–1

40. Fiher C, Kahn E, Edwards A, *et al*. A psychophysiological study of nightmares and night terrors, I: physiological aspects of the stage 4 night terror. *J Nerv Ment Dis* 1973;157:75–98

41. Kales A, Soldatos C, Bixler EO, *et al*. Hereditary factors in sleepwalking and night terrors. *Br J Psychiatry* 1980;137:111–18

42. Ebner A, Dinner DS, Noachtar S, *et al*. Automatisms with preserved responsiveness: a lateralizing sign in psychomotor seizures. *Neurology* 1995;45:61–4

43. Armstrong SC, Watters MR, Pearce JW. A case of nocturnal gelastic epilepsy. *Neuropsychiatr Neuropsychol Behav Neurol* 1990;3:213–16

44. Luciano D, Devinsky O, Perrine K. Crying seizures. *Neurology* 1993;43:2113–17

45. D'Cruz OF, Vaughn BV. Nocturnal seizures mimic REM behavior disorder. *Am J Electroneurodiagn Technol* 1997;37:258–64

46. Lugaresi E, Coccagna G, Mantovani M, *et al.* The evolution of different types of myoclonus during sleep: a polygraphic study. *Eur Neurol* 1970;4:321–31

47. Guilleninault C, Silvestri R. Disorders of arousal and epilepsy during sleep. In Sterman MB, Shouse MN, Passouant PP, eds. *Sleep and Epilepsy.* New York: Academic Press, 1982: 513–31

48. Billiard M, Echenne B, Besset A, *et al.* All-night polygraphic recordings in the child with suspected epileptic seizures, in spite of normal routine and post-sleep deprivation EEGs. *Electoencephalogr Clin Neurophysiol* 1981;11: 450–60

49. Stores G, Zaiwalla Z. Misdiagnosis of frontal lobe complex partial seizures in children. *Epileptol* 1989;17:288–90

50. Fusco L, Iani C, Faedda MT, *et al.* Mesial frontal lobe epilepsy: a clinical entity not sufficiently described. *J Epilepsy* 1990;3:123–35

51. Stores G, Zaiwalla Z, Bergel N. Frontal lobe complex partial seizures in children: a form of epilepsy at particular risk of misdiagnosis. *Dev Med Child Neurol* 1991;33:998–1009

52. Sussman NM, Jackel RA, Kaplan LR, *et al.* Bicycling movements as a manifestation of complex partial seizures of temporal lobe origin. *Epilepsia* 1989;30:527–31

53. Masselli RA, Rosenberg RS, Spire J-P. Episodic nocturnal wanderings in non-epileptic young patients. *Sleep* 1988;11:156–61

54. Spire J-P, Masselli R. Episodic nocturnal wandering: further evidence of an epileptic disorder. *Neurology* 1983;33(Suppl 2):215

55. Lugaresi E, Cirignotta F. Hypnogenic paroxysmal dystonia. In Sterman MB, Shouse MN, Passouant PP, eds. *Sleep and Epilepsy.* New York: Academic Press, 1982:507–11

56. Meierkord H, Fish DR, Smith SJM, *et al.* Is nocturnal paroxysmal dystonia a form of frontal lobe epilepsy? *Move Disord* 1992;1: 38–42

57. Hirsch E, Sellal F, Maton B, *et al.* Nocturnal paroxysmal dystonia: a clinical form of focal epilepsy. *Neurophysiol Clin* 1994;24:207–17

58. Wroe SJ, Sandercock P, Bamford J, *et al.* Diurnal variation in incidence of stroke: Oxfordshire community stroke project. *Br Med J* 1992;304:155–7

59. Marsh EE, Biller J, Adams HP, *et al.* Circadian variation in onset of acute ischemic stroke. *Arch Neurol* 1990;47:1178–80

60. Andreotti F, Davies GJ, Hackett DR, *et al.* Major circadian fluctuations in fibrinolytic factors and possible relevance to time of onset of myocardial infarction, sudden cardiac death and stroke. *Am J Cardiol* 1988;62:635–7

61. Trofler GH, Brezinski D, Schafer AI, *et al.* Concurrent morning increase in platelet aggregability and the risk of myocardial infarction and sudden cardiac death. *N Engl J Med* 1987;316:1514–18

62. Koskenvuo M, Kaprio J, Telakivi T. Snoring as a risk factor for ischaemic heart disease and stroke in men. *Br Med J* 1987;294:16–19

63. Palomaki H, Partinen M, Juvela S, *et al.* Snoring as a risk factor for sleep-related brain infarction. *Stroke* 1989;20:1311–15

64. Wilcox I, Grunstein RR, Hedner JA, *et al.* Effect of nasal CPAP during sleep on 24-hour blood pressure in obstructive sleep apnea. *Sleep* 1993;16:539–44

65. Partinen M, Guilleminault C. Daytime sleepiness and vascular morbidity at 7 years followup in obstructive sleep apnea patients. *Chest* 1990; 97:27–32

66. Linberg E, Janson C, Gislason T, *et al.* Snoring and hypertension. *Eur Respir J* 1998;11: 884–9

67. Nieto FJ, Young TB, Lind BK, *et al.* Association of sleep-disordered breathing, sleep apnea, and hypertension in a large community-based study. *J Am Med Assoc* 2000;283:1829–36

68. Dean RT, Wilcox I. Possible atherogenic effects of hypoxia during obstructive sleep apnea. *Sleep* 1993;16:S15–22

69. Fischer AQ, Chaudhary BA, Taormina MA, *et al.* Intracranial hemodynamics in sleep apnea. *Chest* 1992;102:1402–6

70. Passchier J, Boo M, Quaak HZA, *et al.* Health-related quality of life of chronic headache patients is predicted by the emotional component of their pain. *Headache* 1996;36:556–60

71. Rasmussen BK. Migraine and tension-type headache in a general population: precipitating factors, female hormones, sleep pattern and relation to lifestyle. *Pain* 1993;53: 65–72

72. Wilkonson M, Williams K, Leyton M. Observations on the treatment of acute attacks of migraine. *Res Clin Study Headache* 1978;6: 141–6

73. Blau JN. Sleep deprivation headache. *Cephalalgia* 1990;10:157–60

74. Paiva T, Hering-Hanit R. Headache and sleep. In Olesen J, Tfelt-Hansen P, Welch KMA, eds. *The Headaches,* 2nd edn. Philadelphia: Williams & Wilkins, 2000:969

75. Kudrow L. The pathogenesis of cluster headache. *Curr Opin Neurol* 1994;7:278–82

76. Kudrow L, McGinty DJ, Philips ER, Stevenson M. Sleep apnea in cluster headache. *Cephalalgia* 1984;4:33–8

77. Raskin NH. The hypnic headache syndrome. *Headache* 1988;28:534–6

78. Dodick DW, Mosek AC, Campbell JK. The hypnic ("alarm clock") headache syndrome. *Cephalalgia* 1998;18:152–6

79. Marazziti D, Toni C, Pedri S, *et al*. Headache, panic disorder and depression: co-morbidity or a spectrum? *Neuropsychobiology* 1995;31: 125–9

80. Paiva T, Batista A, Martins I. The relationship between headaches and sleep disturbances. *Headache* 1995;35:590–6

81. Diener HC, Dahlof CGH. Headache associated with chronic use of substances. In Olesen J, Tfelt-Hansen P, Welch KMA, eds. *The Headaches*, 2nd edn. Philadelphia: Williams & Wilkins, 2000:871–7

82. Bassiri AG, Guilleminault C. Clinical features and evaluation of obstructive sleep apnea–hypopnea syndrome. In Kryger MH, Roth T, Dement WC, eds. *Principles and Practice of Sleep Medicine*, 3rd edn. New York: WB Saunders, 2000:869–78

83. American Sleep Disorders Association. *The International Classification of Sleep Disorders of the American Sleep Disorders Association. Diagostic and Coding Manual*. Rochester, MN: American Sleep Disorders Association, 1997

84. Sahota PK, Dexter JD. Sleep and headache syndromes: a clinical review. *Headache* 1990; 30:80–4

22

Fibromyalgia syndrome, chronic fatigue syndrome and sleep

Bill McCarberg

Fibromyalgia syndrome (FMS) is a common musculoskeletal pain syndrome characterized by complaints of widespread pain. Diagnostic criteria were first established by the American College of Rheumatology (ACR) in 1990 and include widespread pain involving areas above and below the waist, the right and left sides of the body, the axial skeleton (cervical spine or anterior chest or thoracic spine or lower back), and lasting more than 3 months. In addition, the patient must have 11 or more of 18 specifically identified tender points, produced by digital pressure of at least 4 kilograms (Figure 22.1)[1]. In 1992 a consensus document on fibromyalgia was produced at the Second World Congress on Myofascial Pain and Fibromyalgia in Copenhagen. In addition to the ACR criteria, the document added a number of symptoms to the definition, including persistent fatigue, generalized morning stiffness, non-refreshing sleep, headaches, irritable bladder, dysmenorrhea, extreme sensitivity to cold, restless legs, odd patterns of numbness and tingling, and intolerance to exercise[2].

Prevalence rates of FMS in the general population range from 2 to 5%, females being affected more often than males at an approximate ratio of 9:1[3]. Multiple etiologies have been advanced – a viral infection[4], a genetic predisposition[5], hypothalamus–pituitary–adrenal axis dysregulation[6], Chiari type I malformation[7] and pain modulation abnormality[8] – among many others.

Chronic fatigue syndrome (CFS) was defined by the Center for Disease Control (CDC) in 1988 as:

(1) A new, unexplained, persistent or relapsing chronic fatigue which is not a consequence of exertion, is not resolved by bed rest, and which is severe enough to significantly reduce daily activity.

(2) The presence of four or more of the following symptoms for at least 6 months:

   (a) headache

   (b) concentration and short-term memory impairment

   (c) muscular pain

   (d) multiple joint pain not accompanied by swelling or redness

   (e) poor and unrefreshing sleep

   (f) post-exertional malaise lasting more than 24 hours

   (g) tender lymph nodes in the neck or axilla

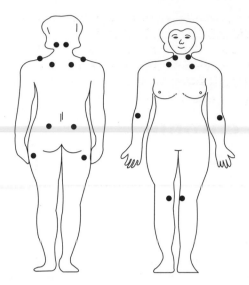

Figure 22.1   Pain points in fibromyalgia

Approximately 70% of patients who meet the CDC criteria for CFS also meet the ACR diagnostic criteria for FMS. For purposes of this chapter, FMS and CFS are discussed together and the difference between the two with regard to sleep is stressed when this distinction is either known or important.

SLEEP, FMS AND CFS

Wakefulness and awakening feeling unrefreshed are common complaints in FMS[9]. Compared to controls, FMS patients complain of perceiving their sleep to be of poor quality[10]. Reported cognitive disturbances may relate to sleep quality[11] and increasing pain[12]. Primary sleep disorders, most notably sleep apnea and periodic leg movement in sleep (PLMS) also occur in FMS patients. Sleep apnea is present in as many as 44% of men with the syndrome[13] and must be aggressively managed as symptoms may improve or disappear.

Multiple polysomnographic abnormalities are reported in FMS and CFS. Compared to healthy controls, patients have lower amounts of slow-wave sleep corrected for age, rapid eye movement (REM) sleep and total sleep time, as well as a higher number of arousals and awakenings, longer awakenings (> 10 minutes), phasic K alpha cycling and an electroencephalogram (EEG) pattern of alpha activity superimposed on delta waves known as alpha–delta anomaly[14] (Figure 22.2).

Several studies suggest that the alpha–delta anomaly may have pathophysiological implications. First reported in 1972 by Hauri and Hawkins in psychiatric patients[15] with malaise and fatigue, it was later described by Moldofsky and colleagues in FMS patients[16]. This abnormality was broadened to include alpha intrusion into all stages of non-REM sleep[17]. Alpha–delta frequency was subsequently correlated with overnight pain scores, fatigue and mood[18]. Spectral EEG patterns show more power in the higher frequency band and a decrease in the lower frequency throughout all non-REM sleep stages compared to controls[19]. Phasic alpha sleep activity (simultaneous with delta activity) correlates best with clinical manifestations[20]. The decreased power in the low-frequency range might reflect a disorder in homeostatic and circadian mechanisms during sleep and would support patients' complaints of non-restorative sleep and higher arousal rates which fragment sleep[5,21]. Daytime hypersomnolence was also linked to greater severity of FMS symptoms and to more severe polysomnographic alterations[22,23]. Although the alpha–delta anomaly is the most frequently encountered sleep abnormality found in FMS as well as CFS, inconsistent results preclude use of the results of the polysomnogram for legal or forensic purposes.

Healthy control subjects monitored in sleep laboratories were artificially aroused in stage 4 sleep using an auditory stimulus. After two nights of auditory intrusion, subjects reported muscle aching and tenderness as well as mood disturbance[11]. Disrupted slow-wave sleep without reducing total sleep or sleep efficiency increased discomfort and fatigue in healthy controls[24]. A sleep disturbance may be an important factor in the genesis of symptoms in FMS or may only be an epiphenomenon or surrogate marker for other central nervous system changes. In a

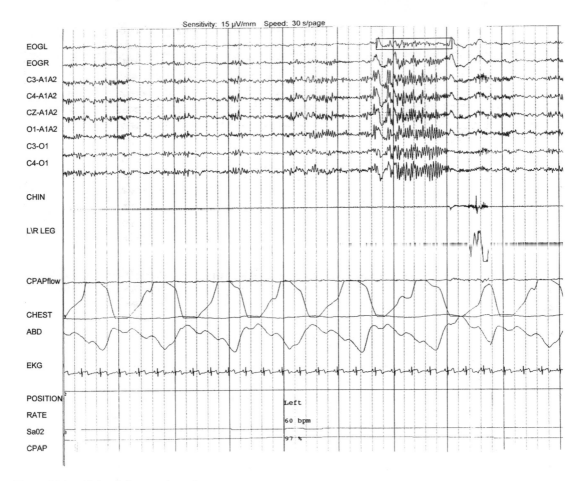

Figure 22.2 Alpha–delta wave intrusions

study looking at elicited pain during sleep, muscle and joint pain increased arousal, and increased alpha and decreased delta activities in normal controls[25].

PLMS is the presence of repetitive, stereotyped jerks in one or both legs which cause brief arousals, usually initiated by sleep. Insomnia, unrefreshing sleep and daytime hypersomnolence can be presenting complaints, symptoms that mimic many sleep complaints in FMS. Finestone and colleagues performed overnight polysomnography to determine the prevalence of PLMS in 15 FMS patients[26]. They found that 47% of the patients had PLMS; polysomnography had been necessary to establish the presence of PLMS since the patients did not report this difficulty. Treatments for these two conditions

may vary, suggesting the need to be alert to the coexistence of the syndromes.

Multiple biochemical abnormalities are present and may relate to the reported sleep disturbance. Decreased cerebrospinal fluid and serum levels of serotonin[27,28], elevated cerebrospinal fluid levels of substance P[29], distinctive disruption of the growth hormone–somatomedin C neuroendocrine axis[30], interleukin-1[31] and lower growth hormone[32] have all been reported. Serotonin may be responsible for delta sleep abnormalities[26], and substance P for arousal[28]. Growth hormone is secreted during stage 4 sleep and may relate to a nighttime deficiency. Although each of these biochemical abnormalities suggests possible treatment strategies, even therapy targeted at the supposed deficiency fails to relieve the symptoms of pain or fatigue.

Neuroimaging using regional cerebral blood flow shows decreased flow to the thalamus and caudate nucleus compared to controls[33]. These structures are involved in pain transmission and pain modulation. Ablation of the thalamus in cats results in persistent and severe insomnia[34].

EVALUATION AND TREATMENT

FMS and CFS treatment should ideally focus on underlying etiology. As noted previously, etiology is uncertain and targeted treatment would be at best speculative. A thorough history must be elicited at the outset to document the patient's sleep habits, environmental disturbances, sleep apnea and PLMS. Once a patient produces a detailed sleep diary the sleep environment can be analyzed. Common issues include widely varying sleep hours, insufficient amounts of sleep, noise from sources such as a snoring spouse or other household member, and disruptive bed partners such as a restless child. The sleep diary may lead to discussions and increased awareness of potentially negative bedtime rituals which may include elements as seemingly innocuous as reading, discussing the work day or watching television. Stimulant intake may interfere with a fragile sleep pattern (caffeine, nicotine) or a mistaken belief that alcohol will improve sleep quality. Although exercise is generally advised for most patients including those with FMS and CFS, those suffering from sleep deprivation may be wise to avoid exercise too near to bedtime, as it may increase sleep latency.

Modifying a patient's behaviors can have positive results; symptomatic relief may be the only approach where definitive pathology is not present and may be more effective than immediately resorting to pharmacological agents. Addressing many of the deficiencies and problems mentioned above may be accomplished through straightforward behavior modification. A patient may quickly enhance the quality of sleep through minor changes, such as establishing a regular schedule for both going to bed and time for rising. Alcohol, caffeine and food should be restricted close to bedtime. The sleep environment should be arranged to be conducive to sleep, minimizing, as far as possible, any disruptive elements such as the snoring family member or restless child. In order to reinforce the concept that the purpose for being in bed is to allow for needed sleep, a patient should not engage in activities such as reading or watching television while in bed. A darkened room with a comfortable temperature also increases the likelihood of restful sleep.

While pharmacotherapy may help sleep, currently no medication is available to improve the EEG sleep arousal disorder including phasic (alpha–delta), tonic alpha non-REM sleep disorder[35]. Traditional hypnotic agents, while helpful in initiating and maintaining sleep and reducing daytime tiredness, do not provide restorative sleep or reduce pain. Tricyclic drugs such as amitriptyline and cyclobenzaprine may not have a continuing benefit beyond 1 month for reducing pain and may precipitate or intensify PLMS. Serotonin reuptake inhibitors are frequently prescribed for the mood disorders accompanying FMS and CFS, but may exacerbate abnormalities already present in the deep stages of sleep. Trazodone at 150 mg to doubles stage 3 and 4 sleep, reducing alpha activity without affecting sleep latency, efficiency or percentage of wake time[36]. Zopiclone increases delta sleep, improves subjective sleep quality and decreases awakening during the night[37]. While 90% of patients reported improvement on zopiclone, 60% of the placebo group also improved, casting doubt on its efficacy. Trials with amitriptyline have been encouraging on self-reported sleep[38,39]. Treatment with both amitriptyline and fluoxetine result in significant improvement in general sleep scores and are superior to either drug alone[40].

CONCLUSION

Fibromyalgia syndrome and chronic fatigue syndrome affect the quality of life for patients. The most distressing symptom for many is disrupted sleep. Multiple aberrations in sleep have been identified from subjective complaints of poor sleep quality to a variety of polysomnographic abnormalities, the most consistent of which is the alpha–delta sleep anomaly. Special attention to sleep history, improved sleep hygiene and judicious use of pharmacological agents can ameliorate symptoms but will not cure the syndromes or change the observed sleep abnormality.

References

1. Wolfe F, Smythe HA, Yunus MB, et al. The American College of Rheumatology 1990 Criteria for the Classification of Fibromyalgia: report of the multicenter criteria committee. Arthritis Rheum 1990;33:160–72
2. Consensus document on FMS: the Copenhagen declaration. Lancet 1992;340
3. Wolfe F, Anderson J, Ross K, et al. Prevalence of characteristics of fibromyalgia in the general population. Arthritis Rheum 1993;36:S48
4. Buckwald D, et al. A chronic illness characterized by fatigue, neurologic and immunologic disorders and active human herpesvirus type 6 infection. Ann Intern Med 1992;116:103–13
5. Pellegrino M. Familial occurrence of primary fibromyalgia. Arch Physical Med Rehab 1989;70
6. Goldenberg D. Fibromyalgia and chronic fatigue syndrome. J Musculoskeletal Pain 1994;2:51–5
7. Moldofsky H. Rheumatic pain modulation syndrome. Abstract #953, presented at the 1997 American College of Rheumatology Meeting
8. Goldstein J. Betrayal of the Brain: the Neurological Basis for FMS and CFS and Related Neural Network Disorders. New York: Haworth Medical Press, 1996
9. Campbell SM, Clark S, Tindall EA, et al. Clinical characteristics of fibrositis I: a "blinded" controlled study of symptoms and tender points. Arthritis Rheum 1983;26:817–25
10. Schaefer KM. Sleep disturbances and fatigue in women with fibromyalgia and chronic fatigue syndrome. JOGNN 1995;24:229–33
11. Jennum P, Drewes AM, Andreasen A, et al. Sleep and other symptoms in primary fibromyalgia and in healthy controls. J Rheumatol 1993;20:1756–9
12. Affleck G, Urrows S, Tennen H, et al. Sequential daily relations of sleep, pain intensity, and attention to pain among women with fibromyalgia. Pain 1996;68:363–8
13. May KP, West SG, Baker MR, et al. Sleep apnea in male patients with the fibromyalgia syndrome. Am J Med 1993;94:505–8
14. Shapiro CM, Devins GM, Hussain MRG. Sleep problems in patients with medical illness. Br Med J 1993;306:1532–5
15. Hauri P, Hawkins D. Alpha-delta sleep. Electroencephalogr Clin Neurophysiol 1973;34;233–7
16. Moldofsky H, Scarisbrick P, England R, et al. Musculoskeletal symptoms and non-REM sleep disturbance in patients with "fibrositis syndrome" and healthy subjects. Psychosom Med 1975;37:341–51
17. Anch AM, Lue FA, MacLean AW, et al. Sleep physiology and psychological aspects of fibrositis (fibromyalgia) syndrome. Can J Exp Psychol 1991;45:179–84
18. Moldofsky H, Lue FA. The relationship of alpha delta EEG sleep frequencies to pain and mood in "fibrositis" patients with chlorpromazine and L-tryptophan. Electroencephalogr Clin Neurophysiol 1980;50:71–80
19. Drewes AM, Nielsen KD, Taagholt SJ, et al. Sleep intensity in fibromyalgia: focus on the microstructure of the sleep process. Br J Rheumatol 1995;34:629–35
20. Roizenblatt S, Moldofsky H, Benedito-Silva AA, et al. Alpha sleep characteristics in fibromyalgia. Arthritis Rheum 2001;44:222–30
21. Molony RR, MacPeek DM, Schiffman PL, et al. Sleep, sleep apnea and the fibromyalgia syndrome. J Rheumatol 1986;13:797–800
22. Sarzi-Puttini P, Rizzi M, Andreoli A, et al. Hypersomnolence in fibromyalgia syndrome. Clin Exp Rheumatol 2002;20:69–72
23. Agargun MY, Tekeoglu I, Gunes A, et al. Sleep quality and pain threshold in patients with fibromyalgia. Compr Psychiatry 1999;40:226–8
24. Lentz MJ, Landis CA, Rothermel J, et al. Effects of selective slow wave sleep disruption on musculoskeletal pain and fatigue in middle aged women. J Rheumatol 1999;26:1586–92
25. Drewes AM, Nielsen KD, Arendt-Nielsen L, et al. The effect of cutaneous and deep pain on the electroencephalogram during sleep: an experimental study. Sleep 1997;20:632–40

26. Finestone DH, Sawyer BA, Ober SK, *et al.* Periodic leg movements in sleep in patients with fibromyalgia. *Sleep Res* 1991;3:179–85

27. Russell IJ, Michalek JE, Vipario GA, *et al.* Platelet ³H-imipramine uptake receptor density and serum serotonin levels in patients with fibromyalgia/fibrositis syndrome. *J Rheumatol* 1992;19:104–9

28. Vaeroy H, Helle R, Forre O, *et al.* Cerebrospinal fluid levels of B-endorphin in patients with fibromyalgia (fibrositis syndrome). *J Rheumatol* 1988;15:1804–16

29. Vaeroy H, Helle R, Forre O, *et al.* Elevated CSF levels of substance P and high incidence of Raynaud phenomenon in patients with fibromyalgia: new features for diagnosis. *Pain* 1988;32:22–6

30. Bennett RM, Clark SR, Campbell SM, *et al.* Low levels of somatomedin C in patients with the fibromyalgia syndrome: a possible link between sleep and muscle pain. *Arthritis Rheum* 1992;35:1113–16

31. Moldofsky H. Sleep, neuroimmune and neuroendocrine functions in fibromyalgia and chronic fatigue syndrome. *Adv Neuroimmunol* 1995;5:39–56

32. Bennett RM, Clark SR, Burchkhardt CS, *et al.* A double-blind placebo controlled study of growth hormone therapy in fibromyalgia (abstract). *J Musculoskeletal Pain* 1995;3:110

33. Mountz JM, Bradley LA, Modell JG, *et al.* Fibromyalgia in women: abnormalities of regional cerebral blood flow in the thalamus and the caudate nucleus are associated with low pain threshold levels. *Arthritis Rheum* 1995;38:926–38

34. Villablance J. Role of the thalamus in sleep control: sleep-wakefulness studies in chronic diencephalic and athalamic cats. In Petre-Quadens O, Schlag JD, eds. *Basic Sleep Mechanisms*. New York: Academic, 1974:51

35. Moldofsky H. Management of sleep disorders in fibromyalgia. *Rheum Dis Clin North Am* 2002;28:353–65

36. Branco JC, Martini A, Palva T. Treatment of sleep abnormalities and clinical complaints in fibromyalgia with Trazodone (abstract). *Arthritis Rheum* 1996;39:591

37. Gronblad M, Nykanen J, Konttinen Y, *et al.* Effect of zopiclone on sleep quality, morning stiffness, widespread tenderness and pain and general discomfort in primary fibromyalgic patients. *Clin Rheumatol* 1993;12:186–91

38. Carette S, McCain GA, Bell DA, *et al.* Evaluation of amitriptyline in primary fibrositis. *Arthritis Rheum* 1986;29:655–9

39. Goldenberg DL, Felson DT, Dinerman H. A randomized, controlled trial of amitriptyline and naproxen in the treatment of patients with fibromyalgia. *Arthritis Rheum* 1986;29:1371–7

40. Goldenberg D, Mayskiy M, Mossey C, *et al.* A randomized, double-blind crossover trial of fluoxetine and amitriptyline in the treatment of fibromyalgia. *Arthritis Rheum* 1996;39:1852–9

23

Pain management and the effects of pain on sleep

Robert L. Barkin

Pain is the most significant cause of sleep disruption, forcing the person to seek medical help. Whether acute or chronic, pain becomes debilitating, slows recovery and rehabilitation, interferes with daily activities and severely affects a patient's quality of life. Whereas the aforementioned associations are self-evident, many health-care workers fail to realize that the pressure of pain diminishes opportunities for adequate sleep.

Acute pain is typically associated with a known etiology, such as an identifiable injury or trauma, manifesting with sudden onset, responding to a variety of therapeutic options and resolving in less than 1 month. Chronic pain, on the other hand, is more of a treatment challenge. Chronic pain is not only difficult for the patient and family to tolerate but often equally difficult for clinicians to treat effectively. The pathogenesis of chronic pain is often unclear, making it difficult to predict the course of treatment or the patient's recovery and rehabilitation times. The ambiguous prognosis of chronic pain, added to the accompanying psychosocial and financial stress, may have a devastating impact on the lives of patient and family.

Pain is usually defined as chronic if it lasts longer than 1 month or if it extends beyond the typical recovery period of a specific injury or operation. Chronic pain can be presented in a continuum or be described as episodic, recurrent or persistent. Most often it is lacking in objective biological markers. Chronic pain is commonly accompanied by emotional stress, increased irritability, depression, social withdrawal, financial distress, loss of libido, disturbed sleep patterns, diminished appetite and/or weight loss.

Chronic pain can have a wide-ranging impact; its management must focus on multiple aspects of a patient's life. A multidisciplinary, comprehensive treatment plan is optimal, including:

(1) Individualizing psychosocial counseling (i.e. spiritual, psychological, biofeedback, relaxation, hydrotherapy, hypnosis, guided imagery, cognitive and behavioral therapy) in conjunction with patient/family education;

(2) Non-invasive or minimally invasive procedures, such as massage therapy, physical therapy, acupressure, vibration, ultrasound, transdermal or transcutaneous electrical nerve stimulation (TENS) or acupuncture;

(3) Lumbar or caudal epidural injections, trigger-point injections, facet injections, other anesthetic blocks, pharmacological and/or anesthetic therapies; and, if necessary,

(4) Invasive measures or interventions: implanted pumps or dorsal column stimulators.

Health-care practitioners must consider all options in creating a patient-specific treatment plan, addressing both physiological and psychological symptoms. Pain is a subjective experience unlike vital signs, which are objective parameters.

In the elderly, one or more of the following may provide a health-care provider with an index of suspicion of less than adequate pain relief: bruxism, facial expression of fear, apprehension, frowning, body posture; bracing, rubbing, guarding, restlessness, agitation, physically or verbally striking out at others, inadequate sleep, crying, groaning, moaning, sighs, diminished functional status, resistance to care and caregivers, immobility, changes in gait and deconditioning. Pain behaviors may also lead to drug-seeking motivated behavior with a focus upon achieving euphoric experiences through pharmacotherapy. Assessment and scales of pain are further complicated by delirium, dementia, depression, cognitive deficits and decremental changes in sensory awareness (visual, hearing, verbal). Pain assessment at baseline should include: pain intensity, onset, distribution, duration variability, quality and intensity in addition to the aforementioned indices in the elderly pain patient.

A pharmacotherapeutic pain treatment plan is initiated with a thorough pain and pain medication history to identify the nature of the patient's pain (acute versus chronic, nociceptive versus neuropathic, etc.). The patient and family interview should focus on patient-reported pain descriptors (palliative and provocative factors, quality of pain, radiation, severity, temporal factors), current and past pharmacotherapy utilization (prescription, over-the-counter, phytopharmaceutical, ethanol (quantified) history, and/or social/recreational) and past treatments (including successes/failures, adverse side-effects, and allergic reactions). Questions that help characterize the daily routine of the patient are also essential, from a normal sleep schedule to typical daytime tasks. A complete blood chemistry profile should be considered to determine if dosage changes are warranted, i.e. creatinine clearance, hepatic function tests, hemoglobin/hematocrit to determine anemia, albumin, acid-1glyocoprotein for highly bound drugs, uric acid for crystal arthropathies, hemostasis. Other tests may include imaging studies, cervical, lumbar and spine films for compression fractures, magnetic resonance imaging (MRI) for spinal stenosis, etc. Health-care practitioners should familiarize themselves with the pharmacodynamics, pharmacokinetics, potential drug–drug or drug–food, drug–laboratory interactions and contraindications of any drugs involved, including those already in use by the patient as well as those yet to be prescribed. This chapter is devoted to review pharmacological agents for treatment of chronic pain.

PHARMACOLOGICAL AGENTS

Non-opioid analgesics: aspirin and acetaminophen

The non-opioid analgesics are utilized for management of mild to moderate pain and postoperative pain, and provide an opioid dose-sparing effect.

Aspirin, an anti-inflammatory analgesic and antipyretic, is utilized for male transient ischemic attacks and for myocardial infarction prophylaxis.

Because of the association between the hepatonecrosis of Reye's syndrome and aspirin, it is not routinely prescribed to treat children younger than 16 years for chicken pox or flu symptoms. Caution should also be exercised in treating patients with platelet or bleeding disorders or renal dysfunction. Aspirin irreversibly acetylates platelet cyclooxygenase 1 (COX-1) for the life of the platelet. Patients with a history of nasal polyps, asthma or rhinitis may exhibit aspirin intolerance, leading to severe exacerbation of allergic symptoms, including potentially fatal bronchospasms. Clinical practice has demonstrated that two salicylates (salsalate and choline magnesium trisalicylate) do not have the aspirin platelet aggregation effect.

Acetaminophen (APAP) is an analgesic and antipyretic agent that lacks anti-inflammatory properties. APAP may also have a central activity through nitric oxide, serotonin and/or a COX-III central mechanism. Metabolism occurs in the liver, primarily by cytochrome P-450 (CYP-450) 1A2, 3A5 and 2E1. Protein binding is approximately 5–20%. The half-life is 2–4 h. The minor metabolite of APAP is NAPQI, which is only 4% normally present, but during glutathione depletion this metabolite produces hepatic necrosis. Fasting patients and alcoholics are at risk of hepatic toxicity. Hepatic inducers also place the patient at risk from the metabolite and CYP-450 drug interactions or phytopharmaceutical interactions. Hepatotoxicity may occur with daily doses of more than 7–8 g, sometimes less, and is exacerbated in patients with a history of alcohol abuse. Indeed two to three or more alcoholic beverages daily may produce hepatic dysfunction for APAP metabolism. No more than 4 g of APAP daily is recommended for acute use and the dose should be decreased to ≈ 2600 mg for chronic use. Safe use has been demonstrated in patients with diminished renal function. Supervised use during pregnancy, in the elderly, ill and very young may be accomplished without enhanced toxicity.

Non-steroidal anti-inflammatory drugs

Non-steroidal anti-inflammatory drugs (NSAIDs) are antipyretic, anti-inflammatory and analgesic agents that decrease prostaglandin production through their inhibition of cyclo-oxygenase. NSAIDs inhibit prostaglandin synthesis by blocking one or both isoforms of the cyclo-oxygenase enzyme (COX-1 and COX-2). Traditional NSAIDs have a somewhat linear structure and block both COX-1 and COX-2. This linear structure provides a 'fit' into the COX hydrophilic channel of COX-1 and COX-2, preventing the access of the COX substrate arachidonic acid. In contrast, COX-2-selective inhibitors block COX-2 preferentially. COX-2-selective inhibitors have a non-linear bulky side chain which enters COX-2 but not COX-1. In this case, the sulfur (i.e. sulfonamide on celecoxib and valdecoxib, non-sulfonamide arylfuranone portion of the rofecoxib molecule) fits into the valine side pocket of the hydrophobic COX-2 channel and prevents access of COX active sites by arachidonic acid substrate.

The analgesic action of NSAIDs may be mediated through COX-2 activity in the central nervous system. Additionally the central nervous system analgesic mechanisms may include: interference with prostaglandin formation, transduction, modulation in the nociceptive system; opiate peptides, serotonin inhibition release and inhibition of excitatory amino acids or N-methyl D-aspartate (NMDA) receptors. All NSAIDs have a therapeutic ceiling dose effect for their analgesics and anti-inflammatory effects.

Traditional NSAIDs carry the risk of severe gastrointestinal, hepatic, hematologic and renal side-effects, which should be considered when contemplating their use long-term for pain. Gastrointestinal ulceration, bleeding and perforation occur, often without warning symptoms, in 2–4% of patients treated with NSAIDs for 1 year.

Other adverse effects associated with NSAID use include reduced renal blood flow and glomerular filtration, interstitial nephritis, acute tubular necrosis, papillary necrosis, nephrotic syndrome, sodium and water retention (edema), acute renal failure, hyperkalemia and hypertension.

Two NSAIDs act as 'pro-drugs': nabumetone hepatically metabolized to 6MNA (the active form) and sulindac which is metabolized to sulindac sulfide (the active form). The package insert for celecoxib (the first COX-2 selective agent) and valdecoxib contains warnings about potential gastrointestinal bleeding, gastrointestinal tract ulcerations, skin rash, weight gain or edema and hepatotoxicity. Additional warnings include anaphylactic reactions in asthmatic patients who experience rhinitis with or without nasal polyps or who exhibit severe bronchospasms after taking NSAIDs or aspirin. Celecoxib and valdecoxib are both sulfonamides and are further contraindicated in a 'sulfa'/sulfonamide allergy. Celecoxib is a CYP-450 2D6 inhibitor and valdecoxib is an inhibitor of 3A4, 2D6, 2C9, C19.

Rofecoxib, the newest COX-II isoform selective inhibitor is a long-acting methylsulfonal derivative. It is not a sulfa/sulfonamide drug like celecoxib and valdecoxib. No clinically relevant effects on bleeding time were observed in our clinical practice with rofecoxib concurrent with warfarin administration (International Normalizing Ratio (INR) changes are 8–11%). Gastric mucosal injury is similar to that with placebo. There are no major reported CYP-450 events. Clinical applications of rofecoxib may include dental pain, osteoarthritis, rheumatoid arthritis, postoperative pain, acute short-term pain and dysmenorrhea. Analgesic activity of rofecoxib is indistinguishable from traditional NSAIDs but with much less gastropathy and no platelet effects (platelet cyclo-oxygenase is COX-I).

Centrally acting agents: tramadol

Tramadol is an atypical analgesic with a binary mechanism of action. It combines centrally acting (the enantiomer binds to the μ-receptor) mild opioid activity with an additional spinal mechanism of monamine reuptake inhibition. With its weak affinity for μ-opioid receptors, in synergistic conjunction with serotonin ([+] enantiomer provides serotonin reuptake) and norepinephrine ([–] enantiomer reuptake) blockade, tramadol interferes with central pathways that mediate pain. The spinal analgesia is modulated by descending non-adrenergic and serotonergic pathways effecting laminae I (A-delta fibers and C-fibers project and synapse), II (C-fibers project and synapse), V (A-delta fibers project and synapse) on the dorsal horn of the spinal cord. Tramadol is associated with a lower degree of respiratory depression than opioids. It exhibits a very low potential for tolerance or abuse and is indicated for the management of moderate to moderately severe pain. The concomitant use of tramadol and NSAIDs may offer the therapeutic benefits of both central and peripheral analgesia, although the requisite studies have not yet been conducted. This combination is frequently observed in clinical practice. Tramadol is a good choice for patients who are at risk for the side-effects of NSAIDs but are reluctant to take opioid analgesics.

Tramadol has been studied in elderly populations and for a variety of conditions. It has been well tolerated overall and has proved to be effective in fibromyalgia, osteoarthritis, back pain and neuropathic pain. In patients with a decreased seizure threshold or in patients taking antidepressants, neuroleptics, or other drugs that decrease this threshold, a risk–benefit analysis should be made. Tramadol is not to be used with a monoamine oxidase inhibitor. A combination of acetaminophen and 37.5 mg tramadol and 325 mg APAP is available. These dosage forms have been effectively utilized with copharmacotherapy (NSAIDs, membrane stabilizers, antidepressants, anxiolytics, anticonvulsants, opiates, skeletal muscle relaxants, etc.).

Opiates and opioids

Probably the best known class of medications used to treat moderate to severe pain are the opiates and opioids. Opioids are synthetic narcotics that resemble opiates in action but are not derived from opium. Opiates are any preparation or derivative of opium. Opiates/opioids produce analgesia centrally, through the central nervous system. Opiates/opioids are useful in treating acute painful states, but pose some challenges with adverse events. These agents commonly have adverse effects, including constipation, urinary retention, sedation, drowsiness, nausea, vomiting, and potentially initial transient severe respiratory depression. Tolerance develops and may be negotiated in some patients. Because of the 'tolerance' issue, prescribers, pharmacists and patients often exhibit 'opio-phobia', which leads to unnecessary underutilization of opiates in pain management. 'Opio-phobia' is a triad: clinicians, less than enthusiastic to prescribe; patients, resisting administration; and pharmacists, with resistance to dispense opiates. A comprehensive article discussing long-term opiate/opioid use has been published.

Opiates/opioids are given either orally, rectally, transdermally, intramuscularly, intravascularly, epidurally, intrathecally, transmucosally, or transnasally. Rectal administration is rarely used since absorption can be erratic.

The opiate/opioid analgesics are subdivided into opioid agonists, partial agonists and mixed agonist antagonists, according to the interaction at the specific receptor. Analgesic effects appear to be a function of several factors, including affinity for specific receptor binding sites, intrinsic activity at respective receptors, and the pharmacokinetics and pharmacodynamics of the agents. Various types and subtypes of opiate receptors have been described at sites within the central nervous system as well as at the sites external to it, such as the gastrointestinal tract. The opiate/ opioid agonists (morphine, codeine, hydrocodone, oxycodone, hydromorphone, oxymorphone, meperidine, propoxyphene, methadone, fentanyl and levorphanol) bind to receptors in the central nervous system as well as MU2 receptors in the gastrointestinal tract.

Codeine is metabolized via CYP-450 2D6 to morphine and is thus a prodrug. Most opioids and codeine have side-effects including sedation, nausea, vomiting, pruritus and urinary retention. Because constipation is an adverse effect to which tolerance does not develop, a bowel management program including a stimulant laxative and stool softener should be added to opioid therapy.

Hydrocodone, a phenanthrene derivative, is a dehydrogenated ketone codeine derivative. The duration of analgesic action is 3–6 h with a plasma half-life of 3–5 h. Following hepatic metabolism by CYP-450 2D6 in part to hydromorphone this prodrug is renally excreted. Euphorigenic effects appear more prominent than with codeine. Fixed analgesic combinations include APAP, homatropine and ibuprofen. Hydromorphone has an onset of less than 30 min by the oral route providing 4-h duration of analgesia.

Morphine dosage must be adjusted according to the patient's characteristics. Elderly patients are more sensitive to morphine and have higher, more variable serum levels than younger patients. Dose adjustments are not necessary in mild hepatic disease but excessive sedation occurs in cirrhotic patients. Morphine utilizes phase II glucuronidation metabolic pathways. This is a function of the accumulation of the active analgesic metabolite, morphine 6 glucuronide (M 6 G), which is eliminated by the kidney. M-6-G is four to eight times more potent than morphine in producing miosis and xerostomia, respectively. M-6-G produces analgesia and sedation. M-3-G is responsible for hyperalgesia, antianalgesic, allodynia and myoclonus. Duration of analgesia is 2–4 h and the half-life is 1.5–2 h. A sustained-release capsule with a pellet dose form (17 h) which may be opened and placed in food or tube routes (nasogastric tube, jejunostomy tube) is available. Delayed-release tables are also available.

Oxycodone is an opiate analgesic that is available alone or in combination with aspirin or APAP and it is available in several forms, including immediate and controlled-release dosage forms. Metabolism to form oxymorphone is by the CYP-450 2D6 isoenzyme and the other metabolites and parent are excreted renally. The major metabolite is noroxycodone. Oxymorphone is a minor metabolite of oxycodone. A controlled-release dosage form is available which initially releases 39% of the dose within 2–3 h following ingestion and is subject to abuse.

Meperidine is a synthetic opioid. Normeperidine, a neurotoxic cerebral irritant, is an active non-opioid metabolite that is thus clinically important and is not naloxone-reversible. Resultant effects of normeperidine include respiratory arrest and hyper-excitatory neurotoxicity (mood alterations (i.e. dysphoria, irritability), agitation, tremors, hyper-reflexia, myoclonus and grand malseizures).

The anticholinergic effects of meperidine are serious enough that the patient may have urinary retention and need catheterization; other effects include ventricular response to atrial flutter and supraventricular tachycardia.

Meperidine also blocks the neuronal reuptake of serotonin and norepinephrine and administration to patients receiving a monoamine oxidase inhibitor is contraindicated because this drug interaction leads to hypertensive crisis and serotonin syndrome, with symptoms such as agitation, hyperactivity, seizures, fever, diaphoresis, myoclonus, confusion and even coma. Meperidine use may aggravate pre-existing seizure disorders. Patients with liver disease may have an elimination half-life that is doubled, and thus dosages should be reduced for patients with this condition or renal disease. Use of meperidine for acute and chronic pain states is now highly discouraged.

Levorphanol is also a synthetic analgesic. Because of its long terminal elimination half-life (11–16 h) with relation to the duration of analgesia (6–8 h), repeated dosing leads to accumulation, generally seen on the second or third day of administration. Metabolism is through glucuronidation phase II metabolism. It is not routinely used for chronic pain.

Methadone is a synthetic agent similar to morphine, with a 4–6 h duration of analgesia but a longer half-life of 15–30 h. Oral bioavailability is about 85%. It is used to manage acute pain, chronic pain, chronic pain and cancer pain, in opiate detoxification, and for the chronically relapsing heroin addict. Accumulation does occur, leading to marked sedation. Longer dosage intervals are required to avoid this and other side-effects. The mechanism of analgesia may be achieved additionally, and 5-HT/NE reuptake blockade by NMDA receptor antagonism.

Propoxyphene is a synthetic opiate analgesic chemically similar to methadone. It is available alone or in conjunction with APAP or aspirin and caffeine. It is metabolized in the liver to norpropoxyphene which is not an opioid but has pro-arrhythmic lidocaine-like effects and anesthetic effects similar to those of amitriptyline. Because of its long half-life, norpropoxyphene accumulates if the parent drug is given repeatedly. Norpropoxyphene accumulation is associated with arrhythmias and pulmonary edema, and it is poorly dialyzed. There have also been reports of apnea, cardiac arrest and death. Naloxone does not reverse the effects of norpropoxyphene. Propoxyphene should be avoided in patients with end stage renal disease. Chronic use of this agent is highly discouraged, and use in elderly patients is not recommended. The US General Accounting Office has listed propoxyphene among drugs 'inappropriate for the elderly' and has emphasized that alternative analgesics are both more effective and safer.

Fentanyl is a highly lipophilic opioid analgesic with agonist activity at the μ-opioid receptor in the brain, spinal cord and smooth muscle. The onset and duration of action depend on the route of administration, serum drug level, and delay of entry into and exit from central nervous system sites. The transdermal dosage (an adhesive rate-controlling membrane) form has an onset of 6–8 h, with a peak effect 24–72 h after application. Initially, a 25 μg/h patch is applied to the skin and is replaced every 3 days while the dose is titrated to the patient's specific pain needs. One week should be allowed before altering the dose, because a new equilibration is not reached until 6 days after a dosage change. The use of a short-acting opioid or centrally acting agent within the first 24 h to supplement analgesia is recommended.

This transdermal system is utilized in the management of chronic pain in patients who require continuous opioid analgesic administration for pain that has not responded adequately to opioid combinations or NSAIDs. Elderly and/or confined patients, because of their altered pharmacokinetics due to poor fat stores, muscle wasting, areas of poor skin thickness or altered clearance, should not start with a dosage greater than 25 μg unless they have been receiving more than 135 mg of oral morphine or an equivalent dose of another opioid. Serum concentrations may increase up to 25% with every 3° increase in body temperature so febrile patients should be monitored. A transmucosal dosage form is also available.

Pentazocine, nalbuphine, butorphanol and dezocine are mixed opioid agonist–antagonists. These agents are less constipating than opioid agonists. However, nalbuphine and pentazocine must be used with caution in patients receiving opioids, to avoid precipitating withdrawal and increasing pain.

Use of pentazocine in chronic pain is limited by its short duration of action (3–4 h) and frequent side-effects of nausea, vomiting and dizziness. Dysphoria, nightmares, depersonalization and visual hallucinations are other adverse effects. Caution is recommended for patients who have impaired renal or hepatic function. Pentazocine should not be used to manage pain secondary to myocardial infarction, because it increases pulmonary arterial and central venous pressure and increases cardiac workload. Long-term use of pentazocine is not advised.

Butorphanol is an antagonist–agonist at the μ-receptor. Therapeutic effects also may occur via the κ-receptor. Side-effects of butorphanol include headache, vertigo, a feeling of floating, dizziness, lethargy, confusion, lightheadedness, hallucinations, unusual dreams and depersonalization. Side-effects can be minimized with administration in small doses (a 50% dilution). Abstinence appears to occur with concurrent butorphed and propoxyphene or methadone.

Nalbuphine has both agonist and antagonist properties. The most common adverse reaction is sedation. Diaphoresis, nausea, vomiting, dizziness, vertigo, xerostomia and headache also occur. Central nervous system effects, such as hallucinations, dysphoria, nervousness, depression and confusion, are rare. Nalbuphine is not used to treat chronic pain, since it is available only in injectable form. Duration of analgesia is 3–4 h.

Buprenorphine is a partial agonist at the μ-receptors and an antagonist at the κ-receptors.

It may also have some antagonist activity at the σ-receptor, but lacks dysphoric effects. Buprenorphine is not available for pain by oral administration because of its significant first-pass metabolism, although a sublingual form that bypasses the first-pass hepatic effect is under investigation, as is a transdermal delivery system in the United States which is already available elsewhere. Buprenorphine has been used for analgesia without producing hemodynamic instability in the management of pain as a result of a myocardial infarction. The duration of analgesia is 6 h because of slow dissolution from central nervous system receptor sites. Adverse reactions include drowsiness (especially within the first hour of administration), but it has a lower incidence of nausea and vomiting than other opioids.

Antidepressants

Antidepressants are commonly used in the management of chronic pain. They increase concentrations of norepinephrine, serotonin and/or dopamine in the central nervous system, possibly interfering with spinal pain pathways. On the dorsal horn of the spinal cord within the laminae, serotonin modulates the rostral central medial medullae and norepinephrine modulates the peripheral afferent fibers. Antidepressants relieve pain in patients with and without depression. Substance P inhibition may be a mechanism for antidepressant analgesia. A comprehensive article reviewing antidepressant use in chronic pain has been published elsewhere.

The selective serotonin reuptake inhibitors (SSRIs) currently available include fluoxetine, fluvoxamine, paroxetine, citalopram, escitalopram and sertraline. SSRIs have a serotonin-limited side-effect profile and do not appear to have the noradrenergic, alpha, histamine, cholinergic blockade of receptor effects of tricyclic antidepressants. The most commonly reported adverse effects include headache, insomnia, anxiety, dizziness, tremors, drowsiness, nausea, vomiting, diarrhea, dyspepsia, xerostomia, sexual dysfunction, anorexia and diaphoresis. Serotonin syndrome can occur when using SSRIs in combination with other medications. SSRIs inhibit the CYP-450 enzyme system and cause delayed clearance of certain medications. An intensification of adverse effects occurs when SSRIs are administered concomitantly with other medications that use CYP-450 1A2, 2D6 and 3A4 enzymes as a substrate for their metabolism. All SSRIs can increase serum levels and decrease clearance of other substrate agents by way of these hepatic enzyme systems.

Monoamine oxidase inhibitors act by inhibiting the monoamine oxidase enzyme system and causing an increase in the concentration of endogenous epinephrine, norepinephrine and serotonin in storage sites throughout the central nervous system. Since these chemicals have a wide range of clinical effects and a potential for serious drug–food and drug–drug interactions, monoamine oxidase inhibitors have been reserved for patients who are resistant to other antidepressants. Use in treating chronic pain is limited. As mentioned previously, administration to patients receiving meperidine can lead to potentially fatal side-effects.

Tricyclic antidepressants are commonly used in treating pain, especially neuropathic pain. The complete mechanism of action is not well understood, but current thinking involves spinal receptor site re-regulation. Independent analgesic action may also be present, or the antidepressants may relieve an underlying, masked depression. Antidepressants with a mixed mechanism of action (both serotonin and norepinephrine reuptake inhibition) are more effective than those that are more selective.

The pharmacokinetic changes that occur with tricyclic antidepressants are important. Amitriptyline is hepatically converted to an active metabolite, nortriptyline. Clearance of nortriptyline is reduced in the elderly and with patients who have low creatinine clearance, and therefore dosages must be decreased. Imipramine is transformed by the liver to desipramine. Amoxapine is transformed by the liver to a neuroleptic agent whose antipsychotic pharmacological side-effect profile includes extrapyramidal symptoms, whereby acute overdose may lead to acute renal failure. Trazodone is hepatically converted to *meta*-chlorophenylpiperazine (mCPP); its mechanisms of action include serotonin reuptake blockade and post-synaptic serotonin-2 blockade. The medication is generally given at bedtime because of its α_1 blockade-induced orthostatic hypotension and sedative properties.

In general, the adverse effects of tricyclic antidepressants result mostly from cholinergic blockade, α_1- and α_2-adrenergic blockade, histamine blockade and dopamine-2 blockade. Blockade of muscarinic receptors can cause blurred vision, xerostomia, sinus tachycardia, constipation, urinary retention, and/or memory dysfunction. Blockade of histamine-1 and/or -2 receptors produces sedation, drowsiness, weight gain, hypotension and potentiation of central nervous system depressant agents. Alpha$_1$-adrenergic blockade is often associated with postural hypotension and dizziness. Dopamine-receptor blockade has been associated with extrapyramidal symptoms, dystonia, akathisia, rigidity, tremor, akinesia, neuroleptic malignant syndrome, tardive dyskinesia and endocrine changes. As a group, tricyclic antidepressants lower the seizure threshold, and care should be taken in patients with a history of seizures or with a decreased seizure threshold. At high doses, these agents also tend to cause tachycardia and prolong the PR and QRS intervals by direct membrane stabilization. They block the fast sodium channels of the myocardium in a manner similar to type 1A antiarrhythmic agents. They may also cause orthostatic hypotension and congestive heart failure in patients who have impaired left ventricular function. Trazodone, however, exerts only minor effects on cardiac conduction; it may produce some ventricular irritability. Bupropion blocks reuptake of norepinephrine and dopamine and also has relatively few cardiac side-effects, minimal, if any, effects on cardiac conduction and no production of orthostatic hypotension. Bupropion utilizes CYP-450 2B6 for its metabolism substrate but is a CYP-450 206 inhibitor.

Other receptor-specific antidepressants such as venlafaxine, nefazodone and mirtazapine do not currently fit into any broad antidepressant classification. Venlafaxine has a favorable, complex mechanism of action. It blocks the reuptake of serotonin at low doses (similar to paroxetine), blocks the reuptake of norepinephrine at medium doses, and blocks the reuptake of dopamine at higher doses (similar to bupropion). Venlafaxine provides the therapeutic benefits of tertiary and secondary amine antidepressants without the side-effect profile. It is also beneficial in chronic pain, as it lacks clinically relevant CYP-450 interactions.

Nefazodone is another antidepressant that acts dually on serotonin. Reuptake inhibition for serotonin and norepinephrine occurs, coupled with serotonin-2-receptor blockade. This agent produces two active metabolites: the hydroxy-nefazodone metabolite, which has activity similar to that of nefazodone, and the mCPP metabolite, which is the same metabolite found with trazodone. The mechanism of action of mCPP is that of a serotonin agonist coupled with mild serotonin-2 and -3 antagonism. This agent exhibits zero-order kinetics, and accumulation occurs with long-term dosing. Frequently reported adverse reactions include drowsiness, nausea, dizziness and headache. Other side-effects include tremor, asthenia, insomnia, agitation and anxiety. Relevant CYP-450 3A4 inhibition also occurs. A black box warning of hepatic toxicity accompanies nefazodone.

Mirtazapine is an atypical antidepressant described as a noradrenergic serotonin-specific antagonist (NASSA). This agent produces unique therapeutic antagonism at both presynaptic α_2 auto- and α_2 heteroreceptors, thus facilitating rapid and robust enhanced noradrenergic and serotonin release. No sexual dysfunction, a decrease in migraine headaches, and decreased anxiety, agitation and depression are associated with serotonin-2, histamine-1, α_2 hetero- and α_2 autoreceptor blockade, as facilitated with mirtazapine. Further antagonism occurs at serotonin-2 receptors (decreasing anxiety and cephalalgia agitation) and at serotonin-3 receptors (decreasing nausea and gastrointestinal distress, augmenting antidepressant effects). Histamine-1-receptor antagonism at low doses (≤ 30 mg) produces drowsiness, facilitates sleep and improves appetite. No clinically significant interactions are revealed on the CYP-450 system. Mirtazapine is a useful adjuvant agent in the management of chronic pain and provides multiple treatment opportunities for elderly patients, especially patients with sleep problems.

Anxiolytic, sedative–hypnotic agents

Both benzodiazepines and non-benzodiazepine anxiolytics have been used in the management of chronic pain, particularly in patients with anxiety and insomnia related to ongoing pain. Benzodiazepines exert their therapeutic effect by binding γ-aminobutyric acid (GABA) receptors. Subunit modulation of the GABA receptor chloride channel complex is believed to be responsible for the sedative, anticonvulsant, anxiolytic and myorelaxant effects. The principal modulatory site of the GABA receptor complex is found on its α-subunit and is referred to as the benzodiazepine or ω-receptor. Three subtype ω-receptors have been identified, and it is thought that the ω_1-receptor is associated with anticonvulsant, anxiolytic and myorelaxant effects. The clinical effects of the ω_3-receptor have not yet been thoroughly investigated.

The ω_2-receptors are associated with memory dysfunction such as forgetfulness and/or amnesia. Anterograde amnesic effects are thus produced by modulating this receptor subtype. Zolpidem, a non-benzodiazepine BZ_1 (ω_1) receptor agent, is indicated for sleep and shows a high degree of selective agonist binding at the ω_1 site. This high degree of selectivity decreases BZ_2- and BZ_3-mediated events. The half-life variability (1.4–4.5 h) and bioavailability are increased in elderly patients and in those with hepatic functional impairment and end-stage renal disease. Zolpidem utilizes CYP-3A4 as a substrate for its metabolism; protein binding is extensive at 92.5%. Zolpidem is indicate primarily for short-term treatment of insomnia. Events for which patients discontinue zolpidem include: daytime drowsiness, dizziness, diarrhea, drugged feeling, amnesia and headache. Zolpidem administered later in the night has been associated with morning sedation, delayed reaction time and an anterograde amnesia and delirium.

Zaleplon is chemically a pyrazolopyrimidine, a selective ω_1-receptor agonist interacting with the GABA–BZ$_2$ receptor complex. The time to peak plasma level is 1 h. The half-life is 1 h, the hepatic metabolism is without active metabolites and there is low protein binding ($60 \pm 15\%$). This shorter half-life creates a clinical opportunity for safe dosing later in the evening. Accumulation is not observed with chronic dosing. Metabolism by aldehyde oxidase inhibitors of CYP-3A4 has no clinically important interactions with the minor CYP-3A4 metabolism route. Diphenhydramine and cimetidine inhibited aldehyde oxidase, the enzyme utilized during zaleplan metabolism. Pharmacokinetics in the elderly (≤ 75 years old) do not differ significantly from those in healthy individuals. Renal insufficiency does not influence this drug's pharmacokinetics and it is without necessity for dose adjustments in cases of mild to moderate renal impairment. Daytime sedation is not noted following use of preceding evening dosing. Late-night administration has no more side-effects than placebo.

Clonazepam is indicated in the management of seizure disorders and has been used to treat some chronic pain states, especially neuropathic pain. Lorazepam, temazepam and oxazepam may be especially useful to patients with liver impairment, because these drugs do not have any active metabolites and are metabolized by phase II processes.

Buspirone, an azaspirone, acts as a selective serotonin-1 receptor partial agonist at postsynaptic serotonin-1A autoreceptors and a full agonist at the serotonin-1A presynaptic autoreceptor. It is commonly used as an anti-anxiety agent and can help patients with anxiety related to their pain. Buspirone is extensively metabolized by the liver to a number of metabolites (active metabolite: 1-pyrimidinyl piperazine). A dosage change may be necessary for patients who have renal impairment. Side-effects of buspirone include dizziness, light-headedness, nausea, headache and insomnia, but not sedation. Buspirone is not associated with abuse. Gepirone will be available this year with pharmacotherapeutic advantages.

Membrane stabilizing agents

Anticonvulsants: sodium-channel blocking agents

These agents are used to manage neuropathic pain states such as diabetic polyneuropathy. Anticonvulsants apparently suppress neuronal firing and create membrane stabilization, causing a decrease in the rate and amplitude of conduction and thus decreasing pain.

Carbamazepine has a chemical structure similar to that of the heterocyclic antidepressants (e.g. imipramine). Steady-state kinetics of carbamazepine are not achieved until 2–6 weeks after initiation of therapy, because of its enzymatic autoinduction, and thus there is a substantial increase in the clearance of carbamazepine at the beginning of therapy. After 3–4 weeks of use, however, the half-life may decrease as a result of the cessation of the autoinduction process. Plasma protein binding is 76%, hepatic metabolism is by CYP-50 3A4 (major) and 1A2/28 (minor) and 2D6. Elimination is 70% renal and 30% fecal. Side-effects of carbamazepine are dose-related and include dizziness, drowsiness, nausea, vomiting, ataxia, gait disturbances, weight gain, arrhythmias, hepatic dysfunction and neutropenia.

Phenytoin possesses non-linear pharmacokinetics, and the half-life increases as the dose increases. The complex pharmacokinetics of its hepatic metabolism necessitates careful dose management in patients with severe liver disease. Side-effects of phenytoin include nausea, vomiting, rash, Stevens–Johnson syndrome, systemic lupus erythematosus, elevated liver function test results, reduced complete blood cell count, generalized lymphadenopathy and blood dyscrasia. Acne-like dermatitis, hirsutism and gingival hyperplasia have also been reported. Acute alcohol ingestion can increase the serum level of phenytoin, but long-term alcohol ingestion may decrease it.

Valproic acid, as well as its derivative, is metabolized 30–50% primarily in the liver by microsomal and beta oxidation, so lower doses are needed in patients with liver dysfunction. Enzyme inhibition occurs. Side-effects include nausea, vomiting, diarrhea, abdominal cramps, tremors (Parkinsonism), sedation, behavioral alterations, somnolence in the elderly, coagulation changes, thrombocytopenia, diplopia, alopecia, weight gain, edema and pancreatitis. Neurological effects include tremors and inco-ordination. Hepatotoxicity and anaphylaxis are also possible drug-induced side-effects with the use of valproic acid. Clinical monitoring includes complete blood count, blood chemistry, electrocardiogram, thyroid function, testes, pancreatic and hepatic function tests.

Gabapentin is another anticonvulsant drug useful for chronic neuropathic pain. Multiple receptors modulated by gabapentin include serotonin-1,norepinephrine, GABA, amino acid and transporter systems and sodium and calcium channels. The drug has a low toxicity and causes no clinically significant CYP-450 drug interactions. No monitoring of gabapentin is necessary unless the patient has renal insufficiency. Side-effects include somnolence, fatigue, ataxia, dizziness, diplopia, blurred vision, amnesia, nystagmus and tremors. Other adverse effects include weight gain, lower extremity edema, xerostomia, dyspepsia, constipation and depression.

Oxcarbazepine produces blockade of voltage-sensitive sodium channels, increasing potassium conductance, and modulates high-voltage-activated calcium channels. Following oral administration, it is metabolized to the pharmacologically active form MHD. Plasma protein (albumin) binding is 40%. Metabolism is by reduction with cytosolic hepatic enzymes which is followed by phase II metabolism. The half-life of the parent drug is 2 h but that of MHD is 9 h. About 80% of the dose is renally secreted as MHD (27%), parent (13%) and other metabolites. Oxcarbazepine inhibits CYP-450 2C19 and induces 3A4/5. Warnings include hyponatremia, carbamazepine cross-hypersensitivity, renal/hepatic function, and impairment-mediated dosing changes. Precautions include central nervous system effects, cognitive symptoms, psychomotor slowing, concentration difficulty, speech/language problems, somnolence or fatigue and co-ordination abnormalities (ataxia, gait disturbances), dermatological reactions, multiorgan hypersensitivity and reduced hormonal contraceptive efficacy.

Topiramate

Topiramate has multiple mechanisms of action which include: decreased action potential via sodium channel blockade, potentiation of inhibitory GABA, kinate/AMPA antagonism (a glutamate subtype receptor) and inhibition of carbonic anhydrase. Absorption is rapid, and peak plasma concentration appears in 2 h. Bioavailability is 80% and distribution kinetics are linear; the half-life is 21 h and steady state concentration is attained in 4 days. Plasma protein binding is small ($\leq 17\%$). Metabolism is not extensive (70% eliminated by renal mechanisms as the parent compound) and some renal tubular reabsorption is noted. Only 10–20% of topiramate is metabolized by the CYP-450 system. Topiramate may be removed by hemodialysis. Hepatic impairment will decrease the clearance of topiramate. Hydration is recommended to decrease renal stone formation. Paresthesia may be noted with higher doses. Topiramate may be a 3A4 and β oxidation inducer and enzyme inhibition is described at 2C19. Therapeutic applications in pain have included migraine headache, neuropathic pain and weight loss. Other clinical applications in psychiatry may include bipolar affective disorder.

Skeletal muscle relaxants

Skeletal muscle relaxants are used for the management of spasms related to pain, although they are not useful in spasms related to demyelinating disease, cerebral palsy or cerebrospinal trauma. Their mechanism of action involves depressing spinal polysynaptic reflexes and facilitating neuronal activity to enhance the muscle stretch reflex within the lateral reticular area of the brainstem. The indications for these agents are focused on spasticity and associated pain, full flexor and extensor spasm from central nervous system disorders, for brief periods, or muscle spasms from acute musculoskeletal disorders.

Baclofen acts as a $GABA_B$ agonist and hyperpolarizes membranes. Binding to presynaptic $GABA_B$ receptors in the dorsal horn, brainstem and other central nervous system sites (e.g. spinal cord) may inhibit substance P in the spinal cord and so relieve pain. It is excreted primarily unchanged in the urine. Bladder and colonic function may also achieve pharmacotherapeutic benefits. Rapidly absorbed, the half-life is 4 h, plasma protein binding is 30% and it is deaminated in the liver. Adverse effects include somnolence, ataxia, dizziness, weakness, fatigue, confusion, headache, insomnia, urinary infrequency, respiratory and cardiac depression and hypotension. Abrupt withdrawal of baclofen can cause seizures and hallucinations.

Carisoprodol has no clinically proven direct effect upon skeletal muscles or neuromuscular function. It is metabolized in the liver by CYP-450 2C19 to an active metabolite, meprobamate (which has a sedative effect). It should be avoided in patients with renal or hepatic disease. Side-effects include dizziness, drowsiness, vertigo, ataxia, tremors, agitation, confusion, disorientation, irritability, headache, depressive reaction, syncope and insomnia. With prolonged use, this drug is frequently associated with dependence.

Chlorzoxazone is rapidly absorbed and is extensively metabolized in the liver by phase II metabolism, and it is excreted in the urine. Side-effects include gastrointestinal disturbances, drowsiness, dizziness, lightheadedness, paradoxical overstimulation, hypersensitivity reactions and hepatic damage. Discoloration of the urine to orange or purplish red has also been reported with chlorzoxazone, and there have also been rare occurrences of gastrointestinal bleeding.

Cyclobenzaprine, a frequently used muscle relaxant, is structurally similar to the tricyclic antidepressants with primary actions on the brainstem. The drug provides relief of spasms locally, without interfering with muscle function. Cyclobenzaprine undergoes extensive metabolism in the liver and is excreted by the kidneys. Side-effects include drowsiness, dizziness, confusion, ataxia, xerostomia and anticholinergic effects. Contraindications are similar to those of tricyclic antidepressants, including (but not limited to) concurrent monoamine oxidase inhibitor use, which may result in a hyperpyretic crisis or severe seizures. Long-term cyclobenzaprine should be avoided; the manufacturer recommends that use should not exceed 3 weeks.

Methocarbamol does not directly relax skeletal muscles but can be used with other measures (e.g. physical therapy) to relieve discomfort associated with acute painful skeletal muscle conditions. Its mechanism of action is not thoroughly known, but it is thought that it creates central nervous system depression. Side-effects include light headedness, dizziness, drowsiness, anorexia, nausea, pruritus, rash, blurred vision, headache and fever. The patient's urine color may change to dark brown, black or green.

TIZANIDINE

Tizanidine is a centrally acting α_2-adrenergic agonist (similar to clonidine) which reduces spasticity by increasing presynaptic spinal motor neuron inhibition especially on polysynaptic pathways. Indications are for spasticity management. Following almost complete absorption the half-life is 2–5 h and peak plasma concentration occurs in 1–5 h. Pharmacokinetics are linear, bioavailability is 40%, 95% of the dose is subject to first-pass hepatic metabolism with inactive metabolites and plasma protein binding is 30%. Renal impairment (creatine clearance ≤ 25 ml/min) reduces clearance by 50%, prolonging duration of action. Hypotensive effects are dose related. Reversible hepatocellular injury is noted. Side-effects include xerostomia, asthonia, dizziness, sedation and hallucinations. Psychotic symptoms are reported. Cytochrome P450 inhibition or induction are not mediated by tizanidine.

Transdermal anesthetics

Lidocaine 5% is available in a transdermal patch for ≥ 12-h application with indications which include relief of allodynia (painful hypersensitivity) and for chronic pain in postherpetic neuralgia.

DISCUSSION AND CONCLUSIONS

Chronic pain presents with many faces, requiring multitherapeutic treatment, focused on aspects which include depression, anxiety, anger, somatic sources, in addition to insomnia. The insomnia may be co-morbid with the pain or may be a function of the other pain-related factors. Additionally depression, anger, agitation and panic may be independent of pain. In addition to pain, there may be other co-morbidities which may precipitate insomnia. These include, but are not limited to, chronic obstructive pulmonary disease, congestive heart failure, obstructive sleep apnea, gastroesophageal reflux disease, nocturnal myoclonus, periodic restless leg movement, polysubstance abuse, ethanol abuse, a paucity of physical activity, connective tissue disorders, nighttime enuresis (frequent nocturia), sleep apnea, hypoventilation of obesity and hormonal imbalance, to list a few. The clinician caring for the pain patient must discriminate the reason(s) which precipitate the insomnia and the complaints of insomnia of the patient independent of the pain itself, and the pain–insomnia association. Chronic pain states impede the patient from achieving a state of relaxation that may also block the restful (delta-wave) sleep. Decremental changes in restful sleep amplify a patient's perception of their pain.

Opioid analgesics may relieve pain. In an attempt to facilitate sleep with amitriptyline or flurazepam, a clinician actually decreases delta-wave sleep, which can result in a less restful or restorative sleep producing an increase in daytime fatigue that is also a function of pharmacologically active metabolites.

Non-rapid-eye-movement sleep, also described as a delta-wave or slow-wave sleep, is generally recognized to exist in four stages. The first stage is generally designated as a state of drowsiness. The second stage is described as a light sleep in which the patient can be easily roused. Third and fourth stages demonstrate delta waves on an electroencephalogram. The absence of slow-wave sleep results in increased pain and malaise. Both intra- and interpatient variability exist for the duration of each stage of sleep and this varies additionally from night to night. Pharmacotherapy can increase the duration of stages one and two and prevent delta wave and rapid-eye-movement sleep. The non-benzodiazepines zolpidem and zaleplon are two medications for sleep that have limited to no effect on the stages of sleep. These agents have not been approved yet for chronic use; however, both share a short half-life and in the case of zaleplon, there exists a lack of daytime sedation. Zaleplon can be used to treat the disorders of initiating and maintaining sleep without daytime hangover in the pain patient. Histamine receptor antagonist antihistamines alter the structure of sleep by acting as delta-wave-blocking agents. Their efficacy and effectiveness are lost over a short period of time and the side-effects, such as xerostomia and hangover, make them less appropriate in most pain patients. Herbal preparations include melatonin and valerian root. Melatonin appears to be useful in sleep–wake cycle disorders and has a poor hypnotic effect. Valerian root has been utilized for many years as an anxiolytic and a hypnotic that may induce sleep but produces a hangover.

Treatment options for patients with chronic pain and concurrent sleep disorders should be directed at diminishing the latent phase of sleep but increasing delta-wave sleep and rapid-eye-movement sleep.

Selected references

Barkin RL. Acetaminophen, aspirin or ibuprofen in combination analgesic products. *Am J Ther* 2001;8:433–42

Barkin RL, Barkin D. Pharmacologic management of acute and chronic pain: focus on drug interactions and patient-specific pharmacotherapeutic selection. *South Med J* 2001;94:755–70

McCarberg B, Barkin R. Long acting opioids for chronic pain: pharmacotherapeutic opportunities to enhance compliance, quality of life and analgesia. *Am J Ther* 2001;8:151–3

Barkin RL. Pharmacotherapy for nonmalignant pain. *Am Family Physician* 2001;63:848

Barkin RL, Schwer WA, Barkin SJ. Recognition and management of depression in primary care: a focus on the elderly. A pharmacotherapeutic overview of the selection process among the traditional and new antidepressants. *Am J Ther* 2000;7:205–26

Barkin RL, Barkin DS, Barkin SJ, Barkin SA. Opiate, opioids and centrally acting analgesics and drug interactions: the emerging role of the psychiatrist. *Emergency medicine update, Medical Update for Psychiatrists* 1998;3:172–5

Fawcett J, Barkin RL. A meta-analysis of eight randomized, double-blind, controlled clinical trials of mirtazapine for the treatment of patients with major depressions and symptoms of anxiety. *J Clin Psychiatry* 1998;59:123–7

Fawcett J, Barkin RL. Efficacy issues with antidepressants. *J Clin Psychiatry* 1997;58(Suppl 6):32–9

Huff J, Barkin RL, Lagatuta F. A primary care clinician's and consultant's guide to medicating for pain and anxiety associated with outpatient procedures. *Am J Ther* 1994;1:186–90

Alexander M, Richtsmeier AJ, Broome ME, *et al*. A multidisciplinary approach to pediatric pain: an empirical analysis. *Child Health Care* 1993;22:81–91

Barkin RL, Lubenow TR, Ivankovich AD. Butorphanol nasal spray for non-malignant chronic pain episodes either a sole agent or in combination with adjuvant treatment in the management of pain. Atlanta, GA: *The Danne Miller Foundation Meeting*

Overton M, Barkin RL. Considerations in the use of drugs in the elderly, in bone. In Roger C, ed. *Quick Reference to Internal Medicine*. New York: Igaku Shoid Medical Publisher

Richtsmeier A, Barkin R. Descriptive profile of pediatric patients managed by an interdisciplinary pediatric pain team. *J Pain Symptom Manage* 1991;6:151

Barkin RL, Barkin S, Stein ZLG. Panic disorder... alprazolam is another option to consider. *Hospital Formulary* 1991;26:91

Stein, ZLG, Barkin RL. Drugs and sexuality. *Am Druggist* 1991;82–4

Barkin RL. Drug abuse? Use and misuse of psychotropic drugs in Alzheimer's care. *J Gerontol Nursing* 1991;16:4–10

Stein ZLG, Barkin RL. G E reflux and vocal pitch. *Hospital Practice* 1989;24:20

Barkin RL, Stein ZLG. Drugs with anticholinergic side effects. *South Med J* 1989;82:1547–8

Barkin RL, Stein ZLG. Noncomplainers or non-compliers. *J Clin Psychiatry* 1988;49:38

Barkin RL. Polypharmacy and iatrogenic disease. *Proceedings of the 29th Annual Spring Clinical Conference in Geriatrics of the Southwestern Michigan Area Health Education Center*. Kalamazoo, Michigan: May, 1988

Barkin RL. Treatment challenges in MPD/DS anxiety. In *The Proceedings of the Sixth International Conference on Multiple Personality*.

Richtsmeier A, Barkin RL. Pediatric pain rounds: a multidisciplinary art. Abstract in *Proceedings of the Eleventh Annual Interdisciplinary Health Care Team Conference – Wyndham Milwaukee Center*. Milwaukee: School of Allied Health Professions University of Wisconsin, 1989

Barkin RL, Stein ZLG. The layer cake phenomena or sweet it isn't. *West J Med* 1986;145:2

Barkin RL, Stein ZLG. Drug demands on the patient – a mirror image of compliance. *Drug Intelligence Clin Pharmacy* 1983;17:753–4

Stein ZLG, Barkin RL. Torsade de pointes: a rare tachyrhythmia. *Drug Intelligence Clin Pharmacy* 1983;17:561

Zoltoski RK, Cabeza R de J, Gillin JC. Biochemical pharmacology of sleep. In Chokroverty S, ed. *Sleep Disorders Medicine*, 2nd edn. Boston: Butterworth/ Heinemann, 1999

24

Dementia and sleep disorders

Peter Dodzik

INTRODUCTION

Research on sleep-related disorders in non-reversible dementias has been sparse. This gap in the field is the result of multiple factors, largely related to issues of methodology. The majority of studies have tended to focus on dementia of the Alzheimer's type (DAT) as this accounts for 65% of all dementias[1].

The prevalence of DAT is only one factor in the difficulty of researching other dementing illnesses. Vascular dementia (formerly multi-infarct dementia) accounts for approximately 25% of all dementias, but can be difficult to quantify as a separate entity from DAT. Issues in quantification are related to the location and amount of vascular damage. Several pharmaceutical studies vying for FDA approval for acetylcholinesterase inhibitors (donepezil and galantamine) have used inclusion criteria based on several factors including the temporal relationship of the dementia and the vascular event, percentage of involvement of subcortical white matter, and location and relative involvement of the infarct. These criteria can lead to substantial disagreements as to what exactly constitutes a vascular presentation exclusively, and they may lack clinical utility as mixed presentations (vascular dementia and DAT) are probably more common.

For other dementias, such as Lewy-body dementia, which may account for 5–15% of all dementias, criteria for inclusion have also been problematic. Thus the research on sleep-related disorders is often considered for Parkinson's disease and Alzheimer's, but specific problems related to Lewy-body dementia are difficult to find.

Less frequently occurring dementing disorders, such as Pick's disease, Creutzfeldt–Jakob disease, progressive supranuclear palsy and those related to infectious diseases (AIDS) and metabolic processes (vitamin B12 deficiencies), have also been poorly researched. This lack of research is further maintained by difficulties in the technology used to study stages of sleep (polysomnography) and treatment methods for sleep-related disorders (continuous positive airway pressure; CPAP).

Stages of alertness may also represent areas for further research in the co-morbidity of sleep disorders and dementia. The associated fatigue following vascular insults, as well as the phenomenon of 'sundowning' in DAT, are major clinical issues for physicians and health-care providers working with demented patients and, therefore, they will be given separate consideration in this chapter.

This chapter will discuss the relevant research on sleep disorders and dementia. Although mixed presentations are commonly seen in clinical practice, this chapter will discuss each dementia as a discrete entity for the purposes of clarity. Relevant diagnostic and treatment options will be discussed, as well as global management perspectives. In most cases, age is a common risk factor for dementia, and thus the changes in sleep associated with aging require some descriptive attention prior to any thorough discussion of the effects of the dementing disorder.

SLEEP AND NORMAL AGING

Sleep architecture has been discussed earlier in this text and will not be repeated here. However, the reader should be cautioned that the ability to measure sleep stages in the elderly has been found to be less consistent than in younger populations. Although more recent normative data on sleep architecture in the elderly have been published[2,3], the accuracy of the data has at times been confounded by sleep-disordered breathing and periodic limb movement (PLM). In addition, like any extreme category, normative data in the very young and elderly tended to have higher variances and may make disruptions more difficult to determine.

Sleep architecture in the elderly

In general, how deeply a person sleeps affects their sleep architecture. Middle-aged and elderly people tend to spend less time in deeper sleep than younger people. By age 60 or 70, many adults experience a decrease in the proportion of time spent in delta sleep. This is particularly true for elderly men. According to Bliwise, studies that rely on visual examination and analysis of polysomnographic records indicate that stage 3 and 4 sleep accounts for 5–10% of the total sleep time in healthy elderly subjects[4]. It has also been pointed out that some studies have shown rates as high as 18–20%[5]. The gender effect can be compelling in some studies[6]. Advancing age in men leads to a decreased amount of visually recorded slow-wave sleep (SWS), while the opposite effect has been found in women who advance in age.

Again, the consideration of the amount of SWS in the elderly can be complicated by the method used to score the data. Bliwise suggests that there is a general decrease in the amplitude of the delta waves used for recording procedures in the elderly[4]. This relative difference could account for the frequent finding of less SWS in subjects over 70. Furthermore, this decrease in amplitude becomes more readily apparent in the very old. However, some researchers have speculated that delta waves in elderly women may be better preserved and thus the changes in SWS by gender and age could in fact be an artifact of the scoring method used to interpret the data[7]. Therefore, the amount of SWS in the elderly is still speculative and may increase in accuracy if frequency data alone are considered on EEG[4].

The amount of rapid eye movement (REM) sleep appears to be more stable. In late adulthood, onset of the first REM sleep periods comes faster than in younger years. The percentage of time spent in REM sleep varies slightly with age according to studies performed by the Sleep Heart Health Study[6]. Overall, in this study the amount of REM sleep decreased from 21% in subjects in their 60s to 18% in subjects in their 80s. However, Bliwise and others point out that this might be an artifact of different wake-up times across sleep laboratories[4].

Total sleep time in the elderly

The amount of sleep needed in the elderly has been a common misconception. General clinical lore has suggested a decreased need for sleep among the elderly. However, the research in this area would suggest otherwise[8]. Total sleep time (TST) can be studied in a variety of ways and the following findings have consistently emerged. Sleep deprivation studies have suggested that elderly subjects who have undergone 36 to 64 h of sleep deprivation show similar recovery periods in the nights that follow with predictable compensatory findings[8].

Interestingly, the average TST has actually been shown to increase slightly after age 65. However, reports of difficulty falling asleep are also noted. One study found that after 65, 35–45% had difficulty initiating sleep[9]. This difficulty could be the result of physiological and lifestyle changes. Physiologically; the elderly generally secrete lesser amounts of certain chemicals that regulate the sleep/wake cycle. Both melatonin and growth hormone production decrease with age[10]. There are also changes in the body temperature cycle, which occur with age, and core body temperature findings may also explain the changes in onset of REM sleep in the elderly. These factors may cause, or be a consequence of, sleep problems.

In addition, a decrease in exposure to natural light and a change in diet may exacerbate sleep difficulties. Some researchers theorize that daytime inactivity (lack of exercise)[11] and decreased mental stimulation may also lead to the 'aging' of sleep. However, frequent napping needs to be considered when looking at the TST in the elderly, as this population tends to engage in more frequent napping, which can fragment the sleep architecture and change the TST for the individual.

Causes of sleep disruption in the elderly

Sleep also becomes more shallow, fragmented and variable in duration with age. The elderly wake more frequently than younger adults. Recent research suggests that the aging bladder can contribute to a substantial degree of sleep disturbance in the elderly. Nocturia has been cited as the most frequent cause of nocturnal arousals (63–72% of elderly patients surveyed)[12]. A tendency to feel more sleepy during the day (as compared to younger subjects) was reported by elderly people as a result of these increased nocturnal awakenings. However, this type of self-reported data demands further investigative scrutiny to determine a causal link.

Menopause can also be a causal or related factor to poor sleep in the elderly. Although the results of studies of menopausal women have generally been less compelling as explanatory causes than nocturia, studies have indicated poorer sleep quality and more frequent nocturnal awakenings in this cohort[13]. Vasomotor symptoms are the most frequently cited symptom, although usually these are reported prior to initiation of sleep. Lest it be thought that this was simply an associated, rather than a potential causal factor, research has shown that estrogen replacement therapy has been associated with improved quality of sleep[11]. Estrogen-induced sleep improvement was associated with alleviation of vasomotor symptoms, somatic symptoms (palpitations and muscular pain), and lessening of mood symptoms on estrogen replacement therapy[14].

Sometimes, age-related changes mask underlying sleep disorders. For example, sleep apnea is more common in the middle and elder years. The repeated awakenings caused by a literal lack of breath lead to daytime sleepiness. Cross-sectional studies of ambulatory, acute-care and nursing-home elderly patients (65 and older) have rates of sleep apnea between 24% (for independent living) and 42% (nursing home) with an Apnea Index (AI) cut-off at 5 or higher[15]. In addition, Ancoli-Israel and colleagues found Respiratory Distress Index (RDI) scores of 10 or with higher in 62% of their sample aged 65 and older[15].

Most studies of sleep apnea in the elderly have found age-related risk. However, some researchers including Bliwise have suggested that there are two types of onset sleep apnea, one in middle age and one in the elderly[4]. Of the risk factors associated with sleep apnea and the elderly a thorough review can be found in the *Principles and Practice of Sleep Medicine*. The reader should be cautioned that rates of apnea this high in the elderly will complicate the presentation of a dementing process with higher rates than may have been previously expected.

Snoring is also more prevalent in the elderly and rates have been found upwards of 33% in subjects in their 70s[16]. However, rates have been shown to increase up to age 80, and thereafter the rates actually appear to decline[4]. Although snoring can be benign, Scharf and colleagues found that snoring was the only sleep disorder symptom question that correlated with nocturnal oxygen desaturation (below 90%) during polysomnography[17]. Thus, snoring remains a critical feature during the initial investigation of the patient's presentation.

Several research studies have found age-dependent relationships with PLM and restless leg syndrome (RLS) as well. In fact, in a study on community-dwelling elderly from 1991, Ancoli-Israel and associates found that rates of PLMs may be as high as 45% in subjects over the age of 65[18]. This finding suggests that PLM may actually be a more common sleep disorder in the elderly than sleep apnea, and unfortunately does not show the same decrease in the very old (above 80) that has been noted in apnea studies in the elderly. However, it should be noted that the Ancoli-Israel study used subjective correlates of PLM (including kicking in bed and sleeping alone) and myoclonus index scores (greater than 5)[18]. Thus, true prevalence of PLMs may vary based on methods of assessment.

There has been increased speculation as to the causes of PLMs in the elderly, and the leading hypothesis tends to favor a decrease in central dopaminergic transmission and neuronal deterioration in the basal ganglia[19,20]. Research on the treatment of PLMs by dopamine agonists has supported this hypothesis, although the reader should be cautioned that work in this area is not necessarily definitive. Vascular and metabolic changes as well as osteoarthritis have been linked to PLMs, but their relative contribution to the final common pathway that is the disorder is still unknown. What can be said is that the elderly face a particular risk for sleep disturbance to due PLMs.

Conclusions

This section indicates some of the prominent difficulties in determining the causality of sleep-related disorders in an aging population. The primary difficulty arises from increases in the causes of fragmented or non-restorative sleep. PLMs and sleep-disordered breathing have higher rates in this population, making the identification of true (and solely) age-dependent changes in sleep architecture more difficult to detect. In addition, a number of co-morbid conditions which lead to nocturnal awakening (e.g. nocturia, trochanteric bursitis, orthopnea and gastroesophageal reflux) occur more frequently in the elderly[4], often resulting in increases in daytime sleepiness and napping. The result is a change in the sleep patterns in the elderly to become polycyclic, in that several sleep–wake cycles occur within a 24-h period. This pattern is similar to the normal sleep pattern of infants. As a result, many elderly experience a significant decrease in nocturnal sleep efficiency and sleep satisfaction and increased frequency of sleep complaints.

Sleep hygiene is paramount in this population. Efforts to consolidate the sleep cycle must be multi-modal. Daytime increases in exercise and mental activity have positive effects on levels of alertness, daytime napping and core body temperature changes, which can affect circadian rhythms. In addition, there is some anecdotal evidence that some increased motor activity of the lower limbs (e.g. walking) in the evening can reduce the effects of PLMs and RLS. While these findings require further scientific inquiry, the potential benefits of healthy exercise are well known.

THE DEMENTIAS AND SLEEP DISORDERS

As mentioned earlier in this chapter, the information on sleep-related disorders and dementia is quite limited. However, as Alzheimer's disease, vascular dementia (formerly multi-infarct dementia) and Parkinson's disease account for upwards of 90% of all dementias, they will be given independent attention here. Treatment options will also be given and specific information regarding other types of dementia will be discussed at that point.

Alzheimer's disease

Bliwise[21] and others have suggested that automated systems for scoring of EEGs are of limited clinical utility in staging sleep in the demented patient. Even wakeful EEGs in these patients show evidence of diffuse slow-wave activity[22]. These pathological changes can make the discrimination of sleep from wakefulness and the separation of different stages of sleep problematic. As stated earlier, delta wave activity in the elderly is already problematic on visual interpretation because of decreased amplitude, and thus determining the normative percentages for each stage of sleep as well as the differentiation of pathological fragmentations and hypersomnias can be quite challenging if a dementing process is suspected. However, again, attention to frequency data on EEG can be helpful[18].

Coben and colleagues[23], in a now somewhat dated longitudinal study, demonstrated that increased theta-wave power was thought to be evident in the earlier stages of the dementing process, followed by decreased alpha and then increased delta power. Awareness of these types of changes (seen at 1- and 2.5-year intervals) have been very useful, because they allow inferences to be made in characterizing the duration, severity and progression of the disease. Again, the clinical utility of these findings is very difficult to determine as the typical patient is not necessarily generally followed for serial EEGs on an out-patient basis.

REM sleep as a function of TST has also been shown to be somewhat problematic in the DAT population. It has been generally accepted that lower sleep efficiency, increased stage 1 sleep as a percentage, and more frequent awakenings and arousals are a result of the dementia and have been linked to severity[24]. Regarding the relationship between REM sleep disturbances and DAT, Bliwise[21] has suggested that the abnormalities found in REM sleep in the elderly demented may reflect the integrity of the cholinergic system. Increased REM latency, EEG desynchronization and decreased REM as a function of TST have been observed. However, severity plays an intimate role in the amount of disruption and thus could provide a functional marker of the total acetylcholine system degradation in DAT[21]. It is of note that this functional marker was present even when subjects were treated with acetylcholinesterase inhibitors[25]. Thus, the complex interactions of multiple neurotransmitters in REM sleep as well as the persistence of structural changes secondary to the dementia are noteworthy here.

In general, the possible suggested that findings on EEGs in patients with DAT should be interpreted with caution because of their lack of sensitivity and specificity as a marker of sleep stages in the demented patient. In addition, the inclusion of pathological/abnormal delta sleep found in DAT and the use of summary (percentile) data from polysomnography should be cautioned when conveying findings to other professionals not trained in dementing illnesses.

Aside from the difficulties with the technical aspects of scoring sleep in DAT, functional difficulties are frequently seen in getting patients with DAT to comply with overnight sleep studies. Nocturnal confusion is common in DAT and will be discussed later in this chapter. Demented patients often become more aggressive and confused at night and many have frequent visual hallucinations, possibly as a result of limited sensory input. These factors can make polysomnographic recording difficult and even impossible in some patients. Thus, careful attention should be paid to the notes from the sleep technicians working with demented patients and include relevant behavioral observations with reports to referral sources. Artifacts are more common in these cases and can lead to erroneous conclusions about data and wasted or ineffective interventions. In addition, the stress and its relative benefit to the potential interventions should be carefully considered before ordering these procedures.

Sleep apnea and DAT

It has been well documented that sleep apnea causes impairments in cognitive functioning, especially, but not exclusively, in the elderly. One study from Redline and colleagues using subjects between the ages of 40 and 65 with mild sleep-disordered breathing found neuropsychological impairments in the areas of attention, memory and executive functioning[26]. The average respiratory distress index among the group was 17, 'with little hypoxia observed and less severe sleep fragmentation than that reported in more severe apnea. Cases reported more snoring, breathing pauses, and sleepiness than controls, but didn't differ from controls on MSLT or [Epworth Sleepiness Scale] ESS scores'.

The control and apneic groups were matched for IQ, age and gender and differed in one of four attention measures. On one of the vigilance tests several of the apnea subjects performed worse with the passage of time whereas controls improved. These subjects were also less able to recall digits in reverse order (a test of short-term memory), and made more perseverance errors (indicating difficulty changing their approach to a problem) on the Wisconsin Card Sort Test. Results on the latter test also correlated with sleepiness measured on the MSLT and with sleep fragmentation according to the study[26].

Although it is unclear how much test data impairment, such as in the study above, relates to real-world impairment or to what degree this impairment improves with the treatment of sleep apnea, some scientists and anecdotal observation suggest that there is improvement on test scores with treatment in the non-demented population. What is clear is that impairments in memory and executive function (along with aphasias) are perhaps the most common types of impairments in DAT.

These findings could suggest a causal link between dementia and sleep apnea. It has been well documented in head injury cases, that hypoxia secondary to the injury leads to differential impairments on hippocampal functioning because the hippocampus is more sensitive to disruptions in oxygen caused by hypoxic events. However, research on the effects of hypoxia has primarily been conducted on animals using sustained hypoxia, rather than the intermittent hypoxia seen in sleep apnea[27]. If a causal relationship existed, one would expect to find more cases of sleep apnea among the elderly demented, but this finding has not been shown consistently[21].

What can be said is that sleep apnea is more common in the elderly than in any other age group and it is extremely common in nursing-home patients, with 42% meeting diagnostic criteria[15]. Age is therefore likely to be the most common risk factor for sleep apnea and dementia and could explain the high correlation between the two. However, as previously stated, there is a decrease in apnea in the very old, with an increased rate for dementia within that group. Thus, there may be other mediating variables to consider. Certainly, the co-morbidity would exacerbate the impairments seen in the dementia and even potentially expose an underlying dementing process prematurely.

CPAP is the treatment of choice for obstructive sleep apnea and in central sleep apnea. However, the use of the CPAP in the demented patient can be very problematic. Nocturnal confusion, fragmented sleep and 'sundowning' (discussed later) make this particular intervention quite problematic. Bliwise[21] has indicated that the role of a concerned caregiver can be essential in this intervention.

It should be noted that any cognitive improvement from CPAP treatment is likely to be obscured by the progression of the dementia. However, clinically the issue of quality of life is probably the best guiding factor. Individuals with mild dementia or mild cognitive complaints that are exacerbated by the effects of the apnea are likely to be aware of the improvements in their cognitive functioning as a result of the CPAP treatment and can be convinced to continue. Individuals with more severe dementia may not be able to grasp the significance of the CPAP as treatment of their apnea and thus the intervention will be more difficult to maintain.

Periodic leg movements, restless legs syndrome, myoclonic disorders and DAT

The literature on PLM and RLS in DAT is more sparse than for apnea. PLMs are repetitive, stereotypic leg movements occurring in non-REM sleep. The leg movements occur every 20–40 seconds and can last much of the night[28]. These movements may or may not be associated with arousal. The incidence of PLM increases with age and can be associated with peripheral neuropathy.

RLS is characterized by an uncontrollable urge to move one's legs at night, primarily to relieve the discomfort caused by the disorder. There may be a family history or underlying medical conditions such as renal, neurological or cardiovascular disease. Prevalence increases with age. Occurrence is 2–15% in the general population and up to 24% in the elderly[29]. Approximately 80% of patients with RLS will also have PLM disorder[30]. Causes of the disorder have been linked to genetics in the primary or familial form and to a host of medical conditions in the secondary form.

The pathogenesis of myoclonus (nocturnal or otherwise) would suggest that it can be caused by the dementing process of DAT. Metabolic and toxic encephalopathies, such as renal and hepatic failure and anoxic brain injury, are also likely causes for myoclonus. Prion dementias (Creutzfeldt–Jakob disease) and subacute sclerosing panencephalitis, or familial progressive myoclonic epilepsies, which include a wide range of storage diseases associated with enzyme deficiencies of the gangliosides, are also common neurological disorders associated with myoclonus.

Nocturnal myoclonus, which is characterized by abrupt 'jerks' or twitches that generally last less than 100 milliseconds, is one of several sleep-related movement disorders which, like the potentially related RLS, is most prevalent in the elderly. Prevalence rates range up to 45% according to the Mayo Clinic in Rochester[31]. Thus, like apnea, aging is the common risk factor. The disease may be stable (i.e. non-progressive) in any given individual patient.

The frequent disturbances of sleep, as well as the accompanying daytime fatigue, are compelling factors for treatment of nocturnal myoclonus. As mentioned, the depletion of dopamine in the central nervous system probably plays a critical role in the development of these symptoms, although the actual cause is still unknown.

The prevalence is unclear in the DAT patient, but Alzheimer's disease is considered to be a primary risk factor in the development of these disorders. However, anecdotally, the clinician should consider the likelihood for increased nocturnal arousals and wandering behaviors, as well as the fact that the cascade of events in DAT (seizures, neuronal loss) could lead to increased risk for the development of myoclonus.

Nocturnal agitation, sundowning and dementia

The phenomenon of 'sundowning' in DAT is not a recent finding. The syndrome has been discussed clinically throughout the history of medicine. In DAT, both physiological and environmental causes can be found and are not mutually exclusive. As previously mentioned in this chapter, visual hallucinations may be related to limited sensory input in the evening hours, fatigue, or the onset of sleep. However, Inouye and Charpentier[32] found relationships between the onset of an unspecified delirium and such factors as nursing staff shift changes, four or more medications, infectious disease, malnutrition, restraints and other related factors in nursing-home patients. Physiological causes have also been reported and may exist along two domains. REM dyscontrol mechanisms may explain the agitation associated with the nocturnal hours (sundowning) or the agitation seen upon nocturnal arousals, while agitation in the evening hours not followed by sleep may be related to chronobiological factors, according to Bliwise[21].

The former factor (REM dyscontrol) from Bliwise's hypothesis will be considered in the section on Parkinson's disease. However, his views on 'forced nocturnal arousals' are worth noting. He points out that forced bed checks and noises associated with staff or other patients in nursing-home settings account for many of the nocturnal arousals of demented patients. In addition, these patients were noted to be the most agitated at the time of arousal[21]. Thus, proper sleep hygiene is likely to be in conflict with safety needs at many institutions and creates a strong conflict for staff members and patients, literally and figuratively.

Disruption of circadian rhythms may also be responsible for agitation in the early evening. Bliwise goes on to point out that this period of increased agitation corresponds to the maximum core body temperature along the daily cycle and that this may put demented individuals at risk for agitation during these periods[21]. However, the exact causes for this type of response are less clear.

What is known is that agitation is certainly a major contributing factor to eventual residential placement. Unfortunately, individuals with DAT are likely to decline dramatically after placement into a nursing home. Cognitive stores (long-term spatial memories) for furniture placement, cues for eating and dressing and other safety-related issues are removed upon placement and confusion is heightened. Thus, anything that can be done to delay the placement of the individual, while maintaining the functional capabilities of the caregivers, is essential. In addition, after placement, careful evaluation of the onset, duration and precipitating factors associated with the agitation can lead to more useful and potentially creative interventions.

Vascular dementia and sleep disorders

As stated in the beginning of this chapter, vascular dementia or cognitive impairments secondary to vascular events represent a heterogeneous profile of presentations and avenues for treatment. In this chapter, vascular dementia will refer to the resulting impairment from serial infarcts involving white matter abnormalities. Although specific diagnostic criteria often involve a minimum amount of cerebral involvement to be considered vascular dementia (around 25%), for our purposes this distinction is less relevant. In addition, research in the area of vascular dementia has tended to focus on this as a discrete entity instead of the common overlap between vascular dementia and DAT. Again, for the purposes of this chapter, that distinction will not be considered because of the lack of clinical utility for treatment options and data based on exclusionary criteria. The spectrum considered in this chapter includes the former diagnosis of multi-infarct dementia (most common, resulting from a culmination of mini-strokes or transient ischemic attacks (TIA)), Binswanger's disease (once thought to be rare, a subcortical presentation involving deep white matter demyelination of nerve fibers) and some major strokes.

The progression in these disorders is variable, and the degree of loss of function depends on the area of involvement, number of events, relative recovery and the ability to prevent recurring attacks. Vascular dementia is often associated with depression, mood swings and higher risks for seizures, while Binswanger's disease includes lethargy, ataxia, loss of bladder control and mood swings. Fatigue following vascular events and during recovery periods is common and can be problematic for sleep cycles.

Strokes, which are generally considered to be major events involving larger vascular systems than TIA, have a more intimate relationship with sleep disorders. Ischemic stroke and myocardial infarctions occur most often in the morning hours after wakening. Elliott[33] reviewed 31 publications of over 11 000 strokes and found that 49% occurred between 6:00 a.m. and midday. In addition, 20–40% of ischemic strokes occur during the night and there has been some suggestion that sleep presents a particular risk for some patients with vascular disease. Other studies[27] have pointed out that although no consistent correlation has been found between time of stroke and sleep apnea, cardiovascular changes produced by apneas do precipitate strokes in some cases.

Sleep apnea and vascular dementia

The relationship between strokes and sleep apnea is still under debate in terms of the causality, but the correlation between the two events is not. Earlier epidemiological studies had found an increased risk of stroke in people with all apneas and hypopneas. Bassetti and Aldrich[34] conducted a prospective study of patients with a history of stroke and TIA. In this sample apnea/hypopnea index (AHI) scores did not differentiate the groups 9 days after the vascular event, but were found to differentiate the stroke and TIA patients from controls matched for age, gender and body mass index (62.5% with AHI > 10 for the vascular group, 12.5% for controls). Although the risk of vascular problems is higher in all apneas, most people with this disorder tend to have a predominantly obstructive syndrome with a few central apneas. Blood flow to the brain declines greatly in obstructive hypopnea episodes and obstructive apneas (up to 80%), but much less in central apneas[35].

In addition, patients with acute stroke have premorbid apnea rates from 69 to 95% based on a cut-off AHI of 10 or more, with 30–50% having moderate to severe rates as characterized by AHI >20[36]. The relationship is also found in the other direction; patients with obstructive sleep apnea can develop the symptoms as a result of the vascular event due to infarctions in the medulla, or indirectly as a result of infarctions to other areas of the brain[36]. As the Bassetti and Aldrich study suggests, the rates of apnea in patients with a history of TIA or stroke are as much as five times those of matched controls without a vascular history, though clearly other health factors such as diabetes must be further considered to determine the relative risk of vascular events on the development of apnea or vice versa.

These findings indicate that improvement in the apnea (primarily as a result of CPAP treatment) could lead to improvement in cognitive functioning for patients. This finding is significant in the differential diagnosis, where the onset and progression of the impairments coupled with minimal vascular evidence from imaging are inconsistent with the volume of the cognitive deficits. It is crucial in vascular cases that the informants (bed partners) be interviewed to help gauge information about heavy snoring, breathing cessation and daytime fatigue. It is also important that apnea be considered after vascular events as the presence of the condition has been found to significantly affect the functional outcome following a vascular event[37].

Other sleep-related issues and vascular dementia

Studies on circadian rhythm disorders in vascular dementia have suggested several differences from DAT. In particular a greater disruption was seen in the sleep–wake cycle over a 24-h period. Meguro and colleagues[38] found that greater white matter lucencies, particularly in the internal capsule, the thalamus and the periventricular region, were associated with greater disruptions in the 24-h cycle.

Hypersomnias are also frequently reported in cases with vascular implications. It is often reported with depressed mood and can result from either bilateral (and sometimes unilateral) stroke of the paramedian thalamus and those that affect the reticular formation[39]. In addition, insomnia or periods of alteration between hypersomnia and insomnia have been noted after vascular events.

Parkinson's disease and sleep disorders

Although typically treated by neurologists, patients with Parkinson's disease may present at sleep clinics because of difficulties in maintaining nighttime sleep, sleep fragmentation, diminished TST or daytime fatigue as a result of difficulties in achieving restful sleep. In addition, the nature of the disorder has a longer progression than other dementias. Estimates vary, but on average 25% of patients with Parkinson's disease go on to develop dementia, often after having had the disease for a number of years. Consequently psychiatrists can become involved with these patients early on in the disease because of the co-morbidity of other psychiatric conditions such as depression.

Individuals with Parkinson's disease often show fragmented sleep cycles in which they struggle to maintain sleep. Many actually report little difficulty falling asleep or com-plain that instead they fall asleep too early. Patients then report waking up frequently during the night for a variety of reasons and often find it difficult or impossible to return to sleep. Involuntary movements and pain can cause disruption of sleep. In many cases, patients report an inability to find comfortable positions in bed.

In terms of the overall sleep organization in Parkinson's disease, fragmentation is widely seen on polysomnography. Kales and colleagues[40] reported that studies conducted on patients with Parkinson's disease (not necessarily with dementia) show total wake times of 30–40%. The relationship between the total wake time and the severity of the dis-ease is significant and shows improvement with the use of anti-Parkinsonian medications. As with vascular dementia, nocturnal halluci-nations tend to be a marker for increased disruption of sleep[41] and are suggestive of structural damage directly related to sleep control mechanisms in the brain. Sleep EEGs show increased alpha activity and reduction in the number of sleep spindles, suggesting similar difficulties in the use of this as a diagnostic marker for recording of sleep architecture[42].

Michael Aldrich gives an excellent account of the specific changes associated with motor activity in Parkinson's disease during sleep[43], and his work will be summarized here. Readers interested in more complete infor-mation are referred to his chapter in *Principles and Practice of Sleep Medicine*. Although most scientists (including Parkinson) have noted that typical tremors tend to be less prevalent during sleep, they are not altogether absent. Tremors are generally absent during stage 1 sleep and slow-wave sleep and are not associ-ated with K complexes. However, tremors may appear (in similar form to waking structure) with awakenings, arousals and body move-ments as well as during sleep stage changes as measured by video–EEG telemetry[38]. Increased muscle tone and complex movements are also seen more frequently in Parkinson's disease patients. Tonic contractions of extensor or flexor muscles can be seen, as can increased rates of REM sleep behavior disorders. In fact, Aldrich points out that REM sleep behavior disorders may actually precede the onset of daytime symptoms in early Parkinson's disease[43].

PLMs are a common occurrence in patients with Parkinson's disease. They can occur in up to one-third of patients with the disorder and are seen most often during non-REM sleep[43]. However, motor symptoms are often least severe in the morning, which suggests some benefit from sleep. A subset of patients also show improvement in motor symptoms following napping, which could further emphasize this point[44]. Further studies are necessary to determine the degree of benefit from nocturnal sleep versus daytime naps. Specific treatment recommendations for dyskinesias, tremor and dystonias associated with Parkinson's disease and the medication used for its treatment will be discussed below.

Sleep apnea has been shown to occur in Parkinson's disease, although the types of sleep disorders, breathing and their causal factors can be unique to the disorder. Obstructive sleep apnea is seen in many cases of Parkinson's disease and is the result of a combination of obstruction of the upper airway, abnormal muscle tone and respira-tory inco-ordination[43]. In addition, Aldrich points out that these ancillary problems in muscle strength do not always improve with levodopa.

In a study conducted by Arnulf and col-leagues[45], Parkinson's disease patients who were pre-selected for daytime sleepiness had high rates of moderate to severe obstructive sleep apnea. The prevalence was greater than that found in an elderly American popula-tion. Obesity, which is a risk factor for sleep-disordered breathing, was rare in the study group and consequently could not account for the high prevalence of sleep apnea in these patients with excessive sleepiness. Upper airway difficulty occurred in as many as 24% of Parkinson's disease patients. It should be noted that this group was also currently being treated with levodopa, re-emphasizing the earlier point that anti-Parkinson's disease medications may have little benefit for apnea in this population.

Treatment considerations

Although some specific recommendations for working with patients with dementia have already been stated, specific recommendations for patients with Parkinson's disease must be further elaborated. Involuntary movements and pain can take several forms in Parkinson's disease. Some people experience dyskinesias, usually as a result of the effects of levodopa. A dyskinetic patient may experience writhing movements that are particularly severe at bedtime. In such cases, reducing the evening levodopa dose may be helpful. However, severe tremors can also make it difficult to get to sleep and in those cases an increase in the evening levodopa might be useful.

REM sleep behavior disorder, which is more common in older men with Parkinson's disease, is also seen in higher rates in Parkinson's disease than in normal elderly. Presentations can vary from patient to patient, but many will describe muscle jerks, flinging movements of the limbs, or restlessness through the night. There have been reports of aggressive or violent nocturnal behavior, falling out of bed and sleepwalking. Clonazepam frequently is used to treat these conditions, and careful changes should be made to the amount and delivery of the anti-Parkinsonian medication[46].

Painful muscle cramps (dystonias) can be seen in Parkinson's disease. Typically these involve cramping of the calf muscles and feet, typically worse on the side of the body with more pronounced Parkinson symptoms. This change in symptom severity is usually associated with the benefits of levodopa wearing off. If the dystonia occurs in the morning the treatment of choice may again involve the delivery of the levodopa by sustained release or early morning dosing. Clonazepam may also be useful.

Specific factors related to sleep hygiene, daytime activity, insomnia treatment and other more general interventions will be discussed below in the section on general treatment.

CASE STUDIES

Executive decision

An 81-year-old, Caucasian, widowed male presented at an out-patient sleep clinic accompanied by his youngest daughter. He was a rather unwilling participant and was quite belligerent with his daughter when she tried to describe the presenting problems. She reported that he had had seven car accidents in as many months as a result of falling asleep behind the wheel. Although no serious damage had been done, his family physician had told the family that he could no longer drive until this problem and the root cause had been addressed.

Mr X was a member of the board of the company he had founded and had been showing subtle signs of increasing memory problems for the past couple of years. The family began to notice them more following his wife's death 2 years ago. Mr X vehemently denied any problems with his memory or any difficulties in performing his duties at his office. However, he could not name the correct date, time or season, and gross memory to confrontation was poor. Despite claiming that his daughter was lying about him falling asleep behind the wheel, he nodded off on two occasions during the initial evaluation. He tended to attribute most of his problems to 'boredom', and stated that many things were not worth listening to and so he would take a short nap because he did not sleep well at night.

A sleep study was conducted, which revealed moderate obstructive sleep apnea (AHI = 22), with more infrequent central events and hypopneas. CPAP treatment was recommended initially. However, Mr X reported that he could not sleep with the mask and would 'rip it off in the middle of the night'. He began to become increasingly agitated and hostile at his work and his memory problems became more evident over the next month. He was referred for a neuropsychological evaluation, which had to be repeated because he fell asleep during the first evaluation. He showed global impairment on the Mini Mental State Examination (MMSE; total score of 23) and mild impairment on memory and attention tasks, with more moderate impairment on executive functioning tasks. Soft frontal release signs were evident and he frequently confabulated during testing.

Mr X was tried on donepezil 10 mg, which was initially helpful according to his family and during the first 2 months of treatment. A home health aid was hired to ensure proper nutrition and medication compliance, and he again tried the CPAP device. Cognitive test scores were stable at 6 months, but he continued to show aggressive changes in behavior. He again began driving and was found on the highway at 3:00 a.m. by the police reporting that he was going to work but could not find the way. Upon inquiry, he reported that he would not use the CPAP device and had little insight into the extent of his impairment or the risks he had posed to himself and others. His driving privileges were revoked and the family employed a driver.

Case discussion

The initial presentation was compelling for sleep apnea because of the extreme daytime fatigue and cognitive changes in alertness. Although the memory impairment was also present, his family and attending physician initially were impressed by the possibility that this was a grief reaction to his wife's death. However, the repeated car accidents, anosognosia, behavior changes and insidious onset were more indicative of a primary dementing disorder, in this case DAT.

Although numerous attempts were made to gain compliance with CPAP treatment, ultimately it was abandoned. Mr X lacked a strong caregiver in the home to deal with nocturnal agitation and confusion. Although he frequently stated during his treatment that he believed his sleep problem was the cause of his memory complaints, the data suggested otherwise.

Minimal benefits were achieved with the addition of an acetylcholinesterase inhibitor, which did allow for a brief trial on the CPAP, but ultimately the progressive nature of the dementing disorder and behavioral changes suggested that the level of impairment was probably more moderate (rather than mild) and he was unable to appreciate the need for his own treatment.

Bed battles

A 76-year-old, married, Caucasian male presented at an out-patient sleep center accompanied by his wife with complaints of visual hallucinations (evening onset), increased aggression in the evening with violent outbursts during sleep. Medical history was significant for 'semantic dementia' according to previous dictations from the neurology clinic. He had a history of subcortical infarcts shown on a previous magnetic resonance image (done 5 years ago) and newer infarcts on a recent image.

The patient was treated for hypertension and had been placed on galantamine 6 months ago for memory loss, naming difficulties and executive dysfunction. The patient's wife reported that the galantamine had been mildly helpful in treating his progressive cognitive difficulties, which were much more noticeable over the past year. No major strokes were identified by history, but he had alternating periods of consciousness and recently he had become confused and aphasic for several hours, without concurrent loss of motor functioning, sensory changes or complete loss of consciousness.

Neuropsychological testing was conducted and he was found to be impaired on most global measures (Mattis Dementia Rating Scale, MMSE, Wechsler Memory Scale, Boston Naming Test). The degree of impairment was thought to be mild, without obvious lateralizing effects. No gait abnormalities were observed at initial evaluation, but the family reported loss of balance, which was more transient, as well as urinary incontinence.

A sleep study was requested because of heavy snoring, suspected PLMs and possible cessation of breathing according to his wife, accompanied by daytime fatigue. The initial polysomnography was discontinued after 4 h following a period of arousal that was accompanied by confusion, physical and verbal aggression and subsequent non-compliance. However, in this case no evidence of sleep apnea was obtained and PLMs were thought to be mild.

The patient initially was treated with risperidone in the evening and he and his wife reported less aggression. Nocturnal confusion was still present but less disruptive. Daytime fatigue was treated with sleep consolidation using initial restriction (limiting time in bed to 7 h) and timed naps (at 45 min between 12:00 p.m. and 3:00 p.m.) to prevent cognitive deterioration in the evening hours due to fatigue.

Case discussion

As with the first case, dementia is the predominant causal factor for this patient's nocturnal confusion. Although 'sundowning' such as this is more prevalent in DAT, this case demonstrates the presentation in other types of dementia. Although the specific type of dementia (e.g. vascular dementia, mixed vascular dementia and DAT) was not clearly delineated, treatment of a possible co-morbid sleep disorder was still possible. The polysomnograph, while not ideal in this case, was able to provide information about co-existing conditions to plan treatment (in terms of determining the presence of apnea and PLMs).

Unfortunately, this type of behavioral disturbance can also be a marker of progression of the severity of the dementing process from mild to moderate severity and recent magnetic resonance imaging demonstrated new vascular events. Treatment therefore reflected preventative measures (anti-hypertensive medication) as well as symptom management. The use of behavioral techniques with the family to help stabilize the sleep–wake cycle

and provide 'planned naps' to reduce evening confusion also proved helpful in this case.

GENERAL TREATMENT CONSIDERATIONS

When dealing with the demented patient, proper diagnosis is essential for determining the best treatment options. Unfortunately, as was evident in the case examples, the assessment can be a 'fluid' process. Many patients will not tolerate polysomnography, lengthy neuropsychological testing or medication trials. Consequently, the clinician is often forced to do more with less information. Step-down methods for standards of care are recommended, which involve moving from ideal diagnostic tests to less than ideal in a progressive fashion based on tolerance (by the patient) and clinical value.

Most physicians can make an accurate diagnosis with the technology available today. However, when options are limited, the task of identifying all contributing factors is complicated. Therefore, procedures to be used should be evaluated on a case-by-case basis with a pragmatic drive. If the patient's symptoms are abrupt rather than insidious, or reflect a pattern more consistent with a known sleep disorder (such as PLM, narcolepsy or obstructive sleep apnea), all attempts to obtain laboratory evidence (e.g. through polysomnography or MSLT) should be made. When attempts fail, rescheduling or discontinuing testing should be considered based on the likelihood of success and the relative impact on treatment.

Behavioral treatments should not be overlooked in this population. Sleep fragmentation, daytime fatigue, low levels of cognitive and physical arousal all play a role in the quality of life of the individual and consequently of the family. As most of these disorders involve progressive deterioration, good habits can become the basis for daily routines and provide the family with tangible schedules for their loved ones, in addition to stabilizing disrupted sleep patterns.

Compliance with treatment is a major obstacle in working with this population. However, the family should understand that increased time within the home could prevent an abrupt decline in global functioning often associated with initial nursing home placement. In addition, many patients begin to rely on one family member over the others (usually a spouse), which can lead to major behavioral disruption when the primary caregiver becomes ill or cannot manage the routines for even one day. Thus, we recommend that as many caregivers as possible are used early on to ensure that the resources for the patient are available and to prevent burnout by any one loved one.

Access to daytime activities, such as water-aerobics, bingo and walking, is important for the mildly impaired patient and can be sustained for longer periods with the advent of medications for dementia. However, families should also be cautioned that cases of progressive dementia will continue to show declines in functioning, and planning for the future must also be a reality and a part of the treatment planning for the patient and family.

Non-pharmacological interventions for sleep disorders may also be useful in the elderly population with or without dementia. Ancoli-Israel and colleagues[47] examined the effects of bright light therapy with demented geriatric patients in nursing homes. They found indications of changes to sleep patterns including more time between periods of arousal during the night, which implies greater sleep consolidation in demented subjects using the therapy in the morning. Evening bright light therapy led to increased regularity of sleep/wake cycles. Recent studies such as this suggest increasing avenues for treatment in the demented population.

While the treatment of associated or co-morbid sleep disorders in the demented patient can improve the quality of life, the primary goal of the attending clinician remains the treatment of the dementia. While no therapy has proved effective at halting or reversing the dementing process, pharmacological interventions can lessen the cognitive and behavioral problems in several forms of dementia.

The cholinesterase inhibitors donepezil, rivastigmine and galantamine have all been demonstrated to lessen some of the behavioral problems seen in this population[48-50]. The resulting reductions in nocturnal agitation can have a significant beneficial effect both on sleep and daytime functioning, as well as reducing care-taker burden. In one study, treatment with donepezil delayed nursing home admission placement with DAT patients by nearly 2 years[51]. The resulting increased time at home can delay increased confusion often associated with nursing home placement.

While typically well tolerated, these medications can contribute to sleep dysfunction in some cases. Insomnia and daytime somnolence have been reported with this class of medication. Some patients have also reported increased dreaming. Gastrointestinal problems have also been reported with cholinesterase inhibitors at higher rates compared to placebo. These complaints may also affect sleep maintenance.

References

1. Zec RF. Neuropsychological functioning in Alzheimer's disease. In Parks RW, Zec RF, Wilson RS, eds. *Neuropsychology of Alzheimer's Disease and Other Dementias*. New York: Oxford University Press, 1993:3–80

2. McCall WV, Erwin CW, Edinger JD, *et al.* Ambulatory polysomnography: technical aspects and normative values. *J Clin Neurophysiol* 1992; 9:68–77

3. Hirshkowitz M, Moore CA, Hamilton CR III, *et al.* Polysomnography of adults and elderly: sleep architecture, respiration, and leg movement. *J Clin Neurophysiol* 1992;9:56–62

4. Bliwise DL. Normal aging. In Kryger MH, Roth T, Dement WC, eds. *Principles and Practice of Sleep Medicine*, 3rd edn. Philadelphia: WB Saunders, 2000:26–42

5. Carskadon MA, Dement WC. Respiration during sleep in the aged human. *J Gerontol* 1981;36: 420–3

6. Redline S, Bonekat W, Gottlieb D, *et al.* Sleep stage distributions in the Sleep Heart

Health Study (SHHS) cohort. *Sleep* 1998;21 (Suppl):210

7. Reynolds CF III, Kupfer DJ, Taska LS, *et al.* Sleep of healthy seniors: a revisit. *Sleep* 1986; 8:20–9

8. Bonnet MH, Rosa RR. Sleep performance in young adults and older normals and insomniacs during acute sleep loss and recovery. *Biol Psychol* 1987;25:153–72

9. Foley DJ, Monjan AA, Brown SL, *et al.* Sleep complaints among elderly persons: an epidemiologic study of three communities. *Sleep* 1995;18:425–32

10. Merck Manual of Geriatrics – website www.merck.com/pubs/mm geriatrics/sec8/ch66.htm

11. Monk TH, Reynolds CF, Machen MA, Kupfer DJ. Daily social rhythms in the elderly and their relationship to objectively recorded sleep. *Sleep* 1992;15:522–9

12. Middlekoop HAM, Smilde-van den Doel DA, Neven AK, *et al.* Subjective sleep characteristics of 1,485 males and females aged 50–93: effects of sex and age, and factors related to the self evaluated quality of sleep. *J Gerontol Series A: Biol Sci Med Sci* 1996;51:108–15

13. Moe KE, Larsen LH, Vitiello MV, *et al.* Objective and subjective sleep of postmenopausal women: effects of long-term estrogen replacement therapy. *Sleep Res* 1997; 26:143

14. Polo-Kantola P, Erkkola R, Helenius H, *et al.* When does estrogen replacement therapy improve sleep quality? *Am J Obstet Gynecol* 1998;178:1002–9

15. Ancoli-Israel S, Kripke, DF, Klauber MR, *et al.* Sleep-disordered breathing in community-dwelling elderly. *Sleep* 1991;14:486–95

16. Enright PL, Newman AB, Wahe PW, *et al.* Prevalence and correlates of snoring and observed apneas in 5201 older adults. *Sleep* 1996;19:537–8

17. Scharf SM, Garshick E, Brown R, *et al.* Screening for subclinical sleep-disordered breathing. *Sleep* 1990;13:344–53

18. Ancoli-Israel S, Kripke DF, Klauber MR, *et al.* Periodic limb movements in sleep in community-dwelling elderly. *Sleep* 1991;14:496–500

19. Mendelson WB. Are periodic leg movements associated with clinical sleep disturbance? *Sleep* 1996;19:219–23

20. Bliwise DL, Rye DB, Dihenia BH, *et al.* Periodic leg movements in sleep in elderly patients with parkinsonism. *Sleep* 1998;21(Suppl):196

21. Bliwise DL. Dementia. In Kryger MH, Roth T, Dement WC, eds. *Principles and Practice of Sleep Medicine*, 3rd edn. Philadelphia: WB Saunders, 2000:1058–71

22. Mundy-Castle AC, Hurst LA, Beerstecher DM, *et al.* The electroencephalogram in the senile

psychoses. *Electroencephalogr Clin Neurophysiol* 1954;6:245–52

23. Coben LA, Danzinger W, Storandt MA. A longitudinal EEG study of mild senile dementia of the Alzheimer's type: changes at 1 year and 2.5 years. *Electroencephalogr Clin Neurophysiol* 1985;61:101–12

24. Prinz PN, Peskind ER, Vitaliano PP, *et al.* Changes in the sleep and waking EEGs of nondemented elderly subjects. *J Am Geriatr Soc* 1992;30:86–93

25. Petit D, Montplaisir J, Lorrain D, *et al.* THA that does not effect sleep or EEG spectral power in mild to moderate Alzheimer's disease. *Eur Neurol* 1996;36:197–200

26. Redline S, Strauss ME, Adams N, *et al.* Neuropsychological function in mild sleep disordered breathing. *Sleep* 1997;20:160–7

27. Gibson GE, Pulsinelli W, Blass JP, *et al.* Brain dysfunction in mild to moderate hypoxia. *Am J Med* 1981;70:1247–54

28. Montplaisir J, Nicolas A, Godbout R, *et al.* Restless leg syndrome and periodic limb movement disorder. In Kryger MH, Roth T, Dement WC, eds. *Principles and Practice of Sleep Medicine*, 3rd edn. Philadelphia: WB Saunders, 2000:742–52

29. Nichols DA, Allen RP, Grauke JH, *et al.* Restless legs syndrome symptoms in primary care: a prevalency study. *Arch Intern Med* 2003;163: 2323–9

30. Montplaisir J, Boucher S, Poirier G, *et al.* Clinical, polysomnographic, and genetic characteristics of restless legs syndrome: a study of 133 patients diagnosed with a new standard criteria. *Move Disord* 1997;12:61–5

31. Mayo Clinic – website www.mayo.edu/geriatrics-rst/Sleep

32. Inouye SK, Charpentier PA. Precipitating factors for delerium in hospitalized elderly persons: predictive model and interrelationship with baseline vulnerability. *J Am Med Assoc* 1996;275:852–7

33. Elliott WJ. Circadian variations in the timing of stroke onset. A meta-analysis. *Stroke* 1999; 29:992–6

34. Bassetti C, Aldrich MS. Sleep apnea in acute cerebrovascular diseases: final report on 128 patients. *Sleep* 1999;22:217–23

35. Netzer N, Werner P, Jochums I, *et al.* Blood flow of the middle cerebral artery with sleep-disordered breathing. *Stroke* 1998;29:87–93

36. Bassetti C, Aldrich M, Chervin E. *et al.* Sleep apnea in the acute phase of TIA and stroke. *Neurology* 1996;47:1167–73

37. Kaneko Y, Hajek V, Zivanovic V, *et al.* Relationship of sleep apnea to functional capacity and length of hospitalization following stroke. *Sleep* 2003;26:293–7

38. Meguro K, Ueda M, Kobayashi I, *et al.* Sleep disturbance in elderly patients with cognitive impairment, decreased daily activity and periventricular white matter lesions. *Sleep* 1995;18:109–14

39. Bassetti C, Mathis J, Gruuger M, *et al.* Hypersomnia following thalamic stroke. *Ann Neurol* 1996;39:471–80

40. Kales A, Ansel RD, Markham CH, *et al.* Sleep in patients with Parkinson's disease and normal subjects prior to and following levodopa administration. *Clin Pharmocol Ther* 1971;12: 397–406

41. Comella CL, Tanner CM, Ristanovich RR. Polysomnographic sleep measures in Parkinson's disease patients with treatment-induced hallucinations. *Ann Neurol* 1993;36: 262–6

42. Moret J. Differences in sleep in patients with Parkinson's disease. *Electroencephalogr Clin Neurophysiol* 1975;38:653–7

43. Aldrich MS. Parkinsonism. In Kryger MH, Roth T, Dement WC, eds. *Principles and Practice of Sleep Medicine*, 3rd edn. Philadelphia: WB Saunders, 2000:1051–7

44. Yamamura Y, Sobue I, Ando K, *et al.* Paralysis agitans of early onset with marked diurnal fluctuation of symptoms. *Neurology* 1973;23: 239–44

45. Arnulf I, Konofal E, Merino-Andreu M, *et al.* Parkinson disease and sleepiness: an integral part of PD. *Neurology* 2002;58:1019–24

46. Fish DR, Sawyers D, Allen PJ, *et al.* The effect of sleep on the dyskinetic movements of Parkinson's disease, Gilles de la Tourette syndrome, Huntington's disease, and torsion dystonia. *Arch Neurol* 1991;48:210–14

47. Ancoli-Israel S, Martin JL, Kripke DF, *et al.* Effect of light treatment on sleep and circadian rhythms in demented nursing home patients. *J Am Geriatr Soc* 2002;50:282–9

48. Feldman H, Gauthier S, Hecker J, *et al.* A 24-week, double-blind, study of donepezil in moderate to severe Alzheimer's disease. *Neurology* 2001;57:613–20

49. McKeith I, Del Ser T, Spano PF, *et al.* Efficacy of rivastigmine in dementia with Lewy bodies: a randomized, double-blind, placebo-controlled international study. *Lancet* 2000;356:2031–6

50. Tariot PN, Solomon PR, Morris JC, *et al.* and the Galantamine USA-10 Study Group. A 5 month, randomized placebo-controlled trial of galantamine in AD. *Neurology* 2000;54:2269–76

51. McRae T, Knopman D, Mastey V, *et al.* Donepezil is strongly associated with delayed nursing home placement in patients with Alzheimer's disease [abstract]. *J Neurol Sci* 2001;187:(Suppl 1):S536

Section 5:

Forensic sleep psychiatry

25

Dangerous and destructive sleep

Alexander Z. Golbin and Leonid Kayumov

In all of us, even in good men, there is a lawless, wild-beast nature which peers out in sleep.

Plato, *The Republic* (cited from Mahowald and Schenck,1999[1])

INTRODUCTION

This chapter is devoted to some dangerous and destructive aspects of sleep. It still states the truth that sleep is an active time of healing, but there is another, dangerous and destructive, side to sleep to which we need to pay attention.

We spend our lives cycling through many stages of vigilance from deep slow-wave sleep (stages 3–4 NREM or delta sleep) to the highest levels of wakefulness and alertness. Other states of vigilance include transitional states between sleep and wakefulness as well as altered states of consciousness in normalcy (meditation; hypnotic trances; artistic and sport-related super-focused attention; ecstasy) and pathology (dissociative conditions, drug-related trance, etc).

Each state of vigilance has its own active process of formation and potential for rest and healing, but they also hide significant, destructive forces. Sleep, more than the other states of vigilance, is an active force that can heal, but also can kill.

The section Medical Disasters in Sleep describes those destructive aspects of sleep that can be related to metabolic, emotional or behavioral changes. Those changes could be self-directed: dangerous fluctuations of blood pressure or glucose level; heart arrhythmias; heart attacks; strokes; sudden death; frightening emotions; self-injurious behavior, etc. The section entitled Violent Sleep describes destructive sleep and sleep-related states that could be directed toward others which may be associated with violent outbursts, property damage, and injuries of others including murder.

Sleep disorders by themselves can have destructive consequences in the family environment, including cases of child abuse, industrial accidents and other social catastrophes. The section Etiology and Clinical Pictures describes different causes of destructive and dangerous sleep, emphasizing how important it is to remember that fatigue and sleepiness are not equal conditions, and also that sleeplessness and alertness are not fully reciprocal states[2].

The next section, Serious Sleep-Related Injuries in Children, describes typical scenarios.

The section entitled Pathophysiology is devoted to the search for mechanisms of dangerous and destructive sleep – alertness states in normalcy or pathology that might help to make credible medical–legal evaluations in cases of significant complexity where an internal turbulent metabolism or external violent behavior caused tragic results. Legal consequences of such cases might be enormous and credible evaluations are crucial.

323

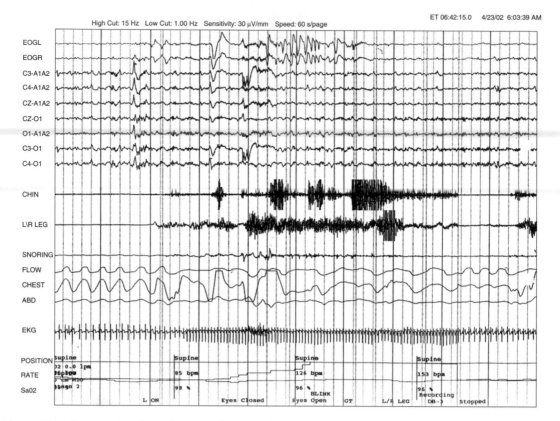

Figure 25.1 Paroxysmal tachycardia in a patient complaining of morning headache

The section entitled Assessing the Role of a Sleep Disorder in Nocturnal Violence mentions several guidelines on how to investigate sleep for forensic applications. In the section on Management a few useful treatment and preventive measures are recommended.

MEDICAL DISASTERS IN SLEEP

When researchers started routinely studying subjects in sleep laboratories, it was quickly observed that subjects might stop breathing during sleep for quite a long time. This forced the immediate inclusion of respiratory monitoring as well as electrocardiography into polysomnography[2–4]. Disorders of body functions causing serious damage to health including death were described for all ages and all stages of sleep[5]. Sudden infant death syndrome (SIDS) and other life-threatening events in infants remain puzzling phenomena.

Recent findings demonstrated a significant decrease of the heart-rate variability and paradoxical breathing in the sleep of infants predisposed to SIDS, which is a phenomenon dependent on sleep and body position[6].

Paroxysmal activity on electroencephalograms (EEGs) and seizures in newborns and infants are frequently considered to be benign phenomena[7], but others have expressed a great deal of concern regarding long-term cognitive, emotional and behavioral consequences of early childhood pathology[8]. This issue might be a focus of disagreement between experts in malpractice cases involving obstetricians and pediatricians. At any age, organs or bodily systems could develop dangerous, potentially destructive symptoms in sleep, such as respiratory symptoms (apneas, upper airway resistance, asthma); cardiovascular symptoms (heart arrhythmias) (Figures 25.1 and 25.2); gastrointestinal symptoms

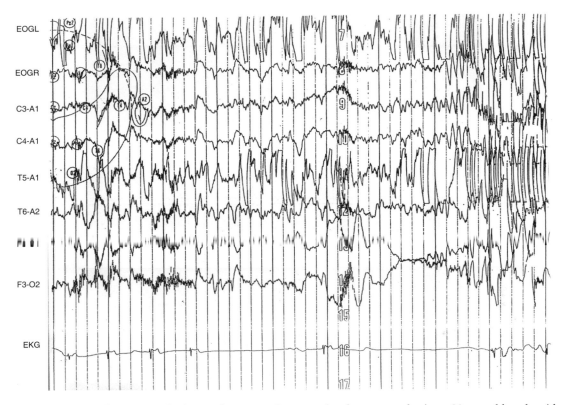

Figure 25.2 Asystole upon awakening: a fragment of nocturnal polysomnography in a 31-year-old male with morning 'seizures'. Speed 30 s/page

(hiccups, abdominal pain, reflux); urinary symptoms (bedwetting); neurological symptoms (convulsions); and skin symptoms (itching), etc. Some symptoms are short-lived and difficult to diagnose, for example paroxysmal tachycardia in the patient complaining of severe headaches upon awakening (Figure 25.1) or heart blocks discovered in a 31-year-old male with morning seizures (Figure 25.2).

It is interesting that there is no direct correlation between age and the severity of a condition. We cannot say, for example, that the younger the child the more dangerous the consequences he/she will have from night terrors or sleepwalking. In some cases of somnambulism and night terrors it is the other way around – adolescents and older people may have more complications (Figure 25.3). The concept of 'critical periods' of increased sensitivity during ontogenetic development might be useful for the explanation of this phenomenon.

Sleep disorders in young children could indirectly cause damage to different body parts or functions. For example, among young orthodontic patients there are an unusually high number of children with a history of significant sleep problems in early childhood, such as multiple awakenings with prolonged screaming at night, reversed day–night sleep and ear infections causing sleep disruptions[8]. It may be that the disruption of slow-wave sleep caused fragmentation in growth hormone release and asymmetric development of growing orofacial areas. Soft neurological symptoms such as mild dysmorphias are frequently found during the neurological examination of patients with chronic childhood onset of sleep disorders[9].

Acute somatic disorders or the exacerbation of chronic conditions (like asthma or sickle cell anemia) may lead to the development of

325

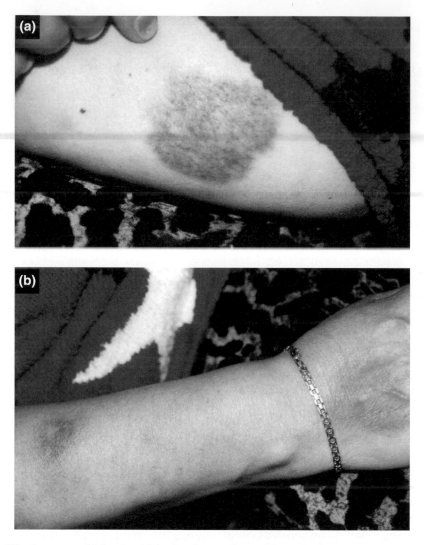

Figure 25.3 Fifty-three-year-old female with bruises from a sleepwalking episode

dangerous symptoms in sleep, such as choking, bleeding, heart arrhythmias, pain, convulsions or even death, and could give rise to questions such as 'who is to blame?'.

Modern disorders, for example fibromyalgia and chronic fatigue syndrome, with their ambiguous and seemingly non-life-threatening symptoms might nevertheless bring a great deal of trouble to the patient and to the treating physicians both clinically and legally (disability issues).

Dreams are a great source of stress in all ages, causing extreme turbulence in autonomic systems with life-threatening results (see Chapter 8).

Self-directed injurious behavior has also been seen in early childhood. Loud screaming in infants may cause asthmatic cough, or cyanosis from hypoxia and apneas. Head banging was also observed with accidental injuries[10]. Among 200 cases of head banging and body rocking, four were involved in litigation, when neighbors bitterly complained about constant disturbing loud noise from the rocking bed in the next apartment or room, and reported possible child abuse from noticing scratches on the child's forehead[9].

Nocturnal eating syndrome in infants and small children might cause profuse vomiting and abdominal pain. In the older population the differentiation between self-injurious behavior and violence toward others is blurred and is typically described together.

VIOLENT SLEEP

The notion that sleep might be violent was not popular until recently. An increased number of sleep centers around the world have found numerous cases of injuries and violent attacks, including homicide, while the litigious nature of our society has brought them to high-profile attention.

Knowledge about the existence and types of injurious behavior is important: (1) to increase awareness among clinicians and the public about this potentially life-threatening phenomenon; (2) to enhance understanding of its pathophysiology and the pathogenesis of human behavior; (3) for practical management and prevention; and (4) for forensic and legal reasons. The body of literature on this subject is growing rapidly and excellent reviews are available[1,11-19].

Increasing reports of serious episodes of violent behavior arising from sleep have changed the perception of these from being extremely rare occurrences to being common disorders with a wide range of types, severity and frequencies of episodes. Moldofsky et al.[11] found that 38 out of 64 (59%) consecutive adult patients with sleepwalking and sleep terrors exhibited some sort of harmful behavior. Twenty-one (46%) showed injuries to themselves and nine (14%) had violent aggressive attacks toward others.

Guilleminault et al.[12] described 41 patients with nocturnal wandering, among whom 29 patients had exhibited violent and aggressive behaviors. Schenck et al.[13] have reported 100 cases. Based on a large epidemiological study of about 5000 non-clinical adults surveyed in the United Kingdom, Ohayon et al.[14]

reported that the rate of those experiencing current episodes of sleep-related violence in the general population is 2%. Cartwright[15] reported 29 patients with violence during arousals from the first hour of sleep. Cartwright estimated that 68 murder cases have been brought to trial in which the defense of sleepwalking has been invoked. Mild and moderate incidents of injurious behavior are probably grossly under-reported and covered up, owing to guilt, shame or simply not knowing to whom to report these stories. Crisp[16] referred to sleepwalking/night terror in adults as a 'closet disorder'.

There is an agreement between sleep specialists that the range of injurious behaviors is extremely wide from night to night, varying from benign acts (such as sudden loud screaming; urinating on a partner; punching the mattress, pillows or the wall; knocking the furniture about) to serious self injury, and attempted/completed murder.

Sometimes it is difficult to find who is to blame for injuries. A 28-year-old woman had a bedwetting episode. Her boyfriend kicked her angrily while sleeping, pushed her out of bed and accidentally poked her eye with his finger.

Leg kicking, head banging, body rocking, thrashing about or vomiting in sleep frequently leads to injury to self or others.

Sleep- and sleepiness-related injuries could be applied to a considerably wider spectrum of incidents, such as forgetting to turn off the stove during nocturnal eating or a sleep-deprived mother bathing her enuretic child in the middle of the night and accidentally scalding the child by turning the hot water knob instead of the cold one. Some patients with severe insomnia use self-injurious rituals (biting, burning, cutting) as a means to release the tension that is preventing them from falling asleep (Figures 25.4 and 25.5). The list of similar cases is infinite. Fatal accidents caused by sleepy drivers have recently been elevated to the status of a major public health issue.

Among dangerous and destructive behaviors related to parasomnia, the most challenging to society and medical science are cases

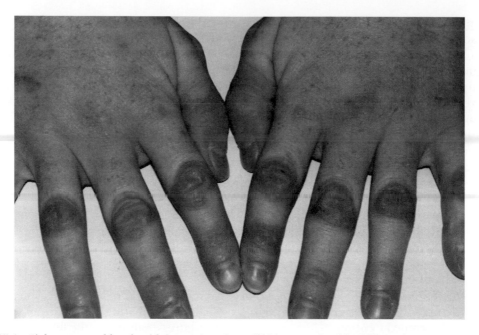

Figure 25.4   Eighteen-year-old male with insomnia, using self-biting as a ritual for falling asleep

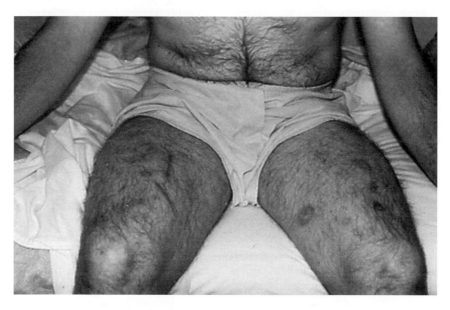

Figure 25.5   Twenty-six-year-old male with self-mutilation (burning and cutting to decrease pre-sleep tension)

of sleep-related homicide. The first documented case of murder committed while asleep happened in medieval times[17–19]. Bernard Schedmazing, a Silesian woodcutter, woke up abruptly after only a few hours of sleep and thought he saw an intruder at the foot of his bed. He picked up his ax and killed his wife who was lying beside him. There are a number of well-documented homicides associated with sleep conditions, most commonly related to sleepwalking or sudden and abrupt arousals in the morning or in the middle of the night. Severe and multiple injuries to oneself and others are typical. Here are two more examples described by Broughton *et al.* which occurred over a century ago. A colonel shot a guardsman on patrol and his own horse. A servant girl stabbed one of her master's children to death during a sleepwalking episode.

Some child abuse cases may be related to confusional conditions due to sleep deprivation, as was described by A. P. Chekhov[20] in a series of short stories, based on real cases. In one of the stories, 'Sleepy Head', he describes the true story of a 12-year-old servant girl with a demeaning nickname 'Varka', who was forced to be a 24-h nanny for an infant. After several sleepless nights, she became confused, started to hallucinate and killed the baby.

At last, tired to death, Varka does her very utmost, strains her eyes, looks up at the flickering green patch, and listening to the screaming, finds the foe who will not let her live.

That foe is the baby.

She laughs. It seems strange to her that she has failed to grasp such a simple thing before. The green patch, the shadows, and the cricket seem to laugh and wonder, too. The hallucination takes possession of Varka. She gets up from her stool, and with a broad smile on her face and wide unblinking eyes, she walks up and down the room. She feels pleased and tickled at the thought that she will be rid directly of the baby that binds her hand and foot...Kill the baby and then sleep, sleep, sleep...

Laughing and winking and shaking her fingers at the green patch, Varka steals up to the cradle and bends over the baby. When she has strangled him, she quickly lies down on the floor, laughs with delight that she can sleep, and in a minute is sleeping as soundly as the dead.[20]

Recently, there were several highly publicized cases of sleep-related homicide[18,21–24] and sexual assault[25] that brought to life a new field: sleep law[22]. The nature of legal defense of sleep-related injuries became very complex because of the issue of insane versus non-insane automatism. In cases of 'non-insane automatism' the accused is entitled to full acquittal, and is therefore set free, which happened in the case

of Kenneth Parks[17,18]. However, if the automatic acts in question are considered to spring from mind disease, they are classified or considered as insane automatism, and the individual is sent to a mandatory institution for the criminally insane for an indefinite period of time.

Despite the diversity, extensive range and various consequences of sleep-related injurious behavior, it has some typical characteristics that distinguish it from similar behavior when awake[1,15,17,18]:

(1) Sleep-related violent behavior contains different degrees of impaired consciousness, defined as the brain function of awareness[17];

(2) The sleeping person has almost completely lost control over his/her behavior;

(3) The appearance of injurious behavior associated with sleep is frequently sudden, with no clear evidence of motivation, and it looks irrational compared to the waking behavior of the same individual;

(4) Acts of violence might not be short but prolonged and well co-ordinated. In one of Cartwright's cases[15] a young man broke his mother's arm by hitting her repeatedly with a baseball bat. Broughton *et al.* reported that Kenneth Parks drove a fair distance prior to the murder[18]. Special orientation and fine motor co-ordination were intact, yet there was no focal recognition at that time and no memory of the event. According to Bonkalo[26] there was 'perplexity and remorse' when these individuals became aware of what they had done; they displayed guilt and tremendous sadness;

(5) Individuals who are violent in sleep are usually described as very nice people and perfect examples of loving husbands, sons and fathers. There is no underlying psychopathology responsible for sleep-related violence;

(6) The person attacked is not usually one with whom there is any ongoing conflict. As one man said of the wife he stabbed

44 times, (she is) 'the only women I ever loved, my best friend'[18]. As Bonkalo[26], who set the criteria for this disorder, stated, the target is anyone who is unlucky enough to be present.

The general agreement is that sleep-related violence is more common in males than in females, typically aged between 15 and 44 years. These people also experience other parasomnias such as night terrors, sleeptalking and bruxism. Seventy-one per cent of those with self-reported violence in the Ohayon study[14] also reported limb jerking. Patients frequently have nocturnal enuresis in their history

ETIOLOGY AND CLINICAL PICTURES

Almost every sleep disorder, and accordingly disorders of alertness, may potentially cause or trigger different degrees of injurious and violent behavior.

Neurological conditions associated with sleep-related violent behavior include disorders of arousal (sleep drunkenness, sleepwalking, sleep terrors, rapid eye movement (REM) sleep behavior disorders, nocturnal seizures and automatic behavior).

Examples of psychogenic sleep disorders are disassociative states (fugues, multiple personality disorder, psychogenic amnesia); malingering; Munchausen by proxy syndrome; medical and primary sleep disorders (obstructive apnea); which might mimic or trigger violent sleep[27]. The most common sleep disorders causing violence are the paroxysmal group of parasomnias such as sleepwalking.

Broughton and Shimizu[17] summarized disorders with potential for sleep-related violence as follows:

Parasomnias are defined as undesirable phenomena during sleep: confusional arousals; sleepwalking; night terrors; REM Behavior Disorder (RBD); paroxysmal nocturnal dystonia; sleep-related epileptic seizures; nocturnal eating syndrome; nocturnal delirium; and overlap parasomnias.

Non-parasomnia disorders: obstructive sleep apnea; idiopathic central nervous system (CNS) hypersomnia; alcoholic/hypnotic related hypersomnia; cerebral degeneration disorders; RLS [restless legs syndrome] and PLM [periodic limb movement] in sleep; intensified sleep starts; waking aggression and malingering.

Confusional and agitated arousals are the most common cause of injuries[28]. As an example, family members described how they tried to awaken the father using a broom, because of his agitation and aggressive reaction to touching or forceful awakening. This ended with multiple blunt traumas to two members of the family, when the 280-pound man inflicted injuries on his wife and older son while they tried to wake him up and forgot, on this occasion, to use a broom. Confusional arousals have been described mainly in slow-wave sleep arousals from the first third of the night, but may appear in the morning during sudden awakening from REM-related unpleasant dreams.

Sleepwalking, or somnambulism, is the next most common condition in which injurious behavior was reported[9,16,18,19,22–24,29–38] and in several cases was directly linked to homicide[23,38]. The most studied example of somnambulistic homicide was Kenneth Parks' case in Canada[18,27]:

While sleepwalking, Kenneth Parks, a 22-year-old 'perfect' son, trampled his wife to death and assaulted his father-in-law. He claimed to have no memory of it in the morning. He was charged with first-degree murder of his wife and an attempted assault on his father-in-law. Based on a thorough evaluation of his history of sleepwalking episodes, he was diagnosed with pathological somnambulism, and after a highly emotional trial, it was concluded that Kenneth Parks committed the violent act unconsciously.

Somnambulism represents a remarkable state, combining some level of 'self awareness' but also having all the symptoms of sleep. It is organized behavior that is sometimes very similar to wakefulness because of its complexity and apparently goal-oriented appearance. Although in sleepwalking episodes the eyes are typically open, the individual does not fully incorporate environmental stimuli. Shakespeare fully recognized this in describing Lady Macbeth's sleepwalking. The Doctor remarked on observing Lady Macbeth that 'her eyes are open', to which the Lady-in-Waiting who had witnessed many such episodes answered 'Aye, but their sense is shot'.

In general it is impossible to distinguish somnambulistic behavior from the person's usual behavior during the daytime, because unconsciously this behavior is pre-programmed and has to 'run itself out'. There is no evidence that a sleepwalker can actually plan during the daytime what he/she will do in sleep and fake in sleep. Similar complex behavior, not remembered afterwards, is seen in a number of medical conditions in which conscious awareness is absent or impaired. This includes some so-called psychotic fugue stages, drug-related dissociated conditions, trance states or epileptic seizures and others.

Sleep terrors (non-REM sleep related agitations) are much less frequently associated with violent behavior; however, a few case reports exist[39]. Sleep terrors usually lead to somnambulism in a single attack[40].

Nightmares (REM sleep dream mentations) and sudden awakenings from a nightmare episode might lead to confusional arousals with agitation and injury[33] (see Chapters 8 and 11).

REM sleep behavior disorder (RBD) is a condition in which the person acts out his dreams that could subsequently lead to complex and, at times, violent behavior. RBD was first described by Japanese authors in patients with organic brain pathology of various types[35] and later elaborated by Schenck et al.

Ferreira et al.[34] reported disorganized behavior in REM sleep in a case of brainstem tumor. Schenck et al.[24,30,36,41,42] found that RBD is a frequent phenomenon among otherwise normal elderly individuals. Injurious behavior among them is quite common, but homicide has not yet been reported.

Sundowning and nocturnal delirium are reported in demented patients with organic brain lesions[17,35]. Injurious behaviors were directed toward themselves, care-takers at home, nursing home attendants or hospital personnel.

Paroxysmal nocturnal dystonia is a condition related to dystonic movements in sleep of either long or short duration. There is evidence, especially for short movements, that such mostly self-injurious episodes may represent frontal lobe seizures[12,17].

The diagnosis of 'episodic nocturnal wandering' was introduced by Pedley and Guilleminault in 1977[43] in reference to a group of conditions in which the person leaves the bed while sleeping and is wandering about in an epileptic episode. Ictal EEG discharges were found in these cases. Epilepsy-related cases of nocturnal wandering are extremely rare, and this phenomenon is more frequently encountered in non-epileptic (by EEG) patients.

Bedwetting can lead to injurious behavior, for example walking into a wall instead of a bathroom, or urinating on another person. It is important to note that enuretic children were frequently ridiculed and attacked by others in closed environments such as the army, school, sport camps, and even by family members[9].

Narcolepsy can lead to amnesic automatic somnambulism[37]. Lethal accidents were reported in narcoleptic drivers[30,31,36]. Narcolepsy might also be associated with RBD[36].

Sleep apnea syndrome and upper airway resistance syndrome may be associated with confusional arousals, sleepwalking and night terrors, which might occur at the initial stages of continuous positive airway pressure (CPAP) treatment[38].

Organic brain syndrome, a significant sleep problem with agitated arousals and daytime confusional states, was reported in brainstem syndromes, alcoholism, brain tumors, olivo-portocerebellar degeneration, progressive supranuclear palsy, Shy–Drager syndrome, Parkinson's disease and Machado–Joseph Azorean disease[17,34,44].

Nocturnal conscious aggression that masquerades as a sleep disorder should always be suspected[15].

SERIOUS SLEEP-RELATED INJURIES IN CHILDREN AND ADOLESCENTS

Sleep-related injuries in children are frequent, and just as significant as they are for adults. In their sleep children and adolescents might run away, have head banging episodes, pull their hair or hurt themselves. The following are anecdotal examples:

(1) A 12-year-old girl ran out of her house into the street in her sleep and was run over by a passing car. As a result she received multiple bruises and head trauma;

(2) An 11-year-old boy jumped out of his bed. He fought with his grandmother who was trying to stop him and calm him down. In a fight he broke his grandmother's leg;

(3) A 10-year-old bedwetter urinated in the closet. On the way back he bumped into the wall, resulting in prolonged nose-bleeding;

(4) A 5-year-old girl, who banged her head in her sleep, accidentally poked her eye with a screw on the bed headboard. The eye was enucleated.

The parasomnias described above are usually associated with arousals from sleep.

Another set of self-injurious behaviors is that related to dissociative conditions and confusional states. Confusional states relate to the person's decreased level of alertness or fragmented alertness due to sleep deprivation, the twilight zone between wakefulness and sleep when the tired person could not fall asleep or between sleep and wakefulness during midnight awakenings or during forceful awakening in the morning.

Self-injurious behavior might be a symptom of certain medical and psychiatric conditions including drug effects where alertness is blurred. One of the relatively benign examples of a self-injurious sleep-related habit is finger sucking, when a child sucks its fingers and damages the skin. As was shown above, many serious bad habits can be conceptualized as self-injurious behavior related to the pathology of alertness.

Another example is adolescents or young adults who repeatedly hold their breath for prolonged intervals or squeeze their neck with a towel to 'hypnotize' themselves – a disorder known as repetitive hanging. They actually choke themselves to achieve these confusional states of mind when the world looks like a dream. These adolescents did not want to commit suicide and they were not depressed, but some of them accidentally choked themselves to death.

PATHOPHYSIOLOGY

A large number of predisposing, facilitating and triggering factors have been indicated in sleep-related violence. Pathophysiological factors, potentially involved in sleep-related violence, are[17]:

(1) Immediate triggers prior to the onset of sleep;

(2) Circadian time of day;

(3) Degree of sleep pressure:

    (a) Total and partial sleep deprivation;

    (b) Sleep microfragmentation;

(4) Speed of arousals from prior sleep;

(5) Physiological level of arousals during violence;

(6) Coexisting microsleeps after arousal;

(7) Incomplete or dissociative sleep–wake states;

(8) Cognitive misperceptions, dreams, hallucinations;

(9) Effects of drugs, alcohol and other substances;

(10) Sleep-related hypoxemia;

(11) Presence of brain lesions;

(12) Epileptic (ictal and post-ictal) confusional states.

Non-REM arousal disorders, such as confusional arousals, sleepwalking and sleep terrors, are considered to be disorders of alertness[17,18,45]. The reason to consider parasomnia as an arousal disorder is that in cases of forced arousal in predisposed individuals it could provoke a full-blown clinical episode. Predisposing triggering factors include family history, gender, physical and sexual abuse, prior sleep deprivation, exogenous environmental stimuli and endogenous dream stimuli.

In RBD the pathophysiology of self-injurious activity is different. Instead of incomplete awakening, episodes arise within the REM sleep stage without atonia. Unlike the REM arousal disorder, genetic predisposition does not appear to be a significant factor. CNS-active substances might induce sleepwalking.

In parasomnias of epileptic origin, ictal or post-ictal confusion almost always appears to be resistant to behavioral restraint during periods of mental confusion.

Overlap diagnoses are of increasing interest. It is well documented that intermediate forms exist between confusional arousals, sleep terrors and full-blown sleepwalking[17]. It is common for an episode that starts as a sleep terror incident to end with the person getting out of bed and sleepwalking.

Both REM and non-rapid eye movement (NREM) sleep might be involved in a single parasomnia. A particular example is a case report of Machado–Joseph Azorean disease with nocturnal wanderings arising in both NREM and REM sleep[17]. There is a general consensus that there is likely to be a genetic flaw involved in the familial parasomnias making the mechanism that switches between deep NREM sleep to REM sleep vulnerable to disruption. Hublin et al.[46] used the Finnish Twin Cohort experiment to conclude that there is a substantial genetic effect in sleepwalking of both children and adults

but that environmental factors are also implicated. Lecendreux et al.[39] have identified a human leukocyte antigen (HLA) class II association in sleepwalkers, which was found significantly more often in this group than in ethnically matched controls.

Among the 'environmental factors' that make this behavior more likely to occur are sleep disruptions secondary to stressful events and prior sleep deprivation. Joncas et al.[40] have demonstrated this in the laboratory. They used sleep deprivation of 36–40 h as a probe in a small group of adult sleepwalkers and controls. They found that the sleepwalkers showed increases in the frequency and the complexity of their events on a recovery night of sleep relative to baseline sleep, and that control subjects showed no such behavioral episodes. These two new studies, although still preliminary, give us hope for more sensitive techniques than presently exist.

Previously, the presence of hypersynchronous delta sleep prior to an arousal from slow-wave sleep had been implicated as a possible diagnostic sign of a parasomnia[47]. Guilleminault et al.[12] found this sign to be present in only seven of their 41 patients. Schenck et al.[41] failed to find 'delta wave build-up' prior to a slow-wave sleep arousal in their sample of 38 adults with injurious sleepwalking and sleep terrors. In re-scoring the sleep studies conducted many months after the attack by a Phoenix man on his wife, only three episodes of hypersynchronous delta sleep prior to an arousal over 4 nights of recorded sleep were found[15]. In contrast, Pressman[48] reports that episodes of hypersynchronous delta bursts (two or more maximum amplitude delta waves within 10 s prior to an arousal) are common in patients being evaluated for sleep apnea. These typically followed a snore or a hypopnea although none had a history of sleepwalking or sleep terrors. This EEG characteristic does not appear to be a sensitive or specific diagnostic sign.

Detailed pathophysiology of sleep-related violent behavior is still not clear. What seems clear is that the visual pathway that terminates in the parietal lobes and controls visually guided movement is functioning normally, but the visual pathway that terminates in the temporal lobe and adds the semantic and affective meaning to what is seen is not operational. Many authors have stated that this is a disorder in which part of the brain is still asleep and part is awake. This difference in the functioning of the two aspects of the visual system is one instance where this is the case. Other senses are also apparently turned off during an episode and return only slowly to full waking levels. Pain perception for self-inflicted wounds or those incurred in a struggle with another person is often delayed, as it may also be in waking during periods of extreme stress. Auditory perception is also shut down. Although a buzzer has been used to stimulate an episode during a laboratory evaluation, during an act of real violence patients have not responded to the cries of their victim or voices calling to them. Nor does cold water wake them up. The higher executive functions of reasoning and planning are clearly not working and the profound amnesia points to a block in memory formation.

Sleep laboratory studies confirm that such patients show some instability of sleep with arousals occurring during the first hour of sleep, prior to the first REM period. Usually this is shown as repetitive arousals from the first delta sleep (stages 3/4), although in some cases arousals may occur in stage 2 as well. The hypnograms of these patients show difficulty in sustaining uninterrupted periods of deep sleep and that they frequently continue to attempt to enter delta sleep persisting into the later hours of the night. However, these late night delta outbursts seldom result in parasomnia events.

Summary

Dangerous autonomic changes in the sleeping person, their injuries and violent behavior, with few exceptions, are not based on the 'structural' damage in one organ or body system. The 'body hardware' is intact. What is wrong is the desynchronization of physiological biorhythms in different systems and, as a result, destructively chaotic or reverse interactions between biorhythms.

Dangerous, injurious and violent sleep are disorders of the 'software'. Successful troubleshooting of these software disorders is based on the development of a general theory of sleep disorders (specifically parasomnias), and methodology of their evaluations.

ASSESSING THE ROLE OF A SLEEP DISORDER IN NOCTURNAL VIOLENCE

Any patient with a history of sleep-related violent behavior requires careful investigation to fully document the condition. A detailed history and physical examination are essential. Most of the information must be obtained from the sleeping partner, the family or other observers, as patients are typically totally unaware and amnesic of their behaviors. Care should be taken to ask about the following: behavioral details; the role of behavioral resistance; any potential motivation for violence; possible facilitating and triggering factors; time of night; presence or absence of recalled mental activity or dreaming; possible involvement of drugs or alcohol; family history of sleep disorders; and other salient features such as bedwetting, night terrors and somnambulism.

Psychological and psychiatric assessment is often indicated. Neuropsychological testing of individuals with possible organic brain syndrome might discover the cognitive deficits, and impaired consciousness, other than those attributable to partial or dissociated sleep states. Personality testing with the Minnesota Multiphasic Personality Inventory (MMPI) or other standardized tests, documentation of depression with the Beck Depression Inventory or other mood inventories, and formal intelligence testing all may be helpful. Detailed psychiatric assessment may reveal an occult motivation for violent behavior. There is the need to examine sleep-related violence as a stress disorder. It differs from post-traumatic stress disorder (PTSD) in the absence of waking symptoms and of nightmares, as these patients have their arousals prior to REM sleep. When the violence is immediate, they do appear to have been startled out of sleep, and to be responding to a heightened sense of threat resulting in a fight or flight response or an attempt to rescue the other person from some impending disaster. Another presentation is a delayed startle response. This is what happened to Kenneth Parks, who while alone took a long uneventful drive before the attack; and similarly, to the Phoenix sleepwalker who arose from bed, walked out to the backyard pool and worked on the defective pool motor for a time before his wife came out to the area. Both men were engaged in doing something they had intended to do next day that their wives had requested – visiting the in-laws, fixing the pool motor. The violence only came when they were interrupted in that task. Both experienced slow recovery of all consciousness following the attack and were without memory of the entire incident according to self reports.

Nocturnal polysomnography (PSG) is an essential step, and more than one study may be necessary. In patients with infrequent parasomnias or with disorders such as sleepwalking and sleep terrors, these events do not frequently appear in a laboratory during PSG testing and, therefore, it is very difficult to document such an event. However, even if an event is not recorded, the PSG may show electrographic and behavior features supportive of the provisional clinical diagnosis. The polysomnograms of persons who sleepwalk may show frequent SWS-to-wake transitions, bursts of hypersynchronous slow waves, and/or frequent micro-arousals or complex behaviors in bed without actual walking. Sleep terror patients may also exhibit frequent SWS-to-wake arousals and autonomic instability independent of episodes. RBD patients often have REM periods without atonia associated with complex gestures in bed without a full-blown episode or before these episodes appear clinically. Of course, patients with sleep-related epileptic seizures may also show inter-ictal EEG discharges, although these are frequently absent in patients with frontal lobe seizures of mesial origin.

New EEG techniques are being developed that may be promising for objective assessment of the level of sleep and sleepiness. One of them is the alpha attenuations task, which can be carried out quickly and easily.

Telemetry is very useful for permitting free movement of the subject unencumbered by wires or cables that lead to a plug-in box. It has been used in the investigation of somnambulism since the 1960s.

Videotape recording, either alone or in association with telemetry, is of great help in objectively documenting the behavioral features for later review and analysis.

Ambulatory monitoring using portable recording devices is another helpful technique. It is particularly useful for parasomnia patients after a traditional PSG has ruled out concomitant sleep disorders (e.g. sleep apnea or periodic limb movement disorder) without recording a parasomnic event, and for patients with infrequent parasomnias. Guilleminault et al.[12] reported it to be particularly useful in determining the final diagnosis in patients presenting with nocturnal wandering.

Neuroimaging techniques such as computerized tomography (CT) scans, magnetic resonance imaging (MRI) and positron emission tomography (PET) scanning may be helpful in localizing structural or functional abnormalities. Particulary well documented is the usefulness of MRI in the localization of lesions in patients with RBD.

Guidelines are needed for determining the role of a sleep disorder in a specific violent act. Mahowald et al.[42] have proposed guidelines which, in our current knowledge, are reasonable. These guidelines apply to a variety of diagnoses and are summarized as follows:

(1) There should be reason in history or investigations to suspect a *bona fide* sleep disorder;

(2) The sleep-related violent action is typically brief (minutes);

(3) The behavior is typically abrupt, immediate, impulsive, senseless and without motivation;

(4) The victim is usually someone who merely happens to be present;

(5) After the action, upon awakening, perplexity and horror are typically present;

(6) Partial or complete amnesia exists for these events;

(7) In the case of sleepwalking, sleep terrors and confusional arousals, the episodes:

    (a) Usually occur in the first third of the night;

    (b) May be precipitated by efforts to awaken the subject;

    (c) May be facilitated by alcohol, sedatives/ hypnotics or prior sleep deprivation.

Sleep-related violence raises difficult ethical problems, as most 'expert witnesses' are retained by either the defense or the prosecution, leading to the tendency for an expert witness to become an advocate or partisan for one side. Frequently, an expert is retained on a contingency based on the outcome of the case. These issues have been grounds for the appearance of what is labelled 'junk science' in the courtroom. Junk science leads to 'junk justice'[1].

The American Academy of Sleep Medicine (previously The American Sleep Disorders Association), with the American Academy of Neurology, have adapted the following guidelines for expert witnesses:

(1) A current, valid, unrestricted license;

(2) A diploma from the American Academy of Sleep Medicine;

(3) Familiarity with the clinical practice of sleep medicine;

(4) Active involvement in clinical practice at the time of the event.

Guidelines for expert testimony include the following:

(1) The witness must be impartial. The ultimate test for accuracy and impartiality is the willingness of the witness to prepare testimony that can be presented unchanged for the use by either the plaintiff or the defendant.

(2) Fees should relate to time and effort and should not be contingent on the outcome of the claim.

(3) The practitioner should be willing to submit his or her testimony for peer review.

(4) To establish consistency, the expert witness should make records of previous expert witness testimony available to the attorneys and expert witnesses of both parties.

(5) The expert witness must not become a partisan or advocate in the legal proceeding.

MANAGEMENT

Pharmacotherapy, using drugs such as benzodiazepines, looks promising by helping to prevent confusional arousals, consolidating sleep architecture and buffering metabolic and blood pressure swings. Anticonvulsive medications (such as gabapentin, topiramate, tiagabin, oxcarbazepine, etc.) may suppress nocturnal movements and act as mood stabilizers.

Psychotherapy with behavioral modification and hypnotherapy might positively modulate the presence of emotional tension, and with post-hypnotic suggestion, full awakening can be induced whenever the person feels like 'hitting the ground'[15].

There is no specific management for sleep-related violence or aggression. Studies have documented that the associated sleep disorder is often present for many months or years before such damaging behaviors appear. This indicates the need for early diagnosis and treatment of the underlying disorder. In many instances facilitating or precipitating factors of the sleep disorder can be identified, and avoiding or minimizing such factors may be extremely helpful. These factors may include various specific stresses, sleep deprivation, intake of alcohol and other CNS-active substances, or other such factors.

Procedures to avoid injury to self or others may be useful, especially in patients with a recurrent predictable pattern of violence. These procedures might include hiding sharp objects, locking doors and other similar strategies. Finally, in many and perhaps most patients, violence or aggression appear only when their behaviors are being restricted. Such restrictions should therefore be totally avoided or at least minimized.

Pharmacotherapy looks promising by helping people get through to the first delta period without arousals. Anticonvulsive medication might suppress nocturnal movement and act as a mood stabilizer. SSRIs may also be helpful.

Psychotherapy, unfortunately often 'post-factum', might help to develop ways of expressing affect in waking and attending to the patient's dream issues that some researches believe to be protective. There are reports that

hypnosis is effective[15] with the post-hypnotic suggestion for full awakening.

CONCLUSION

Sleep can be dangerous. When the 'software' programs in sleep go wrong, destructive Genii might harm the sleeping person's body or jump out to hurt others.

Sleep hides the 'time bombs' of potentially life-threatening disorders and even death, at any age, or causes extreme behavior disorders and violence. The very existence of violent sleep is dramatic proof of the necessity for 'sleep psychiatry' as a field. The forensic sleep psychiatry field is growing out of a public health need. With the increasing knowledge about the mechanisms of sleep–wake disorders the development of new methodologies and technologies make sleep evaluations of forensic cases highly credible.

Sleep is now a serious matter deserving the full attention and alertness of society.

References

1. Mahowald MW, Schenck CH. Sleep related violence and forensic medicine issues. In Chokroverty S, ed. *Sleep Disorders Medicine*. Butterworth/Heinemann, 1999:729–39
2. Guilleminault C, Hoed JVD, Mitler MM. Clinical overview of the sleep apnea syndromes. In Guilleminault C, Dement WC, eds. *Sleep Apnea Syndromes*. New York: Liss, 1978:1
3. Dement WC, Vaughan C. *The Promise of Sleep*. New York: Random House, 1999:462
4. Karacan I, Williams RL, Taylor W. Sleep characteristics of patients with angina pectoris. *Psychosomatics* 1969;10:280
5. Thorpy M. History of sleep in man. In Thorpy M, Yager J, eds. *The Encyclopedia of Sleep and Sleep Disorders*. New York, NY: Facts on File, 1991
6. Guntheroth WG. *Crib Death. The Sudden Infant Death Syndrome*, 2nd revised edn. Mount Kisco, New York: Futura Publishing Co, 1989:165–91
7. Scher MS. Paroxysmal sleep events in the neonate and the young infant: recognizing and treating pediatric parasomnias. In *Recognizing the Treating Pediatric Parasomnias*. APSS 16th Annual Meeting, June 2002. Seattle, Washington, 1–22
8. Shepovalnikov AN. *Activity of the Sleeping Brain*. Leningrad: Nauka, 1971
9. Golbin AZ. *The World of Children's Sleep*. Salt Lake City, UT: Michaelis Medical Publishing Corp, 1995:307
10. Thorpy MJ, Glovinsky PB. Parasomnias. *Psychiatr Clin North Am* 1987;10:623–39
11. Moldofsky H, Gilbert R, Lue FA, *et al*. Sleep-related violence. *Sleep* 1995;18:740–84
12. Guilleminault C, Moscovitch A, Leger D. Nocturnal wandering and violence. *Sleep*, 1995;18:740–84
13. Schenck CH, Milner DM, Hurwitz TD, *et al*. A polysomnographic and clinical report on sleep-related injury in 100 adult patients. *Am J Psychiatry* 1989;146:1166–73
14. Ohayon M, Canlet M, Preist R. Violent behavior in sleep. *J Clin Psychiatry* 1997;58:369–76
15. Cartwright R. Sleep related violence: does the polysomnogram help establish the diagnosis. *Sleep Med* 2000;1:331–5
16. Crisp A. The sleep walking/ night terrors syndrome in adults. *Post Grad Med* 1972;2:569–604
17. Broughton RJ, Shimizu T. Dangerous behaviors by night. In Shapiro C, McCall Smith A,

eds. *Forensic Aspects of Sleep*. Toronto: Willey, 1977:65–84

18. Broughton R, Billings R, Cartwright R, *et al*. Homicidal somnambulism: a case report. *Sleep* 1994;17:253–64

19. Broughton R, Warnes H. Violence in sleep: eleven cases. *Sleep Res* 1989;18:205

20. Chekhov AP. Sleepy head. In *Chekhov Short Stories*. Leningrad: Nauka, 1998:112

21. Fenwick, P. Murdering while asleep. *Br Med J* 1986;293:574–5

22. Nofzinger EA. The Butler sleep apnea homicide. A medico-legal case report. *Sleep Res* 1995;24:312

23. Podolsky E. Somnambulistic homicide. *Med Sci Law* 1960;1:260–5

24. Schenck CH, Milner DM, Hurwitz TD, *et al*. Dissociative disorders presenting as somnambulism: polysomnographic, video and clinical documentation (8 cases). *Dissociation* 1989;2:194–204

25. Fedoroff JP, Brunet Woods V, Gronger C, *et al*. A case controlled study of men who sexually assault sleeping victims. In Shapiro CM, McCall Smith A, eds. *Forensic Aspects of Sleep*. Toronto: Willey, 1997:85–98

26. Bonkalo A. Impulsive acts and confusional states during incomplete arousal from sleep: criminological and forensic implications. *Psychiatry Q* 1974;48:400–9

27. McCall-Smith A, Shapiro CM. Sleep disorders and the criminal law. In Shapiro C, McCall-Smith A, eds. *Forensic Aspects of Sleep*. Toronto: Willey, 1997:29–64

28. Tarsh MJ On serious violence during sleepwalking. *Br J Psychiatry* 1986;148:476

29. Howard C, D'Orbaan PT. Violence in sleep: medico-legal issues and two case reports. *Pyschol Med* 1986;17:915–25

30. Schenck CH, Mahowald MW. A polsomnographically documented case of adult somnambulism with long-distance automobile driving and frequent nocturnal violence: parasomnia with continuing danger as a non-insane automatism? *Sleep* 1995;18:765–72

31. Yellowless D. Homicide by a somnambulist. *J Ment Dis* 1878;24:451–8

32. Lipowski ZJ. Delirium (acute confusional states). *J Am Med Assoc* 1987;258:1789–92

33. Lugersi E, Crignotta F. Hypogenic paroxysmal dystonia: epileptic seizures or a new syndrome? *Sleep* 1981;4:129–38

34. Barros Ferreira DM, Chodkiewizc J, Lairy GC, *et al*. Disorganized relations of tonic and phasic events of REM sleep in a case of brain stem tumor. *Electroencephalogr Clin Neurophysiol* 1975;38:203–7

35. Shimizu T, Sugita Y, Teshima Y, *et al*. Sleep study in patients with OPCA and related diseases. In Koella WP, ed. *Sleep*. Basel: Karger, 1981:435–7

36. Schenck CH, Hurwitz TD, Mahowald MW. REM sleep behavior disorders: an update on a series of 96 patients and review of the world literature. *J Sleep Res* 1993;2:224–31

37. Broughton R, Ghanem Q, Hishikawa Y, *et al*. Life affects of narcolepsy in 180 patients from North America, Asia and Europe compared to matched controls. *Can J Neurol Sci* 1981;8:299–304

38. Millman RP, Kipp GJ, Carskadon MA. Sleepwalking precipitated by treatment of sleep apnea with nasal CPAP. *Chest* 1991;99:750–1

39. Lecendreux M, Mayer G, Bassetti C, *et al*. HLA Class II in sleepwalking. *Sleep* 2000;23(Suppl 2):A13

40. Joncas S, Zarda A, Montplaisir J. Sleep deprivation increases the frequency and complexity of behavioral manifestation adult sleep walkers. *Sleep* 2000;23(Suppl 2):A14

41. Schenck C, Paraja J, Patterson A, *et al*. Analysis of polysmnographic events surrounding 253 slow-wave sleep arousals in 38 adults with injurious sleepwalking and sleep terrors. *J Clin Neurophysiol* 1998;15:159–66

42. Mahowald MW, Bundie SR, Hurwitz TD, *et al*. Sleep violence – forensic implications: polygraphic and video documentation. *J Forensic Sci* 1990;35:413–32

43. Pedley TA, Guilleminault C. Episodic nocturnal wanderings responsive to anticonvulsant drug therapy. *Ann Neurol* 1977;2:30–5

44. Raschka LB. Sleep and violence. *Can J Psychiatry* 1984;29:132–4

45. Broughton R. Human consciousness and sleep/wake rhythms: a review and some neuropsychological considerations. *J Clin Neuropsychol* 1982;4:193–218

46. Hublin C, Kaprio J, Partinen M, *et al*. Prevalence and genetics of sleepwalking: a population based twin study. *Neurology* 1997;48:177–81

47. Blatt I, Peled R, Cadoth I, Levie P. The value of sleep recording in evaluation of somnambulism in young adults. *Electroencephalogr Clin Neurophysiol* 1991;78:407–12

48. Pressman M. Hyposynchronous delta (HSD) activity and sudden arousals from slow-wave sleep (SWS) in adults without NREM parasomnias. *Sleep* 2000;23(Suppl 2):A325

26

Forensic aspects of sleep

Julian Gojer, Leonid Kayumov, Roberta Murphy, Rick Peticca and Colin M. Shapiro

INTRODUCTION

Sleep is a complex phenomenon during which the human mind is at rest and relatively unresponsive to external stimuli[1,2]. People display varying levels of arousability, which vary with many factors including the amount of prior sleep; exposure to stress; ingestion of substances that alter brain function; genetic, social and cultural make-up; and a host of other factors[3,4].

Recent developments in psychiatry and neuropsychiatry in particular underlie a shift from the psychology to the neurology of mind–brain interaction. The year 2003 marks the golden jubilee of the original observation that sleep has alternating cycles defined by the presence or absence of rapid eye movements known as the non-rapid eye movement (NREM) and rapid eye movement (REM) phases[4]. Sleep progresses through four stages beginning with the NREM phase. Stage 1 is the 'lightest' sleep stage and progresses through stages 2 and 3 to stage 4 which is the 'deepest'. During these four stages brain activity slows, and muscle tone, respiratory and cardiac rates decrease. These four stages are known as slow-wave sleep as the frequency of the sleep electroencephalogram (EEG) progressively slows down. REM sleep usually appears after approximately 90 min of slow-wave sleep brain activity. During the night NREM and REM sleep succeed each other. With each recurrence of the cycle the slow-wave period is reduced and the REM stage of sleep is increased. The physiology of sleep is well described in other areas of this book (see Chapters 1, 2 and 3).

Sleep disturbances are well documented and classified by the *International Classification of Sleep Disorders*[5], and many of the diagnostic categories have made their way into the *Diagnostic and Statistical Manual* IV (DSM-IV)[6]. Two important categories are the parasomnias and the dyssomnias. Parasomnias are abnormal behaviors or physiological events associated with sleep. Dyssomnias on the other hand deal with the sleep–wake and timing mechanisms. Both conditions have relevance from a forensic point of view[7,8].

Parasomnias are often associated with motor behaviors that occur in sleep and are a well recognized diagnostic classification. Sleepwalking is one of the most fascinating of the parasomnias. Until recently, most complex motor behaviors in sleep were attributed to sleepwalking or to sleep terror episodes occurring in the NREM stage of sleep[9]. Some episodes were attributed to epileptic attacks, and confusion upon waking[10–12]. Traditionally, it was accepted that REM sleep was associated with muscular atonia. However, it is now known that complex behaviors can occur in the REM phases of sleep[13]. Also of interest are sleep confusional arousals, which are poorly understood, but sometimes associated with motor behaviors of which the individual is not clearly aware[10,14].

Sleepwalking/sleep terrors account for a significant proportion of the reported cases of complex motor behaviors during sleep[11]. Sleepwalking is not an uncommon disorder and is present in 1 to 15% of the community[15]. Sleepwalking is more common in children than in adults[16], in males than in females[17] and in family members of sleepwalkers[18]. Traditionally sleepwalking has been understood as a phenomenon related to sudden arousal from stage 4 NREM sleep, as identified by polysomnography. It can occur spontaneously or in response to triggering mechanisms such as stress, drug and alcohol use, sleep deprivation, pain and as yet unknown factors[18].

In our opinion, sleepwalking has been a loosely defined term to subsume multiple complex motor behaviors occurring in sleep that include walking[19], eating[20], driving[21] and engaging in sexual intercourse[22] to name but a few. Not only has the term become broader, but its primary origins from the NREM stage of sleep have been challenged. We now know that complex motor activity can arise from any stage of sleep, including the REM phase[13].

Complex motor activity during sleep can be amusing or terrifying for onlookers, can be embarrassing for the individual and can result in injury to self or others. Numerous reports of serious physical harm resulting from injuries sustained during sleep exist in the literature[23]. Less frequently reported is harm to a bed partner or some other individual; these incidents include bruising, sexual assaults and even homicides[24,41]. The association between sleep and violence was the focus of an article in the journal *Sleep* in 1995[25].

Many individuals with minor episodes of violence in sleep find their way to sleep clinics and are treated with medication or by environmental manipulation[26]. It can be assumed that these acts result in social disruption and interpersonal strife, but the more sinister acts of violence and those resulting in serious injury and/or death may well become legal issues[27].

The dyssomnias, on the other hand, have relevance from several perspectives. The insomnias are a common reason for referral to a sleep clinic, and hypersomnias along with narcolepsy are equally important. Sleep apneas are often associated with daytime drowsiness and aggressive behavior when the individual is woken[24] (Gojer *et al.*, unpublished).

Treatment of insomnias can lead to individuals falling asleep in the daytime due to hangovers or becoming involved in accidents at home and when driving. The same may be said for narcolepsy[28]. The circadian rhythm sleep disorder also known as the sleep–wake schedule disorder has importance from an employment and social perspective. Prolonged use of hypnotics to treat longstanding sleep disorders can result in medication dependence, and physicians may become liable for a lawsuit.

Parasomnias and dyssomnias can both have legal consequences for the individual and for the treating clinician. The description of the various sleep disorders and their biological and psychological underpinnings are described elsewhere in this book. Here we intend to examine how these disorders interface with the legal system.

THE LAW

Individuals can be held responsible for the acts they commit or the failure to act in a responsible manner. Their behavior may be in violation of the law from a criminal or a civil perspective. This can result in criminal charges being brought by the state or a lawsuit being filed in a non-criminal situation. Sleep behaviors may have implications at the place of work; in personal, business and family relationships; and, more importantly, in the operation of machinery and the driving of vehicles. The physician has a responsibility to the public for ensuring that their patients drive safely. In most jurisdictions this responsibility is codified in provincial or state law.

A criminal act has two components: the *mens rea* and the *actus reus*. An action or a failure to act in a particular situation could carry criminal liability. The concepts of *mens rea* and *actus reus* originate in the development of the criminal common law of England. In order for a person to be convicted of a criminal offence, the state must prove beyond a reasonable doubt that the individual did commit an *actus reus*, a criminal act, and also that the individual simultaneously possessed the *mens rea*, an evil mind or criminal intent, during the commission of the act. It is only the coincidence of *actus reus* and *mens rea* that can lead to a criminal conviction (reviews of these concepts in a forensic context are well addressed by Rogers and Mitchell[29], Rogers[30], Melton and co-workers[31] and Shapiro and Smith[32]).

Any behavior carried out without conscious awareness implies that the *mens rea* or the *actus reus* would be lacking, and the behavior cannot be considered to be criminal. Behaviors occurring during sleep or during partial arousal will be lacking in conscious control. Questions often arise concerning the degree of wakefulness, raising the possibility that such behavior could occur in the context of sleep. In this regard, however, there is often concern about the possibility of feigning sleep when sleep is used as a pretext for denying that an action has occurred.

The courts have wrestled with these ideas and concepts and are unclear how to deal with them. The evolution of actions carried out in a state of altered awareness, diminished level of consciousness or absent consciousness has led to the concept of automatic behaviors. By this it is meant that the behavior was in some way disconnected from the individual's conscious awareness, either wholly or partially. To characterize this behavior, the term automatism entered Anglo-Saxon law.

In a legal context, automatisms refer to a wide variety of conditions that result in behaviors that are essentially criminal in nature but are associated with limited or absent awareness of the act. Fenwick, in his seminal paper, reviewed automatisms and their legal relevance[33]. Organic conditions such as head injuries, seizures, metabolic states, intoxications, medications, etc. have long been accepted as being responsible for automatisms. Similarly

dissociative states of purely psychological origins, with or without coexisting major mental illnesses, have also been accepted by the courts as being the underlying basis for automatisms (*R v. Rabey 1980* – see Appendix for relevant legal cases). Complex sleep-related behaviors, subsumed under the heading of sleepwalking, have been considered to be automatisms (*R v. Parks 1992, R v. Campbell 2000*).

The courts have further divided automatisms into insane and sane automatisms. This distinction has no medical basis, however, appearing to have meaning in only some legal jurisdictions, and has been used to dispose of legal matters accordingly. Sane automatisms are understood to be automatisms that originate from causes outside the individual and/or have a low probability of recurring. Examples of a sane automatism would be a criminal act following a blow to the head or following the administration of insulin with subsequent hypoglycemia-induced altered conscious states. The consequence of a sane automatism would be absolute acquittal, as no crime would have been committed (*R v. Parks 1992*). On the other hand, insane automatisms are caused by conditions that originate from within the individual and/or are likely to recur (*R v. Campbell 2000*). A good example would be epilepsy or epileptic attacks with altered states of consciousness and association with a criminal act. The consequence here would be that the person, though acquitted of the offense, would be liable to be detained in an institution by virtue of being insane or not criminally responsible. Depending on the jurisdiction, the individual may be placed on an ongoing monitoring program by an agency or organization as deemed appropriate by the laws in effect.

In Canada, automatism has been defined in reference to the definition established by the British courts. In *Bratty v. A.-G. Northern Ireland (1961)*, Viscount Kilmuir L.C. in the House of Lords defined automatism as: 'the state of a person who, though capable of action, is not conscious of what he is doing … It means unconscious involuntary action and it is a defense because the mind does not go with what is being done.' In *R. v. Rabey 1980*, the Supreme Court of Canada approved the definition of automatism given by J. Lacourcière in *R. v. Kemp 1957* that is closely modeled to the definition given from Bratty: 'Automatism is a term used to describe unconscious, involuntary behavior, the state of a person who, though capable of action, is not conscious of what he is doing. It means an unconscious, involuntary act, where the mind does not go with what is being done.'

One criticism regarding the above definition is that automatism is characterized in reference to an unconscious state. Legal and medical understandings of unconsciousness often diverge significantly. The medical literature suggests that various different levels of consciousness exist. These levels maintain a hypothetical continuum where the conscious state and the unconscious state are polarized in relation to each other. An 'unconscious' state within the medical literature means that an individual is virtually not arousable, and often this is attributed to organic conditions. Conversely, the legal definition of 'unconscious' connotes that the person did not know what he or she was doing during an automatic episode, and in the legal context both psychological and organic states tend to be lumped together. To avoid this minor confusion, J. Bastarache, writing for the majority of the Supreme Court of Canada in *R v. Stone 1999* supra, defines automatism as: 'A state of impaired consciousness, rather than unconsciousness, in which an individual, though capable of action has no voluntary control over that action.'

The law in Canada recognizes two types of automatism: non-mental disorder automatism and mental disorder automatism. Non-mental disorder automatism occurs when the involuntary action does not stem from a disease of the mind. A verdict of non-mental automatism means that the accused individual would benefit from an absolute acquittal. In contrast, mental disorder automatism occurs when the involuntary action results from a disease of the mind. In

this circumstance, a claim of mental disorder automatism would give rise to a defense of section 16 (1) of the *Canadian Criminal Code* – the defense of mental disorder[34].

Most recently, the Supreme Court of Canada in *R v. Stone 1999* developed a general test that is applicable to all cases involving claims of dissociative states and automatism. The aim of the test focuses on incorporating the various elements of the Court's most recent statements on automatistic behavior in the cases of *Davlault 1994*, *Parks 1992* and *Rabey 1980*. In essence, the test incorporates a two-step approach. The first involves the establishment of a proper foundation for a defense of automatism. To begin, the defense must satisfy the evidentiary burden by proving that the act was involuntary and by adducing expert psychiatric or psychological evidence. The burden is only met where the trial judge concludes that there is evidence upon which a properly instructed jury could find that the accused individual acted involuntarily on a balance of probabilities. In reaching this conclusion, the trial judge must examine psychiatric or psychological evidence and all other available relevant evidence while considering the weight of the foundation and nature of the entire evidence. Examples of other relevant evidence given by the Supreme Court include: the severity of the triggering stimulus; corroborating evidence of bystanders; corroborating medical history of automatistic dissociative states; whether there is evidence of a motive for the crime; and whether the alleged trigger of the automatism is also the victim of the automatistic violence. The trial judge must not rely on any single factor as being determinative and, moreover, the trial judge must weigh all of the evidence on a case-by-case basis.

The second step involves the determination of whether the alleged condition is a mental disorder automatism or a non-mental disorder automatism. If the accused person has laid a proper foundation for a defense of automatism, only then must the trial judge determine whether the condition alleged by the accused person constitutes a mental disorder automatism or non-mental disorder automatism.

If the trial judge concludes that a proper foundation has not been established, then it will be presumed that the alleged condition was a voluntary act and the accused individual would not be able to benefit from either automatism defense. In such a case, the accused person may still claim the defense of mental disorder. Mental disorder is a legal term that is defined in the *Criminal Code* as 'a disease of the mind'.

Whether the accused individual suffered from a disease of the mind is a question of fact that is also to be determined by the trial judge. In determining whether an alleged condition constitutes a disease of the mind, the Court outlines a holistic approach that encompasses the 'internal cause theory' and 'continuous danger theory' from Parks *(R v. Parks 1992)* and the policy concerns in the *Rabey* (1980) decision. The continuous danger theory is not considered to be an exclusive analytical approach to the internal cause theory. Rather, a trial judge, given the context of a case, may find that one or both of these theories are applicable. Furthermore, the trial judge would determine whether and to what extent the theory was useful in each case. Ultimately, the trial judge has the discretion to disregard either theory if its application is not useful.

Under the internal cause theory, the trial judge would consider the nature of the alleged trigger of automatism in order to determine whether a normal person in the same circumstances might have reacted to it by entering a state of automatism. The internal cause theory is considered to be a contextual objective test that is believed to be most useful in cases involving the context of 'psychological blow automatism'. However, this theory is not viewed as a definitive answer to determining the existence of a disease of the mind. Public safety is a policy consideration that also underlies whether a claim of automatism results from a disease of the mind. Such a policy consideration is reflected in the continuous danger theory, which maintains that any condition that is likely to present a

recurring danger to the public should be treated as a disease of the mind. Thus, in examining the possibility for an individual to become a continuing public danger, trial judges will particularly focus on the following two issues: the psychiatric history of the accused, and the likelihood that the trigger alleged to have caused the episode of automatism would recur. Psychiatric evidence revealing a documented history of automatistic dissociative states suggests that the condition alleged by the accused individual is recurring in nature, thus increasing the likelihood that automatism will recur and be classified as a finding of a disease of the mind. Similarly, the likelihood of the trigger that allegedly caused the dissociative episode or a similar episode of equal severity recurring suggests that this would also be classified a disease of the mind.

If the trial judge concludes that the automatistic condition is not a disease of the mind, only then will the defense of non-mental disorder be left with the trial judge. The trial judge must decide whether the defense has proven that the accused individual acted involuntarily on the balance of probabilities. A positive answer will result in an absolute acquittal. On the other hand, if the trial judge concludes that the alleged condition is a disease of the mind, only then will the defense be able to raise section 16 of the *Canadian Criminal Code* – the defense of mental disorder (not criminally responsible on account of mental disorder/insanity). In this event, the trial judge must decide whether the defense has proven, on the balance of probabilities, that the accused individual suffered from a mental disorder which rendered him or her incapable of appreciating the nature and quality of the act in question or knowing that what he or she did was wrong. Wrongfulness, according to the decisions in Chaulk *(R v. Chaulk 1990)* and Oomen *(R v. Oomen)*, is the ability to appreciate moral wrongfulness.

In the USA, the defense of automatism is more commonly referred to as the defense of unconsciousness. In some jurisdictions, such as Oklahoma, the defense of automatism is codified by statute. Similarly, in both Canadian and American criminal law, the defense of automatism maintains, as a general rule, that an individual cannot be held criminally responsible for his or her actions or inactions while in an automatistic or unconscious state. This rule has been affirmed in cases across many state jurisdictions. For example, in *State v. Mercer 1969*, the court argued that 'generally, a person who is unconscious at the time he commits an act which would otherwise be criminal cannot be held responsible for the act.' In *Foster v. State 1983*, the court argued 'the defense of unconsciousness may be used in situations where otherwise criminal conduct of an individual is the result of an involuntary act which is completely beyond the knowledge and control of that individual.' In *State v. Jerrett 1983*, C. J. Branch, writing for the majority, stated 'the rule in this jurisdiction is that where a person commits an act without being conscious thereof, the act is not a criminal act even though it would be a crime if it had been committed by a person who was conscious.' In *State v. Olsen* the situation is similar. In this sense, the defense of automatism is a complete defense to a criminal charge because an automatistic state negates the existence of a mental state and the premise that the criminal act was committed voluntarily. The court in *State v. Jerrett 1983* held that 'the absence of consciousness not only precludes the existence of any specific mental state, but also excludes the possibility of a voluntary act without which there can be no criminal liability.'

The defense of automatism is also an affirmative defense whereby the burden is on the defendant to prove its existence or occurrence to the satisfaction of the judge or jury (*State v. Caddell, NC 1975*). The invocation of the defense of automatism requires the defendant to demonstrate that his or her criminal conduct resulted from an involuntary act completely beyond his or her knowledge. This requirement was expressly stated in *Jones v. State 1982*, *Cartwright v. Maynard 1986* and *Polston v. State 1984*. In the Polston case, the court argued 'a defendant who raises the automatism defense is presumed to be a person with a healthy mind; that the burden is

upon the defendant who raises the defense of automatism to prove the elements necessary to establish defense; and the burden remains with the defendant throughout the trial.'

In some states, such as the state of Wyoming, the defense of automatism is recognized to include abnormal mental conditions resulting from brain injury. However, this defense is separate from the 'defense of insanity' (also referred to as 'the defense of mental illness or deficiency' in some state jurisdictions) in that the defense of automatism is applicable to cases where the automatistic state resulted from a brain injury caused by a concussion. In *Fulcher v. State 1981*, it was held that the 'brain damage' must be only a 'simple brain trauma with no permanent after-effects'; and that brain damage caused a 'serious and irreversible condition having an impact upon the ability of the person to function' momentarily. However, if the impact on the ability of the person to function was 'far more significant than a temporary and transitory condition', then it would be likely to be classified as a 'mental deficiency' and the 'defense of insanity' would then be available to the defendant.

Also, in *Polston v. State 1984*, the court argued that the elements necessary to establish the defense of automatism were the following:

(1) The actor must be a person with a healthy mind;

(2) Who because of a concussion;

(3) Resulting from a brain injury;

(4) That is a simple brain trauma with no permanent after-effects;

(5) Acts in a state of unconsciousness;

(6) In which his actions are devoid of criminal intent.

In *Polston v. State 1984* the court added, 'where unconsciousness results primarily from self-induced intoxication, the defense of automatism is not available but rather the defense is that of intoxication.' Furthermore, the court also argued in this case 'for the purposes of a defense of automatism, a concussion and lack of memory by themselves are not sufficient to establish that the defendant, during the period of time about which he has no recollection, was acting in an automatistic state.'

Sleep disorders with forensic implications

Automatism as a result of sleep disorders

Sleepwalking Sleepwalking has a long history of association with the courts. The literature is replete with examples of all types of offenses[25,27,33,35–38].

The decision of the Supreme Court of Canada in *R v. Parks 1992* set a precedent in addressing the area of automatism as applied to sleepwalking. Evidence was presented that the accused got up in the middle of the night and drove 23 kilometers to the home of his wife's parents. He then entered the house and proceeded to kill his mother-in-law and injure his father-in-law with a knife he found in the kitchen. He then drove to the police station and turned himself in. Uncontradicted psychiatric evidence indicated the accused was sleepwalking. Parks was acquitted of murder charges on the basis of somnambulism. In essence the courts ruled that he was in a state of non-insane automatism and the acquittal was absolute. The courts ruled that the sleepwalking was not a mental disorder[39,40].

The court, however, decided otherwise in *R v. Campbell 2000*[41]. Campbell had been sleeping with his girlfriend with whom he had a good relationship. He had woken in the middle of the night and began to slash at his girlfriend's neck with a knife for a few minutes. Her screams alerted the neighbors who in turn called the police. The episode ended just as the police arrived. Campbell pled guilty to charges of attempted murder and only when an assessment was done at the time of sentencing was the issue of sleepwalking raised. Evidence presented in court resulted in Campbell's initial plea being struck and he was subsequently found to be in a state of

automatism. On this occasion, the presiding judge ruled that his sleepwalking was a disease of the mind and Campbell was acquitted on grounds that he was not criminally responsible on account of mental disorder and the matter was referred to the Ontario Review Board[41].

In *R v. Burgess 1991* the English Court of Appeals upheld the jury decision of the lower court, that Burgess, who hit a friend on the head apparently while asleep, was not guilty by reason of insanity. The appeals court chose to view sleepwalking with violence as not normal and that the causative factor was internal, hence the finding that the condition was a mental disorder, the outcome being insanity.

Sleepwalking and violence are well reported in the literature and outcomes vary[36,37,42–44]. Violent behaviors arising out of sleep or related to sleep disorders have been described by many more authors[23,38,45–48].

Sleep sex (sexsomnia – sexual activity when asleep) Of recent years a new phenomenon has been described, that is: individuals having sexual activity during their sleep. The term sexsomnia has been used to characterize such behavior. The prevalence of sexual activity when either partner is not fully awake is unknown. The reasons for such activity are speculative. Unlike sleepwalking, which has been reported to arise out of slow-wave or NREM stages of sleep, it is suspected that sexual activity during sleep may occur during the REM stage of sleep and may be one of the REM behavior disorders[21,22,43,49,50].

The literature on the phenomenon of sex while sleeping is unclear. Confusion arises about several issues, e.g. whether the victim or the perpetrator was asleep, whether the perpetrator committed the offense in the REM or NREM phase, whether there was memory of the event, etc. Sleep sex or sexsomnia reports generally describe an ill-defined group of individuals. The reader is asked to pay attention to the description of the event and not be carried away by a term used to describe a heterogeneous group of individuals that could also include malingerers.

A report soon to be published by the authors on an individual who was charged with sexually assaulting his daughter is as follows: he had a clearly defined history of sleepwalking, supported by polysomnographic findings and by interviewing three of his adult female sexual partners. His mother also confirmed that he had a childhood history of sleepwalking. What appeared to be a straightforward case of an individual with a history of sleepwalking touching his step-daughter when he was presumed to be asleep was made complicated when phallometric testing was performed in a sexual behaviors laboratory. He showed consistent arousal to pedophilic stimuli on testing and was reported to have an erotic preference for children. Based on this finding he was confronted, and, despite his protestations of innocence, further probing into his background revealed that a former partner acknowledged that he had a history of pedophilic behavior in the past. Faced with this information and with all the evidence of a documented history of sleepwalking, a firm opinion that the offense was a product of that disorder was not offered. The accused reluctantly accepted the findings and on the advice of his counsel pled to lesser charges. To this day, it cannot be said that the individual's behavior was or was not the result of a sleep disorder.

This case then brings into focus yet another case reported by Schenck and Mahowald[51]. Granger *(R v. Granger)* was acquitted on appeal by the Supreme Court of British Columbia on charges related to sexual impropriety with a child. The court acquitted Granger on grounds that the individual had a non-insane automatism. An interesting aspect of this case was the use of alcohol. Schenck and Mahowald[51] address an issue of continuing danger which we will refer to again below.

In a study by Fedoroff and co-workers[22] of men assaulting a sleeping victim, two groups of men who had sexually assaulted a sleeping victim were derived from a legal and a clinical sample and compared to a control sample of men who had sexually offended or had a sexual deviation but had not offended against a sleeping victim. The legal sample had 26 men, the clinical sample had 25 men and the control sample had 25 men. They noted that 2% of sexual assault cases derived from legal records over a 5-year period had committed a sexual assault on a sleeping victim. When a sample of forensic patients referred to a sexual behaviors clinic for sexual assaults were studied, 10% had committed a sexual assault on a sleeping victim.

It was reported that individuals in a clinically derived sample and the controls had more offenses. The legal sample had victims who were generally acquaintances. As compared to the controls, for individuals in the other two groups the sexual act more often involved actual sexual intercourse and intoxication was a more frequent finding. Sexual sadism was more common and so too were sexual dysfunctions. Anxiety disorders were more common.

At our sexual behaviors clinic we sometimes see men accused of perpetrating sexual acts on sleeping victims. The victims often tend to be children or women and very infrequently other men. The overall numbers are small and opinions offered are based on case studies, small cohorts and ill-designed studies.

Referrals to a sleep clinic or a forensic clinic can be complex. The accused may complain of being asleep at the time of the sexual assault, and the victim may or may not have been asleep during the sexual act. In evaluating individuals reported to have exhibited sexual activity with another person, and when one or both individuals claim to have been asleep, several motivating factors need be determined. Such behaviors may fall into one or more of the following domains:

(1) Antisocial and psychopathic individuals who are prepared to take advantage of a sleeping victim;

(2) Individuals with paraphilias (sexual deviations) like pedophilia, coercive rape paraphilia, sexual sadism, necrophilia, exhibitionism, and voyeurism and other paraphilias;

(3) Individuals who are under the influence of drugs and/or alcohol. The victim may be taken advantage of by being intoxicated, because it is speculated that the victim may not remember the act later or not be believed because of extreme intoxication (date-rape situations). The perpetrator may be disinhibited by the intoxicating substance and may not be aware of the sexual act or have a blackout the next day;

(4) Dissociated states when the victim is unable to recall the act or the perpetrator claims to have dissociated at the time of the act (dissociative amnesia or dissociative identity disorder);

(5) Altered states of consciousness other than dissociation which include perpetrators who claim to be genuinely asleep at the time of the sexual act and whose sexual activity reportedly forms part of a parasomnia or a variation of the sleepwalking syndrome (sexsomnia).

Fedoroff and co-workers[22] classified the perpetrators of sleeping victims into three categories:

(1) Men who need to fulfil sadistic or paraphilic fantasies;

(2) Men expressing deviant sexual behaviors to bypass rejection or to avoid detection;

(3) Men who are merely opportunistic.

It is unfortunate that this classification is limited to men who the authors see as perpetrators and are presumed guilty of their offenses, as it does not take into account individuals who also may have had non-criminal motivations for their actions. The classification should have included more categories to reflect other causations for sexual activity while sleeping. We propose adding:

(1) Individuals whose behavior can be explained by a sleep disorder;

(2) Individuals whose behavior can be explained by a major mental disorder;

(3) Individuals who dissociated at the time of the act.

Other researchers have reported cases of a similar nature[43,50–55].

A detailed psychiatric examination, addressing all mental illnesses; personality disorders; triggering and provoking factors; organic and non-organic factors; and intellectual functioning, is extremely important in such cases (Table 26.1).

A word of caution must be given to the individual who is about to venture into the murky field of phallometric testing. The procedures adopted in laboratories across the world vary, and there is no standardized procedure to determine an individual's erotic preference[56]. Many laboratories do not report on their own standardization procedures and their sensitivities and specificities. Phallometric testing tends to be better standardized for pedophilia and less so for the other paraphilias. The procedure has not been accepted in courts as a diagnostic tool or for profiling (*R v. Mohan, Daubert v. Merrell Dow Pharmaceutical 1993, State v. Porter 1997*) in the determination of guilt, but has found its way in influencing sentencing recommendations in Canadian courts.

Sleep apnea, confusional arousal, sleep drunkenness and violence Sleep apnea is a condition that has received little attention in the literature in its association with violence.

Nofziner and Wettstein[24] reported a case where a man shot his wife dead. The experts for the defense argued that the accused had a severe sleep apnea problem as determined by polysomnography. They stated that the sleep apnea resulted in a confusional arousal and he accidentally shot his wife. On the other hand, the prosecution was able to show that there was a motive for the shooting and a history of spousal and child abuse. The individual was found guilty of first-degree murder.

While major mental illnesses are not commonly associated with sleep apnea, we are in

Table 26.1 Investigation of a case of sexual activity when the individual claims to be asleep

Review the police records of the charges and victim/witness statements

Interview the client taking an exhaustive psychiatric and medical history

Arrange for a thorough physical examination along with a full biochemical and hematological screen

Obtain past medical and psychiatric records

Arrange for an electroencephalogram and brain scanning

Interview relatives of the client

Obtaining the victim's account of the event or interviewing the victim is very important

Arrange for polysomnography

Consider phallometric (erotic preference) testing

Consider a blood or urine screen for drug abuse

Psychological testing with a special emphasis on personality testing

Psychodiagnostics looking at all DSM-IV axes*

Look for psychopathy

Generate a differential diagnosis and rule out malingering

Consider a second opinion

*See American Psychiatric Association. Diagnostic and Statistical Manual IV. 1994

the process of reporting a case where a major depression was associated with sleep apnea and violent behavior. Our client was a newly married man and had been diagnosed as suffering from a major depression. He was living with a relative who, in the early hours of the morning, heard screams and on approaching the bedroom of the accused found him to have stabbed his wife many times; she subsequently died from her injuries. Our client was confused at the time of his arrest, did not recall stabbing his wife and would repeatedly ask to see his wife after the event. He was diagnosed with a major depression and based on that diagnosis it was opined that he was not criminally responsible on account of mental disorder. The evidence was not challenged and he made his way into the mental health system under the purview of a review board. This review board, in exploring the individual's history, opined that his prior complaints of insomnia indicated that in addition to his depression a sleep disorder may be present. They recommended, as part of their disposition, that he have a sleep laboratory evaluation. This was conducted at a university sleep laboratory and a definite diagnosis of sleep apnea was made by a sleep specialist.

In retrospect we opined that it was more likely that this individual had a confusional arousal that was associated with the stabbing and that the depression may have had an aggravating influence. This individual has been depression free for the last 4 years and has not had any subsequent confusional arousal problems. At the time of writing this report, the individual in question remains detained in a forensic hospital at the order of the review board.

Dennis and Crisham[57] recently reported that chronic assaultive behavior can be improved with sleep apnea treatment. Pressman and co-workers[58] have also reported a case and have briefly reviewed how parasomnias can be triggered by sleep apnea.

Nofzinger and Wettstein[24] offer some guidelines in determining the role sleep apnea may have in association with violence. They suggest that the presence of sleep apnea can be confirmed by a sleep specialist in conjunction with a detailed history and polysomnographic evaluation. A prior history of automatic behavior should be elicited and such could be provoked in a laboratory setting with obvious precautions. They note that absence of polysomnographic evidence of a violent behavior does not rule out its potential. One should review the violent behavior in light of prior aggressive potential. Presence of complicating factors such as drugs or alcohol, stress, sleep deprivation and forced arousal should be determined. Psychiatric assessment may help with a differential diagnosis and neuropsychological changes could be looked for. Other factors addressed are dealt with below.

Sleep drunkenness (confusional arousal) occurs during the transition between sleep and wakefulness. Roth[10] reported on several aspects of hypersomnia and sleep drunkenness and considers it to be a separate entity. If motor function returns before awareness, complex behaviors may take place without conscious awareness. This state can sometimes be provoked by forced arousals[14]. Confusional arousals are associated with mental disorders, which in turn can be treated with psychotropic medication. Psychotropic drugs, on the other hand, are known to have a depressive effect on the central nervous system and have a propensity to produce confusional arousal[59,60]. Ohayon and co-workers[11] have reported that individuals with confusional arousals have a high association with stressful incidents, mental disorders and sleep apnea.

Kushida and co-workers[12] have described an interesting case of an individual with a degenerative brain disorder who also had a problem with obstructive sleep airway syndrome. It was reported that he showed aggressive behaviors and wandered around the house; this was associated with confusion on arousal.

The literature is essentially unclear on the issue of violent behavior and its association with sleep drunkenness or confusional arousals. Whether these confusional states are sleep disorders, related to organic brain pathology or epilepsy, or are medication induced is not clear. What appears to be important is the act of forced awakening and an aggressive response. A history of such should be sought for. Each case must be evaluated on its own merits.

Epileptic phenomena in sleep The association between epilepsy and aggression is well described in both the general context and the forensic context[61,62]. Treiman states that the diagnosis of epilepsy should be made by a neurologist with a special competence in epilepsy along with CCTV–EEG[61,62]. The aggression should be characteristic of a prior pattern of the seizure disorder. The presence of epileptic automatism needs to be verified in video-recording. The act should be sudden, short-lived, not in response to external stimuli, except in response to restraint. Treiman states that potentially aggression could occur during the seizure, inter-ictally, post-ictally and as a result of an ictal psychotic episode[61,62].

The occurrence of aggression ictally is very rare. Post-ictal violence is more common if the person is being restrained. Ictal psychotic episodes may be associated with aggression, but this aggression is more likely to be directly related to psychological factors and not ictal factors.

For the purposes of this chapter we are more concerned with events that arise out of nocturnal seizures. It is conceivable that a person sleeping next to an individual who suddenly has a seizure may be injured. The aggression is ill-directed and related to the tonic–clonic movements.

Zucconi and co-workers[63] studied a cohort of 34 patients complaining of nocturnal motor agitation or behaviors and compared them to a group of 12 healthy controls. All patients exhibited some degree of motor behaviors ranging from scratching or rubbing of face or nose, some pelvic thrusting or swinging attacks. Fifty-three per cent had major episodes, for example elevation of the head and trunk from the bed and complex behaviors occurring in the NREM phase of sleep. In 80% of the individuals, epileptiform abnormalities were noted, but no reference is made to the nature of the abnormalities, nor do they tell us if any of the individuals had any history of aggression. These authors postulate that the behaviors probably represent aspects of nocturnal frontal lobe epilepsy. Similarly, Silvestri and co-workers[64] followed six children with either sleepwalking or sleep terrors and found all of them to exhibit clear-cut nocturnal seizure activity. None of them, however, had a history of aggression. Similarly, Piazzi and co-workers[65] have shown how four patients who had episodic nocturnal wanderings had clear-cut seizure activity related to them.

The authors of this chapter are uncertain as to the association between nocturnal epileptic attacks and actual directed violent behavior. Because complex nocturnal motor activity can be a concomitant of nocturnal seizures, all cases of violence during the sleep period are worth investigating from an electrophysiological point of view.

Dissociative episodes arising from sleep

In all cases of motor activity arising from sleep, the possibility of a dissociative episode accounting for the behavior exists. Dissociative disorders are notoriously difficult to diagnose and, in a forensic setting, malingering must be ruled out. The literature on dissociative disorders or psychogenic states arising from the sleep state is sparse and limited to case reports[23,66,67]. A summary is provided by Mahowald and Schenck in 1992[68] and Schenck and co-workers[23]. Dissociative disorders are difficult to establish in courts unless there is a prior history of dissociative episodes or documented treatment for such a condition. If one can be convinced about the diagnosis and in turn is able to convince the court that the case at hand is indeed a dissociative disorder, then a defense may be available, whether the diagnosis is a parasomnia or a dissociative disorder.

The *DSM-IV*[6] lists the various dissociative disorders and these include dissociative amnesia, dissociative fugue, dissociative identity disorder, and dissociative disorders not otherwise specified. It is conceivable that a person may not recall what happened the night before because of an amnesic episode. They way wander away from a particular location and have no memory of their past as in a fugue, or have no recollection of the past and assume a new identity as in a dissociative identity disorder. A thorough understanding of these disorders will help to distinguish them from a parasomnia or any complex sleep-related movement disorder.

Clinical studies often indicate that sleep disorders may be associated with an underlying mental disorder. Major depressive disorders are more common in confusional arousal and night terrors[11]. Panic disorders and generalized anxiety disorders occur more frequently in night terrors. Sleepwalkers have high levels of mental stress. That there are many co-morbid disorders responsible for triggering a parasomnia or a dissociative disorder should alert the clinician to obtain a thorough psychiatric history.

REM sleep behavior disorder

In REM sleep behavior disorder, the somatic muscle atonia usually present during REM sleep is absent. This enables the person to move about during his/her dreaming, thus causing injury to persons or property. Motor behaviors including violence and sexual activity have been reported in the REM phase of sleep[8,69–71]. Under such circumstances, REM sleep behavior disorder should be considered when parasomnias are investigated.

Legal liability and driving, operating machinery, etc.

The presence of a sleep disorder like narcolepsy and sleep apnea can pose a problem for the individual when operating any machinery or driving an automobile. Driving is a privilege, and the responsibility for driving safely clearly rests with the individual driver. Falling asleep at the wheel is a major cause for motor vehicle accidents. Several jurisdictions require commercial drivers to maintain logs of driving hours and are restrictive to driving beyond a fixed number of hours. Legal issues arise for the individual, the employer or the physician who sees an individual with a sleep disorder[28]. Ellis and Grunstein[28] review the concepts of foreseeability and proximity in the context of legal liability. In particular, they highlight issues related to falling asleep at the wheel and whether or not the courts would consider this a voluntary act, and also whether the falling asleep was foreseeable. The other issue is proximity, which addresses the liability someone else has for the person responsible for an event that is the result of a sleep-related accident. This brings into focus the responsibility an employer has to an individual, to co-workers, the quality of the goods produced or delivered and society as a whole.

Shuman[72] recently reviewed civil liability interfaces with sleep deprivation and sleep disorders. Shuman categorizes this liability into four areas: (1) The liability directly

Table 26.2 Malingering and sexual activity during sleep – key points to consider in legal cases

Presence of a history of a parasomnia does not necessarily rule out malingering. The individual may actually take advantage of the fact that they have a sleep problem

Presence of an abnormal polysomnography testing does not necessarily rule out malingering

There is no specific factor that can help one establish or rule out malingering in a situation where a parasomnia is an issue

Clinical opinion is buttressed by laboratory findings and any opinion given will be a composite of all factors evaluated

Table 26.3 Factors that raise the index of suspicion of malingering

Presence of legal situation

Presence of an antisocial personality disorder or psychopathy

Presence of a paraphilia in the history

Presence of a paraphilia on phallometric testing

Vague or atypical symptomatology

Absence of a history of a parasomnia

Absence of a history of a parasomnia in childhood

Absence of abnormal findings during polysomnography

Prior history of sexual offending

Absence of medical/neurological causes for cognitive dysfunctioning

Absence of any triggering factor for a parasomnia

Presence of a courtship disorder, sexual dysfunction or an anxiety disorder

Presence of an illegal situation where there may be some purpose for not taking responsibility or avoiding a situation

caused by an individual with sleep deprivation or a sleep disorder. This encompasses all acts, be they driving, operating machinery, or otherwise. (2) The liability to a third party on the part of a health care giver. This could involve two issues: the treatment causing drowsiness, inattention, reduced reaction time and resulting injury and the failure to warn of such risk. (3) The issue of proximity, in that the net responsibility or liability spreads to include an employer or an agent who employs an individual, who either has a sleep disorder or, due to sleep deprivation or fatigue, causes injury to a third party. Adequate medical evaluations, maintenance of driving logs, and policies for drivers that are reviewed by company management with legal input help to minimize this. (4) The most important category is the degree of responsibility of the claimant towards the injury suffered by the individual, as a result of the sleep-related problem (contributory negligence).

A medical practitioner has a duty to warn a client in several situations: the risk that a parasomnia or sleep disorder poses to the individual; the risk it poses to others associated with this individual; available treatments; effect of certain medications on alertness or tendency to cause drowsiness; or what medications can do to slow down reaction times – all can become live legal issues. Reporting laws are diverse, and one is referred to the medical association or society that governs a particular jurisdiction[73]. There

is a liability involved in prescribing hypnotics and sedatives apart from the risk of initiating dependence on the medication. Due caution should be taken in reviewing such risks with a client. Documentation of risk–benefit discussion is essential.

Malingering and sleep disorders

Malingering is the conscious fabrication or gross exaggeration of physical and/or psychological symptoms for an external goal[6] (Tables 26.2–26.4). It is distinguished from factitious disorders in that the malingered presentation extends beyond a patient role and is understandable in light of the individual's circumstances. In factitious disorders, the primary goal is to seek medical help.

The issue of malingering arises with all legal cases. Automatism due to a sleep disorder is no exception. Malingering is an important differential diagnosis to be considered in any case where there is legal involvement[74]. In any case where sleepwalking is put forward as a defense, malingering should be considered and ruled out.

The probability that an offense is the product of a sleepwalking episode or a sleep-related event becomes higher the more one

Table 26.4 Factors that suggest genuine sleep sex problems (sexsomnia)

Absence of any motivating factor
Legal situation inconsequential or absent
Behavior out of character
Prior history of a parasomnia
Childhood history of a parasomnia
Abnomalities on polysomnography testing suggestive of a parasomnia
No prior sex-offending history
No history of paraphilia
No history of abnormalities on phallometric testing
Triggering factors present for a parasomnia
Absence of an antisocial personality disorder or psychopathy
Presence of underlying medical or neurological disorder contributing to cognitive impairment
Prior history of healthy sexual functioning

can establish factors that are well founded as being related to the sleep event. Similarly, the more bizarre the case, the more it deviates from well known patterns, and the presence of a motive tends to make malingering a probable diagnosis.

In particular one should look for the following:

Clinical features

(1) The nature of the sleep event;

(2) Timing of the event: sleepwalking episode in the first third of the night;

(3) Onset of sleepwalking or other parasomnias in childhood;

(4) Past history of sleepwalking/parasomnias, confusional arousals, sleep apnea;

(5) Family history of sleepwalking;

(6) Male gender;

(7) Associated known triggers, e.g. substance abuse, alcohol abuse, sleep deprivation, night shift, irregular sleep, stress and pain;

(8) Presence or absence of amnesia of the event;

(9) Personality factors, e.g. antisocial and psychopathic traits in an individual should

alert the examiner to the possibility of manipulation and deception.

Legal issues

(1) The nature of the plea;

(2) Who brings the defense forward – the prosecution or the defense;

(3) What possible consequences the acquittal may result in.

Victim-related factors

(1) Observations of the victim;

(2) Relationship of the victim to the accused;

(3) Motives for the victim.

Investigative procedures

(1) Laboratory findings (polysomnography);

(2) Sleep video recordings;

(3) Telemetry;

(4) Cerebral imaging studies.

Collateral support of clinical factors by

(1) Spouse;

(2) Victim;

(3) Bed partners;

(4) Parents;

(5) Friends;

(6) Other medical records;

(7) Legal records;

(8) Jail records.

The greater is the degree of corroboration of clinical and non-clinical features from external sources the greater is the credibility of the diagnosis.

That an individual has a history of sleepwalking, of other parasomnias, or an abnormal

Table 26.5   Investigation of a case of violence related to sleep should follow a systematic process. The authors recommend the investigative processes detailed below

The history of the violent episode
   Birth history
   Childhood history
   Schooling
   Work history
   Relationships, marital and sexual history
   Legal history
   Medical history
   Drug and alcohol history
   Hobbies, interests and pastimes
   (The history should be corroborated by parents, siblings, spouse, sexual partners or roommates)

Violence risk assessment (the clinical evaluation should involve a detailed neurological work-up

Collateral information
   Eyewitness accounts
   Victim account
   Police reports
   Criminal record

An extensive account of the events that led up to the incident should include
   Eyewitness accounts
   Duration of the episode
   Reaction of the accused on discovery
   Amnesia
   Onset and termination of the episode
   Motives
   Relationship to the victim
   Behavior of the accused hours and days before the event
   Review of police records

Laboratory investigations
   Complete blood count, electrolytes, urea, creatinine, liver function tests and thyroid function tests
   Routine EEG, sphenoidal EEG
   CT scan
   MRI
   Sleep EEG, with videotaping

EEG, electroencephalography; CT, computed tomography; MRI, magnetic resonance imaging

sleep event and has a laboratory finding that suggests the presence of a parasomnia does not negate criminal responsibility for an alleged act. It must be established that the individual was indeed experiencing a sleep event that was directly related to the time period of the offense in question.

In arriving at one's conclusions, the offense in question has to be clinically analyzed in depth as described above. The laboratory evaluations can weaken or strengthen the case. Finally, the offender characteristics, the victim's characteristics, and other environmental circumstances should complete the picture.

Only then can one offer an opinion qualifying one's degree of certainty.

The clinician's duty is first to identify as many relevant factors as possible, put them together and arrive at a clinical opinion as to whether a specified behavior could be the result of a parasomnic act. Secondly, if it were, then was the person's level of consciousness impaired to such a degree that the individual was not aware of his or her actions?

It is left to the courts to decide whether to accept the clinician's opinion as to whether the act in question was the result of a sleep-related event, whether or not the event resulted in an altered level of awareness of the act and finally whether the event constitutes a mental disorder. A detailed understanding of the concepts of malingering and deception along with its assessment has been detailed in a book by Richard Rogers[30] and the reader is well advised to refer to that text.

Appendix: relevant legal cases

McNaughten. K 130, 4 St. Tr. NS.847, 1843

Bratty v. Attorney General of Northern Ireland. 46 CR.App. R.1. (H.L.), 1961;7–8

R v. Rabey (Psychological Blow) 2S.C.R. 513, aff g (1977), 17 O.R. (2d) 1,1980

R v. Cognen

R v. Watkins

R v. Schwarz (Legal Wrongfulness)

R v. Chaulk (Moral Wrongfulness). 3 S.C.R. 1303, 1990

R v. Swain (Not Criminally Responsible Defence)

R v. Parks (Sleepwalking Not a Mental Disorder and Absolute Acquittal) 2 S.C.R. 871, 1992

R v. Burgess (Sleepwalking a Mental Disorder). 2 All, ER 769, 1991

R v. Campbell (Sleepwalking a Mental Disorder and Not Criminally Responsible). 2000

R v. Stone (Dissociation in a Legal Context). 134 C.C.C. (3d) 353, 1999

R v. Winko (Significant Risk and Detention of Not Criminally Responsible Acquittees)

R v. Revelle

R v. Mohan

HM Advocate v. Cunningham lC 80.1963

HM Advocate v. Frarer. 4 Coupcr 78,1878

R v. Dhlamlni. SALR (1) 120,1955

R v. Kemp I. QB 399,1957

R v. Ngang. SALR (3) 363,1960

R v. Nhete. SR1,1941

R v. Quick. 3 All ER 347,1973

R v. Smith. 3 All ER 605,1979

R v. Sullivan. 3 WLR 123,1983

R v. Daviault. 3 S.C.R. 63,1994

R v. Oomen

R v. Granger

State v. Mercer. 275 N.C. 108, 116; 165 S.E.2d 328, 334, 1969

Foster v. State. 657 P.2d 166, 171 (Okl.Cr.), 1983

State v. Jerrett. 307 S.E.2d 339 (N.C.), 1983

State v. Olson. (North Dakota) 356 N.W.2d 110.

State v. Caddell. (North Carolina) 287 N.C. 266, 215 S.E.2d 348, 1975

Jones v. State. (Oklahoma) 648 P.2d 1251 (Okl.Cr.), 1982

Cartwright v. Maynard. (Oklahoma) 802 F.2d 1203 (10th Cir.), 1986

Polston v. State. (Wyoming) 685 P.2d 1 (Wyo.), 1984

Fulcher v. State (Wyoming) 633 P.2d 142, 1981

Daubert v. Merrel Dow Pharmaceutical, 509 U.S. 579, 113 S.Ct.2786,125 L.Ed.2d 469,1993

State v. Porter. 241 Conn. 57, 698 A.2d 739,1997

References

1. Ogilvie RD, Wilkinson RT. The detection of sleep onset: behavioral and physiological convergence. *Psychophysiology* 1984;21:510–20

2. Coenen AM. Neuronal phenomena associated with vigilance and consciousness: from cellular mechanisms to electroencephalographic patterns. *Conscious Cogn* 1998;7:42–53

3. Roehrs T, Papineau L, Rosenthal L, Roth T. Ethanol as a hypnotic in insomniacs: self-administration and effects on sleep and mood. *Neuropsychopharmacology* 1999;20:279–86

4. Carskadon MA, Dement WC. Normal human sleep: an overview. In Kryger M, Roth T, Dement W, eds. *Principles and Practice of Sleep*

Medicine, 3rd edn. Philadelphia: WB Saunders, 2000:15–25

5. American Sleep Disorders Association. *The International Classification of Sleep Disorders, Revised: Diagnostic and Coding Manual.* Rochester, MN: American Sleep Disorders Association, 1997

6. American Psychiatric Association. *Diagnostic and Statistical Manual*, 4th edn. Washington, DC: American Psychiatric Association, 1994

7. Mahowald MW, Schenck CH. Complex motor behavior arising during the sleep period: forensic science implications. *Sleep* 1995;18: 724–7

8. Mahowald MW, Bundie SR, Hurwitz TD, *et al.* Sleep violence – forensic implications: polygraphic and video documentation. *J Forensic Sci* 1990;35:413–32

9. Broughton R. Sleep disorders: disorders of arousal? Enuresis, somnambulism, and nightmares occur in confusional states of arousal, not in 'dreaming sleep'. *Science* 1968;159:1070–8

10. Roth B, Nevsimalova S, Rechtschaffen A. Hypermania with 'sleep drunkenness'. *Arch Gen Psychiatry* 1972;26:456–62

11. Ohayon MM, Guilleminault C, Priest RG. Night terrors, sleepwalking, and confusional arousals in the general population: their frequency and relationship to other sleep and mental disorders. *J Clin Psychiatry* 1999;60:4

12. Kushida CA, Clerk AA, Kirsch CM, *et al.* Prolonged confusion with nocturnal wandering arising from NREM and REM sleep: a case report. *Sleep* 1995;18:757–66

13. Mahowald MW, Schenck CH. REM sleep behavior disorder. In Kryger MH, Roth T, Dement WC, eds. *Principles and Practice of Sleep Disorders Medicine*. Philadelphia: WB Saunders, 1989:389–401

14. Bonkalo A. Impulsive acts and confusional states during incomplete arousal from sleep: criminological and forensic implications. *Psychiatric Q* 1974;48:400–9

15. Guilleminault C. Disorders of arousal in children: somnambulis and night terrors. In Guilleminault C, ed. *Sleep and its Disorders in Children*. New York: Raven Press, 1987:243–52

16. Aldrich MS. Cardinal manifestations of sleep disorders. In Kryger M, Roth T, Dement W, eds. *Principles and Practice of Sleep Medicine*, 3rd edn. Philadelphia: WB Saunders, 2000: 526–33

17. Hublin C, Kaprio J, Partinen M, Heikkila K, Koskenvuo M. Prevalence and genetics of sleepwalking: a population-based twin study. *Neurology* 1997;48:177–81

18. Broughton RJ. NREM arousal parasomnias. In Kryger M, Roth T, Dement W, eds. *Principles and Practice of Sleep Medicine*, 3rd edn. Philadelphia: WB Saunders, 2000:693–706

19. Guilleminault C, Leger D, Philip P, Ohayon MM. Nocturnal wandering and violence. Review of a sleep clinic population. *J Forensic Sci* 1997;43:158–63

20. Roper P. Bulimia while sleepwalking: a rebuttal for sane automatism? *Lancet* 1989; 2:796

21. Schenck CH, Mahowald MW. A polysomnographically documented case of adult somnambulism with long-distance automobile driving and frequent nocturnal violence: parasomnia with continuing danger as a noninsane automatism. *Sleep* 1995;18:765–72

22. Fedoroff JP, Brunet A, Woods V, *et al.* A case-controlled study of men who sexually assault sleeping victims. In Shapiro CM, Smith M. eds. *Forensic Aspects of Sleep*. Chichester, UK: John Wiley and Sons, 1997:85–98

23. Schenck CH, Milner DM, Hurwitz TD, *et al.* Dissociative disorders presenting as somnambulism: polysomnographic, video and clinical documentation (8 cases). *Dissociation* 1989;2:194–204

24. Nofzinger EA, Wettstein RM. Homicidal behavior and sleep apnea: a case report and medicolegal discussion. *Sleep* 1995;18:776–82

25. Broughton RJ, Shimizu T. Sleep related violence: a medical and forensic challenge. *Sleep* 1995;18:727–30

26. Mahowald MW, Schenck CH, Rosen GM, Hurwitz TD. The role of a sleep disorder center in evaluating sleep violence. *Arch Neurol* 1992;49:604–7

27. Mahowald MW, Schenck CH. Parasomnias: sleepwalking and the law. *Sleep Med Rev* 2000;4:321–39

28. Ellis E, Grunstein R. Medicolegal aspects of sleep disorders: sleepiness and civil liability. *Sleep Med Rev* 2001;5:33–46

29. Rogers R, Mitchell CN. *Mental Health Experts and the Criminal Courts*. Toronto: Carswell, 1991:406

30. Rogers R, ed. *Clinical Assessment of Malingering and Deception*, 2nd edn. New York: Guilford Press, 1997

31. Melton GB, Petrila J, Poythress NG. *Psychological Evaluation for the Courts. A Handbook for Mental Health Professionals and Lawyers*, 2nd edn. New York: Guilford Press, 1997:794

32. Shapiro C, Smith AM. *Forensic Aspects of Sleep*. Chichester, England: John Wiley and Sons Ltd, 1997

33. Fenwick P. Automatism, medicine and law. *Psychol Med* Monograph 1990;17:1–27

34. *Martin's Annual Criminal Code*. Ottawa: Canada Law Books Inc, 2002

35. Fenwick P. Murdering while asleep. *Br Med J* 1986;293:574–5
36. Fenwick P. Somnambulism and the law: a review. *Behav Sci Law* 1987;5:343–57
37. Howard C, D'Orban PT. Violence in sleep: medico-legal issues and two case reports. *Psychol Med* 1987;17:915–25
38. Moldofsky H, Gilbert R, Lue FA, *et al.* Forensic sleep medicine: violence, sleep, nocturnal wandering. *Sleep* 1995;18:731–9
39. Broughton R, Billings R, Cartwright R, *et al.* Homicidal somnambulism: a case report. Sleep 1994;17:253–64
40. Broughton R, Shimizu T. Sleep related violence: a medical and forensic challenge. *Sleep* 1995;18:727–30
41. Gojer *et al.* 2003;in press
42. Guilleminault C, Moscovitch A, Leger D. Nocturnal wandering and violence. *Sleep* 1995;18:740–8
43. Guilleminault C, Moscovitch A, Yuen K, Poyares D. Atypical sexual behavior during sleep. *Psychosom Med* 2002;64:328–36
44. Guilleminault C, Moscovitch A, Leger D. Forensic sleep medicine: nocturnal wandering and violence. *Sleep* 1995;18:740–8
45. Lee MK, Guilleminault C. Rapid eye movement sleep-related parasomnias. *Curr Treat Options Neurol* 2002;4:113–20
46. Hartmann E. Two cases reports: night terrors with sleepwalking: a potentially lethal disorder. *J Nerv Ment Disord* 1983;171:503–5
47. Oswald I, Evans J. On seious violence during sleep walking. *Br J Psychiatry* 1985;147:688–91
48. Patterson JF. Non-rapid eye movement parasomnias with behavior disorder. *South Med J* 1989;82:802–3
49. Alves R, Aloe F, Tavares S, *et al.* Sexual behavior in sleep, sleepwalking and possible REM behavior disorder: a case report. *Sleep Res Online* 1999;2:71–2
50. Olson EJ, Boeve BF, Silber MH. Rapid eye movement sleep behaviour disorder: demographic, clinical and laboratory findings in 93 cases. *Brain* 2000;123:331–9
51. Schenck C, Mahowald MW. An analysis of a recent criminal trial involving sexual misconduct with a child, alcohol abuse and a successful sleep-walking defence. *Med Sci Law* 1998; 38:147–52
52. Rosenfeld DS, Elhajjar AJ. Sleep sex: a variant of sleepwalking. *Arch Sex Behav* 1998;27:269–78
53. Jovanovic D, Fedoroff JP, Kayumov L, Shapiro CM. The co-occurrence of sleep and paraphilic sexual behavior. *Sleep* 2000;23:361

54. Shapiro CM, Fedoroff JP, Trajanivic N. Sexual behaviour in sleep: a newly described parasomnia. *Sleep Res* 1996;25:181–2
55. Shapiro CM, Trajanovic N, Fedoroff JP. Sexomnia – a new parasomnia? *Can J Psychiatry* 2003;48:311–17
56. Howes RJ. A survey of plethysomographic assessment in North America. *Sexual Abuse: J Res Treatment* 1995;7:9–24
57. Dennis JL, Crisham KP. Chronic assaultive behavior improved with sleep apnea treatment. *J Clin Psychiatry* 2001;62:571–2
58. Pressman MR, Meyer TJ, Kendrick-Mohamed J, *et al.* Night terrors in an adult precipitated by sleep apnea. *Sleep* 1995;18:773–5
59. Llorente MD, Currier MB, Norman SE, *et al.* Night terrors in adults: phenomenology and relationship to psychopathology. *J Clin Psychiatry* 1992;53:392–4
60. Montfort JC, Manus A, Levy-Soussan P. Automatic actions with amnesia induced by taking hypnotic drugs. Association with personal and familial history of somnambulism and epilepsy. *Ann Med Psychol* 1992;150:371–4
61. Treiman DM. Psychobiology of ictal aggression. In Smith D, Treiman D, Trimble M, eds. *Advances in Neurology.* New York: Raven Press, 1991;55:341–56
62. Treiman DM. Aggressive behavior and violence in epilepsy: guidelines for expert testimony. In Rosner R, ed. *Principles and Practice of Forensic Psychiatry.* New York: Chapman and Hall, 1994:451–60
63. Zucconi M, Oldani A, Ferini-Strambi L, Bizzozero D, Smirne S. Nocturnal paroxysmal arousals with motor behaviors during sleep: frontal lobe epilepsy or parasomnia? *J Clin Neurophysiol* 1997;14:513–22
64. Silvestri R, de Domenico P, Mento G, *et al.* Epileptic seizures in subjects previously affected by disorders of arousal. *Neurophysiol Clin* 1995;25:19–27
65. Piazzi G, Timper P, Montagna P, Provini F, Lugaresi E. Epileptic nocturnal wanderings. *Sleep* 1995;18:749–56
66. Molaie M, Deutsch GK. Psychogenic events presenting as parasomnia. *Sleep* 1997;20:402–5
67. Fleming J. Dissociative episodes presenting as somnambulism: a case report. *Sleep Res* 1987; 16:263
68. Mahowald MW, Schenck CH. Dissociated states of wakefulness and sleep. *Neurology* 1992;42:44–52
69. Schenck CH, Bundlic SR, Ettinger MG, *et al.* Chronic behavioral disorders of human REM sleep: a new category of parasomnia. *Sleep* 1986;9:293–308

70. Schenck CH, Mahowald MW. REM sleep para-somnias. *Neurol Clin* 1996;14:697–720
71. Schenck CII, IIurwitz TD, Mahowald MW. Symposium: Normal and abnormal REM sleep regulation: REM sleep behaviour disorder: an update on a series of 96 patients and a review of the world literature. J Sleep Res 1993;2:224–31
72. Schuman DW. Civil liability issues arising out of sleep deprivation and sleep disorders. In Shapiro CM, Smith M, eds. *Forensic Aspects of Sleep*. Chichester, England: John Wiley and Sons, 1997
73. Pakola SJ, Dinges DF, Pack AI. Review of regulations and guidelines for commercial and noncommercial drivers with sleep apnea and narcolepsy. *Sleep* 1995:18:787–96
74. Resnick PJ. In Rosner R, ed. *Principles and Practice of Forensic Psychiatry*. Chapman and Hall, 1994:417–26

Section 6:

Treatment methods in sleep psychiatry

27

Pharmacology of sleep

Henry W. Lahmeyer

INTRODUCTION

The pharmacology of sleep has been studied since antiquity. Ancients used alcohol, herbs and animal extracts to try to induce sleep, and teas, coca, coffee and many other herbs to promote wakefulness. Over the past 50 years rapid progress has been made in our understanding of the mechanisms by which hypnotics, stimulants and other drugs affect sleep architecture and the brain's own endogenous sleep and alerting mechanisms. The science of sleep has profited from progress in brain molecular biology in general.

Rapid progress has also been made in neuroanatomy and neuropharmacology of chronophysiology, which allows more sophisticated use of pharmacological agents. This chapter will focus on sleep pharmacology of hypnotics, stimulants, psychotropic drugs, drugs that disrupt sleep and wakefulness and a brief review of chronopharmacology.

Over the past 100 years more potent and specific drugs have been developed that promote sleep or enhance wakefulness. Each new generation of drugs is more selective and generally produces fewer unwanted side-effects.

NEUROPHYSIOLOGY AND MOLECULAR BIOLOGY OF SLEEP AND WAKEFULNESS

Sleep and wakefulness are thought to be regulated by two endogenous processes:

(1) Process C – endogenous biological clock which drives the circadian rhythm of sleep and wakefulness. Process C is an endogenous rhythm with a period of about 24 h. The suprachiasmatic nucleus (SCN) generates most of the afferent pathways for regulating circadian rhythms and receives most of its efferent input from the retina. Sunlight is the source of the 24-h rhythm although clocks and other social rhythms also play an important role in adapting the SCN[1].

(2) Process S – homeostatic process that increases as a function of prior wakefulness. One measure of process S is the intensity of stage 3/4 sleep right after sleep onset. Stage 3/4 sleep-pressure dissipates rapidly after the onset of sleep. The intensity of process S can also be measured at any time of day by measuring latency to sleep onset.

Process S also plays a significant role in the timing of sleep onset and particularly sleep offset and the propensity for rapid eye movement (REM) sleep. Sleep latency is the most rapid during the falling phase of core body temperature and sleep is least likely to occur when core body temperature is rising. Falling body temperature occurs during the first half of the night, achieving a nadir around 4:00 a.m. for most entrained sleepers. Temperature rises until about 11:00 a.m., then begins to fall again in mid-afternoon when increased sleepiness occurs. REM sleep is more closely linked to process C. The peak of REM sleep propensity peaks at the nadir of core body temperature or about 4:00 a.m.[2].

RETICULAR ACTIVATING SYSTEM

Components of the ascending reticular activating system are critically important for the generation and maintenance of waking states or arousal. They reside in the pontine and mesencephalic tegmentum, including both noradrenergic cell bodies such as the locus ceruleus and the cholinergic cell bodies such as the pedunculopontine tegmental and lateral dorsal tegmental nuclei and the thalamus, hippocampus, hypothalamus and cingulate cortex. In addition, histaminergic neurons and posterior hypothalamic neurons project into the cortex and maintain arousal. Glutaminergic neurons and subcortical and cortical structures may also play an important role in wakefulness and arousal[3].

At least five anatomical sites have been implicated in the generation of non-REM sleep: (1) basal forebrain area; (2) thalamus; (3) hypothalamus; (4) dorsal raphe nucleus; and (5) nucleus solitarius of the medulla. Immediately prior to and during REM sleep when cholinergic activity in the lateral dorsal tegmental and pedunculopontine tegmental nuclei is high the electroencephalogram (EEG) becomes gradually desynchronized. While histaminergic cells in the posterior hypothalamus maintain arousal, ventrolateral preoptic neurons in the inferior hypothalamus may be involved in the induction of slow-wave sleep[3].

Monosynaptic projections from the dorsal raphe nucleus to the cholinergic neurons in the tegmentum produce a hyperpolarization of the 'REM-on cells' through serotonin (5-HT$_{1A}$) receptors and finally inhibit REM sleep. On the other hand, activation of the self-inhibitory 5-HT$_{1A}$ auto-receptors and the dorsal raphe nucleus leads to the disinhibition of REM sleep.

PHARMACOLOGY OF SLEEP HYPNOTICS

There is a widespread perception among physicians that insomnia is a relatively benign complaint. As a result, thousands of Americans are untreated or under-treated for insomnia. Data from a 1985 survey reinforced this perception: 35% of the 3161 Americans surveyed nationwide reported having insomnia at some time during the study year. However, only a minority reported being treated for their insomnia, with either prescription or over-the-counter (OTC) drugs. Fifty per cent of the individuals who experienced insomnia described it as serious, and 85% of these individuals did not receive treatment[4].

Similarly, a 1991 Gallup Organization report indicated that only 5% of people who suffer from insomnia see a physician specifically for that problem, and 69% never discuss it with their doctors[5]. Poor sleepers have reduced daytime alertness[6,7]. Many physicians apparently fail to ask their patients if they have any difficulty sleeping, and unless a patient brings up the subject, insomnia is not discussed.

Despite the recent progress in the use of non-benzodiazepine hypnotics, physicians remain reluctant to prescribe drugs because the risks of dependence and addiction are perceived to be too high[8]. This perception seems to be based on concern over issues of tolerance and addiction that was a significant problem with hypnotic drugs developed and used during the 1950s and 1960s. During this period the hypnotics that were available included alcohol derivatives and the short-acting barbiturates[9]. More recently, sporadic but significant adverse events have been reported when triazolam was used in high dosages[10]. This review will focus on progress made in recent years in using benzodiazepines more effectively and on the use of more recently developed hypnotics that are more receptor-specific than benzodiazepines.

The treatment of transient and short-term insomnia is the single most appropriate use of hypnotics[11]. Such patients only require hypnotic support for a night or two. If the circumstances that provoked the transient insomnia are with some certainty likely to recur, the patient may use the medication only on those nights and does not have to worry about rebound insomnia on drug-free nights. The same guidelines apply in the treatment of short-term insomnia. Furthermore, nightly use should be limited to not more than 4 weeks[12].

Individuals with short-term insomnia precipitated by acute stress can benefit from hypnotics used sparingly while the stress remains high. Most patients do best if they use short or intermediate half-life hypnotics only on nights when they have significant sleep disruption or anticipate a poor night of sleep[13].

Patients suffering from chronic insomnia, without co-morbid psychiatric disorders, may benefit greatly from adjunctive hypnotic therapy, although primary therapy for these patients should be behavioral[14]. Virtually all sleep specialists agree that long-term treatment with hypnotic drugs is ill-advised in this population because of short- and long-term memory impairment, tolerance, withdrawal and falls in the elderly[15–19].

Long-term use of hypnotics in patients with severe insomnia, parasomnias or co-morbid psychiatric disorders has been demonstrated to be effective and rarely associated with abuse. Hypnotics with a longer half-life maintain effectiveness longer[20]. Insomnia is extremely common in patients with psychiatric disorders, particularly depression. Depression is almost always accompanied by insomnia. Evidence suggests that the arrow can go the other way. In one study of 1000 individuals suffering from insomnia, but not complaining of depression, 50% of those who continued to suffer from insomnia a year later had developed a major depressive disorder[21]. Chronic insomnia associated with chronic mental illness often requires adjunctive use of hypnotics[22], although it is generally recommended that psychotropic drugs appropriate for the condition be fully exploited as sleep agents before hypnotics are added.

Benzodiazepine hypnotics

The benzodiazepines swept in a new era of hypnotic use because of their safety, effectiveness and lack of significant side-effects compared to all previously developed hypnotics. However, as the popularity of benzodiazepines increased and physical surveillance waned, patients experienced significant side-effects[15]. Virtually all hypnotic drugs work by potentiating the inhibitory actions of the γ-aminobutyric acid (GABA) receptor complex. Specifically, benzodiazepines interact with $GABA_A$ but not $GABA_B$ receptors. Benzodiazepine receptors are part of a large complex of proteins at the synapse in the target neuron. Benzodiazepines bind to this complex close to the GABA binding site and the chloride channels close to, but distinct from, the binding site for barbiturates and alcohol. When a benzodiazepine molecule binds to this synaptic complex, the chloride channels open, facilitating the inhibitory effects of GABA[23,24].

Benzodiazepines increase total sleep time primarily by prolonging stage 2 sleep, but at the 'expense' of suppressing stage 3 and 4 sleep and REM sleep to a variable degree[20].

In the USA, five benzodiazepines are indicated for the treatment of insomnia. Flurazepam was the first benzodiazepine indicated for the treatment of insomnia, and it is still widely regarded as the standard of effectiveness against which new drugs should be compared. It has a long half-life of 47–100 h, and several doses are required to achieve steady-state plasma levels. The drug maintains its efficacy with long-term use unlike the older hypnotics such as pentobarbital, secobarbitol and chloral hydrate, etc.[20,25]. The persistence of active metabolites may affect next-day alertness, an attribute that can prove useful in the treatment of anxious individuals but can also lead to diminished daytime alertness. In one study, daytime sleepiness measured by the multiple sleep latency test (MSLT) the next day was much worse in patients with insomnia treated with flurazepam than in those patients receiving placebo[26].

The major active metabolite of quazepam is identical to that of flurazepam. It has a similar half-life (48–120 h), rendering the two drugs similar in their clinical effects. However, quazepam is more lipophilic than flurazepam and enters the brain somewhat more rapidly. Therefore, in a single dose, quazepam acts more like an intermediate-acting benzodiazepine, while repeated doses produce similar negative effects on daytime alertness to those of flurazepam[27].

The gel capsule preparation of temazepam dissolves more slowly than that of other benzodiazepines, rendering it somewhat less effective in patients who have difficulty falling asleep even if the drug is given an hour prior to bedtime. Temazepam has a half-life of 9.5–13 h. It may aid patients with sleep-maintenance problems; however, the 30 mg dosage can produce a decrement in reaction time and alertness the next day[28,29].

Estazolam is intermediate in its kinetics, with a half-life of 12–15 h, thus providing some of the benefits of relatively rapid onset hypnotics, although daytime impairment is similar to that of temazepam[26,30].

Triazolam, by virtue of its rapid absorption and elimination, and a half-life of about 3.5 h, does not cause next-day sedation. It produces rapid sleep onset and increased total sleep time and significant REM suppression. In two major studies of insomnia patients, triazolam was found to be superior to flurazepam in preventing the symptoms of next-day fatigue associated with insomnia and long-acting benzodiazepines[31,32].

However, reports of rebound insomnia, tolerance and anterograde amnesia are more common with triazolam than with other hypnotics[33,34]. This appears to be mostly due to using the drug in excessively high dosages. These adverse events regularly occur at doses of 0.5 mg, but not at 0.125 mg per night. Abrupt drug discontinuation rather than gradual withdrawal clearly produces rebound insomnia (by definition less total sleep time than prior to drug initiation)[35]. The severity of the rebound insomnia is a function of the dose and duration of prior therapy. In one study, a single triazolam dose of 0.25 mg at bedtime was associated with next day 'nervousness' in 4.6% of subjects. They also experienced headaches, paresthesias, visual disturbances and tinnitus[36].

Anterograde amnesia, or amnesia for events occurring usually during the night after a drug is ingested, is more common with triazolam use than with other benzodiazepines. In one study, anterograde amnesia with triazolam was found at 0.5 mg but not at 0.25 mg[37,38]. Somnambulism or sleepwalking or other motor movements during sleep have also been reported with triazolam.

In general, while most patients are likely to prefer shorter-acting hypnotics, there are many patients with chronic insomnia for whom a longer-acting benzodiazepine will remain the drug of choice[32,39].

Anxious patients or patients with somnambulism or REM behavioral disorder may benefit from the persisting anxiolytic effects of long-acting benzodiazepines such as clonazapam, for example. Although this drug has little effect on sleep latency, it increases total sleep time without affecting next-day memory function[40,41]. Lorazepam is useful in some patients with evening anxiety but objective increases in total sleep time are modest. Alprazolam is similar in most respects to lorazepam for short-term use in anxious insomniacs, although it can produce a more serious withdrawal syndrome than clonazepam, with increased anxiety being particularly intense. Alprazolam is a strong REM suppressant and withdrawal produces significant REM rebound and rebound insomnia. Diazepam will produce improved sleep in most cases but, just like flurazepam, its active metabolites have very long half-lives which can produce daytime impairment and falls, particularly in the elderly[42]. Alprazolam and lorazepam have been well documented to produce short-term memory impairment when used in doses of 4 mg or more for lorazepam and in dosages of 2 mg or more in the case of alprazolam[33,34]. There is a much greater risk of memory impairment when these drugs are used in the elderly. Furthermore, this patient group is also at an increased risk of falls when taking benzodiazepines because of the myorelaxant properties[38,43]. Reduced psychomotor co-ordination can occur in individuals who have to handle complex machinery[44].

Non-benzodiazepine hypnotics

For many patients with insomnia, the newer non-benzodiazepine hypnotics such as the imidazopyridine zolpidem and the pyrazolopyrimidines cyclopyrrolone, zaleplon and zopiclone may prove to be superior alternatives to the benzodiazepines. (As zopiclone has not yet been approved in the USA, it will not be discussed further.) Both zaleplon and zolpidem are short-acting, have a rapid onset of action, and selectively bind to the omega-1 benzodiazepine GABA$_A$ receptor. This is in contrast with the benzodiazepines, which bind to omega-1 and -2 receptors in the brain and omega-3 receptors in the periphery. This receptor-binding selectivity is presumed to account for the relatively specific hypnotic action of these two drugs[45].

These drugs share some of the hypnotic properties of the benzodiazepines without having the myorelaxant, anticonvulsant or anxiolytic properties. Because zolpidem has a half-life of around 3 h it shares the short duration of action of triazolam. Both drugs offer the same freedom from next-day sedation. Zolpidem and triazolam produce comparable hypnotic effects. Zolpidem taken within the therapeutic dosage range does not produce tolerance, rebound insomnia, REM rebound or next-day anxiety[46–48]. Zolpidem causes the next-day psychomotor or memory impairment that can complicate treatment with some of the other benzodiazepines[49,50]. While occasionally patients feel some drowsiness on waking when given zolpidem, this rapidly dissipates in an hour or less and does not affect next-day alertness. In laboratory studies, next-day impairment of alertness and performance was virtually undetectable after zolpidem treatment[50].

Unlike the benzodiazepines, which prolong stage 2 sleep at the expense of stages 3 and 4, electrophysiological studies have found that the sleep elicited by zolpidem and zopiclone is similar to the normal sleep profile, with a normal sleep stage distribution despite increased total sleep time[51,52]. At doses higher than the recommended 10 mg adult dose, REM sleep may be reduced. Zolpidem's superiority in inducing a normal sleep pattern was demonstrated in a study of the drug's effect on markers for arousal instability, indicated by cyclical patterns of alternating EEG activity during periods of sleep with no REM[53]. In insomnia patients who received placebo, the arousal instability rate was 68.6%, compared with 38.5% in healthy controls. This finding indicates that people with insomnia have a high level of arousal instability. Zolpidem treatment significantly reduced the arousal instability rate to 25% in the insomnia group. In the control group, zolpidem reduced that arousal instability rate to 31%[54]. Although the clinical importance of the sleep profile remains uncertain, a more normal sleep profile is generally considered to be desirable.

Like other hypnotics and central nervous system (CNS) depressants, zolpidem can exacerbate obstructive sleep apnea. However, zolpidem does not seem to affect breathing adversely in older people who are in good health or have mild-to-moderate chronic obstructive pulmonary disease (COPD).

In clinical trials zolpidem did not demonstrate evidence of tolerance or withdrawal[46,55,56]. Complex patients with severe insomnia and co-morbid psychiatric disorders can tolerate zolpidem and an occasional substance abuser will abuse zolpidem, but the overall abuse potential of zolpidem appears to be less than that of benzodiazepines[57]. Tolerance with repeated administrations does not occur. Rebound insomnia is not evident in most clinical trials. Zolpidem is chosen much less frequently by patients with drug abuse histories than other benzodiazepines in a 'free choice' experiment[58]. Zolpidem has no effect on next-day cognitive performance[59].

Finally, preliminary evidence suggests that tolerance and rebound insomnia do not occur with the extended use of zolpidem as they can with triazolam. Zolpidem may therefore prove to be the drug of choice for the treatment of chronic insomnia. Nevertheless, the efficacy and safety of zolpidem with extended use remain to be firmly established[60].

Zaleplon has a half-life of around 1 h. This ultra-short acting hypnotic significantly reduces sleep latency but does not increase total sleep time. It also improves sleep efficacy early in the night. Zaleplon is therefore useful in patients with sleep-onset insomnia and may prove useful in helping shift workers take daytime naps[61], because of its very rapid onset and clearance and lack of residual sedation, and appears helpful in treating patients with middle insomnia[56,62].

In a head-to-head comparison of zolpidem and zaleplon, there was a trend for shorter sleep latency with zaleplon, but total sleep time and sleep efficiency were significantly better in the zolpidem group compared to either placebo or the zaleplon group[63].

Precautions with hypnotic therapy

Although hypnotics are not contraindicated in the elderly, it should be kept in mind that this population metabolizes hypnotics more slowly, and therefore lower doses should be prescribed. Falls and hip fractures are significantly increased in the elderly who have been prescribed long-acting benzodiazepines[64]. Drug metabolism is further compromised in patients with liver disease, and elimination of the drug and its metabolic by-products may be impaired in patients with kidney disease; both conditions are common in the elderly[31,43,65,66]. Long-term use of drugs with intermediate or long half-lives can produce cumulative cognitive impairment, which is more pronounced in the elderly[17].

In general, hypnotic doses of benzodiazepines have little or no influence on respiration during wakefulness or sleep in asymptomatic subjects. The likelihood of respiratory depression with orally administered benzodiazepine hypnotics is affected by a number of factors including: presence of respiratory impairment, dose level and elimination half-life. Clinical experience indicates that benzodiazepine use in obstructive sleep apnea (OSA) patients is associated with a worsening of breathing abnormalities. This is supported by studies or case reports which showed that apneas become more frequent in symptomatic apneics. Hypnotics will also affect oxygen saturation at night in patients with COPD or in any other chronic respiratory condition.

Hypnotics are generally inappropriate for children. Furthermore, people who may need to be alert at a moment's notice, such as firefighters and other emergency workers, should not be given hypnotics of any kind. The safety of hypnotics in pregnant women has not been established. Similarly, nursing mothers should not be given hypnotic drugs, as these medications and their active metabolites have been detected in breast milk[11].

Rebound insomnia is dependent on the type of drug, dosage and length of prior usage[67]. The symptoms of withdrawal are distinct from those symptoms that led to the use of the medication in the first place. For example, tinnitus, high levels of anxiety, headaches and nightmares are symptoms of benzodiazepine withdrawal, as distinct from anxiety that was the original symptom. True withdrawal symptoms are a sign of an abstinence syndrome and imply that the use of the drug has resulted in persisting physiological changes[22].

DRUG DEPENDENCE

Other contraindications for the use of hypnotics include people with alcoholism, because of additive sedative effects caused by the fact that both the hypnotic and the alcohol are GABA agonists, which produces an additive effect with regard to psychomotor impairment resulting in an increase in accidents. Former alcoholics or drug addicts of any kind are particularly susceptible to the abuse of any scheduled drug, including hypnotics[68]. Caution should also be exercised in co-administration with other GABA drugs such as anticonvulsants.

Much of the abuse of benzodiazepines reported in the medical literature does not represent recreational use *per se* but unsupervised therapeutic use at or above prescribed dosages[68]. A frequent scenario is one in which a patient discontinues the hypnotic, cannot tolerate the withdrawal symptoms and then continues use of the drug. As hypnotic use continues, tolerance develops. The patient increases the dosage and subsequent attempts to withdraw become progressively more difficult. Hypnotics users rarely increase their own dosage[22,69]. Although the alleviation of symptoms reinforces the taking of any drug to a slight degree, recreational drug abuse occurs only with greater reinforcement. Physicians may be held liable if patients are not adequately monitored, attempts are not made to discontinue hypnotic and anxiolytic use and the patients are not adequately informed of the abuse potential of these drugs[9].

MEDICATIONS FOR EXCESSIVE SLEEPINESS

Psycho-stimulants have been used for years in 'diet pills' and other preparations to treat weight gain, fatigue and sleepiness. The psycho-stimulants are indicated for the treatment of narcolepsy and hypersomnia. Caffeine is the most common stimulant now in general use in the USA. Ephedrine, derived from the ephedra root, has been used since antiquity for stimulating euphoria and was an early treatment for narcolepsy. In the 1930s the amphetamines were developed, first as an inhalant for asthma and then for narcolepsy. Methylphenidate was approved by the Food and Drug Administration (FDA) in 1956.

The armamentarium for the treatment of narcolepsy and excessive daytime sleepiness (EDS) has been significantly enhanced by the FDA approval of modafinil, a stimulant drug with little abuse potential, and the approval of γ-hydroxybutyrate (GHB) for insomnia associated with narcolepsy and cataplexy[70].

Narcolepsy

Narcolepsy is a clinical condition in which the individual usually has multiple 'sleep attacks' during the day that are overwhelming and difficult to resist[71]. Sleep attacks occur throughout the day with varying intensity. In some individuals these attacks can be nearly constant and produce total impairment, while in others the attacks may require considerable sedentary activity before they occur.

Most narcoleptics also have intrusions of REM sleep into wakefulness in the form of sleep paralysis, hypnogogic or hynopompic hallucinations that can occur just before sleep or during arousal. The hallucinations can occur in any sensory modality. Frequently the hallucinations are very frightening because the individual drifts in and out of sleep/wake while seeing frightening images and experiencing the paralysis simultaneously. Cataplexy is another form of REM intrusion and is characterized by sudden muscle weakness or paralysis that is precipitated by strong emotions such as fear, excitement or laughter[72].

Indirect sympathomimetics

Most clinically useful compounds available for the treatment of EDS act indirectly on dopaminergic and, to a lesser extent, on adrenergic neurons. Methylphenidate and cocaine are structurally similar to each other. Amphetamines have been used by the military for many years to combat fatigue.

This class of drugs which includes amphetamines and methylphenidate acts primarily by increasing the amount of monoamines available within the synaptic cleft of monoamine synapses in the CNS, and by blocking reuptake and enhancing release of norepinephrine, dopamine and serotonin[73]. Amphetamines are also weak inhibitors of monoamine oxidase (MAO). The midbrain dopamine systems include two major pathways that project to the forebrain and appear to be responsible for different aspects of psychomotor stimulant actions.

Pharmacokinetics and pharmacological action

Amphetamines are rapidly absorbed in the gastrointestinal tract. D-Amphetamine has a half-life of approximately 12 h, methylphenidate of 2–4 h and methylamphetamine of 6–8 h. All of these drugs increase blood pressure, heart rate and alertness, energetic vitality, talkativeness and aggressiveness, decrease appetite and inhibitions and improve motor performance and muscle strength.

Amphetamines and methylphenidate given at night decrease sleepiness, increase the latency to falling asleep, increase latency to the onset of REM sleep, reduce the proportion of REM and decrease stage 3 and 4 sleep. Amphetamines when administered during the day for narcolepsy, idiopathic hypersomnia or in sleep-deprived individuals decrease sleep propensity.

The classic way to measure the daytime sleepiness is the MSLT[74]. In this test, patients are given the opportunity to sleep for 20 min every 2 hours during the day for a total of five naps that begin at 10:00 a.m. The MSLT is used to diagnose narcolepsy and also to compare the relative potency of alerting drugs. Mitler and co-workers also developed a test that measured the ability to stay awake while sitting in a chair, the 'maintenance of wakefulness test' (MWT)[75], which more closely approximates a typical task that someone with narcolepsy or sleep deprivation must be able to perform.

Using the MWT, Mitler found that methylamphetamine was the most potent stimulant followed by D-amphetamine and methylamphetamine. These drugs brought the score of narcoleptics on the MWT to over 60% of normal patients. The majority of patients with narcolepsy can function adequately with this considerable improvement on the MWT.

Side-effects of stimulants

Common side-effects of amphetamines include headaches, irritability, nervousness or tremulousness, anorexia, insomnia, gastrointestinal complaints, dyskinesias and palpitations. In a study of 100 patients, 10% discontinued stimulants because of failure to respond, tolerance or side-effects[76]. Some studies have reported that the incidence of tolerance and side-effects is less in narcoleptics than in others taking methylphenidate or methylamphetamine, but the basis for this belief is unclear. There is little evidence that stimulants cause a clinically significant increase in blood pressure with commonly used doses in normotensive individuals. Increases in diastolic and particularly systolic blood pressure can occur in older or hypertensive patients.

Psychosis and hallucinations are rare in narcoleptics treated with stimulants. There have been only isolated cases of amphetamine psychosis, hallucinations and addiction, especially in patients with co-existing psychiatric conditions. Unwanted side-effects and amphetamine abuse can produce a variety of effects. Major symptoms of amphetamine toxicity are agitation, hallucinations, suicidal behavior and chest pain. Seizures and strokes can occur with use or 'freebasing' of cocaine. Tolerance to the alerting effects of stimulants in narcoleptics appears to occur with variable frequency, in the 10–30% range.

Modafinil

Modafinil, a novel stimulant that has been postulated to be a centrally active α_1-adrenergic agonist, may also affect caffeine or adenosine receptors. Moreover, it may also have some effect on dopamine reuptake and may also work at hypothalamic sites subserving wakefulness. The actual mechanism of action is unknown. Unlike the amphetamines, it has minimal peripheral sympathomimetic side-effects[77]. A 200–500 mg dose administered to narcoleptic patients produces reduced sleepiness and increased alertness but has minimal abuse potential[78]. One reason for this is that it has no euphoric effects and when used in excess produces headaches. Modafinil is less effective than amphetamines. Some clinicians use amphetamines with modafinil, although there is no research to support this practice.

GHB has been studied extensively in France and Canada as a treatment for narcolepsy and is now available in the USA under 'orphan drug' status. Given at night, GHB increases slow-wave sleep and sleep continuity. Since it has a short half-life, the drug needs to be re-administered if the first dose is taken before bedtime. GHB has been recreationally abused as a 'date rape' drug[70].

Antidepressants

Since the mid-1970s, the use of stimulants has been revolutionized by the introduction of tricyclic antidepressants for the collateral symptoms in narcolepsy. Protriptyline and chlormipramine have demonstrated efficacy for cataplexy and also help suppress nightmares and sleep paralysis. The serotonergic antidepressants such as fluoxetine are now used more frequently than the tricyclic antidepressants.

CIRCADIAN RHYTHM DISORDERS

Antidepressants, e.g. lithium, MAO inhibitors and tricyclic antidepressants, have been shown to have direct pharmacological effects on the circadian pacemaker in the superchiasmic nucleus by lengthening the period of the circadian rhythms. Tricyclics and antidepressants in general can cause rapid cycling in women with bipolar disorder prior to menopause, producing periods of sleeplessness with periods of depression and depressive sleep disturbance including insomnia.

Effects of antidepressants on sleep

There has been interest in the effects of antidepressants on sleep for many years because of the early observation that over 85% of depressed patients have insomnia, and around 10% of depressed patients have hypersomnia. Insomnia tends to be more severe in the melancholic and more severely depressed patients, and in patients with mixed anxiety and depression. Hypersomnia occurs in the 'atypical' depressives or in bipolar patients in the depressed phase and in seasonal affective disorder (SAD). Reduced total sleep time and sleep need occurs during the hypomanic or manic phase of bipolar illness.

Antidepressant drugs are generally classified by structure (for example the tricyclic antidepressants), or by mechanism of action (such as selective serotonin reuptake inhibitors (SSRI) or the MAO inhibitors, that specifically inhibit the breakdown of serotonin, norepinephrine and dopamine). There are other antidepressants that do not fit in these categories such as buproprion, which functionally potentiates the effects of norepinephrine, dopamine and nefazadone, which has 5-HT$_{IA}$ agonist properties.

Antidepressants can also be classified as sedating and non-sedating, or as selective and non-selective. In general, drugs that have high antihistaminic activity will cause weight gain and sedation[80]. Drugs with α_1 activity may produce hypotension and sexual dysfunction. SSRIs also are associated with nausea, insomnia and sexual dysfunction. Drugs that increase norepinephrine or dopamine may lead to activation, insomnia and an increase in muscle tone. Strong anticholinergic activity produces the side-effects of dry mouth, blurred vision and sedation.

Studies by Kupfer[80,81] and others have found that sleep during depression is associated with longer sleep latency, middle insomnia and early-morning awakening. Most depressed patients have reduced stage 3 and 4 sleep, especially in the first non-REM period, and a reduced latency from sleep onset to the first REM period than expected for their age. Sleep in a depressed person is thus similar to sleep in much older non-depressed people. Frequently, the first REM period is longer than normal and REM density, or number of eye movements during a REM cycle, is often increased. These characteristics of sleep in depression are further accentuated in the more severely depressed individuals[82].

Several lines of evidence suggest that REM sleep deprivation may be a biological process underlying the antidepressant properties of drugs which improve depression. Vogel[83] demonstrated that after 3 consecutive weeks of REM sleep deprivation by selective awakenings, patients during REM sleep were significantly less depressed than patients undergoing non-REM sleep deprivation. Another argument in favor of the hypothesis is the statistical comparison across studies indicating that in terms of hospital discharge rates and reduction in depression scores, REM sleep deprivation and imipramine have similar efficacy. Kupfer and associates[84] found that when depressed subjects were given amitriptyline, those subjects who had the greatest increase in REM latency on the first three nights of therapy had the most robust response to the drug. In general these subjects also had a reduction of REM time, significantly improved sleep efficiency and increased stage 3 and 4 sleep.

The REM suppression hypothesis, however, appears to be an oversimplification because there are other REM-reducing drugs such as barbiturates and amphetamines, for example, that do not have antidepressant action. In addition, there are certain antidepressant drugs such as trimipramine, trazodone and nefazadone which do not have significant REM-suppressing activity, yet are relatively effective antidepressants in some patients[85].

Heiligenstein and co-workers[86] used the known facts about the effects of antidepressants on sleep to predict a drug response to fluoxetine in individuals with moderate to severe depression. Subjects obtained two baseline sleep recordings to determine their REM latency and then were treated for 8 weeks with 20 mg of fluoxetine per day. Those subjects who had shortened REM latency of less than 60 min responded significantly better to fluoxetine than those whose REM latency was greater than 60 min, even though the severity of depressive symptoms did not differ between the two groups. This study indicated that depressed patients who have this biological marker for depression are biologically distinct in sleep. So distinct, in fact, that the long REM latency group did not respond any better than depressed patients taking placebo while the short REM latency group had a much more robust response to 20 mg of

fluoxetine than the pooled sample of depressed subjects.

Most antidepressant drugs are thought to increase REM latency through blocking the reuptake of monoamines in presynaptic neurons. Some drugs, such as desipramine and buproprion, act more on norepinephrine and dopamine, while the SSRIs produce the same effect on REM by blocking the reuptake of serotonin. The tricyclic antidepressants also have antihistaminic and anticholinergic effects that also suppress REM sleep.

The MAO inhibitors are powerful REM suppressors and very effective antidepressants[87,88]. Kupfer studied the effects of two selective inhibitors of MAO-A, in 20 depressive patients. After a single morning dose of cimoxaton he observed a significant decrease of REM sleep and prolongation of REM latency during the subsequent night[88]. However, after 300 mg of moclobemide (given in three portions, last dose at 5:00 p.m.), there was only a tendency toward suppression of REM sleep and prolongation of REM latency.

If shortened REM latency is found in the sleep of depression, can this be experimentally produced? Gillin has demonstrated that when depressed patients are given a cholinergic drug such as physostigmine, REM sleep is rapidly induced and this is accompanied by the rapid onset of dysphoria.

The SSRIs suppress REM sleep, comparable to tricyclic antidepressants. They also reduce total sleep time, cause sleep fragmentation, reduce sleep efficiency and early in the treatment often result in insomnia. However, as the patient's depression improves, insomnia improves dramatically in most patients who have significant antidepressant effect. When acute insomnia occurs with activating SSRIs such as fluoxetine and citalopram, it has been demonstrated that zolpidem given during the first 3 weeks of fluoxetine therapy enhances patient acceptance of fluoxetine but ultimately leads to lowered depression ratings early in treatment, fewer insomnia complaints and outcome measures comparable to those of patients using fluoxetine alone. The activating SSRIs such as fluoxetine and citalopram are often given in the morning initially, but if the dosage is increased fatigue may result and they can be given at night-time. Sertraline and paroxetine are usually given at night initially, which can reduce the daytime sedation that is sometimes seen with these drugs.

Significant sleep disruption and relapse from depression can occur during acute withdrawal from antidepressants. This is quite pronounced with the tricyclic antidepressants and the SSRIs and occurs most commonly with paroxetine, followed by venlafaxine and sertraline. Fluoxetine has no significant withdrawal symptom apparently because of its very long half life.

The effects of chronic administration

The effects of chronic administration of antidepressants on sleep are similar to those of acute administration, e.g. sustained REM sleep suppression and prolongation of REM, although REM sleep returns toward baseline to some degree. An early return of 'REM pressure' as manifested by short REM latency may precede a depressive relapse.

Use of antidepressants in sleep-related disorders

Some antidepressants, principally the sedative antidepressants, improve sleep continuity. Based on this observation 17 insomniacs were administered trimipramine for 4 weeks[89]. Then the active drug was discontinued and replaced by placebo for the subsequent 2 weeks. A significant improvement of total sleep time (TST) and sleep efficiency (SE), a diminution of wake time and an increase in stage 2 sleep were observed after 4 weeks of treatment. REM sleep remained unaltered, i.e. it seemed that treatment with trimipramine restored a physiological sleep architecture. Subjective reports of patients agreed with the objective data. After drug discontinuation a progressive deterioration of sleep continuity was noted, but the values did not exceed baseline values, so that no rebound insomnia occurred. Other sedating antidepressants can increase total sleep time as well but are poorly tolerated in patients with uncomplicated insomnia.

Trazodone is a potent α_1-andrenergic receptor blocker. Trazodone has less effect on REM sleep than most antidepressants, but in clinical use it is less effective than most antidepressants and poorly tolerated because of the excessive daytime sleepiness when used in therapeutic dosages. However, in dosages of 25–100 mg, trazodone increases total sleep time and has been widely used to treat chronic insomnia associated with anxiety and depression.

Adverse effects of antidepressants on sleep

Antidepressants have also been reported to produce occasional somnambulism. More frequently nocturnal myoclonus, restless leg syndrome, hypnogogic hallucinations, sleep paralysis REM behavior disorder, dreaming and nightmares have been noted.

MOOD-STABILIZING DRUGS

Kupfer and co-workers[90] demonstrated an increase in slow-wave sleep and a decrease in REM with lithium treatment. REM latency increased significantly and the increase correlated with serum lithium levels. Despite the considerable reduction in REM sleep during the treatment period, abrupt discontinuation of lithium is associated with an immediate restoration of REM sleep or a compensatory REM rebound.

Adverse effects of lithium include reduced daytime alertness, but no increase in sleepiness and slowed cognition. Lithium, when combined with neuroleptics, has been associated with somnambulism or sleepwalking[91].

ANTICONVULSANT DRUGS

Carbamazepine produces an improvement in parameters of sleep continuity. The impact on slow-wave sleep is prominent, doubling baseline values after 5 days of treatment.

Carbamazepine appears to have no negative effects on sleep in treated patients. Sleep structure was almost unaltered and sleep stability was actually improved. Daytime fatigue and cognitive slowing can also be bothersome side-effects. Oxycarbamazepine (Trileptl), an isomer of carbamazepine, has no apparent association with daytime fatigue.

Phenobarbital shares with other barbiturates hypnotic and sedative properties, and has similar effects on sleep architecture. Phenobarbital reduces sleep latency, wakefulness and REM sleep, and increases stage 2 sleep[92]. Valproic acid appears to have little or no long-term effects on sleep; indeed, studies in patients receiving the drug have variably reported a slight increase in stages 1, 3 and 4 or a sleep structure no different from that of control subjects; furthermore, it has little adverse effect on daytime alertness.

Impaired daytime alertness is, however, among the major side-effects of the anticonvulsants. Its impact on the quality of life of patients is sometimes marked enough as to interfere with the occupational or learning spheres of the patient's life. Thus, with phenobarbital, sedation is one of the main adverse events.

NEUROLEPTICS

Phenothiazines

The aeiphatic phenothiazines are characterized by excessive daytime sedation but tolerance increases significantly with time. Chlorpromazine and thioridazine produce more sedation and affective blunting than the non-aliphatic phenothiazines such as trifluoperazine and fluphenanzine.

Butyrophenones

It appears that there may be a bimodal effect of butyrophenones on sleep. Thus, low doses of these drugs were shown to increase indices of nocturnal wakefulness, whereas higher dosages have a sedating effect[93,94]. The effects of butyrophenones on sleep stages were quite inconsistent.

Clozapine

Clozapine antagonizes D1 more than D2 receptors, while it is also a potent antagonist of D4 receptors[95]. Furthermore, many other neurotransmitter systems (adrenergic, serotonergic, cholinergic, histaminergic) are also influenced by clozapine[95]. A sedative effect was reported on the first night of administration of the 25 mg dose[96], while slight sedation was suggested even with 12.5 mg at the beginning of a 2-week drug administration period[97]. The effects of clozapine on sleep stages are inconsistent[94,98], but REM sleep was suppressed both in humans[97] and in animals[94,98].

ANTIHISTAMINES

Sedative antihistamines

In this group, 13 drugs are included. Five of them (chlorpheniramine, doxylamine succinate, diphenhydramine, hydroxyzine and promethazine) were found to have quite sedative effects in sleep laboratory studies[99–102]. Moreover, neuropsychological studies demonstrated that they lower alertness and impair psychomotor performance to a considerable degree[103,104]. They were also found to shorten sleep latency more than placebo on the MSLT[105–108]. However, it should be emphasized that tolerance was shown to develop after the first day of administration of diphenhydramine. Since diphenhydramine is the most common constituent of OTC sleep aids it is clear that it would only be effective if taken occasionally. Epidemiological studies have shown that antihistamine users are overrepresented among a group of fatally injured drivers who were deemed responsible for their automobile accidents. Among older antihistamines, chlorpheniramine is least likely to cause sedation[109]. Finally, diphenhydramine and promethazine were found to suppress REM sleep.

Non-sedative antihistamines

Examples of this class of drugs include astemizole, cetirizine, loratadine, mepyramine, temelastine and terfenadine. Neuropsychological studies showed that *none* of these drugs in the usual dose range impaired performance[104] or shortened sleep latency in the MSLT[105,106].

CORTICOSTEROIDS

When steroids are used on a short-term basis (14 days), sleep disturbance is one of the most common side-effects. The degree of sleep disturbance is somewhat dependent on dosage. Persistant insomnia can occur often accompanied by euphoria or depression[85,110,111].

BRONCHODILATORS

Because of their stimulant effects on the CNS, bronchodilating drugs, which contain ephedrine, theophylline and norepinephrine, can lead to sleep difficulties. However, studies suggest that stimulatory effects of bronchodilators are mild and, in asthmatics, the enhancement in breathing from the therapeutic effects of the drug may result in an overall improvement in sleep despite stimulatory side-effects.

ANTIHYPERTENSIVES

Some beta-blockers are lipid-soluble, easily enter the brain and have high sympatholytic activity. Therefore, they have a greater probability of affecting sleep than less lipophilic beta-blockers. This is consistent with a sleep laboratory finding of increased wakefulness during the night with pindolol, a lipophilic drug with partial beta-agonist effect. Effects of both the lipophilic and non-lipophilic beta-blockers have been reported either to suppress REM sleep or cause no significant change. Sedation from beta-blockers has been linked to indirect effects on the CNS, i.e. the reticular formation responds to a reduction in blood pressure by decreasing CNS activity. Somnambulism has been reported occasionally with lipophilic beta-blockers[85]. The use of angiotensin converting enzyme inhibitors such as captopril and enalapril has been associated with nightmares[112].

OTHER DRUGS

Methylsergide, a serotonin-blocking drug that is used to prevent severe migraine, has been shown to cause over-stimulation and insomnia. The use of amantadine has been associated with insomnia in 10 of 295 hospital employees taking the drug[113] and in 49 of 430 Parkinson's disease patients[114]. Similarly, mefloquine, an antimalaria agent, has been associated with insomnia as the initial symptom of an acute major depressive disorder that can occur with this drug.

NARCOTICS

Oral analgesics containing codeine and other morphine derivatives are excitatory and can produce insomnia and nightmares. Heavy use of morphine or heroin produces light alpha sleep with diminished REM and slow-wave sleep. Withdrawal from opiates produces insomnia that is poorly alleviated with benzodiazepines[115].

Narcotic analgesia, compared to local anesthetic analgesia, produces considerable sleep-disordered breathing with a higher number of apneic events and a greater degree of oxygen desaturation. Thus, an additive effect in producing sleep-disordered breathing may occur in patients given both narcotics and general anesthesia.

Furthermore, in a recent study, pre-existing sleep apnea syndrome was shown to be a risk factor associated with the occurrence of respiratory depression following the parenteral use of opiates. Extreme caution is recommended in the use of narcotics in patients with sleep apnea.

ANESTHETICS

It has been commonly observed that asymptomatic subjects develop upper airway obstruction during anesthesia. These effects are more pronounced in obese individuals and patients with OSA.

Preoperative sedation should be administered with caution. In those patients to whom general anesthesia is administered, careful monitoring in the recovery room for respiratory depression and upper airway obstruction is essential. Further, monitoring in the intensive care unit should be utilized for patients with sleep apnea who have had major surgery, prolonged anesthesia or received narcotic drugs. Whenever possible, local analgesia is preferred over general anesthesia.

ANTI-PARKINSONIAN MEDICATIONS

A variety of dopamine agonists are used in the treatment of Parkinson's disease, restless legs periodic syndrome and limb movements in sleep (PLMS). In one report, a paradoxical leg restlessness, which was treatment-emergent, developed in eight out of 47 patients with L-dopamine at bedtime, seven of whom required daytime medication for relief. Generally, patients with Parkinson's disease experience daytime fatigue, but dopamine agonists exacerbate fatigue and promote daytime sleepiness as a function of dosage.

CHRONOPHARMACOLOGY

Antidepressants (e.g. lithium, MAO inhibitors and tricyclic antidepressants) have been shown to have a direct pharmacological effect on the circadian pacemaker in the SCN by lengthening the period of circadian rhythms[116]. MAO inhibitors and tricyclic antidepressants given prophylactically may cause a rapid cycling between depression and mania, indicating a drug-induced circadian rhythm disorder. This effect may be accounted for by the finding that, in animals, both MAO inhibitors and tricyclic antidepressants, in contrast to lithium, have been shown to induce a dissociation of the activity components of the rest–activity cycle from body temperature rhythms. This pattern is strikingly similar to that seen in humans in free-running conditions, as well as in manic-depressive patients, when they undergo spontaneous or drug-induced switches from depression to mania. The finding that lithium does not induce this dissociation[116] may explain why this drug, in contrast to MAO inhibitors and tricyclic antidepressants, is a good prophylactic agent in the treatment of most bipolar patients.

CONCLUSIONS

All drugs that cross the blood–brain barrier affect sleep. No drug has been definitively shown to improve sleep in normal people, although daytime alertness can be enhanced with stimulants in the short term. Pharmacological progress in the treatment of sleep disorders has been profound but slow. We are a long way from realizing highly specific pharmacology of sleep. Drugs produce sleep that is similar to normal sleep but these effects are often transient or weak. Similarly, drugs are now available that enhance daytime alertness but these effects are still too unreliable and produce too many side-effects. Now that particular genetic defects have been identified in depression and narcolepsy, more specific drugs should start to be developed.

References

1. Daan S, Beersma DG, Borbely AA. Timing of human sleep: recovery process gated by a circadian pacemaker. *Am J Physiol* 1984;246: R161–83
2. Czeisler CA, Weitzman E, Moore-Eda MC, *et al.* Human Sleep: its duration and organization depend on its circadian phase. *Science* 1980; 210:1264–7
3. Gillin JC, Seifreitz D, Zoltoski RK, Salin-Pascual RJ. Basic science of sleep. In Sadock BJ, Sadock VA, eds. *Comprehensive Textbook of Psychiatry*. Philadelphia, PA: Lippincott, Williams and Wilkins, 2000:1999–208
4. Mellinger GD, Balter MB, Uhlenhuth EH. Insomnia and its treatment: prevalence and correlates. *Arch Gen Psychiatry* 1985;42:225–32

5. The Gallup Organization, Inc. *Sleep in America*. Princeton, NJ: 1991

6. Johnson LC, Spinweber CL. Good and poor sleepers differ in Navy performance. *Mil Med* 1983;148:727–31

7. Mendelson WB, Garnett D, Linnoila M. Do insomniacs have impaired daytime functioning? *Biol Psychiatry* 1984;19:12691–64

8. The Gallup Organization, Inc. *Doctor's Experience and Behavior with Insomnia Patients*. Princeton, NJ: 1993

9. Petursson H, Laddr M. *Dependence on Tranquilizers*. Oxford: Oxford University Press, 1984

10. Roth T, Roehrs T, Vogel G. Zolpidem in the treatment of transient insomnia: a double-blind, randomized comparison with placebo. *Sleep* 1995;18:246–51

11. Dement W, Seidel W, Carskadon M. Issues in the diagnosis and treatment of insomnia. *Psychopharmacology* 1984;1(Suppl):11–43

12. Consensus Conference. Drugs and insomnia: the use of medications to promote sleep. *J Am Med Assoc* 1984;251:2410–14

13. Bixler EO, Kales A, Sodatos CR, *et al*. Effectiveness of emazepam with short, intermediate- and long-term use: sleep laboratory evaluation. *J Clin Pharmacol* 1978;18:110–18

14. Stepanski EJ. Behavior therapy for insomnia. In Kryger MH, Roth T, Dement WC, eds. *Principles and Practice of Sleep Medicine*, 2nd edn. Philadelphia: WB Saunders Co., 1994:535–41

15. Gillin JC, Mendelson WB. Sleeping pills: for whom? When? How long? In Paler GC, ed. *Neuropharmacology of Central Nervous System and Behavioral Disorders*. New York: Academic Press, 1980:285–316

16. Kales A, Bixler EO, Tan TL, *et al*. Chronic hypnotic use: ineffectiveness, drug withdrawal insomnia, and hypnotic drug dependence. *J Am Med Assoc* 1974;227:513–17

17. Kales A, Kales JD. Sleep laboratory studies of hypnotic drugs: efficacy and withdrawal effects. *J Clin Psychopharmacol* 1983;3:140–9

18. Subhan Z. The effects of benzodiazepines on short-term memory processing and information processing. In Hindmarch, *et al*. eds. *Psychopharmacology* (Berlin) 1984;(Suppl 1): 174–81

19. Ray WA, Griffin MR, Schaffner W, *et al*. Psychotropic drug use and the risk of hip fracture. *N Engl J Med* 1987;316:363–9

20. Kales A, Kales JD, Bixler EO, Scharf MB. Effectiveness of hypnotic drugs with prolonged use: flurazepam and pentobarbital. *Clin Pharm Ther* 1975;18:356–63

21. Ford DE, Kamerow DB. Epidemiologic study of sleep disturbances and psychiatric disorders: an opportunity for prevention? *J Am Med Assoc* 1989;262:1479–84

22. American Psychiatric Association. *Benzodiazepine Dependence, Toxicity, and Abuse: A Task Force Report of the American Psychiatric Association*. Washington, DC: American Psychiatric Association, 1990

23. Zorumski CF, Isenberg KE. Insights into the structure and function of GABA-benzodiazepine receptors: ion channels and psychiatry. *Am J Psychiatry* 1991;148:162–73

24. Squires RF, Braestrup C. Benzodizepine receptors in rat brain. *Nature* 1974;266:732–4

25. Dement WC, Carksadon MA, Mitler MM, *et al*. Prolonged use of flurazepam: a sleep laboratory study. *Behav Med* 1978;5:25–31

26. Balter MB, Uhlenhuth EH. The beneficial and adverse effects of hypnotics. *J Clin Psychiatry* 1991;52:16–23

27. Mamelak M, Csima A, Price V. A comparative 29 night sleep laboratory study on the effects of quazepam and triazolam on chronic insomniacs. *J Clin Pharmacol* 1984;24:64–75

28. Fuccella LM. Bioavailability of temazepam in soft gelatine capsules. *Br J Clin Pharmcol* 1979;8:31S–35S

29. Lahmeyer HW. Insomnia: *how to get a good night's sleep*. *Consultant* 1995;January:108–11

30. Allen MD, Greenblatt DJ, Arnold JD. Single and multiple dose kinetics of estazolam, a triazolo benzodiazepine. *Psychopharmacology* 1979;66:267–74

31. Greenblatt DJ, Divoll M, Abernethy DR, *et al*. Benzodiazepine kinetics: implication for therapeutics and pharmacogeriatrics. *Drug Metab Rev* 1983;14:251–92

32. Lahmeyer HW, Roth T, Jenning DJ, *et al*. Predictors of somnolence to flurazepam, temazepam, triazolam and estazolam. *Sleep Res* 1990

33. Roehers T, Zorick FJ, Sicklesteel JM, *et al*. Effects of hypnotics on memory. *J Clin Psychopharmacol* 1983;3:310–13

34. Roth T, Hartse KM, Saab PG, *et al*. The effects of flurazepam, lorazepam, and triazolam on sleep and memory. *Psychopharmacology* 1980; 70:207–10

35. Kales A, Scharf MB, Kales JD. Rebound insomnia: a new clinical syndrome. *Science* 1978;201:1039–41

36. Roth T, Roehrs TA. A review of the saftey profiles of benzodiazepine hypnotics. *J Clin Psychiatry* 1991;52:38–41

37. Spinweber CL, Johnson LC. Effects of triazolam (0.5 mg) on sleep, performance, memory and arousal threshold. *Psychopharmacology* (Berlin) 1982;76:5–12

38. George KA, Dundee JW. Relative amnesiac actions of diazepam, flunitrazepam and lorazepam in man. *Br J Clin Pharmacol* 1977; 4:45–50

39. Wheatley D. Prescribing short-acting hypnosedatives: current recommendations

from a safety perspective. *Drug Safety* 1992;7: 106–15

40. Schenck CH, Mahowald MW. A polysomnographic, neuralgic, psychiatric and clinical outcome report on 70 consecutive cases with REM sleep behavior disorder (RBD): sustained clonazepam efficacy in 89.5% of 57 treated patients. *Cleve Clin J Med* 1990; 57(Suppl):10–24

41. Kales A, Mafredi RL, Vgontzas AN, *et al.* Clonazepam: sleep laboratory study of efficacy and withdrawal. *J Clin Psychopharmacol* 1991; 11:189–93

42. Fillingim JM. Double blind evaluation of temazepam, flurazepam and placebo in geriateric insomniacs. *Clin Ther* 1982;4:369–80

43. Marttila JK, Hammel RJ, Alexander B, Zustiak R. Potential untoward effects of long-term use of flurazepam in geriatric patients. *J Am Pharm Assoc* 1977;17:692–5

44. Nicholson AN. Impaired performance. In D'Arcy PF, Griffin JP, eds. *Latrogenic Diseases*, 3rd edn. Oxford: Oxford University Press, 1986:671–9

45. Langer SZ, Arbilla S, Scatton B, *et al.* Receptors involved in the mechanism of action of zolpidem. In Sauvanet JP, Langer SZ, Morselli PL, eds. *Imidazopyridines in Sleep Disorders*. New York: Raven Press, 1988

46. Lahmeyer HW, Wilcox CS, Kann FJ, Leppik I. Subjective efficacy of zolpidem in outpatients with chronic insomnia. *Clin Drug Invest* 1997;13:

47. Scharf MB, Roth T, Vogel GW, *et al.* A multicenter, placebo-controlled study evaluating zolpidem in the treatment of chronic insomnia. *J Clin Psychiatry* 1994;55:192–9

48. Walsh J, Hartman P, Kowall JP. Insomnia. In Chokroverty S, ed. *Sleep Disorders Medicine: A Comprehensive Textbook*. Stoneham, MA: Butterworth, 2000

49. Morselli PL, Larribaud J, Guillet P, *et al.* Daytime residual effects of zolpidem: a review of available data. In Sauvanet JP, Langer SZ, Morselli PL, eds. *Imidazopyridines in Sleep Disorders*. New York: Raven Press, 1988:183–91

50. Monti JM. Effect of zolpidem on sleep in insomniac patients. *Eur J Clin Pharmacol* 1989; 36:461–6

51. Monti JM. Concluding remarks: toward a third-generation of hypnotics. In Sauvanet JP, Langer SZ, Morselli PL, eds. *Imidazopyridines in Sleep Disorders*. New York: Raven Press, 1988:363–8

52. Wright NA, Belyavin A, Borland RG, Nicholson AN. Modulation of delta activity by hypnotics in middle-aged subjects; studies with a benzodiazepine (flurazepam) and a cyclopyrrolone (zopiclone). *Sleep* 1986;9: 348–52

53. Kryger MH, Steljes D, Pouliot Z, *et al.* Subjective versus objective evaluation of hypnotic efficacy; experience with zolpidem. *Sleep* 1991;14:399–407

54. Terazono MG, Parrino L, Fioriti G, *et al.* Modifications of sleep structure induced by increasing levels of acoustic perturbation in normal subjects. *Electroencephalogr Clin Neurophysiol* 1990;76:29–38

55. Holm KJ, Goa KL. Zolpidem an update of its pharmacology, therapeutic efficacy and tolerability in the treatment of insomnia. Adis Drug Evaluation. *Drugs* 2000;59:865–89

56. Walsh J, Hartman P, Kowall JP. Insomnia. In Chokroverty S, ed. *Sleep Disorders Medicine: A Comprehensive Textbook*. Stoneham, MA: Butterworth, 1994:219–39

57. Woods JH, Katz JL, Winger G. Use and abuse of benzodiazepines; issues relevant to prescribing. *J Am Med Assoc* 1988;260:3476–80

58. Evans SM, Funderburk FR, Griffiths RR. Zolpidem and tiazolam in humans: behavioral and subjective effects and abuse liability. *J Pharm Exp Ther* 1990;225:1246–55

59. Lahmeyer HW. Pharmacological management of insomnia. In Chase MH, Roth T, eds. *Management of Insomnia in Psychiatric Populations. Advances in Sleep Medicine* 1993;3

60. Schlich D, L'Heritier C, Coquelin J, *et al.* Long-term treatment of insomnia with zolpidem. *J Int Med Res* 1991;19:271–9

61. Ware JC, Allen R, Scharf MB, *et al.* An evaluation of residual sedation following nighttime administration of 10 or 20 mg of zaleplon, 30 mg of flurazepam, or placebo in healthy subjects. *Sleep* 1998;21(Suppl):263

62. Fleming J, Moldofsky J, Walsh JD, *et al.* Comparison of the residual effects and efficacy of short term zolpidem, flurazepam and placebo in patients with chronic insomnia. *Clin Drug Invest* 1995;9:303–13

63. Fry J, Scharf MB, Berkowitz DV, *et al.* A phase III, 28 day, multicenter, randomized, double-blind, comparator- and placebo-controlled, parallel-group safety, tolerability, and efficacy study of 5, 10, 20 mg of Zelaplon, compared with 10 mg of Zolpidem or placebo, in adult outpatients with insomnia. *Sleep* 1998; (Suppl):262

64. Ray WA, Griffin MR, Downey W. Benzodiazepines of long and short elimination half-life and the risk of hip fracture. *J Am Med Assoc* 1989;262:3303–7

65. Divoll M, Greenblatt DJ, Harmatz JS, Shader RI. Effect of age and gender on disposition of temazepam. *J Pharm Sci* 1981;70:1104–7

66. Carskadon M, Seidel WF, Greenblatt DJ, *et al.* Daytime carryover of triazolam and flurazepam in elderly insomniacs. *Sleep* 1982;4: 361–71

67. Roehrs TA, Zorick FJ, Wittig RM, *et al*. Dose determinants of rebound insomnia. *Br J Clin Pharmacol* 1986;22:143–7

68. Ladewig D. Abuse of benzodiazepines in Western European society – incidence and prevalence motives, drug acquisition. *Pharmacopsychiatry* 1983;16:103–6

69. Balter MD, Manheimer DI, Mellinger GE, *et al*. A cross-national comparison of anti-anxiety/sedative drug use. *Curr Med Res Opin* 1984;8(Suppl):5–20

70. Broughon R, Mamelack VI. The treatment of narcolepsy, cataplexy with nocturnal gammahydroxybutyrate. *Can J Neurol Sci* 1979;12:1–6

71. Dement W. Daytime sleepiness and sleep 'attacks'. In Guilleminault C, Dement W, Passaouant, eds. *Progress in Behavior Modification*. New York: Academic Press, 1978;6:1–45

72. Daly D, Yoss R. Narcolepsy. In Vinken PJ, Bruyn GW, eds. *Handbook of Clinical Neurology*. Vol. 15: *The Epilepsies*. Amsterdam: North-Holland, 1974:chap 43, 836–52

73. Shindler J, Schachter M, Brincat S, Pares JD. Amphetamine, mazindol, and fencamfamin in narcolepsy. *Br Med J (Clin Res Ed)* 1985;290:1167–70

74. Milter MD. The multiple sleep latency test as an evaluation for excessive somnolence. In Guilleminault C, ed. *Sleeping and Waking Disorder: Indications and Techniques*. Reading, MA: Addison-Wesley, 1982

75. Mliter MM, Aldrich MS, Koob GF, Zarcone VP. Narcolepsy and its treatment with stimulants. *Sleep* 1994;17:352–71

76. Parkes JD. Narcolepsy. *Nurs Times* 1975;71:881–3

77. Lyons TJ, French J. Modafinil: the unique properties of a new stimulant. *Aviat Space Environ Med* 1991;62:432–5

78. US Modafanil in Narcolepsy Multicenter study group. Randomized trial of modafanil as a treatment for excessive daytime somnolence of narcolepsy. *Neurology* 2000;54:1166–75

79. Ware JC. Tricyclic antidepressants in the treatment of insomnia. *J Clin Psychiatry* 1983;44:25–8

80. Kupfer DJ. REM latency: a psychobiological marker for primary depressive disease. *Biol Psychiatry* 1976;11:159–74

81. Kupfer D, Brondy D, Coble P, Spiker D. EEG sleep and affective psychosis. *J Affect Disord* 1980;2:17–25

82. Kupfer DJ, Spiker DG, Neil JF, McPartland RJ. EEG sleep. A longitudinal placebo study. *J Affect Disord* 1979;1:131–8

83. Vogel G, Thurmond A, Gibbons P, Edwards K, Sloan KB, Sexton K. The effect of triazolam on the sleep of insomniacs. *Psychopharmacology* 1975;41:65–9

84. Kupfer DJ, Hanin I, Spiker D, *et al*. Amitriptyline plasma levels and clinical response in primary depression: II. *Commun Psychopharmacol* 1978;2:441–50

85. Bootzin RR, Lahmeyer HW, Lilie JK, eds. *Integrated Approach to Sleep Management; The Healthcare Practitioner's Guide to the Diagnosis and Treatment of Sleep Disorders*. Cahners Healthcare Communications, 1994

86. Heiligenstein JH, Faries DE, Rush AJ, *et al*. Latency to rapid eye movement sleep as a predictor of treatment response to fluoxetine and placebo in non psychotic depressed outpatients. *Psychiatr Res* 1994;52:327–39

87. Cohen R, Pickar D, Garnett D, *et al*. REM sleep supression induced by selective monoamine oxidase inhibitors. *Psychopharmacology* 1982;78:137–40

88. Hoff P, Golling H, Kapfhammer R, *et al*. Climoxaton and moclobemid. Two new MAO-inhibitors: influence of sleep parameters in patients with major depressive disorders. *Pharmacopsychiatry* 1986;19:249–50

89. Hohagen F, Montero RF, Weiss E, *et al*. Treatment of primary insomnia with trimipramine: an alternative to benzodiazepine hypnotics? *Eur Arch Psychiatry Clin Neurosci* 1994;244:65–72

90. Kupfer DJ, Reynolds CF, Weiss BL, Foster FC. Lithium carbonate and sleep in affective disorders: further considerations. *Arch Gen Psychiatry* 1974;30:79–84

91. Charney DS, Kales A, Soldatos CR, Nelson JC. Somnambulistic-like episodes secondary to combined lithium-neuroleptic treatment. *Br J Psychiatry* 1979;135:418–24

92. Kales A, Kales JD, Scharf MB, Tan TL. Hypnotics and altered sleep and dream patterns. II. All-night EEG studies of chloral hydrate, flurazepam and methaqualone. *Arch Gen Psychiatry* 1970;23:219–25

93. Cookson IB, Wells PG. Haloperidol in the treatment of stutterers [Letter]. *Br J Psychiatry* 1973;123:491

94. Sayers AC, Kleinlogel H. [Neuropharmacological findings after chronic administration of haloperidol, K loxapine and clozapine.] *Arzneimittelforschung* 1974;24:981–3

95. Coward DM. General pharmacology of clozapine. *Br J Psychiatry* 1992;17(Suppl):5–11

96. Touyz SW, Beumont PJ, Saayman GS, Zabow T. A psychophysiological investigation of the short-term effects of clozapine upon sleep parameters of normal young adults. *Biol Psychiatry* 1977;12:801–22

97. Touyz SW, Saayman GS, Zabow T. A psychophysiological investigation of the long-term effects of clozapine upon sleep patterns

of normal young adults. *Psychopharmacology (Berl)* 1978;56:69–73

98. Spierings EL, Dzoljic MR, Godschalk M. Effect of clozapine on the sleep pattern in the rat. *Pharmacology* 1977;15:551–6

99. Brannon JO, Jewett RE. Effects of selected phenothiazines on REM sleep in schizophrenics. *Arch Gen Psychiatry* 1969;21:284–90

100. Adam K, Oswald I. The hypnotic effects of an antihistamine: promethazine. *Br J Clin Pharmacol* 1986;22:715–17

101. Rickels K, Ginsberg J, Morris RJ, *et al.* Doxylamin succinate in insomniac family practice patients: a double blind study. *J Clin Pharmacol* 1983;23:235–42

102. Rickels K, Morris JR, Newman H, *et al.* Diphenhydramine in insomniac family practice patients: a double-blind study. *Curr Ther Res* 1984;35:532–40

103. Carruthers SG, Shoeman DW, Hignite CE, Azarnoff DL. Correlation between plasma diphenhydramine level and sedative and antihistamine effects. *Clin Pharmacol Ther* 1978;23:375–82

104. Clarke CH, Nicholson AN. Performance studies with antihistamines. *Br J Clin Pharmacol* 1978;6:31–5

105. Roehers T, Lamphere J, Paxton C, *et al.*, Temazepam's efficacy in patients with sleep onset insomnia. *Br J Clin Pharmacol* 1984; 17:691–6

106. Roth R, Roehrs T, Koshorek G, Sicklesteel J, Zorick F. Sedative effects of antihistamines. *J Allergy Clin Immunol* 1987;80:94–8

107. Seidel WF, Cohen S, Bliwise NG, Dement WC. Direct measurement of daytime sleepiness after administration of cetirizine and hydroxyzine with a standardized electroencephalographic assessment. *J Allergy Clin Immunol* 1990;86: 1029–33

108. Nicholson AN, Pascoe PA, Turner C, *et al.* Sedation and histamine H1-receptor antagonism: studies in man with the enantiomers of chlorpheniramine and dimethindene. *Br J Pharmacol* 1991;104:270–6

109. Meltzer EO. Antihistamine- and decongestant-induced performance decrements. *J Occup Med* 1990;32:327–34

110. Lahmeyer HW. Comments on M.D. Majewska's paper: Actions of steroids on neuron: role in personality, mood, stress, and disease. *Integrative Psychiatry* 1085;5:267 8

111. Lahmeyer HW. Sleep in two depressed patients with Cushing's syndrome. *J Neuropsychiatry* 1989;

112. Haffner CA, Smith BS, Pepper C. Hallucinations as an adverse effect of angiotensin converting enzyme inhibition. *Postgrad Med J* 1993;69:240

113. Flaherty JA, Bellur SN. Mental side effects of amantadine therapy: its spectrum and characteristics in a normal population. *J Clin Psychiatry* 1981;42:344–5

114. Schwab RS, Poskanzer DC, England AC Jr, Young RR. Amantadine in Parkinson's disease. Review of more than two years' experience. *J Am Med Assoc* 1972;222:792–5

115. Rogalski CJ, Lahmeyer HW. Effects of the hypnotic flurazepam on sleep of pentazocine and heroin addicts during withdrawal. *Int J Addict* 1983;18:407–18

116. Wirz-Justice A, Krauchi K, Morimasa T, Willener R, Feer H. Circadian rhythym of [3H]imipramine binding in the rat suprachiasmatic nuclei. *Eur J Pharmacol* 1983;87: 331–3

28

Alternative therapies in sleep medicine

Leonid Kayumov, Raed Hawa, Colin M. Shapiro, Howard D. Kurland,
Marc Oster, Joel Bornstein and Alexander Z. Golbin

INTRODUCTION

Interest in alternative medicine nowadays is not just the curiosity of lay people, but an urgent necessity for medical professionals that reflects a crisis in modern medicine and especially in health care. Sleep medicine, despite being a young discipline, is not an exception.

Advances in modern medicine tend to focus on acute medical and surgical care and less on the treatment of chronic illnesses. In addition, the significant increase in the cost of medication and health care in general, the skyrocketing cost of malpractice insurance for doctors and the public's fear of medication side-effects generated by the media have all contributed to physicians as well as the public wanting to know more about alternative (non-prescription) treatment techniques. Alternative medicine has become a fashionable and confusing field.

When someone uses the phrase 'alternative medicine', it is important to clarify what they mean: (1) an alternative approach to understanding the nature of a particular disorder, or (2) an alternative treatment for a conventional problem (i.e. non-prescription medications, either remedies from the past such as herbal treatments or modern state-of-the-art techniques such as sound therapy). The first use of the phrase 'alternative medicine' is 'anti-doctors' (anti-traditional), denying current medicine altogether and proclaiming a 'new' approach. This group accuses traditional medicine of focusing on a 'war' on disease (war on cancer, chemotherapy as cell killing, war on infections, etc.), while doctors practicing alternative medicine do not fight disease, but 'repair' the body. On the other hand, both researchers and clinicians are very interested in the second definition of 'alternative medicine' mentioned above. The study of the positive and negative effects of any non-prescription technique to control symptoms or treat disorders is a welcome method and considered as a complementary tool.

This chapter is based on the understanding that alternative medicine is very helpful, but only as an adjunct to conventional medicine.

There are endless non-drug medical techniques ranging from ancient acupuncture, herbal medicine and yoga to relatively new treatments like energy medicine, biofeedback, hypnotherapy, neurolinguistic programming, magnetic field therapy, light therapy, applied kinesiology and sound therapy. Some non-prescription techniques are proven to be helpful, while the claims of others are yet to be substantiated.

In this chapter we present the available research and clinical data on some alternative (non-prescription) treatments related to sleep and alertness disorders.

This survey will include such treatments as acupuncture, yoga, meditation, music therapy, phytotherapy or herbology, hypnotherapy, dream and phototherapy. Herbology or phytotherapy is a term used to cover the many different herbs used as sleep aids such as valerian, catnip, chamomile, gotu kola, hops, lavender, passionflower, skull cap, kava and many others.

Many aspects of alternative treatment remain controversial and questionable. The role of placebo mechanisms (patient expectations), the optimal duration and the cost-effectiveness of the treatment still have not been convincingly settled by any single study; hence they are often disputed. Many clinical studies suffer from methodological weaknesses such as small sample size and differentially designed or poorly controlled protocols, making them difficult to interpret. Furthermore, the results of these studies are not consistent across all outcome measures. Above all, there are no consensus guidelines available for the use of 'complementary' or 'alternative' medicine (CAM) therapies for sleep disorders such as insomnia.

The purpose of this chapter is to facilitate and evolve a set of consensus guidelines to produce clinically feasible and scientifically meaningful evidence-based recommendations.

ALTERNATIVE MEDICINE AND SLEEP

Music (sound) therapy

Music therapy can be defined as the therapeutic use of music in patient health and well-being[1]. Historical evidence shows even Florence Nightingale recognized the healing power of music in the care of the sick[2]. A recent article by Chlan[2] elegantly reviewed the practical and theoretical implications (cautions, concepts, methods and recommendations) of music therapy that are being used to alleviate symptoms of discomfort and anxiety, offer relaxation and promote restful sleep.

Bonnet and Arand[3] found, based on daytime nap studies (both multiple sleep latency test and maintenance of wakefulness test) in normal young adult subjects ($n = 12$), that music may play a small beneficial role that helps to maintain arousal. Moreover, Mornhinweg and Voignier[4] offered further beneficial effects of music on sleep disturbances in the aged population ($n = 25$). Results of this particular study revealed that 96% of these aged subjects reported improved sleep using self-administered intervention. Williamson[5] found that playing taped ocean sounds throughout the night to patients who had undergone coronary artery bypass surgery after they left the critical care unit resulted in an improvement in depth of sleep, fewer episodes of nocturnal awakening, easier return to sleep, better quality of sleep and higher total sleep scores, indicating a better sleep.

Recently developed brain music therapy has attracted a great deal of attention both in scientific and media circles[6-8]. The multidisciplinary team of researchers includes computer programmers, music therapists, composers, neurophysiologists and psychiatrists. The most intriguing part of this treatment modality is the use of computers and synthesizers to create sequences of notes that are customized for each patient, who then listens to the music while trying to sleep. After documenting a patient's subjective complaints and taking objective measurements to determine the nature of the problem, the brain electrical activity is recorded by means of an electroencephalogram (EEG) at several points on the surface of the brain during various states of consciousness, such as alert concentration and deep relaxation. The EEG signals are sent to a computer for fast-Fourier-transform (FFT) analysis, after which a specially designed algorithm generates musical instrument digital interface (MIDI) note data based on the FFT. This is not a direct conversion of the frequency spectrum of the electrical waveforms from the brain; the music arises from the relationships between the various EEG signals, which form a map of the brain's electrical activity in different areas.

The MIDI messages are sent to a synthesizer, and the resulting audio is recorded onto CD-ROM, which the patient can take home and play according to personalized instructions. Listening to these sounds stimulates the electrical activity associated with the state of consciousness on which they are based; if the sounds are derived from theta and delta waves, those waves are induced in the patient's brain, which helps the person to sleep.

In a recent double-blind study, Kayumov and co-workers[6,7] generated custom 'sleep music' for 40 volunteers who had experienced at least 2 years of anxiety- or stress-related insomnia. The subjects were divided into two groups: the experimental group got CDs of music based on their own brain oscillations, while the control group got CDs of music based on other people's 'brain music'. After 4 weeks of use at home, the experimental group showed clear signs of objective (polysomnographic measures and endogenous melatonin secretion values) and subjective improvement (variety of psychometric scales) in the quality of their sleep, while the control group exhibited no objective improvement.

Another route of investigation being pursued by Kayumov's team is to have a human musician compose music while a patient is connected to the EEG machine; this is a variation of biofeedback. The composer plays music while watching an FFT display with the patient in real time. When the composer finds music that consistently affects the FFT in the desired manner (usually increased power in theta and delta activity) over 2 or 3 min, that music is recorded to be used by the patient at home.

Music-based solutions for insomniacs have advantages over hypnotics, with virtually no side-effects or dependency issues. This research is in its infancy, but it holds great promise for non-pharmacological management of insomnia.

Acupuncture

Overview

Acupuncture is one of the major pillars of traditional Chinese medicine. Acupuncture therapy focuses on the repair of faulty interconnected systems in the entire body. It is an energy-based, holistic system. Acupuncture in China has a history spread over five millennia[9]. The utilization of stone needles began many centuries before being documented during the Han dynasty (206 BC to AD 220) in the Analytical Dictionary of Characters. With more sophisticated production techniques, stone needles were replaced by those made of bone, followed by bamboo and then bronze. Metal needles were in use by the time of the compilation of the Huangdi Nei Jing (known as the Canon of Medicine and as The Yellow Emperor's Textbook of Medicine) during the period from 175 to 221 BC. This treatise detailed the use of acupuncture techniques and described the current concepts of energy channels and viscera. The conceptualization that 'the ear is the place where all channels meet' introduced the integration of macrosystems (body points) with microsystems (such as ear points).

Throughout the centuries, techniques were developed for stimulating needles, which included twirling and multiple rapid insertion and removal (called pecking). Stimulation with heat was done with a burning herb called moxa, and termed moxibustion.

In more recent times, stimulation with electric currents was developed. Systems of variable intensity of energy, variable wave forms and variable frequencies were developed. Delivery systems for the stimulation of acupuncture points without the use of needles were developed and labeled with the acronym TENS (transcutaneous electric neurostimulation systems).

The stimulation of acupuncture points without needles was developed many centuries before the discovery of electricity. Utilization of acupuncture therapy principles was adapted throughout the ancient oriental world with the use of massage techniques. Practitioners developed the use of fingers, hands, and occasionally elbows and knees as substitutes for needles. The diverse methods of oriental massage are commonly referred to as acupressure techniques. The Japanese version of finger pressure therapy was popularized with the name Shiatsu. In recent times, Western systems of self-administered acupressure were developed to facilitate 'auto-acupressure'[10].

Low Reactive-Level Laser Therapy (LRLLT) was the twentieth and the twenty-first century technological development for exploiting the potential of bioregulating acupuncture strategies. It was enabled by the pioneering work of Nogier with ear acupuncture (auriculotherapy) through the identification of frequencies of tissue groups.

Following the lead of the World Health Organization, the US National Institutes of Health issued a 1997 consensus statement, which concluded that in a variety of medical and pain disorders 'acupuncture may be useful as an adjunct treatment or an acceptable alternative or be included in a comprehensive management program'[11]. Several excellent reviews of the subject are available.

Physiology

In his classic textbook, Jayasuriya[12] presents a concise summary of a plethora of theories that attempt to explain acupuncture effects. Among the highlights are neurological theories such as Melzack and Wall's Gate Control Theory[13] and Mann's Somatovisceral Theory[14]. A landmark humoral theory was that of endorphin release formulated by Pomeranz and Chiu[15].

Electroacupuncture may produce long-lasting pain relief, which demonstrates increased endorphin indices[16] and morphine cross-tolerance[17]. The pain relief is diminished and/or reversed by opiate antagonists[18] and serotonin antagonists[19] and substantially abolished by the creation of lesions in areas associated with the descending inhibitory pathways[20].

The ability of acupuncture lasers to affect internal organ function involves the pro-opiomelanocortin system in cutaneous neuroimmunomodulation[21]. This complex system in the skin has key roles in the coordination of neuroendocrine–immune interactions that maintain homeostasis and control stress-induced tissue damage. Skin has long been recognized as the classical target organ for adrenocorticotropic hormone (ACTH). The skin immune system is involved in reactions to noxious stimuli, such as solar radiation (ultraviolet light) and thermal, biological and chemical insults[21].

Laser-mediated analgesia has been investigated extensively in both human and animal models. Clinical responses include an impressive spectrum of biological and physiological responses that are obtained from multiple wavelength and energy outputs[22]. Laser irradiation has effects on neural activity[23], is able to initiate a lasting analgesic response[24], and some of the analgesic mechanisms are non-endorphin mediated[25,26].

Acupuncture-related treatment strategies need to be integrated into comprehensive treatment programs. In the current practice of American and European physicians who utilize acupuncture, it is ordinarily combined with the concomitant use of allopathic and/or homeopathic medications. Unrealistic expectations of permanent cure are often caused by successful outcomes with laser biostimulation (acupuncture).

Pain has been reported to be a leading cause of insomnia in medical illnesses, where more than 70% of the patients complain of sleep difficulties[27]. Patients can utilize pain-relieving auto-acupressure techniques, and use TENS units for modest relief. Acupuncturists can administer classic acupuncture treatments. Physicians can administer twenty-first century medical acupuncture techniques offering non-drug, non-surgical, non-physically invasive interventions utilizing optical energies to initiate internal biochemical cascades producing analgesic, regenerative and muscle-relaxing effects.

The clinical effects of pain relief are frequently very dramatic, but need to be viewed in the light that if the underlying disorder is chronic, it will usually cause difficulty again. Acute pain and spasm generally respond with more lasting relief, but relieving sciatica pain will not eliminate spinal stenosis. Relieving a migraine headache will not ensure a lifetime free of another migraine. Alleviating fibromyalgia pain and spasm will not abolish all further episodes. Relaxation responses with resolution of acute panic attacks will not confer a lifetime immunity from anxiety. Endorphin levels increased by acupuncture may eliminate the physical need for opiates, but addictions can persist even with methadone maintenance.

Clinical implications

For a quick and precise review of acupuncture concepts, techniques and clinical implications, we would refer the reader to Meng and co-workers[28].

Acupuncture techniques are unusually well-suited to reduce, control and/or resolve pain problems that interfere with restful sleep. Patients can utilize established techniques of auto-acupressure to treat painful conditions such as migraine[10] and back pain[29]. Patients can also employ TENS units for modest pain-relieving effects. Acupuncturists can employ classic acupuncture techniques utilizing needles enhanced with stimulation by the heat of burning herbs (moxibustion) and/or electric stimulation. Physicians can employ medical low-level laser therapy utilizing optical energy with pulsed frequencies to enhance the therapeutic effect of acupuncture techniques. Frequently treated pain problems that are significantly responsive to acupuncture techniques (and especially to laser biostimulation) include tension headaches, migraine headaches, muscle spasm, whiplash, tennis elbow, lumbago, sciatica, radiculopathies and local areas of arthritis and fibromyalgia.

Commonly employed low-level therapeutic lasers utilize infrared radiation with wavelengths of 904 nm. Energy pulses usually do not exceed 200 ns (0.2 millionth of a second). Individual Nogier frequencies are utilized, but commonly devices have three programs of grouped frequencies: analgesic, regenerating and muscle-relaxing. Analgesic frequencies are E (4672 Hz) and G (146 Hz). Regenerating frequencies are A (292 Hz), B (584 Hz) and F (73 Hz). Muscle-relaxing frequencies

are C (1168 Hz), D (2336 Hz) and G (146 Hz). Individual areas are usually stimulated in 40-s epochs. Lasers are not used for patients with a cardiac pacemaker. Analgesic and muscle-relaxing effects are usually obtained from the first session. Treatment sessions usually last from 15 to 30 min, depending on the number of body areas that require attention. The number of sessions required is often one for acute conditions and acute exacerbations of chronic conditions, but may be six or more for chronic disorders that present with persistent pain.

Many health care practitioners use acupuncture as an alternative therapy to pharmacological interventions mostly for localized pain relief and induction of sleep[28].

Evidence supporting acupuncture's utility as a treatment for insomnia has come from a variety of sources, including the non-Western scientific literature. Among these, investigations by Nan and Qingming[30], Jiarong[31], Cangliang[32] and Yi[33] nearly all showed positive results. The shortcoming of these studies, however, is that their dependent measures were usually inexact, relying mainly on subjective accounts of sleep experience or duration, and consequently, despite the consistency of their support for acupuncture, they are difficult to evaluate. Several European studies[34–36] used polysomnography to measure acupuncture effects on sleep disorders, but all failed to monitor nocturnal neurochemical changes, which would have strengthened their experimental design.

Spence and colleagues recently completed an open trial study to determine if acupuncture would affect nocturnal melatonin production and alleviate symptoms of insomnia and anxiety[34].

Eighteen adult subjects who complained of insomnia and who met test criteria for above-normal anxiety on the Zung Anxiety Scale were assessed in an open clinical trial design. The subjects had sub-syndromal depressive symptoms, i.e. did not meet formal criteria for a depressive disorder. Their response to 5 weeks of acupuncture treatment (two treatments per week, ten treatments in total) was evaluated on a before and after basis. This included their responses to psychometric measurement of depressive and anxious symptomatology, polysomnographic recordings of their sleep profile, and 24 h readings of urinary melatonin secretion. Acupuncture treatment was associated with significant improvements in depressive symptoms on the CES-D ($p = 0.001$). Both state and trait anxiety scores were significantly improved ($p = 0.049$ and $p = 0.004$). Changes in urinary melatonin levels were also found. Post-test analysis showed a significant increase ($p = 0.002$) of nocturnal urinary 6-sulfa-toxymelatonin (aMT6s) levels over baseline values, while daytime (morning and early afternoon) levels dropped to below baseline ($p = 0.037$), both changes representing a trend toward physiological normalization. Improvements were found in most polysomnographical parameters of sleep architecture and continuity. Sleep onset latency and the arousal index dropped significantly ($p = 0.003$ and $p = 0.001$, respectively). The total sleep time and sleep efficiency were similarly improved ($p = 0.001$ and $p = 0.002$, respectively). Some improvement in sleep quality was confirmed by the increase in the amount of time spent in stage 3 sleep ($p = 0.023$), but the amount of time spent in stages 1, 2 and 4 sleep did not significantly change in the before–after comparison. Additionally the percentage of rapid eye movement (REM) sleep and REM sleep latency did not change following acupuncture.

Objective findings of sleep improvement and the parallel reductions in depression and anxiety scores support the conclusion that acupuncture may represent an alternative to pharmaceutical therapy for some categories of patients with depressive and anxiety symptoms.

Medical hypnosis

Hypnosis is an altered state of vigilance with a unique combination of sleep-like absence of self-awareness and unusual physiological and behavioral flexibility. The word 'hypnosis' means 'sleep' in Greek.

There is substantial evidence appearing in the literature that supports the use of clinical hypnosis in a variety of medical settings[37]. This section presents a brief overview of these data as well as the range of clinical situations in which hypnosis has been shown to be effective in and beneficial to patients. Finally, there will be a discussion of the relationship between hypnosis and sleep and hypnotherapeutic methods for treating certain sleep disorders.

An overview of medical hypnosis

Hypnosis is probably one of the most researched modalities in psychoimmunology. There is an ever-increasing literature demonstrating that the nervous system is capable of modulating the immune response. Ruzyla-Smith and co-workers[38], for example, determined that there are significant increases in the number of lymphocyte cell types, B cells and T cells, in highly hypnotizable patients.

Hannigan has stated that 'a review of research in the area of hypnosis and the immune system indicates that, generally, hypnotic intervention can moderate immune system functioning... Trends indicate that hypnotizability is positively correlated with the degree of immune system changes'[39]. The puzzling placebo effect has hinted at mind/body healing systems, which defy convention medical drug models. It has been this effect that has stimulated research into the use of hypnosis to modulate the body's immune function. In her review, Hannigan cites research showing that even children who were taught self-hypnosis were capable of significantly increasing IgA (immunoglobulin) levels. Once again, these studies emphasized that significant changes occur only in highly hypnotizable people; hence high hypnotizability is positively correlated with immune system changes. Yet here, as above, even highly hypnotizable subjects under relaxation or control conditions showed no significant changes to their immune systems.

Freeman[37] has reviewed a wealth of literature demonstrating the utility of hypnosis, either as an adjunct or as primary intervention, for surgical and medical procedure outcomes, dermatological conditions, pain (especially acute and procedural pain), gastrointestinal disorders (especially irritable bowel syndrome (IBS)), control of nausea and vomiting in oncology treatment, post-surgery and in obstetrics and gynecology, asthma and obesity and smoking cessation.

Immunological dysregulation has been shown to be associated with acute stressors. This logically leads to the assumption that those who experience acute stress are more inclined to be susceptible to disease. Kiecolt-Glaser and co-workers'[40] experimental data provide encouraging evidence that hypnotic interventions may reduce the immunological dysregulation associated with acute stressors.

Bejenke[41] states that cancer patients, in general, are highly susceptible to suggestion.

Hypnosis has repeatedly been shown to be of great value in patients who experience acute and chronic pain[41,42]. Peter reported that the reduction of pain through hypnosis goes well beyond mere reduction of unpleasantness, and demonstrates significant attenuation of spinally mediated pain processes[42]. Similar to the medical uses of hypnosis mentioned above, successful hypnotic analgesia correlates with the ability of the patient to be hypnotized. When compared to control groups, hypnotized patients reported significantly less pain in one study of patients with metastasized breast cancer. In yet another study, hypnosis was more effective than behavioral interventions in experiencing less pain associated with bone marrow aspiration.

Peter refers to three techniques involved in hypnotic pain control[42]. Dissociative techniques attempt to separate or isolate the pain from the rest of the healthy body.

Associative techniques necessitate very good rapport with the therapist, and require that the patient pay attention to his or her radiating pain, which initially will have a reinforcing effect.

The third technique involves symbolic information processing. Here the total pain, or certain aspects of it, are transformed into symbolic or synesthetic representations (acoustic or visual hallucinations).

Large, in an earlier review[43], concluded that hypnosis is an effective therapy in the management of chronic pain. In a study involving children with leukemia and non-Hodgkin's lymphoma, Hawkins and co-workers found that hypnotic intervention resulted in a statistically significant reduction in pain and anxiety during lumbar spinal punctures[44].

Hypnosis has also been used successfully in the management of some chronic medical conditions. Here we see an alteration in physiological functioning ostensibly mediated through hypnotic techniques used on patients. Galovski and Blanchard[45] demonstrated significant improvement in symptomatology in a patient with both IBS and generalized anxiety disorder. After only six treatment sessions, the patient showed marked improvement, and continued with self-hypnosis beyond that point. Future follow-ups continued to demonstrate retained improvement in symptoms.

Crasilneck[46] developed his bombardment technique of hypnosis to treat patients with intractable organic pain, such as headache, backache and arthritic pain. Six diversified methods of hypnotic inductions are used consecutively within 1 h. These include: (1) relaxation; (2) displacement; (3) age regression; (4) glove anesthesia; (5) hypno-anesthesia; and (6) self-hypnosis[53]. One-year re-evaluations provided evidence of sustainability of effect, reported as 80–90% relief. Relaxation allows the patient to control muscle spasm, which can reduce the cycle of pain. Displacement involves transferring pain from one area of the body to another. Age regression allows the patient to return to a time prior to the onset of pain, and allows him or her to become aware of freedom from discomfort. Glove anesthesia may be transferred to other parts of the body, creating freedom from discomfort. Hypno-anesthesia is used to reduce anxiety, for sedation, to increase peace of mind and permit post-hypnotic suggestion. Self-hypnosis is a method that is essential in the long-term management of pain and discomfort[46,47].

Dissociative techniques, such as hand levitation, are used to treat pain from whiplash injury[47]. Trance states are concluded with self-hypnosis, followed by post-trance discussions of individuals' experiences.

Other medical aspects of hypnosis include improved wound healing and faster post-surgical recovery rates. Mauer and co-workers[48] found that hypnotic intervention in patients undergoing orthopedic hand surgery not only reduced pain and anxiety, but also resulted in significantly fewer medical complications and enhanced post-surgical recovery and rehabilitation. Brooks demonstrated in her study that clinical hypnosis could accelerate post-surgical wound healing. According to nursing assessments, the hypnotic intervention group exhibited significantly accelerated appearance of soft tissue wound resolution compared to the control group[49]. Greenleaf and Fisher[50] found that the recovery sequence following cardiac surgery was enhanced in patients who were hypnotized.

Physiological relationships between hypnosis and sleep

Evans' review[51] of the literature indicates that there are no basic similarities between hypnosis and sleep in terms of well documented EEG characteristics that typically define sleep. Hypnosis is characterized by waking EEG patterns; those of sleep are not. Evans has demonstrated that both hypnotizability and the control of sleep are related to the voluntary control of absorption, such as becoming engrossed in a book or movie, but not involuntary absorption, such as being emotionally overwhelmed by an event.

Further, Evans[51] concludes that the ability to achieve deep hypnosis and the ability to fall asleep easily share some common mechanism. This mechanism involves individual differences and the ability to maintain control over the level of functioning for the state of consciousness that seems appropriate to the person at the time. This control mechanism apparently involves the ability to change readily from one kind of psychological state or activity to another, or to maintain flexibility in changing psychological sets. The control system that allows a person to allow entry into hypnosis, and presumably other states, may be a very general ability possessed by some people and may manifest itself in any of a number of circumstances.

If it does appear that hypnotizable subjects have the ability to fall asleep easily and in a wide variety of circumstances, while this finding does not imply any basic similarity of sleep and hypnosis, it does indicate that there may be a common underlying mechanism involved in the capacity to experience hypnosis and the ability to fall asleep and easily maintain control of basic sleep processes.

There is hope that advances of new high-tech methodologies in EEG analysis and radiology will uncover brain mechanisms of hypnosis as a separate and distinct physiological state.

Hypnotherapy for sleep disorders

Hammond[52] indicates that the sleep patterns of a significant proportion of insomnia patients' are disturbed by: (1) cognitive over-activity and condition habit patterns incompatible with sleep; and (2) central nervous system excitation and underlying or unconscious conflicts or fears that disrupt sleep. These patients are likely to receive substantial benefit from hypnotherapeutic intervention.

Hammond goes on to say that hypnosis strategies may involve several elements: (1) self-hypnosis to facilitate deep muscle relaxation; and (2) the use of additional self-hypnosis methods to control cognitive over-activity. Hammond concludes that when the first two approaches are not successful within four or five sessions, a third approach involving unconscious exploration of underlying functions or conflicts associated with sleep disturbance should be considered.

Stanton[53] reported on three typical cases of hypnotherapy for insomnia (initial, middle and failure to daytime nap) in which he found success rates of 85%. The treatment model he describes includes two sessions with follow-up as needed. Stanton's model utilizes hypnosis in the following ways. (1) Visualization of a soft curtain which has a warm comfortable feel about it. As thoughts enter the patient's mind during the session they allow those thoughts to drift across the curtain and disappear out the other side of their mind. They are then able to return to a contemplation of the curtain. (2) Visualization of a scene in which subjects imagine themselves on the veranda or patio of a lovely house which has ten steps leading down to a beautiful garden below. For each step downward they allow themselves to let go more and more. At the bottom of the steps, peaceful and relaxed, they enter the garden, attention being drawn to the colors, flowers, drifting clouds, birds singing, leaves rustling and the pleasant warmth of the sun. The final phase (3) of this model is referred to as a 'special place'. After letting go of problems, subjects are able to remain in the garden, or, if they prefer, 'go away' to a special place where they are able to feel peaceful and content.

There are several reports of successful use of hypnotherapy for parasomnias, specifically for head and body rocking, bedwetting and somnambulism[54–56]. Evidently, hypnotherapy has significant therapeutic potential. This potential should be seriously explored as well as the physiology of the hypnotic state *per se*.

Herbal medicine

Herbal medicine is the most ancient form of health care known to humankind. Herbs have been used to treat all kinds of diseases in all cultures throughout history. The word 'drug' comes from the old Dutch word *drogge* meaning 'to dry'. Ancient healers or modern pharmacists dried plants for use as medicines. In fact, the World Health Organization notes that of 119 plant-derived pharmacotherapeutic medicines, about 74% are used in modern medicine in ways that correlate directly with their traditional uses as plant medicines by native cultures.

The word 'herb' as used in herbal medicine (also known as botanical medicine or phytotherapy) means a plant suitable to make medicine. A herb could be a leaf, a flower, a stem, a root, a seed, a fruit, bark or any other part. Only an estimated 5000 of 500 000 existing plants are believed to be studied for medical use. In general, herbal medicine works in much the same way as do conventional pharmaceutical drugs, i.e. via their chemical make-up. In the past 150 years, chemists and pharmacists have been isolating and purifying the 'active' compounds from plants to produce reliable drugs. Examples include such drugs as digoxin (from foxglove (*Digitalis purpurea*)), reserpine (from Indian snakeroot (*Rauwolfia serpentina*)), morphine (from the opium poppy (*Papaver somniferum*)), etc.

The qualities of herbs that make them beneficial in treating the human body (in relation to sleep medicine) include the following:

(1) Adaptogenic: These herbs are believed to increase resistance and resilience to stress, enabling the body to adapt to the condition or situation and avoid collapse. Adaptogens work by supporting the adrenal glands. An example would be Siberian ginseng.

(2) Alternative: Herbs that gradually restore proper functioning of the body, increasing health and vitality (e.g. *Echinacea*).

(3) Anti-inflammatory: Herbs that soothe inflammation and reduce inflammatory responses of the tissue.

(4) Antispasmodic: Herbs that ease cramps in smooth and skeletal muscles, alleviate muscle tension and decrease psychological tension.

(5) Hypotensive: Herbs that lower blood pressure.

(6) Nerve relaxants: Herbs that ease anxiety, produce tranquil mood and induce sleep.

(7) Tonic and stimulating herbs.

There are many reviews, and detailed references are available[57,58].

A list of most commonly used herbal products for sleep, alertness, mood and performance

Caffeine Caffeine, probably the most consumed stimulant in the world today, is used by 80% of people in the United States. Many adults ingest enough caffeine to cause some type of clinical symptom, for example restlessness, nervousness, excitement, diverse agitation, insomnia, etc. 'Caffeinism' is a term used to describe the clinical syndrome produced by acute or chronic overuse of caffeine. The risk in developing serious side-effects from caffeine becomes high when intake exceeds 500 mg per day. In terms of cups of coffee, how much is too much?

The average cup of coffee contains 85–100 mg of caffeine, while teas can contain 60–110 mg of caffeine. Caffeine is contained in many other items like soft drinks, prescription drugs and chocolate. As little as 85–250 mg of caffeine or 1–3 cups of coffee can alter one's motor skills or stimulatory reaction.

Taken 3–4 h before sleep, it will shorten sleep time, increase sleep latency and make sleep poorer. Its effects are correlated with the amount of caffeine consumed.

Sleep laboratory testing results revealed that caffeine increases sleep and MSLT latency (preventing sleep), increases the ability to stay awake and improves subjective alertness. In contrast, in narcolepsy patients 2–8 cups of coffee decrease the ability to stay awake.

Caffeine ingestion varies, depending on culture and nation, from 80 to 400 mg per person per day. In the United States, the average intake is 200–240 mg per day.

Caffeine is a drug without any governmental regulation. Interestingly, some caffeine formulations can be obtained only by prescription.

Caffeine can cause dependence and withdrawal or even addiction. Caffeine may interfere with sleep in non-tolerant individuals. Once tolerance has developed, people are much less likely to self-report abnormalities or they may sense insomnia has disappeared.

Nonetheless, it is prudent to avoid caffeine at least 3–6 h (or more) before bedtime.

Cayenne (Capsicum annuum) Cayenne or red pepper is the most useful of the systemic stimulants. It stimulates blood flow and strengthens the heartbeat and metabolic rate. A general tonic, it is helpful specifically for the circulatory and digestive systems. In some sports it is used to increase prefight alertness. The effect on sleep is unknown.

Chamomile (Matricaria recutita) Chamomile flower is used in many cultures for its pleasant tasting tea and is consumed as an after-dinner beverage to help digestion. Chamomile is noted as a mild sedative, for insomnia and for its anti-inflammatory property, especially in over-the-counter preparations for oral hygiene and skin creams. Chamomile is accepted as an over-the-counter drug for internal use against gastrointestinal spasms; externally, it is used as an external bath for relaxation.

Chasteberry (Vitex agnus-castus) Chasteberry is becoming widely used as a herb that addresses various hormonal imbalances in women. The clinical results are thought to be due to some regulatory effect on the pituitary gland. Chasteberry is believed to help restore a normal estrogen-to-progesterone balance. It is indicated for irregular or painful menstruation, premenstrual syndrome and other disorders related to hormone function, such as hot flashes during menopausal changes especially at night[57].

Echinacea (Echinacea angustifolia) Often called purple coneflower, the genus *Echinacea* contains several species of plants that are generally found in the Great Plains region of North America. It was the most widely used medicinal plant of the Native Americans of this area. Native Americans often exploited echinacea for its external wound-healing and anti-inflammatory properties. Echinacea seeds were introduced into Europe by Dr Gerhard Madaus, who initiated the first modern scientific research on the immunostimulating properties of this plant. Echinacea has become one of the most important over-the-counter remedies and it is employed as a mild central nervous system (CNS) stimulant.

Ephedra or ma-huang (Ephedrasineca) Ephedra is a medicinal plant that has been cultivated for over 5000 years in China, where it was used for asthma and hay fever-like conditions. Also known as ma-huang, the stems contain two primary alkaloids, ephedrine and pseudoephedrine, which are now approved for use in over-the-counter decongestant and bronchial drugs. Ephedrine has a marked peripheral vasoconstricting (causing constriction of the blood vessels) action. Pseudoephedrine is a bronchodilator, approved for use in asthma and certain allergy medicines. Ma-huang and its extracts are found in a number of herbal formulas that are designed to increase energy and reduce appetite. Both ephedrine and pseudoephedrine have CNS-stimulating properties, ephedrine being more active. The CNS activity of these alkaloids has been characterized as being stronger than caffeine and weaker than methamphetamine. This herb should be used with caution or avoided by those with high blood pressure, diabetes, glaucoma and related conditions where hypertensives are contraindicated. Several deaths have been reported by overdose of ephedra products.

Feverfew (Tanacetum parthenium) Feverfew is a herbal remedy that dates back to Greco-Roman times. It was formerly employed as a remedy for difficulties associated with young women's menstrual cycles (the word parthenium is derived from the Greek word *parthenos*, meaning 'virgin') and was later used in European herbalism to reduce fevers (the common name feverfew being a corruption of the Latin word *febrifuga*, an agent that lowers fevers). Interest in this herb has been generated because feverfew leaves have been found to bring relief in a significant number of migraine patients who have not responded

positively to conventional medications; it also helps to prevent the onset of additional episodes. Recently, the Canadian government's Health Protection Branch (equivalent to the United States' FDA) has approved feverfew leaf extract for migraine prevention, as long as the products contain a minimum of 0.2% parthenolide. Effect on sleep is unknown.

Ginger (Zingiber officinalis) In addition to its very popular food flavoring qualities, ginger is widely used as a medicinal herb in Chinese and Ayurvedic medicine as a nervous system stimulant and is often added to herbal formulas to increase digestion and the activity of other herbs. Ginger has become best known for its anti-nausea and anti-motion sickness activity. Unlike the leading over-the-counter drug, Dramamine®, ginger does not relieve nausea by suppressing CNS activity. Rather, the effect is explained by the anti-emetic (preventing or relieving nausea and vomiting) effects of this herb, which are well documented, although more research is needed. Ginger is also known to have cardiotonic properties. The herb has been used in traditional medicine for migraine relief, and fresh ginger juice has been used for increasing physical performance.

Ginkgo (Ginkgo biloba) Ginkgoes are the oldest living trees on earth. They first appeared about 200 million years ago and, except for a small population in northern China, were almost completely destroyed in the last Ice Age. Ginkgo leaves contain several compounds called ginkgolides that have unique chemical structures. The leaves were mentioned in a major Chinese herbal text of the Ming dynasty in 1436. A standardized extract is used to treat a number of conditions associated with peripheral circulation, and for the treatment of cerebral dysfunction, with: difficulty in memory, dizziness, tinnitus, headaches and emotional instability coupled with anxiety. Ginkgo leaf extracts are also used for heart diseases, and accidents involving brain trauma. Volumes of technical papers on the chemistry, pharmacology and clinical studies of *Ginkgo biloba* extract have been published. Recent studies, however, did not find any measurable benefits for memory or related cognitive functions to healthy elderly people.

Ginseng (Panax ginseng, Oriental ginseng; Panax quinquefolius, American ginseng) Ginseng has an ancient history and as such has accumulated much folklore about its actions and uses. The genus *Panax* is derived from the Latin word *panacea* meaning 'cure all'. Many of the claims that surround ginseng are exaggerated, but it is clearly an important remedy, receiving attention from researchers around the world. It is a powerful adaptogen, aiding the body to cope with stress, primarily through effects upon the functioning of the adrenal gland. Ginseng has antioxidant, antihepatotoxic (liver-protecting) and hypoglycemic effects. Thus, there is a wide range of possible therapeutic uses. The main application is with weak, debilitated, stressed or elderly people, where these properties can be especially useful. In addition, ginseng may lower blood cholesterol and stimulate a range of immune system and endocrine responses. If ginseng is abused, however, serious side-effects can occur, including headaches, skin problems and other reactions. For this reason, the proper dosage for the individual should be determined.

Ginseng creates particular problems for consumers, because all forms of the herb are not equal. Different forms of ginseng have been found to have different active ingredients and chemical properties. Asian ginseng (*Panax ginseng*), which produces the strongest stimulation, probably holds the public's most common understanding of the uses for ginseng as an energy enhancer. American ginseng (*Panax quinquefolius*) is more useful for soothing and Siberian ginseng (*Eleutherococcus senticosus*), which is technically not ginseng, is used as a stamina booster.

Korea produces red ginseng, a processed form of ginseng stronger than the white, unprocessed form exported from China. Both of these forms stimulate and are reported to speed up metabolism and circulation to help boost energy. These benefits are believed to stem from ginseng's saponins (chemicals similar to human hormones), as well as the herb's traces of essential oils, vitamins, minerals and amino acids along with a smattering of carbohydrates and antioxidants. Research on efficacy is mixed, but this form has been found to be the most potent for energy enhancement.

Similar to the other ginseng varieties, American ginseng (*Panax quinquefolius*) has been found to increase mental acuity and fertility. American ginseng is also used to relieve fevers and night sweats and its reputation for lubricating and increasing fluids, while strengthening the body, influences the choice for alleviation or soothing dry lung problems like smoker's cough. Siberian ginseng, named for its native habitat in Siberia, prefers a cool climate. This type of ginseng produces similar physiological effects to true ginseng products and thus is sold to consumers under the name 'ginseng'. During the 1960s, Soviet scientists[59] studied Siberian ginseng's effects on factory workers and athletes. Athletes were found to run faster, factory workers worked quicker and everyone recovered rapidly after exertion and dealt with stress more easily. Siberian ginseng is considered ideal for increasing stamina and life endurance. Thus, while the Asian form may increase energy more substantially, Siberian forms produce more benefits to stress and fatigue.

Goldenseal (Hydrastis canadensis) One of the most widely used American herbs, goldenseal is considered to be a tonic remedy that stimulates the immune response and is directly antimicrobial itself. In addition, because of its bitter effects it can help in many digestive problems, from peptic ulcers to colitis. Its bitter stimulation helps in loss of appetite, and the alkaloids it contains stimulate production and secretion of digestive juices. The antimicrobial properties are due to alkaloids, such as berberine.

Hawthorn (Crataegus oxyacantha) Europeans have employed both the edible fruit as well as the leaves and flowers, primarily for their beneficial effects on the cardiovascular system. Hawthorn is one of the primary heart tonics in traditional medicine. Fruit and leaf extracts are known for their cardiotonic, sedative and hypotensive activities. In Germany, hawthorn extracts are used clinically for a number of heart-related conditions, often in conjunction with digoxin, the primary conventional pharmaceutical drug. Hawthorn has been extensively tested on animals and humans and is known to decrease blood pressure with exertion; increase contractility (ability to contract or shorten) of the heart muscle; increase blood flow to the coronary muscle; decrease heart rate, and decrease oxygen use of the myocardium. Hawthorn extracts are used in Europe for declining heart performance, sensations of pressure or restrictions in the heart area, senile heart in cases where digitalis is not yet required and mild forms of bradyarrhythmia[60].

Hops (Humulus lupulus)   Hops are a mild CNS tranquilizer. Hops are used for anxiety as well as sleep disorders, due to their calming and sleep-inducing properties, and for emotional tension, excitability and restlessness, due to their calming effect on vagal control of the heart.

Kava   Kava is a mild sedative and widely used, including as a ceremonial beverage in the South Pacific to achieve a higher level of consciousness during meditation. It has anesthetic effects and produces mild euphoria, but is mostly used as an anxiolytic. It is a strong L-type calcium channel inhibitor and weak sodium channel blocker. Kava increases also outward potassium current with hyperpolarization and may increase γ-aminobutyric acid (GABA) transmissions. This mechanism is similar to traditional antiepileptic medications that are used as mild tranquilizers and mood stabilizers. If a patient is not responding well to anticonvulsants, he/she is not likely to be helped by kava. Adverse effects include hepatotoxicity, sedation, ataxia, hypertension, lymphopenia, thrombocytopenia and hematuria.

Nettle (Urtica dioica)   Throughout Europe, nettle, a mild stimulant, is used as a spring tonic and detoxifying remedy. If used regularly over the long term it can be helpful in cases of rheumatism and arthritis. A lectin (plant protein) found in a nettle's leaf stimulates the proliferation of human lymphocytes. It is traditionally used in the treatment of allergic rhinitis (hayfever) and before sleep to improve nasal breathing and decrease snoring.

Passion flower (Passiflora incarnata)   Passion flower, a mild CNS tranquilizer, is taken for its mildly sedative properties. Passion flower is often added to other calming herbs, usually valerian and hawthorn, for anxiety and restlessness. Passion flower and hawthorn are often used together as antispasmodics for digestive spasms in cases of gastritis and colitis.

Peppermint (Mentha piperita)   Peppermint has been a popular folk remedy for digestive disorders and is currently one of the most economically significant aromatic food/medicine crops produced in the United States. In Europe, peppermint leaf is recognized as a digestive aid due to the carminative (gas-preventing) and cholagog (bile increasing) action of the aromatic oil. It could be used for pain- or itching-related insomnia.

St. John's Wort (Hypericum perforatum)   A remedy long used for its mild sedative and pain-reducing properties, St. John's Wort has recently regained medical attention. Taken internally, it has traditionally been used to treat neuralgia, anxiety, tension and similar problems. In addition to neuralgic pain, it is believed to ease fibrositis, sciatica and rheumatic pain. It is especially regarded as a herb to use in the case of menopausal changes triggering irritability and anxiety. It was recommended in the treatment of depression, but the recent research does not support these claims. Its components, hyperforin and hyperacid, inhibit synaptosomal serotonin, adrenaline and dopamine intake. In high dosages and in association with valerian extract it might induce insomnia and acute mania.

Saw palmetto (Serenoa repens)   Saw palmetto, a stimulant, is a herb that acts to tone and strengthen the male reproductive system. It is used for a boost to the male sex hormones and to boost physical performance. It can help in cases of prostatitis (inflamed prostate gland) if combined with echinacea and bearberry.

Senna (Cassia angustifolia)   Senna is a mild CNS stimulant. It is a laxative from the leaves and pods of the senna plant, a member of the pea family, that is derived from ancient Arabic medicine. In Europe and in the United States, extracts from senna are approved in over-the-counter stimulant laxative products. Long-term use or misuse can result in dependency and electrolyte loss. Like other stimulant laxatives, senna should not be used during pregnancy or lactation unless professionally supervised. Its effect on sleep is unknown.

Valerian (Valeriana officinalis)   Valerian root, its teas and extracts are used as over-the-counter medicines for anxiety, insomnia, nervousness and depression. Sedative properties of valerian are due to hydroxypinoresinol that binds at the γ-aminobutyric acid (GABA)–benzodiazepine receptor complex. James and Mendelson in their excellent review[61] concluded that extract of valerian improves slow-wave sleep and decreases wake time after sleep onset, thus improving sleep perception. There were no changes on polysomnography and no REM improvements. Concerns about valerian are related to its potentiation of barbiturates and benzodiazepines, increasing of vivid dreams, mutagenic effect *in vitro* and post-withdrawal cardiac symptoms.

*Some herbal sleep products lack
the key claimed ingredient*

As an example, ConsumerLab.com, an independent evaluator of dietary supplements and nutrition products, recently released the results of its Product Review of valerian supplements used primarily as sleep aids and minor tranquilizers. Sales of valerian more than doubled over the past year, making it the fastest growing herbal product in the United States according to the research firm Information Resources, Inc.

ConsumerLab.com purchased 17 products claiming to contain *Valeriana officinalis* root, the species for which most supporting clinical evidence exists, and tested them for key compounds to evaluate the identity and quantity of the herb present. Only nine of the 17 valerian products passed ConsumerLab.com's testing. Four products completely lacked the marker compounds that identify the presence of *Valeriana officinalis* and four others had roughly half of the expected levels. Results were confirmed in a second independent laboratory.

Of additional concern is the possibility that products which totally lacked the expected marker compounds were made from an inappropriate species of valerian – particularly since these products had the characteristic smell of valerian root. Products made from some species other than *Valeriana officinalis* can be rich in a compound called didrovaltrate, which laboratory testing shows to be toxic to cells.

Similar information is available online from ConsumerLab.com for Asian and American ginseng, calcium, chondroitin, CoQ10, creatine, echinacea, ginkgo biloba, glucosamine, multivitamins/multiminerals, saw palmetto, St. John's Wort and vitamins C and E.

Abuse of illegal narcotics of herbal origin is a separate topic. In the context of this chapter it is appropriate to mention marijuana, which is up to now widely used recreationally, for pain and mood elevation. Its legality is still in debate. Prenatal exposure to marijuana is tied to later hearing problems. Children prenatally exposed to marijuana are two times more likely than unexposed children to fail a standard hearing test.

Over-the-counter sleep aids

Over-the-counter sleep aids comprise mostly antihistamines (H_1 receptor antagonists), and left serotonergic, cholinergic and central L-adrenergic antagonists[58,61]. The original H_1 blockers (chlorpheniramine and diphenhydramine) cross the blood–brain barrier causing daytime sedation. Second-generation agents (loratadine and fexofenadine) penetrate the blood barrier much less and induce less daytime sedation.

The nighttime hypnotic effects from antihistamines were greater in patients who were not treated previously. Daytime sedation from the first generation of antihistamines continued to be somewhat less after a long treatment time, although still significant. It is important to note that daytime sedation decreases performance without the patient's knowledge. For example, a study using position emission tomography showed that D-chlorpheniramine reduces effectiveness in attention-demanding tasks even though subjects deny any changes in alertness[61].

In addition to daytime sedation, several other side-effects are important to mention, such as effects on respiration in young children and the elderly, interfering with the swallowing reflex, potential increase of sleep apneas, cardiotoxicity and anticholinergic confusional states. Another problem might arise from drug interaction. Antihistamines, such as diphenhydramine, as a cytochrome P45 2D6 inhibitor, could alter the half-life of some medications like metoprolol.

Yoga and sleep

For those devoted to the practice of Hatha yoga, sleep is not just a state of unconsciousness – good sleep should be trained just like any waking experience. The following are several recommended yoga techniques for sleep[62–67].

Going to sleep – relaxation

As the person lies in bed, he gently slows down the rate of exhalation until he exhales for twice as long as he inhales. Focus is on the smoothness and evenness of breath, gradually eliminating any jerks and pauses.

Falling asleep – position techniques

Lying on the back can be a good way to start the night if it does not cause problems. The first reason, according to yoga instructors, is linked to the digestive system. Lying on the back will avoid compressing the stomach and allow free movement of food during digestion. The second reason is linked to awareness. The classical yoga 'corpse' position is one in which awareness is maximized. Stresses on the body are reduced, and one finds it easier to breathe, and to relax deeply.

Time of sleeping

Another yoga recommendation is to go to bed before 10 p.m. The reasoning is that between the hours of 6 and 10 p.m., the energy of the body will be more 'earthy, heavy, slow and quiet', so it is the easiest and best time to go to sleep. Being awake after midnight can arouse hunger.

Advanced yogis claim that they can go directly to the state of deep sleep and stay there, thus avoiding other parts of the sleep cycle, including the dream stages[62,63].

There are reports that yoga confers measurable improvements in mental and physical health[62–65].

There is considerable anecdotal evidence regarding the utility and power of yoga, recognizing that for over 5000 years it has been shown to be beneficial as a potential therapeutic tool for better health and sense of well-being. Today in the United States, the practice boasts about 20 million followers, which more than triples the 6 million enthusiasts in 1994[64].

Clinical observations of psychosomatic patients indicate that their distorted somatopsychic functioning necessitates their practice of yoga-like therapy[65]. There is also cause to believe that there are beneficial effects of regular practice of yoga on subjective well-being and quality of life[66].

In traditional yoga, the whole theory is to bring the parasympathetic nervous system into dominance. Yoga relaxes and, by relaxing, heals[67].

CONCLUSION

The popularity of alternative medicine treatments is exponentially growing. It is important to emphasize that people who use alternative therapies are well-informed, more highly educated, and have a tendency for self-treatment similar to the popularity for the patient-initiated diagnostic scanning procedures. There is no question that many alternative sleep aids could be useful, but the danger is that many such agents are not fully benign, and might have side-effects or interactions with other medications or therapies. Another danger is that users of alternative therapies might reject or neglect scientific treatment. For these reasons it is important to investigate thoroughly each therapy or product and educate ourselves and our patients.

References

1. Chlan L. Effectiveness of a music therapy intervention on relaxation and anxiety for patients receiving ventilatory assistance. *Heart Lung* 1998;27:169–76

2. Chlan L. Music therapy as a nursing intervention for patients supported by mechanical ventilation. *AACN Clin Issues* 2000;11:128–38

3. Bonnet MH, Arand DL. The impact of music upon sleep tendency as measured by the multiple sleep latency test and maintenance of wakefulness test. *Physiol Behav* 2000;71:485–92

4. Mornhinweg GC, Voignier RR. Music for sleep disturbance in the elderly. *J Holistic Nurs* 1995;13:248–54

5. Williamson 1991 (cited in reference 6)

6. Kayumov L, Soare K, Serbine O, *et al*. Brain music therapy for treatment of insomnia and anxiety. APSS 16th Annual Meeting, Seattle, WA, June 8–13, 2002. *Sleep* 2002;25:241

7. Kayumov L, Hawa R, Lowe A, *et al*. Increases in evening-and-night-time melatonin levels following brain music therapy for anxiety-associated insomnia. APSS 17th Annual Meeting, Chicago, IL, June 3–8, 2003. *Sleep* 2003;26:99

8. Shapiro CM, Strygin A, Levin Y, *et al*. The effects of patterned neurofeedback on sleep continuity. APSS 17th Annual Meeting, Chicago, IL, June 3–8, 2003. *Sleep* 2003;26:397

9. Hoizey D, Hoizey MJ. *A History of Chinese Medicine*. Edinburgh: Edinburgh University Press, 1988

10. Kurland H. *Quick Headache Relief Without Drugs*. New York: William Morrow, 1977:291

11. US National Institutes of Health Consensus Statement on Acupuncture. 1997;15:1–34

12. Jayasuriya A. *Clinical Acupuncture*. Kalubowila, Sri Lanka: Chandrakanthi Press, 1967

13. Melzack R, Wall P. Pain mechanisms: a new theory. *Science* 1965;150:971–9

14. Mann F. *Acupuncture: The Ancient Chinese Art of Healing*. London: William Heinemann Medical Books, 1960:248

15. Pomeranz B, Chiu D. Naloxone blockade of acupuncture analgesia: endorphin implicated. *Life Sci* 1976;19:157–62

16. Toda K. Neurophysiological basis of acupuncture analgesia. *J Tokyo Dental Assoc* 1983;31:7–16

17. Han JS, Zhang YZ, Zhou ZF. Potentiation of acupuncture analgesia by d-phenylalanine in the rabbit. *Acta Zool* 1981;27:133–7

18. Pomeranz BH, Cheng R. Supression of noxious responses in single neurons of ca spinal cord by electroacupuncture and its reversal by the opiate antagonist naloxone. *Exp Neurol* 1979;64:327–41

19. Jin GZ, Zhang ZD, Yu L, *et al*. Role of serotonergic and catecholaminergic systems in acupuncture analgesia. In Xiangtong Z, ed. *Research on Acupuncture, Moxibustion and Acupuncture Anagesia*. Beijing: Science Press, 1986:316–31

20. Takeshiga C, Sato T, Mera T, *et al*. Descending pain inhibitory system involved in acupuncture analgesia. *Brain Res* 1992;28:379–91

21. Luger TA, Paus R, Lipton JM, Slominski. Cutaneous neuroimmunomodulation: the proopiomelanocortin system. *Ann NY Acad Sci* 1999;885

22. Karu T. Photobiology of low-power laser effects. *Health Physics* 1989;56:691–704

23. Fork RL. Laser stimulation of nerve cells in aplysia. *Science* 1971;171:907–8

24. Ponnudural RN. Laser photobiostimulation-induced hypoalgesia in rats is not naloxone reversible. Acupuncture electro-therapeutics *Res Int J* 1987;12:93–100

25. Walker JB, Katz RL. Non-opioid pathways suppress pain in humans. *Pain* 1981;11:347–54

26. Rusakov DA. The effect of spinal cord irradiation by low-intensity laser on the characteristics of synaptic transmission in the dorsal horn. *Neurofiziologiia* 1987;5:545–8

27. Kryger M, Shapiro CM. Pain and distress at night. *Sleep Sol* 1992;5:1–20

28. Meng FQ, Luo HC, Halbreich U. Concepts, techniques, and clinical applications of acupuncture. *Psychiatr Ann* 2002;32:45–9

29. Kurland HD. *Back Pains: Quick Relief Without Drugs*. New York: Simon and Schuster, 1981

30. Nan L, Qingming Y. Insomnia treated by auricular pressing therapy. *J Trad Chin Med* 1990;10:174–5

31. Jiarong L. Ten cases of somnambulism treated with combined acupuncture and medicinal herbs. *J Trad Chin Med* 1989;9:174–5

32. Cangliang Y. Clinical observation of 62 cases of insomnia treated by auricular point imbedding therapy. *J Trad Chin Med* 1988;83:190–2

33. Yi R. Eighty-six cases of insomnia treated by double point needling – Daling through to Waiguan. *J Trad Chin Med* 1985;5:32

34. Spence DW, Kayumov L, Chen A, *et al*. Acupuncture increases nocturnal melatonin secretion and reduces insomnia and anxiety: a preliminary report. *J Neuropsychiatr Clin Neurosci* 2004;in press

35. Montakab H, Langel G. The effect of acupuncture in the treatment of insomnia. Clinical study of subjective and objective evaluation. *Schweizerische Medizinische Wochenschrift – Supplementum*. 1994;62:49–54

36. Dallakian IG, Vein AM, Kochetkov VD, *et al*. Relation between clinico-physiologic indices of sleep and the nature of stress and reflexotherapy application. [Russian] *Zhurnal Nevropatologii i Psikhiatrii Imeni S-S – Korsakova* 1985;85:534–9

37. Freeman LW. *Complementary and Alternative Medicine: An Evidence Based Approach*. Aspen, CA: Aspen Publishing, 2002

38. Ruzyla-Smith P, Barabasz A, Barasz M, Warner D. Effects of hypnosis on the immune system: B-cells. T-cells, helper cells and suppressor cells. *Am J Clin Hypnos* 1995;38:71–9

39. Hannigan K. Hypnosis and immune system functioning. *Hypnosis* 2001;28:76–81

40. Kiecolt-Glaser JK, Marucha PT, Atkinson C, Glaser R. Hypnosis as a modulator of cellular immune dysregulation during acute stress. *J Consult Clin Psychol* 2001;69:674–82

41. Bejenke CJ. Benefits of early interventions with cancer patients: a clinician's 15-year observations. *Hypnosis* 2000;27:75–81

42. Peter B. Hypnosis in the treatment of cancer pain. *Hypnosis* 1996;23:99–108

43. Large RG. Hypnosis for chronic pain: a critical review. *Hypnosis* 1994;21:234–7

44. Hawkins PJ, Liossi C, Ewart BW, *et al*. Hypnosis in the alleviation of procedure related pain and distress in pediatric oncology patients. *Contemp Hypnos* 1998;15:199–207

45. Galovski TE, Blanchard EB. Hypnotherapy and refractory irritable bowel syndrome: a single case study. *Am J Clin Hypnos* 2002;45:31–7

46. Crasilneck HB. The use of the Crasilneck Bombardment Technique in problems of intractable organic pain. *Hypnos* 1996;23:19–29

47. Finer B. Whiplash injury and hypnotherapy. *Hypnos* 1995;2:32–8

48. Mauer MH, Burnett KF, Ouellette E, *et al*. Medical hypnosis and orthopedic hand surgery: pain perception, postoperative recovery, and therapeutic comfort. *Int J Clin Exp Hypnos* 1999;47:144–61

49. Brooks P. The use of clinical hypnosis to accelerate the appearance of soft tissue wound resolution and patient recovery in post-surgical patients. *Dis Abstr Int* 2002;62:3412

50. Greenleaf M, Fisher S. Hypnotizability and recovery from cardiac surgery. *Am J Clin Hypnos* 1992;35:119–28

51. Evans FJ. Hypnosis and sleep: the control of altered states of awareness. *Sleep Hypnos* 1999;4:232–7

52. Hammond DC. *Handbook of Hypnotic Suggestions and Metaphors*. New York: W.W. Norton & Co, 1990:220–1

53. Stanton HE. Hypnotic relaxation and insomnia: a simple solution? *Sleep Hypnos* 1999;1:64–7

54. Rosenberg C. Elimination of a rhythmic movement disorder with hypnosis: a case report. *Sleep* 1995;18:608–9

55. Koe GG. Hypnotic treatment of sleep terror disorder: a case report. *Am J Clin Hypnosis* 1989;32:36–40

56. Kohen DP, Mahowald MW, Rosen GM. Sleep terror disorder in children: the role of self-hypnosis in management. *Am J Clin Hypnosis* 1992;34:233–44

57. Akerele D. Summary of WHO guidelines for the assessment of herbal medicines. *HerbalGram* 1992:28:13–16 (available as Classic Botanical Reprint 234)

58. Strohecker J, Trivieri L, Lewis D, *et al*., eds. *Alternative Medicine: The Definitive Guide 1995*. Fife, WA: Fortune Medicine Publishing, 1995:838–48

59. Brekhman II, Dardymov IV. Pharmacological investigation of glycosides from ginseng and eleutherococcus. *Lloydia* 1969;32:46–51

60. Hobbs C. Hawthorn: a literature review. *HerbalGram* 1990;21:19–33

61. James SP, Mendelson WB. Herbal and OTC sleep remedies. *Psychiatric Times* November 2003:72–5

62. Sherman D. *Yoga and Sleep. Sleep and Health.* Chicago: Des Plaines Publishing, 2003;3:6–7

63. Sherrill DL, Kotchou K. Association of physical activity and human sleep disorders. *Arch Intern Med* 1998;158:1894–8

64. Feuerstein, Lamb T. Yoga Research and Education Center, International Association of Yoga Therapists, California, 2002, January

65. Goyeche JR. Yoga as therapy in psychosomatic medicine. *Psychother Psychosom* 1979;31:373–81

66. Malathi A, Damodaran A, Shah N, *et al.* Effect of yogic practices on subjective wellbeing. *Ind J Physiol Pharmacol* 2000;44:202–6

67. Bera TK, Gore MM, Oak, JP. Recovery from stress in two different postures and in Shavasana – a Yogic relaxation posture. *Ind J Physiol Pharmacol* 1998;42:473–8

Conclusion

When I thought I had all the answers,
They changed all the questions.

Lev Landau, PhD (physicist)

It was not that long ago that research on sleep was considered a scientific desert, a field that many felt did not deserve the investment of money or time. In a relatively short period of time, researchers have discovered that sleep is a dynamic world of amazing complexity, controlled by elaborate and precise mechanisms with intimate effects on our maturation. Scientists are becoming more aware of the restorative process that sleep has for our body's 'hardware', and the ways in which sleep aids in programming and reprogramming the 'software' of our body functions and mental activity. The ultimate conclusion of this awareness is that we are born in, and grow from (out of), sleep. Truly, the past 50 years have been tremendous in the paradigm shift of the importance of sleep.

Evolutionary, ontogenetic and physiological investigations have demonstrated that mechanisms of sleep develop first in the organism, preparing and enforcing the development of wakefulness. The normal development of physiological mechanisms of sleep serve as a 'foundation' for the development of normal alertness, wakefulness, attention, learning and otherwise productive mental and physical performance. There is much evidence confirming the supportive and enhancing role that different stages of sleep play in consciousness, memory, emotions, decision-making and creative thinking. These changes have made sleep research an area of paramount importance.

If the normal development of sleep cycles and sleep–wake circadian rhythms ensure normal psychomotor maturation, deviation in the development of sleep mechanisms in early ontogenesis may lead to deviation in alertness, as well as attention, activity levels, learning, emotion and behavior later in life. Thus, the advent of sleep research has brought about fundamental changes in our perceptions of stages of alertness.

Sleep, once thought to be a state of rest, peace and healing, has been discovered to have a darker side as well: approximately 82 disorders related to sleep are now known and more are yet to be discovered. We have learned that some sleep disorders are life-threatening and may trigger sickness or even death. We have learned about the existence of dangerous behavior patterns in sleep that can be destructive to oneself or to others. The emergence of these findings related to disordered sleep has evoked an urgent need to develop the practice of sleep medicine within all disciplines of medicine. This book began with the concept of bridging the gap between the fields of psychiatry and sleep medicine. Each field has a dynamic nosology that has been closely refined with the advent of new technologies for the assessment, classification and treatment of disorders within their respective purview. However, the bulk of the data available to readers in secondary sources has been correlational, without a firm emphasis toward the practicing clinician. Our hope was not to redefine either field, but rather to provide readers with a broad understanding of the impact that each field has on the other.

The psychiatric impact of disordered sleep is large enough to warrant attention as a separate field. We have learned also that disordered sleep could be an essential component and/or underlying part of the pathophysiology of major psychiatric problems such as depression, schizophrenia, obsessive–compulsive disorders, anxiety and certain personality deviations. There are data to show that some of our habits may be 'born' from parasomnias which have served as tools for self-soothing or self-stimulation, and no data that show psychiatric problems in which sleep deviations are considered to be a factor. Indeed, one might be so bold as to say that there are sleep disorders without psychiatry, but there is no psychiatry without sleep disorders.

The more we learn about the inter-relationships between sleep and mental functions, the more questions arise. Should we expect to find concrete physiological markers for each mental disorder? Probably not. History is rich with this type of 'stereo-tactic' failure. However, certain pathogno-monic patterns probably do exist for several disorders and should continue to be sought by science.

What about the other spectra of human activity, namely creative, religious, healing, altered states from sleep like nirvana, relaxation, meditation, hypnosis and more, on up to ecstatic states of vigilance? Some are related to physical performance. During these, yet 'untouchable' by the strict science states of human vigilance, at some point, sleep and alertness become mixed and produce the highest performance or the worst disease.

Our list of contributing authors is both multidisciplinary and multinational.

Our hope was to provide a broad continuum of thought to readers who might not otherwise have had exposure to the leading researchers and clinicians around the world. This effort has proved a challenge and an asset to this text in terms of the wealth of ideas. Some authors' manuscripts were painstakingly translated, and close collaboration was required to ensure the accuracy of their thoughts. We hope that the breadth of their ideas is novel and provocative.

The fields of sleep medicine and psychiatry continue to grow and, in the 2 years since we began this production, many new studies have emerged. Every effort has been made to include the latest advances, but some works were no doubt missed. It is our hope that we will be able to integrate new findings in later editions of this text.

Secrets of daytime physical and mental activity, both normal and abnormal, are hidden in deep sleep. Uncovering these secrets is the mission of sleep psychiatry.

There are sleep disorders without psychiatry, but there is no psychiatry without sleep disorders.

Alexander Z. Golbin
Howard M. Kravitz
Louis G. Keith

Index